WORLD HEALTH ORGANIZATION

INTERNATIONAL AGENCY FOR RESEARCH ON CANCER

# MODELS, MECHANISMS AND ETIOLOGY OF TUMOUR PROMOTION

Proceedings of a Symposium organized by
the Hungarian Cancer Society and the IARC,
held in Budapest,

16–18 May 1983

EDITORS

M. BÖRZSÖNYI
N.E. DAY
K. LAPIS
H. YAMASAKI

IARC Scientific Publications No. 56

INTERNATIONAL AGENCY FOR RESEARCH ON CANCER
LYON
1984

The International Agency for Research on Cancer (IARC) was established in 1965 by the World Health Assembly, as an independently financed organization within the framework of the World Health Organization. The headquarters of the Agency are at Lyon, France.

The Agency conducts a programme of research concentrating particularly on the epidemiology of cancer and the study of potential carcinogens in the human environment. Its field studies are supplemented by biological and chemical research carried out in the Agency's laboratories in Lyon and, through collaborative research agreements, in national research institutions in many countries. The Agency also conducts a programme for the education and training of personnel for cancer research.

The publications of the Agency are intended to contribute to the dissemination of authoritative information on different aspects of cancer research.

Oxford University Press, Walton Street, Oxford OX2 6DP

London New York Toronto
Delhi Bombay Calcutta Madras Karachi
Kuala Lumpur Singapore Hong Kong Tokyo
Nairobi Dar es Salaam Cape Town
Melbourne Auckland

and associated companies in
Beirut Berlin Ibadan Mexico City Nicosia

Oxford is a trade mark of Oxford University Press

Published in the United States
by Oxford University Press, New York

ISBN 0 19 723058 X
ISBN 92 832 1156 1 (Publisher)


The authors alone are responsible for the views expressed in the signed articles in this publication.



PRINTED IN SWITZERLAND

# TABLE OF CONTENTS

## TUMOUR PROMOTION IN OTHER ORGANS



## MEMBRANE INTERACTION OF TUMOUR-PROMOTING AGENTS



## CELLULAR RESPONSE TO TUMOUR-PROMOTING AGENTS

## INTERACTION OF TUMOUR PROMOTERS WITH HOST GENES, VIRUSES AND THE IMMUNE SYSTEM



## MODELS OF MULTI-STAGE CARCINOGENESIS IN EPIDEMIOLOGY



## EXPERIMENTAL MODELS TO STUDY ETIOLOGICAL FACTORS IN MULTI-STAGE CARCINOGENESIS



## ETIOLOGY OF HUMAN MULTI-STAGE CARCINOGENESIS

## INHIBITION OF TUMOUR PROMOTION



## CONCLUDING REMARKS

# FOREWORD

Both epidemiological and laboratory studies indicate that most malignant tumours result from the interaction of target cells with multiple endogenous and exogenous factors and that their development is the result of a succession of steps occurring over a considerable part of the host's life span. Environmental factors are considered to play major roles at different stages during the development of human cancers.

One of the main goals of the research activities of the Agency is the primary prevention of human cancer, and the identification of environmental risk factors in carcinogenesis is an important aspect. In order to fulfill this goal, it is also essential to understand the mechanisms underlying different stages of carcinogenesis. Mechanisms of later stages of carcinogenesis – especially tumour promotion in two-stage models of carcinogenesis – are now being studied widely; however, much less is known about the later stages than about the earlier stage of carcinogenesis – including tumour initiation.

This volume is the first IARC publication devoted specifically to multi-stage carcinogenesis. It is my hope that it will not only summarize the state of present knowledge but also encourage further investigations for a better understanding of tumour promotion and multi-stage carcinogenesis.

The hospitality of the Hungarian Cancer Society, Budapest, is gratefully acknowledged. The meeting was cosponsored by the European Association for Cancer Research and was financed in part by donations made by a number of individual firms in the Federal Republic of Germany, France, Hungary, Italy, Switzerland, the UK and the USA.

L. Tomatis, MD
Director
International Agency for Research on Cancer

# INTRODUCTION

Following the first observation of two-stage carcinogenesis on mouse skin in the 1940s, many studies of tumour promotion were carried out, with mouse skin as the target organ and with phorbol esters as model tumour promoters. More recently, work with other species, at other sites and with other agents has led to acceptance that the multi-stage process is a general mechanism of carcinogenesis. In parallel, but almost independently, multi-stage models have been developed to explain a wide variety of epidemiological observations. An abundance of data has accumulated, both epidemiological and experimental, in support of the idea that the development of many cancers is multi-stage.

In order to understand the nature of the multi-stage process of carcinogenesis, and to identify risk factors involved in the causation of cancer, multi-disciplinary approaches are essential. However, epidemiologists and laboratory investigators often take separate and independent approaches to the very same problem. In the study of tumour promotion, cooperation between experimentalists and epidemiologists is especially desirable, since the elimination of risk factors that act in the later stages of carcinogenesis should lead to rapid reductions in human cancer mortality.

The present symposium was planned to stimulate a dialogue between epidemiologists and experimentalists in order to advance our knowledge of multi-stage carcinogenesis. Thus, this volume contains descriptions of human models of multi-stage carcinogenesis and models for possible identification of etiological factors in terms of multi-stage or multi-factorial carcinogenesis, as well as models and cellular and molecular mechanisms of experimental tumour promotion.

The interaction of epidemiologists and laboratory experimentalists in studies of the mechanism of multi-stage carcinogenesis and in the identification of environmental risk factors in terms of multi-stage carcinogenesis is still in an initial phase. It is our sincere hope that this volume will stimulate more such interaction in order to attain our mutual goal – cancer prevention.

The Editors

# PARTICIPANTS

E. Amtmann
Institute of Virus Research,
German Cancer Research Center,
Im Neuenheimer Feld 280,
6900 Heidelberg, FRG

C.L. Ashendel
McArdle Laboratory for Cancer
Research, University of Wisconsin,
Madison, WI 53706, USA

S. Bardócz
Department of Biochemistry,
University Medical School,
4012 Debrecen, Hungary

G. Bauer
Institute of Virology, University of
Freiburg, Hermann-Herder Strasse 11,
78 Freiburg, FRG

C.S. Baxter
Department of Environmental Health
University of Cincinnati, 3223 Eden
Avenue, Cincinnati, OH 45267, USA

A. Bisshop
Laboratory for Carcinogenesis and
Mutagenesis, National Institute of
Public Health, 3720 BA Bilthoven,
The Netherlands

P.M. Blumberg
Laboratory of Cellular Carcino-
genesis and Tumor Promotion,
National Cancer Institute, Bethesda,
MD 20205, USA

M. Boeva
Institute of Oncology, Medical
Academy, Sofia, Bulgaria

F. Boján
Department of Hygiene, University
Medical School, 4012 Debrecen,
Hungary

M. Börzsönyi
National Institute of Hygiene
Gyáli út 2–6, 1966 Budapest, Hungary

R.K. Boutwell
McArdle Laboratory, University of
Wisconsin, Madison, WI 53706, USA

A. Buchmann
Institute of Biochemistry,
German Cancer Research Center,
Im Neuenheimer Feld 280,
6900 Heidelberg, FRG

R.D. Bulbrook
Imperial Cancer Research Fund,
Lincoln's Inn Fields, London
WC2A 3PX, UK

B.I. Carr
Department of Medicine, City of Hope
Medical Center, 1500 East Duarte
Road, Duarte, CA 91010, USA

S.M. Cohen
Pathology and Laboratory Medicine
Department, University of Nebraska
Medical Center, Omaha, NE, USA

N.H. Colburn
Laboratory of Viral Carcinogenesis,
National Cancer Institute, Bldg.
560, Room 12–89, Frederick,
MD 21701, USA

M. Collins
Imperial Cancer Research Fund,
Lincoln's Inn Fields, London
WC2A 3PX, UK

O. Csuka
Research Institute of Oncopathology,
Ráth Gy.u.7., 1122 Budapest, Hungary

N.E. Day
Unit of Biostatistics, International
Agency for Research on Cancer,
150 cours Albert Thomas, 69372 Lyon,
Cédex 08, France

W. Davis
Research Training and Liaison Unit,
International Agency for Research on
Cancer, 150 cours Albert Thomas,
69372 Lyon, Cédex 08, France

C. Delescluse
International Centre for
Dermatological Research, Sophia
Antipolis, 06565 Valbonne, France

E. Deml
Department of Toxicology, Institute
of Toxicology and Biochemistry,
Society of Radiation and
Environmental Research,
8042 Neuherberg, FRG

T.A. Dragani
Division of Experimental Oncology A,
National Tumour Institute, Via G.
Venezian 1, 20133 Milan, Italy

P.E. Driedger
LC Services Corporation, 165 New
Boston Street, Woburn, MA 01801,
USA

S. Eckhardt
National Institute of Oncology, Ráth
Gy.u. 7., 1122 Budapest, Hungary

L. Eliasson
Department of Tumor Biology,
Karolinska Institutet, 104 01
Stockholm, Sweden

J.M. Elwood
Department of Community Health,
University of Nottingham, Queen's
Medical Centre, Clifton Boulevard,
Nottingham, NG7 2UH, UK

T. Enomoto
Division of Environmental Carcino-
genesis, International Agency for
Research on Cancer,
150 cours Albert Thomas,
69372 Lyon, Cédex 08, France

P. Fabian
Neustadt, FRG

G. Fürstenberger
Institute of Biochemistry,
German Cancer Research Center,
Im Neuenheimer Feld 280,
6900 Heidelberg, FRG

H.St C. Gainer
Paterson Laboratories, Christie
Hospital and Holt Radium Institute,
Manchester M20 9BX, UK

D. Gemsa
Pharmacology, Medical School of
Hanover, Hanover, FRG

H. Greim
Department of Toxicology,
Society of Radiation and
Environmental Research, 8042
Neuherberg, FRG

M. Gschwendt
Institute of Biochemistry,
German Cancer Research Center,
Im Neuenheimer Feld 280,
6900 Heidelberg, FRG

E. Hamel
International Agency for Research on
Cancer, 150 cours Albert Thomas,
69372 Lyon, Cédex 08, France

E. Hecker
Institute of Biochemistry,
German Cancer Research Center,
Im Neuenheimer Feld 280,
6900 Heidelberg, FRG

M. Hergenhahn
Institute of Biochemistry,
German Cancer Research Center,
Im Neuenheimer Feld 280,
6900 Heidelberg, FRG

E. Heseltine
Editorial and Publications Services,
International Agency for Research on
Cancer, 150 cours Albert Thomas,
69372 Lyon, Cédex 08, France

Y. Hiasa
First Department of Pathology, Nara
Medical University, Kashihara-shi,
Nara 634, Japan

E. Hidvégi
Frédérick Joliot-Curie National
Research Institute for Radiobiology
and Radiohygiene, Pentz K.u. 5.,
1775 Budapest, Hungary

K.H. Horn
Department of Chemical
Carcinogenicity, Central Institute
of Cancer Research Berlin-Buch,
Lindenberger Weg 80,
1115 Berlin-Buch, GDR

N. Ito
Department of Pathology, Nagoya City
University Medical School,
Nagoya 467, Japan

L. Juhász
Cancer Registry of
Szabolcs-Szatmár County,
4401 Nyiregyháza,
Hungary

S. Kimura
Department of Food Chemistry,
Tohoku University, 1–1 Tsutsumidori
Amamiyacho, Sendai, Japan

A.R. Kinsella
Paterson Laboratories, Christie
Hospital and Holt Radium Institute,
Manchester M20 9BX, UK

V. Kinzel
Institute of Experimental Pathology,
German Cancer Research Center,
Im Neuenheimer Feld 280,
6900 Heidelberg, FRG

A.J.P. Klein-Szántó
The University of Texas System
Cancer Center, Science Park Research
Division, Smithville, TX 78957, USA

L. Komáromy
Department of Biology, University
Medical School, 7643 Pécs, Hungary

Y. Konishi
Department of Oncological Pathology,
Cancer Center, Nara Medical College,
840 Shijo-cho, Kashihara, Nara 634,
Japan

M. Kramer
Hoechst AG, Pharma Forschung
Toxikologie, 6230 Frankfurt/Main 80,
FRG

T. Kubasova
Frédérick Joliot-Curie National Research Institute for Radiobiology and Radiohygiene, Pentz K.u. 5., 1775 Budapest, Hungary

H.W. Kunz
Institute of Biochemistry, German Cancer Research Center, Im Neuenheimer Feld 280, 6900 Heidelberg, FRG

M. Lafaurie
Laboratoire d'Histologie, INSERM U210, UER Médecine, 06034 Nice, France

K. Lapis
First Institute of Pathology and Experimental Cancer Research, Semmelweis Medical University, 1085 Budapest, Hungary

C. Lasne
Institute for Scientific Research on Cancer, 94802 Villejuif, France

A. Likhachev
Unit of Mechanisms of Carcinogenesis, International Agency for Research on Cancer, 150 cours Albert Thomas, 69372 Lyon, Cédex 08, France

F. Marks
Institute of Biochemistry, German Cancer Research Center, Im Neuenheimer Feld 280, 6900 Heidelberg, FRG

E. Matsunaga
Department of Human Genetics, National Institute of Genetics, Mishima, Shizuoka-ken, 411, Japan

F.M. Michiels
LRACC, Institute for Scientific Research on Cancer, 94802 Villejuif, France

A.W. Murray
School of Biological Sciences, Flinders University, South Australia, 5042

Y. Moulé
Institute for Scientific Research on Cancer, 7 rue Guy Moquet, 94802 Villejuif, France

P. Nettesheim
National Institute of Environmental Health Sciences, Research Triangle Park, NC 27709, USA

H.-G. Neumann
Institute of Pharmacology and Toxicology, University of Würzburg, Versbacher Strasse 9, 8700 Würzburg, FRG

D. Oesterle
Department of Toxicology, Institute of Toxicology and Biochemistry, Society of Radiation and Environmental Research, 8042 Neuherberg, FRG

A.F. Pelfrene
Rhône-Poulence Agrochimie, 14–20 rue Pierre Baizet, 69263 Lyon, France

C. Peraino
Division of Biological and Medical Research, Argonne National Laboratory, Argonne, IL 60439, USA

M. Petkova
Governmental Hospital, 1199 Sofia, Bulgaria

J. Peto
Institute of Cancer Research,
Division of Epidemiology,
Clifton Avenue, Sutton,
Surrey SM2 5PX, UK

V.G. Pinchouk
Cytology and Virology Departments,
Institute for Oncology Problems,
Kiev, USSR

A. Pintér
National Institute of Hygiene, Gyáli
út 2–6, 1966 Budapest, Hungary

M. Poirier
Bldg. 37, Room 3A23, National Cancer
Institute, Bethesda, MD 20205, USA

J. Pot-Deprun
Institute for Scientific Research on
Cancer, 94802 Villejuif, France

L. Pylev
Cancer Research Center, Academy of
Medical Sciences, Moscow 115478,
USSR

P. Rády
Department of Biochemistry,
University Medical School,
4012 Debrecen, Hungary

G. Ragnotti
General Pathology, Faculty of
Medicine, University of Brescia,
25100 Brescia, Italy

M. Reinacher
Veterinary-Pathology Institute
Frankfurter Strasse 96,
6300 Giessen, FRG

E. Rivedal
Laboratory for Environmental and
Occupational Cancer, Norwegian
Radium Hospital, Montebello, Oslo 3,
Norway

H. Roeser
Institute of Biochemistry,
German Cancer Research Center,
Im Neuenheimer Feld 280,
6900 Heidelberg, FRG

T. Sanner
Laboratory for Environmental and
Occupational Cancer, Norwegian
Radium Hospital, Montebello, Oslo 3,
Norway

E. Scherer
Division of Chemical Carcinogenesis,
Antoni Van Leeuwenhoek-Huis,
The Netherlands Cancer Institute,
121 Plesmanlaan, 1066 CX Amsterdam,
The Netherlands

R. Schmidt
Institute of Biochemistry,
German Cancer Research Center,
6900 Heidelberg, FRG

M. Schönfelder
Surgical Clinic of the
Karl-Marx University, Liebigstrasse 20,
7010 Leipzig, GDR

R. Schulte-Hermann
Institute of Toxicology and
Pharmacology of the
Philipps University Marburg,
Pilgrimstein 2, 355 Marburg, FRG

M. Schwarz
Institute of Biochemistry,
German Cancer Research Center,
Im Neuenheimer Feld 280,
6900 Heidelberg, FRG

J. Schweizer
Institute of Experimental Pathology,
German Cancer Research Center,
Im Neuenheimer Feld 280,
6900 Heidelberg, FRG

J. Sugár
Research Institute of Oncopathology, Ráth Gy.u. 7., 1122 Budapest, Hungary

G. Sydow
Central Institute of Cancer Research, Academy of Sciences of the GDR, 1115 Berlin-Buch, GDR

S. Szondy
Department of Biochemistry, University Medical School, 4012 Debrecen, Hungary

S.-W. Teigen
The State Pollution Control Authority, P.O. Box 8100 Dep., Oslo 1, Norway

H.A. Tennekes
Institute of Biochemistry, German Cancer Research Center, Im Neuenheimer Feld 280, 6900 Heidelberg, FRG

E.B. Thorling
The Institute of Cancer Research, Radium Stationen, Nörrebrogade 44, 8000 Aarhus C, Denmark

A. Tompa
National Institute of Occupational Health, Nagyvárad tér 2., 1096 Budapest, Hungary

A. Tigyi
Department of Biology, University Medical School, 7643 Pécs, Hungary

G. Török
National Institute of Hygiene, Gyáli út 2–6, 1966 Budapest, Hungary

J.E. Trosko
Department of Pediatrics/Human Development, Michigan State University, East Lansing, MI 48824, USA

V. Turusov
Cancer Research Center, Academy of Medical Sciences, Moscow 115478, USSR

F. Waechter
Ciba-Geigy Limited, 4002 Basel, Switzerland

I.B. Weinstein
College of Physicians and Surgeons, Columbia University, New York, NY 10032, USA

U. Willnow
Clinic for Children's Surgery of the Karl-Marx University, Liebigstrasse 32, 7010 Leipzig, GDR

I.P. Witz
Department of Microbiology, The George S. Wise Faculty of Life Sciences, Tel Aviv University, Ramat Aviv 69978, Israel

V. Wunderlich
Central Institute of Cancer Research, Academy of Sciences of the GDR, 1115 Berlin-Buch, GDR

H. Yamasaki
International Agency for Research on Cancer, 150 cours Albert Thomas, 69372 Lyon, Cédex 08, France

S.H. Yuspa
National Cancer Institute, Bethesda, MD 20205, USA

# MODELS AND MECHANISMS OF SKIN TUMOUR PROMOTION

# ON THE ROLE OF TUMOUR PROMOTION IN CHEMICAL CARCINOGENESIS

R.K. BOUTWELL

*McArdle Laboratory for Cancer Research, University of Wisconsin-Madison, Madison, WI 53706, USA*

This symposium is very timely, because we are in a period of rapid advances in our understanding of carcinogenesis and the role of promoters in the process. This is one of the first meetings designed to explore the role of promoters in human as well as experimental carcinogenesis.

When dealing with a process as complex as carcinogenesis, it is advantageous to simplify investigations into the mechanism of the process by dividing the process into its components. Within a few years of the first demonstration of the experimental production of cancer in mouse and rabbit skin, it was found that the process had multiple components. Thus, the mouse-skin model that I will discuss was pioneered by Berenblum (1941), Mottram (1944) and others. I will restrict myself largely to the phorbol ester tumour promoters which became available through the work of Hecker (1967). Emphasis will be placed on the biological and biochemical responses of mouse skin treated with the tumour-promoting phorbol esters and on receptors. Some areas of future research will be noted.

The initiation-promotion model in mouse skin is characterized by the following criteria:

(1) For all carcinogens, there is a dose that is sufficiently small that no skin tumour develops as a result of that dose, at least for practical purposes. Some agents are quite free of cytotoxic and/or pleiotropic effects at initiating doses, for example benzo-[*a*]pyrene and 7,12-dimethylbenz[*a*]anthracene, the initiator used in all of the experiments that are described below (Slaga *et al.*, 1974). Other agents, such as β-propiolactone, accomplish little, if any, initiation without inducing severe cytotoxic effects (Colburn & Boutwell, 1968; Slaga *et al.*, 1973).

Skin tumours may be initiated by the systemic administration of some skin carcinogens as well as by agents not carcinogenic for the skin, such as 2-acetylaminofluorene. It is of interest that pretreatment of the skin with agents that cause increased DNA synthesis/cell division increase the effectiveness of a given dose of initiator (Hennings & Boutwell, 1970; Hennings *et al.*, 1969). An analogous phenomenon is observed in liver (Pitot *et al.*, 1980), and perhaps the phenomenon plays a role in human cancer formation.

(2) There also exists a class of agents known as 'promoters'. These may be regarded generally as not carcinogenic, but when applied to mouse skin that has been initiated, both benign and malignant skin tumours appear. This is the classical initiation-promotion protocol. However, treatment of mouse skin with the promoter alone may result in the slow development of a few benign and malignant tumors (Boutwell, 1964; Astrup *et al.*, 1980). The reason is unknown. The promoting agent may possess some initiating activity. Alternatively, the promoter may reveal the presence of an oncogene or of a spontaneous error in DNA replication, assuming that a specific alteration in DNA is the essential characteristic of the initiated cell. Moreover, the occasional tumour that develops may be the result of initiation by background ionizing radiation (a demonstrable initiator), by the endogenous formation of carcinogens such as *N*-nitrosamines, or by unavoidable exposure to traces of exogenous carcinogens, such as aflatoxin, and by the carcinogens present in natural foodstuffs at levels that are sufficient to initiate the carcinogenic process but that only rarely cause cancer (Ames, 1983).

(3) Promoting agents cause the early appearance of large numbers of skin tumours only when administered after initiation, Reversing the order of application is no more effective than applying either agent alone (Berenblum & Haran, 1955; Roe, 1959). Clearly, a defect is introduced into a cell by the initiator which is made manifest by treatment with the promoter.

(4) Furthermore, the defect is permanent for all practical purposes. Tumours appear rapidly and in large numbers in mouse skin even if an interval as long as one year intervenes between initiation and the start of promotion (Van Duuren *et al.*, 1975).

(5) In contrast, the interval between applications of the promoter is critical (Boutwell, 1964). If the applications are spaced closely (e.g., twice per day) or too far apart (once a month), little or no tumour response is seen if the total dose is not different from that which is effective if applied in the usual, twice weekly, format. The recent work of Takigawa *et al.* (1983a) may provide an explanation for the loss of promoting activity by frequent applications of TPA. They found that a refractory period for the induction of epidermal ornithine decarboxylase activity exists if applications of the promoter, 12-*O*-tetradecanoylphorbol-13-acetate (TPA), are spaced at intervals of 36 hours or less.

The initiation-promotion regimen utilizing a single application to the skin of 7,12-dimethylbenz[*a*]anthracene followed by twice-weekly applications of the promoter yields large numbers of papillomas, depending on dosages and strain of mice (Boutwell, 1964; DiGiovanni *et al.*, 1980; Verma & Boutwell, 1980). After about 18–20 weeks of promotion, malignant tumours begin to appear, but the incidence may not exceed 50% after one year (Verma & Boutwell, 1980). In contrast, multiple applications of appropriate doses of 7,12-dimethylbenz[*a*]anthracene are less effective at eliciting papillomas, but they are more effective at eliciting carcinomas than the initiation-promotion protocol.

The reason for the relative inefficiency of carcinoma formation by the initiation-promotion protocol is unknown but is being investigated by Strickland *et al.* (1982).

Furthermore, Hennings *et al.* (1983) found that progression of papillomas to carcinomas was independent of promoter treatment but that a second exposure of papilloma-bearing mice to an initiator hastened the appearance of carcinomas in a larger number of mice. We have found that the yield of carcinomas at 49 weeks after the start of promotion was largely independent of the duration of treatment with the promoter (Verma & Boutwell, 1980). Those mice treated with TPA only during the first six weeks of the 49-week observation period developed a 14% incidence of carcinomas. Only at the time promotion was discontinued did the first papillomas begin to appear. Other groups of mice received phorbol ester promotion for 12, 18, 24, 30 or 36 weeks, and the carcinoma incidence in the mice ranged from 20–30%, with one exception. Carcinomas began to appear between 20 and 25 weeks, and, in the groups in which promotion was discontinued, carcinomas appeared in larger numbers. It is possible that continuous treatment with phorbol esters suppresses progression to carcinomas. In general, papilloma incidence is indicative of the ultimate yield of carcinomas, but it may not be true in all cases. These issues need additional study.

The effects of TPA on the epidermis that are deemed relevant to the process of tumour promotion include elevation of putrescine levels (essential for tumour promotion but not sufficient in itself), increased DNA synthesis and hyperplasia, inhibition of maturation as shown by the activation of otherwise dormant genes, elimination of metabolic cooperation, and the formation of dark cells. These effects are compatible with the concept that tumour promotion causes normal cells to take on some of the characteristics of tumour cells in a reversible mode. Moreover, one may postulate that the characteristics of the tumour cell phenotype are maintained in an initiated cell because of a gene deletion resulting in the loss of a specific control mechanism. This concept is compatible with the blocked ontogeny hypothesis of Potter (1981). Furthermore, a number of examples have been cited of increased gene read-out

Table 1. Some effects of treatment with 12-*O*-tetradecanoylphorbol-13-acetate on mouse epidermis

| |
|---|
| Increased levels of cyclic nucleotides |
| Increased phosphatidylcholine turnover |
| Increased prostaglandin synthesis |
| Increased chromatin phosphorylation |
| Increased RNA, protein and DNA synthesis |
| Induction of ornithine decarboxylase activity |
| Increased levels of putrescine |
| Increased protease activity |
| Production of active forms of oxygen |
| Chromatin changes |
| Increased numbers of dark cells |
| Inhibition of intercellular communication[a] |
| Altered patterns of differentiation[a] |

[a] Best demonstrated in cultured cells

consequent to phorbol-ester treatment, in addition to those shown in Table 1. These include the stimulation by TPA of the production of human chorionic gonadotropin and progesterone as well as the increased production of Epstein-Barr virus by Burkitt lymphoma cells treated with TPA.

There is no direct way of proving the relevance to the mechanism of promotion of the many effects of TPA on epidermis that are listed in Table 1. Correlative evidence, however, may be obtained in the skin model by varying the dose of the promoter, by imposing structural variations, and by observing the effect of modifying factors on the tumour incidence *vis-à-vis* the effect under study. The correlative approach has been used to establish the relevance of the induction of ornithine decarboxylase activity and the resultant increase in putrescine level to tumour promotion. Thus, the degree of induction of ornithine decarboxylase activity correlates very closely with tumour incidence as the dose of TPA is varied (Verma & Boutwell, 1980). Using optimal doses of TPA, an induction of 200-fold or more is accomplished within five hours after treatment (O'Brien *et al.,* 1975). The degree of induction is even greater after multiple applications of TPA (Verma *et al.,* 1979), and the resulting tumours show elevated levels of ornithine decarboxylase (Astrup & Boutwell, 1982). Likewise, structural changes to the phorbol ester molecule have identical effects on induction of the enzyme and on tumour incidence.

A number of agents also inhibit both the induction of ornithine decarboxylase activity and tumour promotion by TPA. These include a number of retinoids, prostaglandin synthesis inhibitors, specific inhibitors of ornithine decarboxylase and certain polyamines. In all cases, the degree of inhibition of enzyme induction and tumour incidence are equivalent as the dose or structure of the inhibitor is changed. Moreover, the induction of the first enzyme in the polyamine biosynthesis pathway, ornithine decarboxylase, is inhibited without detectable inhibition of the induction of the second enzyme, *S*-adenosylmethionine decarboxylase.

Because of its specificity for ornithine decarboxylase, the irreversible inhibitor of the enzyme, α-difluoromethylornithine, was tested as an inhibitor of tumour promotion. First, an appropriate dose and time of application was determined on the basis of the ability of α-difluoromethylornithine to inhibit the level of ornithine decarboxylase activity in the epidermis. The promoting activity of TPA is effectively inhibited by α-difluoromethylornithine administered by any one of three routes: direct application to the skin in the same area to which TPA is applied, by intraperitoneal injection, and by addition to drinking-water (Takigawa *et al.,* 1982, 1983b). The inhibition of tumour formation occurred with the same dose-response relationship as the inhibition of enzyme activity. Because of the specificity of α-difluoromethylornithine for the enzyme, ornithine decarboxylase, the results with the inhibitor provide convincing evidence for an essential role for increased ornithine decarboxylase activity or an elevated level of putrescine or a putrescine metabolite in the mechanism of tumour promotion. However, although essential, increased ornithine decarboxylase activity alone is not sufficient to accomplish tumour promotion. There is evidence for an essential role in promotion of a number of other responses to tumour promoters, including increased rates of DNA synthesis, the appearance of dark cells (Klein-Szanto *et al.,* 1980) and the inhibition of intercellular communication (Murray & Fitzgerald, 1979; Yotti *et al.,* 1979).

Other inhibitors of tumour promotion exist, including protease inhibitors and steroid hormones. Yavelow *et al.* (1982) reported recently that the increase in the level of superoxide radical caused by TPA is inhibited by protease inhibitors.

Combinations of inhibitors of tumour promotion were tested for possible additive and synergistic effects on papilloma incidence for at least three reasons. First, sequential blocks of metabolic pathways may lower the level of the ultimate product of that pathway in a synergistic manner. Second, it is likely that a number of changes must be accomplished in a cell that are not on a common metabolic pathway (see Table 1), and, if more than one change is blocked by imposing two or more inhibitory agents, an additive or synergistic effect on tumour inhibition is likely. And, finally, by using two or more inhibitors in combination, lower levels of each may be effective, thereby lessening the possibility of undesirable effects. An example of an apparent synergistic action of two inhibitors, retinoic acid and dexamethasone, is shown in Table 2. The control animals had an average of about 10 papillomas per mouse at 20 weeks; the number was reduced by approximately 50% by either agent alone, but an average of only 0.8 papillomas per mouse developed in the mice treated with the combination. Combinations of retinoic acid and a protease inhibitor were more effective than either alone (Table 3); and the same was true of the combination of retinoic acid and indomethacin (Table 4). This approach holds great promise for practical applications for prophylaxis in human populations.

As a start, we have found that ornithine decarboxylase is inducible in epidermis prepared from human skin obtained from amputations. Incubation with TPA induces the enzyme, and the induction by TPA is inhibited if the incubation is done in the presence of retinoic acid. In addition, we have shown that, in mice, orally administered all-*trans* retinoic acid inhibits the induction of ornithine decarboxylase in the skin as well as skin tumour promotion. Thus, it was considered reasonable to determine if orally administered retinoic acid is capable of inhibiting induction of the enzyme in people, using punch biopsies of skin. We have found that ornithine decarboxylase can be induced by incubating punch biopsies in the presence of TPA. In this way, a dosage schedule for 13-*cis*-retinoic acid will be established. It is anticipated that the dose will not cause undesirable side-effects. In contrast, until now,

Table 2. Inhibition of tumour promotion by retinoic acid and dexamethasone, alone and in combination

| Initiator (once) | Promoter (twice/week) | Inhibitor (twice/week) | Papillomas/mouse (20 weeks) |
|---|---|---|---|
| DMBA[a], 0.1 μmol | TPA[b], 5 nmol | None | 9.8 |
| DMBA, 0.1 μmol | TPA, 5 nmol | Retinoic acid, 1.7 nmol | 3.8 |
| DMBA, 0.1 μmol | TPA, 5 nmol | Dexamethasone, 45 μg | 5.1 |
| DMBA, 0.1 μmol | TPA, 5 nmol | Retinoic acid and dexamethasone | 0.8 |

[a] 7,12-Dimethylbenz[*a*]anthracene
[b] 12-*O*-Tetradecanoylphorbol-13-acetate
All agents were applied to the skin of the backs of CD-1 mice in 0.2 ml of acetone. Retinoic acid and dexamethasone were applied one hour before each application of TPA.

Table 3. Inhibition of tumour promotion by retinoic acid and a protease inhibitor, tosyl lysine chloromethyl ketone (TLCK), alone and in combination

| Initiator (once) | Promoter (twice/week) | Inhibitor (twice/week) | Papillomas/mouse (20 weeks) |
|---|---|---|---|
| DMBA[a], 0.1 μmol | TPA[b], 5 nmol | None | 13.7 |
| DMBA, 0.1 μmol | TPA, 5 nmol | Retinoic acid, 1.7 nmol | 0.6 |
| DMBA, 0.1 μmol | TPA, 5 nmol | TLCK, 10 ng | 4.1 |
| DMBA, 0.1 μmol | TPA, 5 nmol | Retinoic acid and TLCK | 0.0 |

[a] 7,12-Dimethylbenz[*a*]anthracene
[b] 12-*O*-Tetradecanoylphorbol-13-acetate
TLCK was applied to the skin two hours before each application of TPA. Other details are as described in the footnote to Table 2. The original data on the inhibitory effect of TLCK on tumour promotion were published by Troll *et al.* (1970).

Table 4. Inhibition of tumour promotion by retinoic acid and indomethacin, alone and in combination

| Initiator (once) | Promoter (twice/week) | Inhibitor (twice/week) | Papillomas/mouse (20 weeks) |
|---|---|---|---|
| DMBA[a], 0.1 μmol | TPA[b], 10 nmol | None | 7.3 |
| DMBA, 0.1 μmol | TPA, 10 nmol | Retinoic acid, 1.7 nmol | 3.2 |
| DMBA, 0.1 μmol | TPA, 10 nmol | Indomethacin, 100 ng | 2.3 |
| DMBA, 0.1 μmol | TPA, 10 nmol | Retinoic acid and indomethacin | 0.5 |

[a] 7,12-Dimethylbenz[*a*]anthracene
[b] 12-*O*-Tetradecanoylphorbol-13-acetate
Indomethacin was applied to the skin two hours before each application of TPA. Other details are as described in the footnote to Table 2.

the approach used was to give the maximum tolerated dose in attempting to prevent cancer in people at high risk for the disease. Using the same approach, appropriate dose schedules for other inhibitors of ornithine decarboxylase will be determined, e.g., indomethacin and α-difluoromethylornithine. It is anticipated that combinations of agents will be more effective in people, just as in mice (Tables 2–4) and that, by using combinations of agents, effective inhibition will be possible with lower levels of each.

Another variable has a profound effect on the tumour response in an initiation-promotion experiment: We have bred mice for susceptibility and resistance (Boutwell, 1964; DiGiovanni *et al.*, 1980), and remarkable differences have been obtained (Fig. 1). After only seven weeks of promotion with 2 μg (3.3 nmol) of TPA in 0.2 ml of acetone twice a week, the susceptible mice averaged more than eight papillomas per mouse. None appeared in a widely used strain of commercially available mice (CD-1) by that time. The CD-1 strain of mice is more responsive to the initiation-promotion regimen than most other strains (Boutwell, 1964), and it provided half of the gene pool for both the most responsive mice ($B^2S$) and the SENCAR mice (DiGiovanni *et al.*, 1980).

Recent evidence reported by Castagna *et al.* (1982) shows that TPA activates a calcium- and phospholipid-dependent protein kinase. Following this clue, Neidel and coworkers (1983) found that the phorbol ester receptor in the brain-particulate fraction co-purifies with protein kinase C activity. Concurrently, Ashendel *et al.*

Fig. 1. Incidence of papillomas, expressed as average number of papillomas per mouse, in groups of CD-1 (Charles River Breeding Labs, NY, USA) (△), SENCAR (●) and B²S (○) mice.
All mice were initiated by a single application to the skin of 10 nmol 7,12-dimethylbenz[*a*]anthracene (DMBA) in 0.2 ml acetone. After one week, promotion was begun by twice-weekly applications of 3.3 nmol 12-*O*-tetradecanoylphorbol-13-acetate (TPA) in 0.2 ml acetone. The B²S mice were removed from the experiment at seven weeks for breeding; no tumour had appeared in the CD-1 mice at seven weeks at the doses of initiator and promoter that were used.

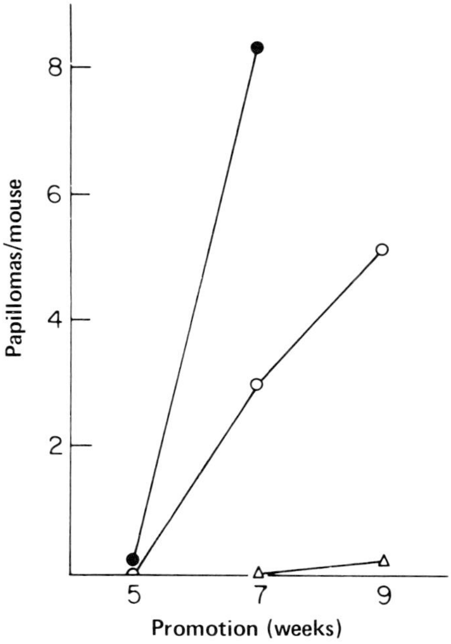


(1983) reached the same conclusion. Thus, a whole new area of research is open to determine directly if a role for protein phosphorylation exists in tumour promotion. A convergence in the mechanisms of chemical carcinogenesis and viral carcinogenesis may well be brought about by research on protein phosphorylation. The subject was reviewed recently by Weinstein (1983).

Thus, one may conclude that research on tumour promotion is playing a vital role in solving the problem of the mechanisms involved in chemical carcinogenesis.

## REFERENCES

Ames, B.N. (1983) Dietary carcinogens and anticarcinogens. *Science,* ***221,*** 1256–1264

Ashendel, C.L., Staller, J.M. & Boutwell, R.K. (1983) Protein kinase activity associated with a phorbol ester receptor purified from mouse brain. *Cancer Res.,* ***43,*** 4333–4337

Astrup, E.G. & Boutwell, R.K. (1982) Ornithine decarboxylase activity in chemically induced mouse skin papillomas. *Carcinogenesis,* ***3,*** 303–308

Astrup, E.G., Iversen, O.H. & Elgjo, K. (1980) The tumorigenic and carcinogenic effect of TPA when applied to the skin of BALB/CA mice. *Virchows Arch. B.*, ***33***, 303–304

Berenblum, I. (1941) The mechanism of cocarcinogenesis: A study of the significance of cocarcinogenic action and related phenomena. *Cancer Res.*, ***1***, 807–814

Berenblum, I. & Haran, N. (1955) The significance of the sequence of initiating and promoting actions in the process of skin carcinogenesis in the mouse. *Br. J. Cancer*, ***9***, 268–271

Boutwell, R.K. (1964) Some biological aspects of skin carcinogenesis. *Prog. exp. Tumor Res.*, ***4***, 207–250

Castagna, M., Takai, Y., Kaibuchi, K., Sano, K., Kikkawa, V. & Nishizuka, Y. (1982) Direct activation of calcium-activated, phospholipid dependent protein kinase by tumor-promoting phorbol esters. *J. biol. Chem.*, ***257***, 7847–7851

Colburn, N.H. & Boutwell, R.K. (1968) The binding of β-propiolactone and some related alkylating agents to DNA, RNA, and protein of mouse skin; relation between tumor-initiating power of alkylating agents and their binding to DNA. *Cancer Res.*, ***28***, 653–660

DiGiovanni, J., Slaga, T.J. & Boutwell, R.K. (1980) Comparison of the tumor-initiating activity of 7,12-dimethylbenz[*a*]anthracene and benzo[*a*]pyrene in female SENCAR and CD-1 mice. *Carcinogenesis*, ***1***, 1381–1389

Hecker, E. (1967) Phorbol esters from croton oil. Chemical nature and biological activities. *Naturwissenschaften*, ***11***, 282–284

Hennings, H. & Boutwell, R.K. (1970) Studies on the mechanism of skin tumor promotion. *Cancer Res.*, ***30***, 312–320

Hennings, H., Bowden, G.T. & Boutwell, R.K. (1969) The effect of croton oil pretreatment on skin tumor initiation in mice. *Cancer Res.*, ***29***, 312–320

Hennings, H., Shores, R., Wenk, M.L., Spangler, E.F., Tarone, R. & Yuspa, S.H. (1983) Malignant conversion of mouse skin tumors is increased by tumor initiators and unaffected by tumor promoters. *Nature*, ***304***, 67–69

Klein-Szanto, A.J.P., Major, S.M. & Slaga, T.J. (1980) Induction of dark keratinocytes by 12-*O*-tetradecanoylphorbol-13-acetate and mezerein as an indicator of tumor-promoting effeciency. *Carcinogenesis*, ***1***, 399–406

Mottram, J.C. (1944) A developing factor in experimental blastogenesis. *J. Pathol. Bacteriol.*, ***56***, 181–187

Murray, A.W. & Fitzgerald, D.J. (1979) Tumor promoters inhibit metabolic cooperation in cocultures of epidermal and 3T3 cells. *Biochem. biophys. Res. Commun.*, ***91***, 395–401

Neidel, J.E., Kuhn, L.J. & Vandenbark, G.R. (1983) Phorbol diester receptor copurifies with protein kinase C. *Proc. natl Acad. Sci. USA*, ***80***, 36–40

O'Brien, T.G., Simsiman, R.C. & Boutwell, R.K. (1975) Induction of the polyamine biosynthetic enzymes in mouse epidermis and their specificity for tumor promotion. *Cancer Res.*, ***35***, 2426–2433

Pitot, H.C., Goldsworthy, T., Campbell, H.A. & Poland, A. (1980) Quantitative evaluation of the promotion by 2,3,7,8-tetrachlorodibenzo-*p*-dioxin of hepatocarcinogenesis from diethylnitrosamine. *Cancer Res.*, ***40***, 3616–3620

Potter, V.R. (1981) The present status of the blocked ontogeny hypothesis of neoplasia: the thalassemia connection. *Oncodev. Biol. Med.*, ***2***, 243–266

Roe, F.J.C. (1959) The effect of applying croton oil before a single application on 9,10-dimethyl-1,2-benzanthracene (DMBA). *Br. J. Cancer*, ***13***, 87–91

Slaga, T.J., Bowden, G.T., Shapas, B.G. & Boutwell, R.K. (1973) Macromolecular synthesis following a single application of alkylating agents used as initiators of mouse skin tumorigenesis. *Cancer Res.*, ***33***, 769–776

Slaga, T.J., Bowden, G.T., Shapas, B.G. & Boutwell, R.K. (1974) Macromolecular synthesis following a single application of polycyclic hydrocarbons used as initiators of mouse skin tumorigenesis. *Cancer Res.*, ***34***, 771–777

Strickland, J.E., Hennings, H., Jetten, A.M., Yuspa, S.H., Allen, P.T., Hellmann, K.B. & Strickland, A.G. (1982) *Susceptibility determinants for mouse epidermal carcinogenesis*. In: Bartsch, H. & Armstrong, B., eds, *Host Factors in Human Carcinogenesis (IARC Scientific Publications No. 39)*, Lyon, International Agency for Research on Cancer, pp. 258–268

Takigawa, M., Verma, A.K., Simsiman, R.C. & Boutwell, R.K. (1982) Polyamine biosynthesis and skin tumor promotion: Inhibition of 12-*O*-tetradecanoylphorbol-13-acetate-promoted mouse skin tumor formation by the irreversible inhibitor of ornithine decarboxylase, α-difluoromethylornithine. *Biochem. biophys. Res. Commun.*, ***105***, 969–975

Takigawa, M., Simsiman, R.C. & Boutwell, R.K. (1983a) The difference between the effects of single and double applications of 12-*O*-tetradecanoylphorbol-13-acetate, a potent tumor promoter, on polyamine metabolism and nucleic acid synthesis in the mouse epidermis. *Carcinogenesis*, ***4***, 5–7

Takigawa, M., Verma, A.K., Simsiman, R.C. & Boutwell, R.K. (1983b) Inhibition of mouse skin tumor promotion and of promoter-stimulated polyamine biosynthesis by α-difluoromethylornithine. *Cancer Res.*, ***43***, 3732–3738

Troll, W., Klassen, A. & Janoff, A. (1970) Tumorigenesis in mouse skin: inhibition by synthetic protease inhibitors. *Science*, ***169***, 1211–1213

Van Duuren, B.L., Sivak, A., Katz, C., Seidman, I. & Melchionne, S. (1975) The effect of aging and the interval between primary and secondary treatment in two-stage carcinogenesis in mouse skin. *Cancer Res.*, ***35***, 502–505

Verma, A.K. & Boutwell, R.K. (1980) Effects of dose and duration of treatment with the tumor-promoting agent, 12-*O*-tetradecanoylphorbol-13-acetate, on mouse skin carcinogenesis. *Carcinogenesis*, ***1***, 271–276

Verma, A.K., Shapas, B.G., Rice, H.M. & Boutwell, R.K. (1979) Correlation of the inhibition by retinoids of tumor promoter-induced mouse epidermal ornithine decarboxylase activity and of skin tumor promotion. *Cancer Res.*, ***39***, 419–425

Weinstein, I.B. (1983) Protein kinase, phospholipid, and control of growth. *Nature*, ***303***, 750

Yavelow, J., Gidlund, M. & Troll, W. (1982) Protease inhibitors from processed legumes effectively inhibit superoxide generation in response to TPA. *Carcinogenesis*, ***3***, 135–138

Yotti, L.P., Chang, C.C. & Trosko, J.E. (1979) Elimination of metabolic cooperation in Chinese hamster cells by a tumor promoter. *Science*, ***206***, 1089–1091

# STAGES OF TUMOUR PROMOTION IN SKIN

F. MARKS & G. FÜRSTENBERGER

*Institute of Biochemistry, German Cancer Research Center, 6900 Heidelberg, Federal Republic of Germany*

## INTRODUCTION

Skin is the classical target organ of experimental multi-stage tumorigenesis. As early as the 1920s, the observation was made that wounding or chemical irritation promotes the growth of tumours induced by chemical carcinogens (Deelman, 1924; Twort & Ing, 1928).

The terms 'initiation' and 'promotion' were first introduced by Peyton Rous and coworkers (Rous & Kidd, 1941; Friedwald & Rous, 1944). At about the same time, Berenblum and Shubik (1947), as well as Mottram (1944), developed an experimental, standard approach of two-stage skin tumorigenesis by treating mouse skin with 7,12-dimethylbenz[*a*]anthracene (DMBA) as an initiator and croton oil as a promoter. The isolation of phorbol esters from croton oil by Hecker (for a review see Hecker & Schmidt, 1974) and Van Duuren and Orris (1965) has enabled investigators to perform experiments under strictly controlled conditions, using chemically well-defined compounds. Today, multi-stage skin tumorigenesis may be considered the most advanced method for artificial generation of benign and malignant tumours. This method seems to reflect the human situation, more than any other approach, and every hypothesis or theory on cancer must take into account the facts we have learned from it.

We cannot explain the phenomenon of transformation and malignant growth unless we understand the definitions of 'initiation' and 'promotion'.

## THE ROLE OF CELLULAR PROLIFERATION

Promotion of skin tumours is always accompanied by inflammatory reactions and by epidermal hyperproliferation. Therefore, from the beginning, promotion was thought to be due to enhanced cellular proliferation – for example, that stimulation of tissue growth may enable the initiated cell to form a mini-tumour. It was thought that when this tumour reached a certain size it might become independent of local growth restraints, thus acquiring developmental autonomy.

This is a rather simplistic view that does not tell us the whole truth, for the simple reason that induction of cellular proliferation is not sufficient in itself to promote tumour development in initiated skin. Indeed, we know of many agents and manipulations that induce epidermal hyperplasia plus inflammation, but only a few of them are tumour promoters.

Consequently, investigations of the mechanism of action of tumour promoters concentrated on the biochemical events occurring in skin after promoter treatment. It was hoped that a reliable biochemical parameter of promotion could be found, if the investigator only looked closely enough.

In skin, a tumour promoter such as 12-*O*-tetradecanoyl-phorbol-13-acetate (TPA) has been shown to bring about the following sequence of events (a still far from detailed elucidation):

(1) Interaction with binding sites (probably membrane-bound), called receptors (see Hergenhahn & Hecker, 1981; Blumberg *et al.,* this volume, p. 139)

(2) Translocation of calcium ions across the plasma membrane (Ganss *et al.,* 1982)

(3) Activation of two calcium-dependent enzymes: protein kinase C (Castagna *et al.,* 1982) and phospholipase A2 (Ganss *et al.,* 1982; Ganss, 1983)

(4) Enhanced phospholipid turnover (Kreibich *et al.,* 1971; Rohrschneider & Boutwell, 1973; Balmain & Hecker, 1974, 1976), especially a release of arachidonic acid from cellular phospholipids catalysed by phospholipase A2 (Fürstenberger *et al.,* 1981a)

(5) Formation of prostaglandins and lipoxygenase products from arachidonic acid; prostaglandin $E_2$ has been shown to be an essential mediator of the hyperplastic response (Marks *et al.,* 1981; Fürstenberger *et al.,* 1982), whereas lipoxygenase products may play a role in inflammation. Thus, the whole complex of events consisting of inflammation and hyperplastic growth, which has been called 'hyperplastic transformation' (Marks *et al.,* 1978), is probably triggered by the arachidonic acid cascade

(7) Induction of ornithine decarboxylase, followed by enhanced polyamine formation (O'Brien, 1976; Boutwell *et al.,* 1979; Marks *et al.,* 1979)

(8) Stimulation of protein, RNA and DNA synthesis and mitotic activity (Baird *et al.,* 1971, 1972; Hennings & Boutwell, 1970; Krieg *et al.,* 1974)

(9) Desensitization of epidermis for chalone inhibition and catecholamine- (Grimm & Marks, 1974; Marks, 1980) or prostaglandin E-induced (Marks *et al.,* 1982a) cAMP synthesis, as well as breakdown of intercellular communication (Fitzgerald & Murray, 1980). Such tachyphylactic processes seem to reflect a general weakening of local growth restraints which results in a disturbance of tissue homeostasis, i.e., the steady-state between cell gain and cell loss. As a result of such a disturbance, more cells are generated than are lost, i.e., hyperplasia develops.

All these responses are evoked not only by tumour promoters, but also by non-promoting hyperplasiogenic agents.

Within the phorbol ester series, an interaction with a cellular receptor [probably identical with protein kinase C (Castagna *et al.,* 1982; Niedel *et al.,* 1983; Blumberg *et al.,* this volume, p. 139] seems to be obligatory, although we are still awaiting final proof that receptor occupation is directly and causally related to an early response, such as calcium ion displacement or arachidonic acid release.

The whole sequence of events can also be induced, however, without receptor occupation, for example by mechanical damage of skin (Marks *et al.*, 1982b) or by non-phorbol ester mitogens such as the ionophore A 23187 (Marks *et al.*, 1981). Thus, all biochemical reactions observed so far following TPA treatment must be considered a reflection of the mitogenic properties of the phorbol ester rather than true parameters of promotion. It has been concluded that hyperplastic transformation of skin is not a sufficient condition of promotion.

## HYPERPLASTIC TRANSFORMATION IS A NECESSARY CONDITION OF PROMOTION

Although hyperplastic transformation is not sufficient for promotion, it seems to be a necessary condition. We can now provide experimental evidence that this assumption is indeed correct. This has become possible, since the long-term process of skin tumour promotion has been found to consist of at least two separate steps. As long as promotion could be achieved only by repeated TPA treatment over a period of at least 8–10 weeks, the investigator was faced with a bewildering mixture of inflammatory reactions, acute mitogenic responses, sustained hyperplasia and events probably releated to promotion, which was almost impossible to follow up. The first evidence that promotion could be subdivided was provided by Boutwell in 1964.

Recently, Slaga *et al.* (1980) introduced a more clearly defined approach to two-stage promotion, using SENCAR mice and a combined treatment with TPA and the non-promoting irritant mezerein.

In our hands, i.e., using NMRI mice and a semisynthetic TPA derivative, this method gave highly satisfactory results. The derivative was obtained by replacing the $C_{14}$ fatty acid side-chain of TPA by retinoic acid, a well-known anti-promoting agent (Sorg *et al.*, 1982). By this chemical manipulation, the tumour-promoting activity of the phorbol ester was practically abolished, whereas its efficacy as an irritant mitogen was not altered (Fürstenberger *et al.*, 1981b). 12-Retinoylphorbol-13-acetate (RPA) turned out to be a very effective 'incomplete' tumour promoter, in that it enhanced the effect of limited TPA treatment, probably by inducing sustained epidermal hyperplasia when applied chronically to mouse skin.

Since TPA treatment can now be limited to a single application, we are able to take a closer look at events relevant to promotion which are normally completely camouflaged by chronic processes and pleiotropic reactions. At present, there are two lines of evidence for an obligatory role of hyperplastic transformation not only in the second but also in the first stage of promotion.

In the first series of experiments, it was shown that an interruption of DNA synthesis by hydroxyurea, occurring 18 h after TPA treatment of mice in the first stage of promotion, not only prevents the development of epidermal hyperplasia but, in addition, leads to a complete inhibition of tumour promotion which is not due to cytotoxicity (Kinzel *et al.*, this volume, p. 253).

The second approach is a little more sophisticated. Ten years ago, we observed that baby mouse epidermis does not respond to TPA or other mitogenic treatments by hyperplastic transformation (Bertsch & Marks, 1974). Hyperplastic transformation seems indeed to be a physiological response to damage which is subject to ontogenetic development (Bertsch & Marks, 1974, 1978, 1982). It appears 1–2 weeks after birth. If the first stage of tumour promotion depends on hyperplastic transformation, it should exhibit a similar time course of ontogenetic development.

Table 1. Two-stage skin tumour promotion with newborn mice

| Initiation | Promotion | | Tumour formation after 18 weeks | |
|---|---|---|---|---|
| | 1st stage (day) | 2nd stage | Tumour-bearing animals (%) | No. of papillomas/ survivor |
| DMBA | – | – | 0 | 0 |
| Acetone | 3× TPA (1, 3, 5) | – | 0 | 0 |
| Acetone | 3× acetone (1, 3, 5) | RPA | 4 | 0.02 |
| DMBA | 1× TPA (1) | RPA | 18 | 0.22 |
| DMBA | 2× TPA (1, 3) | RPA | 20 | 0.45 |
| DMBA | 3× TPA (1, 3, 5) | RPA | 61 | 1.4 |
| DMBA | 3× TPA (1, 3, 5) | TPA | 76 | 2.0 |
| Control experiment with adult mice (7-weeks old): | | | | |
| DMBA | 1× TPA | RPA | 63 | 3.9 |

Animals were initiated prenatally by intragastric administration of 60 mg/kg body weight 7,12-dimethylbenz[*a*]-anthracene (DMBA) to pregnant mice at day 19 of gestation. 12-*O*-Tetradecanoylphorbol-13-acetate (TPA) was applied locally 1–3 times on days 1, 3 and 5 after birth (4 nmol/0.02 mL acetone each) followed by twice weekly administration of acetone (0.05 mL), TPA (5 nmol/0.05 mL acetone each) or retinoyl phorbol-13-acetate (RPA) (5 nmol/0.05 mL acetone each) beginning at day 10 after birth. From day 21, the phorbol ester doses were increased to 10 nmol/0.1 mL acetone each. For treatment of adult animals (control experiment) see footnote to Table 2. At the end of the experiment $\geq$90% of the animals were alive.

Table 2. Age-dependent stimulation of mitotic activity by 12-*O*-tetradecanoylphorbol-13-acetate (TPA) in the back skin of female NMRI mice

| Treatment on postnatal day | Mitoses/visual field after treatment with: | |
|---|---|---|
| | Acetone | TPA |
| 1 | $0.90 \pm 0.25$ | $1.05 \pm 0.28$ |
| 3 | $0.65 \pm 0.2$ | $1.0 \pm 0.2$ |
| 5 | $0.80 \pm 0.3$ | $2.70 \pm 0.55$ |
| 50 | $0.22 \pm 0.07$ | $1.95 \pm 0.35$ |

A single topical application of TPA (4 nmol/0.02 mL acetone on day 1, 3 or 5 or 10 nmol/0.1 mL acetone on day 50) or acetone (controls) was made, and the mitotic activity was determined 27 h later following treatment with vincristine for 4 h (i.p. injection of 1 mg/kg body weight). The skin was fixed in 10% formaldehyde, and 5-µm sections were made and stained with haematoxylin-eosin. Each value was obtained by counting 20 sections prepared from 5 animals ($\pm$SD).

Table 3. Age-dependent induction by 12-*O*-tetradecanoylphorbol-13-acetate (TPA) of ornithine decarboxylase activity in the back skin of female NMRI mice

| Treatment at postnatal day | ODC activity (pmol $CO_2$/mg protein per h) after treatment with: | |
|---|---|---|
| | Acetone | TPA |
| 1 | 12±5 | 10± 4 |
| 3 | 4±2 | 6± 4 |
| 5 | 6±2 | 46± 18 |
| 7 | 10±4 | 200± 40 |
| 50 | 5±3 | 1 160±340 |

For details on TPA treatment, see footnote to Table 2. Ornithine decarboxylase (ODC) activity was measured 4 h after treatment, according to the method of O'Brien (1976). Each value is the mean (±SD) of 12 determinations (6 mice).

In Tables 1–3 it is shown that the efficacy of TPA in causing stage 1 of promotion in newborn mice indeed parallels the ability of the animals' skin to respond to the phorbol ester by increased DNA synthesis and induction of ornithine decarboxylase.

Our conclusion is, therefore, that hyperplastic transformation of skin is an obligatory condition for both stages of promotion.

## THE IRREVERSIBLE COMPONENT OF TUMOUR PROMOTION

The results shown above indicate that, besides promotion itself, the responses of skin during stage 1 of promotion are apparently identical to those during stage 2. But there is one significant and rather spectacular difference between hyperplastic transformation and promotion: the alterations brought about in the tissue during stage 1 seem to be more or less irreversible, whereas hyperplastic transformation is by all criteria an entirely reversible process. This is shown by the finding that the rate of tumour development remains unchanged when the multistage experiment is interrupted for 8 weeks between stage 1 and stage 2 of promotion (Fürstenberger *et al.*, 1983).

## RELATIONSHIPS BETWEEN TUMOUR PROMOTION AND THE WOUND RESPONSE

An acceleration of skin tumour development by local wounding was first observed 60 years ago (Deelman, 1924). More recently, skin wounding was found to mimic the tumour-promoting effect of TPA in the two-stage approach to skin tumorigenesis (Hennings & Boutwell, 1970; Clark-Lewis & Murray, 1978; Argyris, 1982). In these experiments, repeated wounding was necessary to induce visible tumours. When, however, wounding was restricted to the first stage of promotion, followed by repeated RPA treatment in the second stage, a single wound exerted a rather strong tumour-promoting effect in initiated mouse skin (Table 4).

Table 4. First-stage tumour promotion by wounding as compared with the effect of 12-*O*-tetradecanoylphorbol-13-acetate (TPA)

| Promotion | | Tumour-bearing animals (%) after: | | | No. of papillomas/survivor after: | | |
|---|---|---|---|---|---|---|---|
| 1st stage | 2nd stage | 12 | 15 | 18 weeks | 12 | 15 | 18 weeks |
| TPA | TPA | 93 | 93 | 93 | 8.1 | 8.4 | 8.5 |
| TPA | RPA | 44 | 50 | 63 | 2.6 | 3.4 | 3.9 |
| Wounding | RPA | 13 | 50 | 56 | 0.4 | 1.0 | 1.7 |
| RPA | RPA | 0 | 13 | 13 | 0 | 0.3 | 0.3 |

Groups of 16 female NMRI mice (7 weeks old) were initiated by topical application of 100 nmol 7,12-dimethylbenz[*a*]anthracene in 0.1 mL acetone onto the shaven back skin. One week later, the animals were treated topically once with 10 nmol TPA or retinoyl phorbol-13-acetate (RPA), or wounding was performed by six cuts of 1-cm length made into the back skin of anaesthesized animals (1st stage). One week later, treatment was continued by repeated application of either TPA or RPA (10 nmol each, 2nd stage). At the end of the experiment ≥90% of the animals were alive.

## CONCLUSIONS

In stage 1 of promotion, TPA induces a more or less irreversible change which is brought about by means of cellular proliferation and which finally manifests itself in tumour development, i.e., the appearance of a new phenotype which differs from that of normal epidermis, at least by an altered growth pattern. Such change is probably due to a permanent alteration of gene expression.

Phenotypic expression *via* cellular proliferation has been found to play an important role in tissue development. Holtzer (1978) introduced the term 'quantal cell division' and postulated that DNA replication is sometimes or always necessary to fix or 'lock' gene expression.

Provided that gene expression is involved in stage 1 of promotion, we may ask, which gene is expressed? The simplest deviation from normal tissue to neoplastically transformed is the benign tumour. Indeed, 90% of the tumours generated in the course of the multistage approach have been shown to be benign papillomas (Burns *et al.*, 1978). By definition, a benign tumour first differs from normal tissue by an altered growth pattern. Whereas normal tissue stops growing as soon as a steady state between cell gain and cell loss is reached, a tumour remains in disequilibrium. Therefore, the genes whose expression is probably altered in stage 1 of promotion may be engaged first of all in the control of cellular proliferation.

Unfortunately, we are still far from a satisfactory understanding of the mechanisms which control the steady state of tissue homeostasis in living animals, and the many observations on growth control made in cell cultures do not seem to be very helpful in this respect. It is evident that during tissue growth or regeneration – for example, after damage – the mechanisms that control the steady state between cell loss and cell gain must be switched off transiently. Therefore, the relationships between skin wounding and tumour promotion are certainly more than just a coincidence. In this connection, the finding that a cellular oncogene becomes expressed after tissue damage, e.g., during liver regeneration, may become a key observation (Goyette *et al.*, 1983). Although it seems to be still too early even to formulate a meaningful working hypothesis that is just a little more than pure speculation, one fundamental conclusion may be drawn as far as the difference between a normal cell and an initiated cell in terms of growth control is concerned. The simplest possibility would seem to be that, under normal conditions, the critical gene expression is transient – the growth controlling genes are switched off automatically as soon as the requirements of development, defence or tissue repair are fulfilled. In contrast, in an initiated cell, the switch-off mechanism may not work, so that the genes remain active as soon as they have been switched on.

Why then is stage 2 of promotion necessary at all? It may simply be that a breakdown of growth control can proceed in a step-wise fashion rather than following the all-or-nothing principle. In initiated and promoted skin, indeed, all types of tumours can be found, from the benign, reversibly growing type to the benign, autonomous type to the malignant type (Burns *et al.*, 1978).

These tumour types reflect a gradual weakening of growth control devices, accompanied by gradual changes in phenotypic expression. Logically, a reversibly growing benign tumour needs additional growth stimulation in order to become visible. Since the great majority of papillomas generated by multistage tumorigenesis in mouse skin belong to the reversibly growing benign type, it is easy to see that persistent growth stimulation is an obligatory condition for promotion. Stage 2 is probably nothing but persistent growth stimulation.

Thus, the role of stage 2 seems to be quite trivial; but this view may change completely if the progression of a benign to a malignant tumour type is found to take place within the second stage of promotion, perhaps *via* selective pressure. The multistage development of a carcinoma may therefore start with a mutation which subsequently is expressed during stage 1 of promotion and selected for increasing developmental autonomy during later stages.

## REFERENCES


Argyris, T.S. (1982) Tumor promotion by regenerative epidermal hyperplasia in mouse skin. *J. cutaneous Pathol.*, ***9***, 1–18

Baird, W.M., Sedgwick, J.A. & Boutwell, R.K. (1971) Effects of phorbol and four diesters of phorbol on the incorporation of tritiated precursors into DNA, RNA and protein of mouse epidermis. *Cancer Res.*, ***31***, 1434–1439

Baird, W.M., Melera, P.W. & Boutwell, R.K. (1972) Acrylamide gel electrophoresis studies on the incorporation of cytidine-$^{3}H$ into mouse skin RNA at early times after treatment with phorbol esters. *Cancer Res.*, ***32***, 781–788

Balmain, A. & Hecker, E. (1974) Early effects of growth-stimulating phorbol esters on phosphate transport and phospholipid synthesis in mouse epidermis. *Biochim. biophys. Acta*, ***362***, 457–468

Balmain, A. & Hecker, E. (1976) The effects of tumor promoters on [$^3$H]-choline and [$^3$H]-glycerol incorporation into mouse epidermal phosphatidylcholine in relation to their effects on [$^3$H]-thymidine incorporation into DNA. *Z. Krebsforsch.*, ***86***, 251–261

Berenblum, I. & Shubik, P. (1947) A new, quantitative approach to the study of the stages of chemical carcinogenesis in mouse skin. *Br. J. Cancer*, ***1***, 383–391

Bertsch, S. & Marks, F. (1974) Lack of an effect of tumor-promoting phorbol esters and of epidermal $G_1$-chalone on DNA synthesis in the epidermis of newborn mice. *Cancer Res.*, ***34***, 3283–3288

Bertsch, S. & Marks, F. (1978) Removal of the horny layer does not stimulate cell proliferation in neonatal mouse epidermis. *Cell Tissue Kinet.*, ***11***, 651–658

Bertsch, S. & Marks, F. (1982) A comparative study on wound-healing in neonatal and adult mouse epidermis *in vivo*. *Cell Tissue Kinet.*, ***15***, 81–87

Boutwell, R.K. (1964) Some biological aspects of skin carcinogenesis. *Prog. exp. Tumor Res.*, ***4***, 207–250

Boutwell, R.K., O'Brien, T.G., Verma, A.K., Weekes, R.G., de Young, L.M., Ashendel, C.L. & Astrup, E.G. (1979) The induction of ornithine decarboxylase activity and its control in mouse skin epidermis. *Adv. Enzyme Reg.*, ***17***, 89–112

Burns, F.J., Vanderlaan, M., Snyder, E. & Albert, R.E. (1978) *Induction and progression kinetics of mouse skin papillomas*. In: Slaga, T.J., Sivak, A. & Boutwell, R.K., eds, *Carcinogenesis*, Vol. 2, *Mechanisms of Tumor Promotion and Cocarcinogenesis*, New York, Raven Press, pp. 91–96

Castagna, M., Takai, Y., Kaibuchi, K., Sano, K., Kikkawa, V. & Nishizuka, Y. (1982) Direct activation of calcium-activated, phospholipid-dependent protein kinase by tumor-promoting phorbol esters. *J. biol. Chem.*, ***257***, 7847–7851

Clark-Lewis, I. & Murray, A.W. (1978) Tumor promotion and the induction of epidermal ornithine decarboxylase in mechanically stimulated mouse skin. *Cancer Res.*, ***38***, 494–497

Deelman, H.T. (1924) Die Entstehung des experimentellen Teerkrebses und die Bedeutung der Zellregeneration. *Z. Krebsforsch.*, ***21***, 220–226

Fitzgerald, D.J. & Murray, A.W. (1980) Inhibition of intercellular cooperation by tumor promoting phorbol esters. *Cancer Res.*, ***40***, 2935–2937

Friedwald, W.E. & Rous, P. (1944) The initiating and promoting elements in tumor production. *J. exp. Med.*, ***80***, 102–125

Fürstenberger, G., Richter, H., Fusenig, N.W. & Marks, F. (1981a) Arachidonic acid and prostaglandin $E_2$ release and enhanced cell proliferation induced by the phorbol ester TPA in a murine epidermal cell line. *Cancer Lett.*, ***11***, 191–198

Fürstenberger, G., Berry, D.L., Sorg, B. & Marks, F. (1981b) Skin tumor promotion by phorbol esters is a two-stage process. *Proc. natl Acad. Sci. USA*, ***78***, 7722–7726

Fürstenberger, G., Gross, M. & Marks, F. (1982) *On the role of prostaglandins in the induction of epidermal proliferation, hyperplasia and tumor promotion in mouse skin*. In: Powles, T.J., Bockman, R.S., Honn, K.V. & Ramwell, P., eds, *Prostaglandins and Cancer: First International Conference*, Vol. 2, New York, A.R. Liss, pp. 239–254

Fürstenberger, G., Sorg, B. & Marks, F. (1983) Tumor promotion by phorbol esters in skin: Evidence for a memory effect. *Science*, ***220***, 89–91

Ganss, M. (1983) *Zum Wirkungsmechanismus tumorpromovierender Phorbolester und anderer Mitogene in der Epidermis: Untersuchungen über die Rolle von Phospholipasen in vivo und in vitro,* PhD Thesis, University of Heidelberg

Ganss, M., Seemann, D., Fürstenberger, G. & Marks, F. (1982) Calcium-dependent release of arachidonic acid from a murine epidermal cell line induced by the tumor promoter TPA or ionophore A23187. *FEBS Lett.,* ***142,*** 54–58

Goyette, M., Petropoulos, C.J., Shank, P.R. & Fausto, N. (1983) Expression of a cellular oncogene during liver regeneration. *Science,* ***219,*** 510–512

Grimm, W. & Marks, F. (1974) Effect of tumor-promoting phorbol esters on the normal and the isoproterenol-stimulated level of cyclic AMP in mouse epidermis in vivo. *Cancer Res.,* ***34,*** 3128–3134

Hecker, E. & Schmidt, R. (1974) Phorbolesters–the irritants and cocarcinogens of *Croton tiglium* L. *Fortschr. Chemie Organ. Naturst.,* ***31,*** 377–467

Hennings, H. & Boutwell, R.K. (1970) Studies on the mechanism of skin tumor promotion. *Cancer Res.,* ***30,*** 312–325

Hergenhahn, M. & Hecker, E. (1981) Specific binding of the tumor promoter TPA in various mouse organs as measured by a 'cold acetone filter assay'. *Carcinogenesis,* ***2,*** 1277–1281

Holtzer, H. (1978) *Cell lineages, stem cells, and the quantal cell cycle concept.* In: Lord, B.I., Potten, C.S. & Cole, R.J., eds, *Stem Cells and Tissue Homeostasis (British Society of Cell Biology, Symposium 2),* New York, Cambridge University Press, pp. 1–27

Kreibich, G., Hecker, E., Süss, R. & Kinzel, V. (1971) Phorbolester stimulates choline incorporation. *Naturwissenschaften,* ***58,*** 323

Krieg, L., Kühlmann, I. & Marks, F. (1974) Effect of tumor-promoting phorbol esters and of acetic acid on mechanisms controlling DNA synthesis and mitosis (chalones) and on the biosynthesis of histidine-rich protein in mouse epidermis. *Cancer Res.,* ***34,*** 3135–3146

Marks, F. (1980) Prevention of phorbol ester-induced catecholamine refractoriness by inhibitors of protein and RNA biosynthesis in mouse epidermis in vivo. *FEBS Lett.,* ***114,*** 261–264

Marks, F., Bertsch, S., Grimm, W. & Schweizer, J. (1978) *Hyperplastic transformation and tumor promotion in mouse epidermis: possible consequences of disturbances of endogenous mechanisms controlling proliferation and differentiation.* In: Slaga, T.J., Sivak, A.K. & Boutwell, R.K., eds, *Carcinogenesis,* Vol. 2, *Mechanisms of Tumor Promotion and Cocarcinogenesis,* New York, Raven Press, pp. 97–116

Marks, F., Bertsch, S. & Fürstenberger, G. (1979) Ornithine decarboxylase activity, cell proliferation, and tumor promotion in mouse epidermis *in vivo. Cancer Res.,* ***39,*** 4183–4188

Marks, F., Fürstenberger, G. & Kownatzki, E. (1981) Prostaglandin E-mediated mitogenic stimulation of mouse epidermis in vivo by divalent cation ionophore A23187 and by tumor promoter TPA. *Cancer Res.,* ***41,*** 696–702

Marks, F., Fürstenberger, G., Ganss, M. & Seemann, D. (1982a) *Biological effects of phorbol ester tumor promoters in mouse skin.* In: Akoyunoglou, G., Evangelopoulos, A.E., Georgatsos, J., Palaiologos, G., Trakatellis, A. & Tsiganos, C.P., eds, *Cell Function and Differentiation,* Part A, New York, A.R. Liss, pp. 243–259

Marks, F., Berry, D.L., Bertsch, S., Fürstenberger, G. & Richter, H. (1982b) *On the relationship between epidermal hyperproliferation and skin tumor promotion.* In: Hecker, E., Fusenig, N.E., Kunz, W., Marks, F. & Thielmann, H.W., eds, *Carcinogenesis,* Vol. 7, *Cocarcinogenesis and Biological Effects of Tumor Promoters,* New York, Raven Press, pp. 331–346

Mottram, J.C. (1944) A developing factor in experimental blastogenesis. *J. Pathol. Bacteriol.,* ***56,*** 181–187

Niedel, J.E., Kuhn, L.J. & Vanderbark, G.R. (1983) Phorbol diester receptor copurifies with protein kinase C. *Proc. natl Acad. Sci. USA,* ***80,*** 36–40

O'Brien, T.G. (1976) The induction of ornithine decarboxylase as an early, possibly obligatory, event in mouse skin carcinogenesis. *Cancer Res.,* ***36,*** 2644–2653

Rohrschneider, L.R. & Boutwell, R.K. (1973) The early stimulation of phospholipid metabolism by TPA and its specificity for tumor promotion. *Cancer Res.,* ***33,*** 1945–1952

Rous, P. & Kidd, J.G. (1941) Conditional neoplasms and subthreshold neoplastic states. A study of tumors in rabbits. *J. exp. Med.,* ***73,*** 365–389

Slaga, T.J., Fischer, S.M., Nelson, K. & Gleason, G.L. (1980) Studies on the mechanism of skin tumor promotion: Evidence for several stages of promotion. *Proc. natl Acad. Sci. USA,* ***77,*** 3659–3663

Sorg, B., Fürstenberger, G., Berry, D.L., Hecker, E. & Marks, F. (1982) Preparation of retinoic acid esters of phorbol derivatives. *J. Lipid Res.,* ***23,*** 443–447

Twort, C.C. & Ing, H.R. (1928) Untersuchungen über krebserzeugende Agentien. *Z. Krebsforsch.,* ***27,*** 309–351

Van Duuren, B.L. & Orris, L. (1965) The tumor-enhancing principles from *Croton tiglium* L. *Cancer Res.,* ***25,*** 1871–1875

# MODELS AND MECHANISMS OF LIVER TUMOUR PROMOTION

# ALTERATIONS OF MARKERS DURING HEPATOCARCINOGENESIS IN RATS

K. LAPIS, E. UJHELYI, M. GYENES & A. JENEY

*First Institute of Pathology and Experimental Cancer Research,*
*Semmelweis Medical University,*
*Budapest, Hungary*

## SUMMARY

Fischer 344 male rats were treated with *N*-nitrosodiethylamine, and two weeks later promotion was effected by treatment with *N*-2-acetylaminofluorene for 14 days. At midpoint of the promotion protocol, one group of rats was subjected to partial hepatectomy (model A); others were treated with either carbon tetrachloride (model B) or thioacetamide (model C). Alterations in the activities of marker enzymes (glucose-6-phosphatase, γ-glutamyl transpeptidase, cytochrome P-450, *N*-demethylase) during hepatocarcinogenesis were followed biochemically. The highest incidences of liver foci and of hepatocellular carcinomas were observed in model A, and these showed a good correlation with long-lasting elevated γ-glutamyl transpeptidase activity. Analysis of the marker alterations suggests that there are three stages in hepatocarcinogenesis: (1) depression resulting from the toxic action of the initiator; (2) recovery and adaptation to cellular injury; and (3) long-lasting adverse alterations in the activities of the marker enzymes after promotion. The loss of certain non-histone proteins soon after promotion was also observed.

Comparative studies of the individual actions of initiators and promoters on marker enzymes indicated that both contribute to the marker changes during hepatocarcinogenesis.

## INTRODUCTION

Since hepatocarcinogenesis has been described as a multistep process, elucidation of the alteration specific to each stage, i.e., initiation and promotion (Peraino *et al.*, 1973; Farber, 1980; Pitot & Sirica, 1980) is especially worthwhile. Application of the initiator, followed by promotion, gives rise to multiple foci, nodules and, subsequently, to hepatocellular carcinomas. Early lesions could be detected by measuring those phenotypic markers expressed in the initiated hepatocytes that form foci as a result of promotion. The most frequently investigated markers include deficiency of glucose-6-phosphatase (G-6-Pase) and canalicular ATPase, the retention of glycogen upon fasting, and finally the high γ-glutamyl transpeptidase (GGT) activity, relative to that of the surrounding hepatocytes. Histochemical methods make possible determination of the size, number and distribution of foci. Therefore, they are suitable for estimating the extent of the lesions induced by the hepatocarcinogen (Friedrich-Freksa *et al.*, 1969; Fiala *et al.*, 1972; Rabes *et al.*, 1972; Scherer & Emmelot, 1975; Solt & Farber, 1976; Pitot *et al.*, 1978; Lapis, 1982). One way to gain a better understanding of hepatocarcinogenesis is to elucidate the role of initiators and promoters in the formation of markers, by following marker alterations during the complete course of hepatocarcinogenesis. In general, the available data provide information only about the marker alterations occurring after treatment with the complete hepatocarcinogen. In fact, there are only two recent reports in which initiator and promoter actions are discussed separately (Garcea *et al.*, 1982; Capouya & Lindahl, 1983). Although biochemical methods are not suitable for detection of foci and the data were obtained from a mixed liver cell population, it seems important to complete the histochemical observation with quantitative and more sensitive measurements. Biochemical studies may lead to the identification of new markers. In the reports of Garcea *et al.* (1982) and Leonard *et al.* (1982), hepatic drug metabolizing enzymes were considered to be markers for chemical carcinogenesis. Since disorder in gene regulation is implicated in the molecular process of carcinogenesis, we decided to study the alterations of nuclear proteins as well as the phenotypic markers of hepatocarcinogenesis. In this communication, experimental data are presented which show the alterations of G-6-Pase, *N*-demethylase and GGT activities and of the levels of cytochrome P-450 and nuclear proteins, during the course of hepatocarcinogenesis induced according to the protocol described by Solt and Farber (1976).

## MATERIALS AND METHODS

### *Animals*

Male Fischer F344 rats weighing 130 to 150 g were obtained from LATI Breeding Center (Gödöllö, Hungary). Animals were maintained in plastic cages (five per cage) and given laboratory chow (LATI, Gödöllö) and water *ad libitum*.

### *Protocols*

The initiation-promotion system developed principally by Solt and Farber (1976) was utilized to investigate alterations of markers during the course of hepatocarcinogenesis. The animals were sacrificed at different times after *N*-nitrosodiethylamine (NDEA) treatment. NDEA (Eastman, Kodak, Rochester, USA), as initiator, was administered i.p. at a dose of 200 mg/kg body weight. The animals were permitted to recover for two weeks, and then promotion was effected by administration of 5 mg/kg 2-acetylaminofluorene (2-AAF, Serva, Heidelberg, FRG) p.o. daily for two

Fig. 1. Experimental models of hepatocarcinogenesis
■, period of AAF treatment; NDEA, *N*-nitrosodiethylamine; PH, partial hepatectomy; $CCl_4$, carbon tetrachloride; TAA, thioacetamide; AAF, *N*-2-acetylaminofluorene

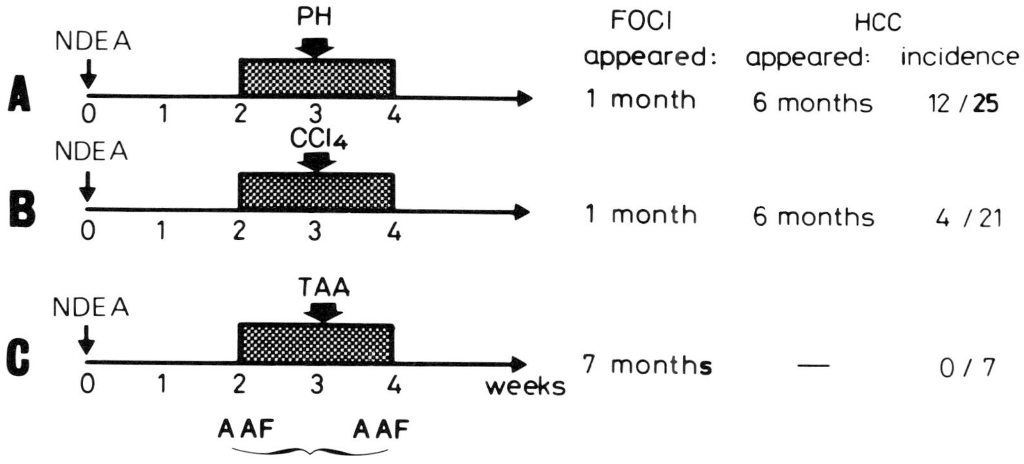


weeks. One week after starting promotion (i.e., 21 days after NDEA initiation), the first group of animals was subjected to partial hepatectomy (model A). The second group was treated with 0.5 ml/kg carbon tetrachloride p.o. (Reanal, Budapest, Hungary) (model B). The third group received 60 mg/kg thioacetamide (TAA, Fluka, Buchs, Switzerland) i.p. (model C). The three initiation-promotion protocols employed and the incidences of hepatocellular carcinoma induced are shown in Figure 1. In order to compare the action of initiator and promoters on marker enzyme activities, animals were sacrificed at day 6 and at day 14 following NDEA treatment, and at day 14 after treatment with 2-AAF including partial hepatectomy (promotion system in model A). In order to study the action of another type of promoter, phenobarbital was administered by adding it to the drinking water (0.5%) for five days; these animals were sacrificed on the sixth day.

*Biochemical procedures*

Livers were removed from the ether-anaesthetized rats and kept frozen at −30 °C until utilization. One gram of the liver samples was washed and homogenized in cold 50 mM Tris-hydrochloric acid (pH 7.4) buffer containing 1.15% potassium chloride. Nuclei were removed by centrifugation at 600 × *g* and mitochondria at 15 000 × *g*. Enzyme measurements were performed on the pellet from the 100 000 × *g* centrifugation (microsomal fraction).

*Cytochrome P-450 concentration:* Microsomes were resuspended in 50 mM Tris-hydrochloric acid (pH 7.6) containing 1 mM ethylenediaminetetraacetic acid. Spectral measurements were performed in a Zeiss Specord UV VIS dual beam spectrophotometer, and cytochrome P-450 concentrations were determined from reduced CO difference spectra as described by Omura and Sato (1964).

N-*Demethylase activity:* Ethylmorphine was used as the substrate, and microsomes were incubated in the presence of an NADPH generating system at 37 °C for 10 min. Formaldehyde, as the reaction product, was measured with Nash reagent in a Farrand spectrofluorimeter (A/F: 405/508), according to the procedure described by Belmon (1963) and Castro and Gilette (1967).

*GGT activity:* Microsomes (200–400 μg protein) were incubated with γ-glutamyl-*p*-nitroanilide as substrate and glycylglycine as acceptor for 15 min at 37 °C as described by Szász (1969). The *p*-nitroaniline released was measured at 405 nm in a Zeiss spectrophotometer. Units of enzyme activity are expressed as μmol *p*-nitroaniline formed per min at 37 °C.

*G-6-Pase activity:* Microsomes in 50 mM Tris-hydrochloric acid (pH 6.8) buffer were incubated with G-6-P (Harper, 1963). The inorganic phosphorus liberated was measured as described by Fiske and Subbarow (1925).

In order to study nuclear proteins, nuclei were isolated using the method described by Hewish and Burgoyne (1973). Histones and acid-soluble non-histones were extracted from the purified nuclei with 0.2N sulfuric acid at 0 °C for one hour, precipitated with five volumes of acetone and vacuum dried. Protein samples were separated according to molecular weights by applying SDS-polyacrylamide-gel electrophoresis as described previously (Jeney *et al.,* 1979). All measurements of protein concentration were performed according to the method of Hartree (1972).

## RESULTS

Following the initiation-promotion protocol according to model A and model B, hyperplastic foci appeared equally in both models one month after promotion. However, more hepatocellular carcinomas were induced in model A than in model B rats. Remarkably, in model C, foci appeared much later (seven months) and no hepatoma was observed (Fig. 1). Studies on the time course of the enzymatic alterations also indicated certain other differences among the three model systems. Treatment for 24 h with NDEA caused a reduction in the activity of most of the enzymatic markers. This depression was followed by a rapid recovery. The amount of cytochrome P-450 began to increase, and GGT, as well as G-6-Pase activities, rose above control values (Figs 2, 3, 4). However, the alterations of the enzyme markers during the later period of hepatocarcinogenesis varied according to the type of promotion protocol applied two weeks after NDEA treatment. The promotion protocol of model A caused a relatively consistent elevation of GGT activity, a decrease in that of G-6-Pase, and a transient increase followed by a substantial reduction in the level of cytochrome P-450 in the liver (Fig. 2).

The replacement of partial hepatectomy by carbon tetrachloride (model B) did not result in this consistent elevation of GGT, and there was no transient rise in the amount of cytochrome P-450 at the end of the promotion (Fig. 3). In model C, particularly, alterations were the same as those observed as in liver treated according to model B, but, soon after promotion, a substantial reduction of G-6-Pase and a late increase in the amount of cytochrome P-450 were also observed (Fig. 4).

Fig. 2 Alterations of markers during hepatocarcinogenesis induced according to the protocol of model A
Enzyme alterations expressed as % of controls. GGT, γ-glutamyl transpeptidase; G-6-Pase, glucose-6-phosphatase; NDEA, *N*-nitrosodiethylamine; PH, partial hepatectomy; AAF, *N*-2-acetylaminofluorene

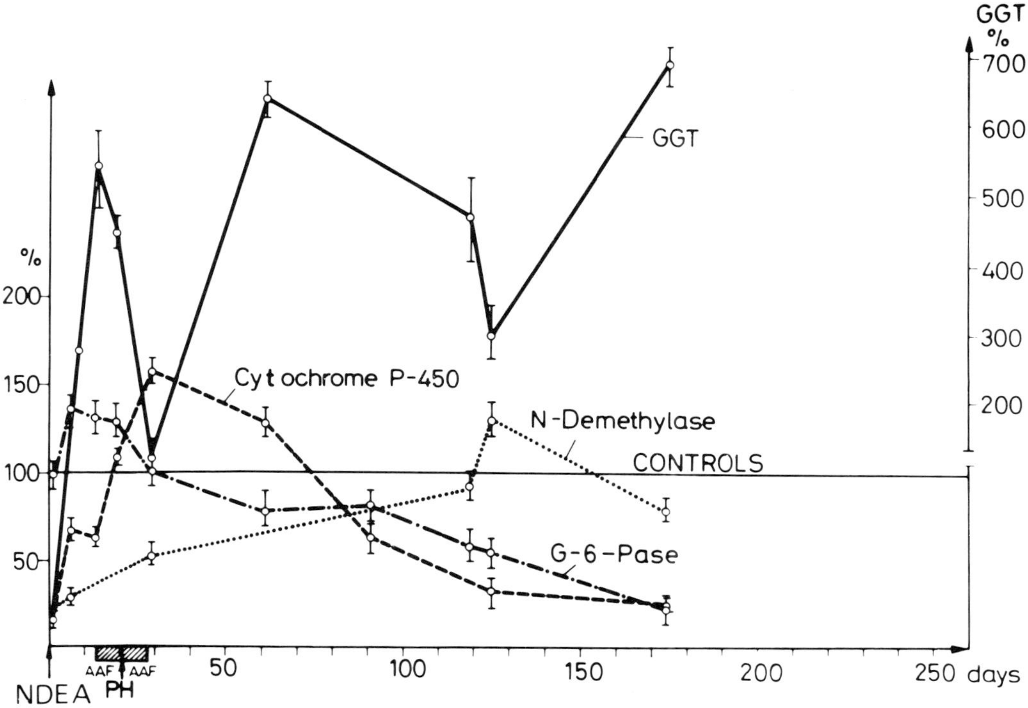


Upon investigation of the polymorphism of the acid-soluble nuclear proteins, definite alterations were observed soon after completion of the promotion protocol. The disappearance of approximately six protein species with low mobility on the SDS-polyacrylamide gel-electropherogram could be seen, especially in rat liver treated according to model A. This change seemed to be specific to the stage of promotion (day 21), because it could not be observed 14 days after NDEA treatment nor one month later (i.e., 60 days) (Fig. 5).

When visible liver lesions appeared, they were isolated, and it was possible to determine enzyme markers in histologically defined and relatively homogeneous samples. The preneoplastic nodules obtained from livers treated according to model A showed a substantially lower amount of cytochrome P-450 and of G-6-Pase activity and a higher GGT activity. In the preneoplastic nodules from model B, the cytochrome P-450 level and G-6-Pase activity changed much less drastically, and no change at all was observed in the activity of GGT. These enzyme changes, however, were evident in all hepatocellular carcinomas, irrespective of whether they originated from livers obtained from animals treated according to model A or B (Fig. 6).

Fig. 3. Alterations of markers during hepatocarcinogenesis induced according to the protocol of model B
Enzyme alterations expressed as % of controls. GGT, γ-glutamyl transpeptidase; G-6-Pase, glucose-6-phosphatase; NDEA, *N*-nitrosodiethylamine; AAF, *N*-2-acetylaminofluorene; $CCl_4$, carbon tetrachloride

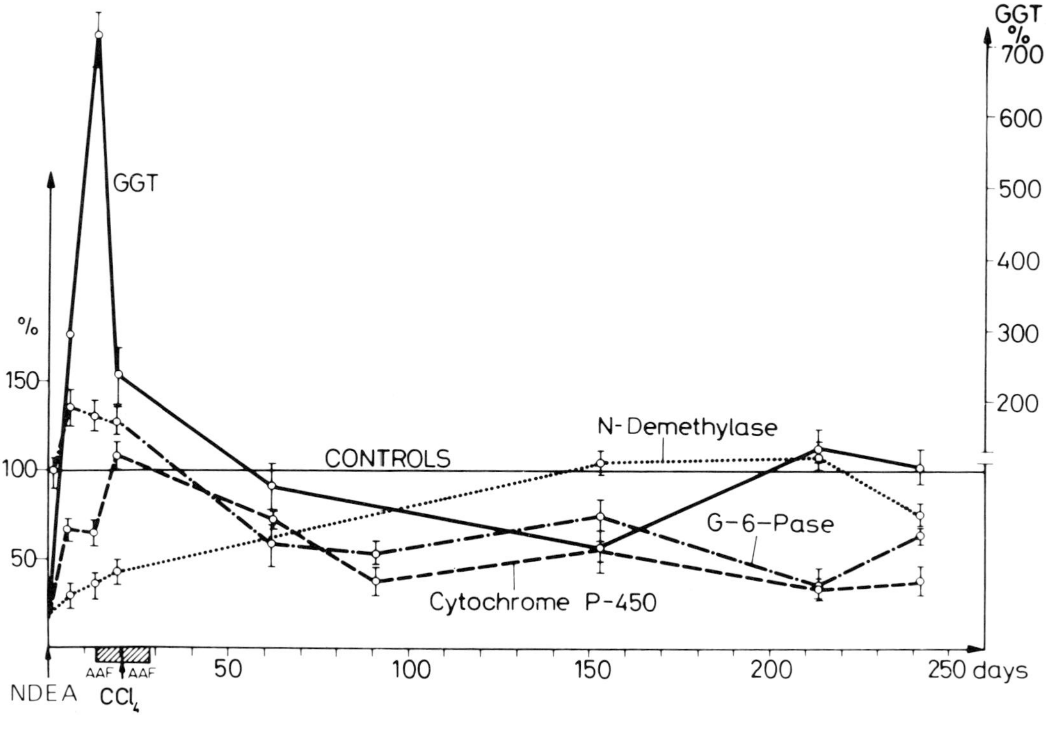


Finally, we attempted to ascertain whether enzymatic markers were also induced by promoters alone. Figures 7 and 8 show that the alterations in hepatocarcinogenic markers could be detected after a single treatment with either NDEA or promoters. Furthermore, there were differences in the responses of livers toward the two promoters: one, the promotion protocol of model A (2-AAF + partial hepatectomy) and the other, phenobarbital. Increase in GGT activity was common to rats treated both by NDEA and by promoters. In contrast, however, the amount of cytochrome P-450 was transiently reduced by NDEA, elevated by phenobarbital and not affected by the promotion protocol of model A (Figs 7 and 8).

## DISCUSSION

Numerous studies have concluded that promotion in the carcinogenic process involves those cellular events which lead to the phenotypic expression of initiation (rare events) by the selective multiplication of the initiated cell population (Farber, 1980). The detection of enzymatic markers in focal arrangement (liver foci) after

Fig. 4. Alterations of markers during hepatocarcinogenesis induced according to the protocol of model C
Enzyme alterations expressed as % of controls. GGT, γ-glutamyl transpeptidase; G-6-Pase, glucose-6-phosphatase; NDEA, *N*-nitrosodiethylamine; AAF, *N*-2-acetylaminofluorene; TAA, thioacetamide

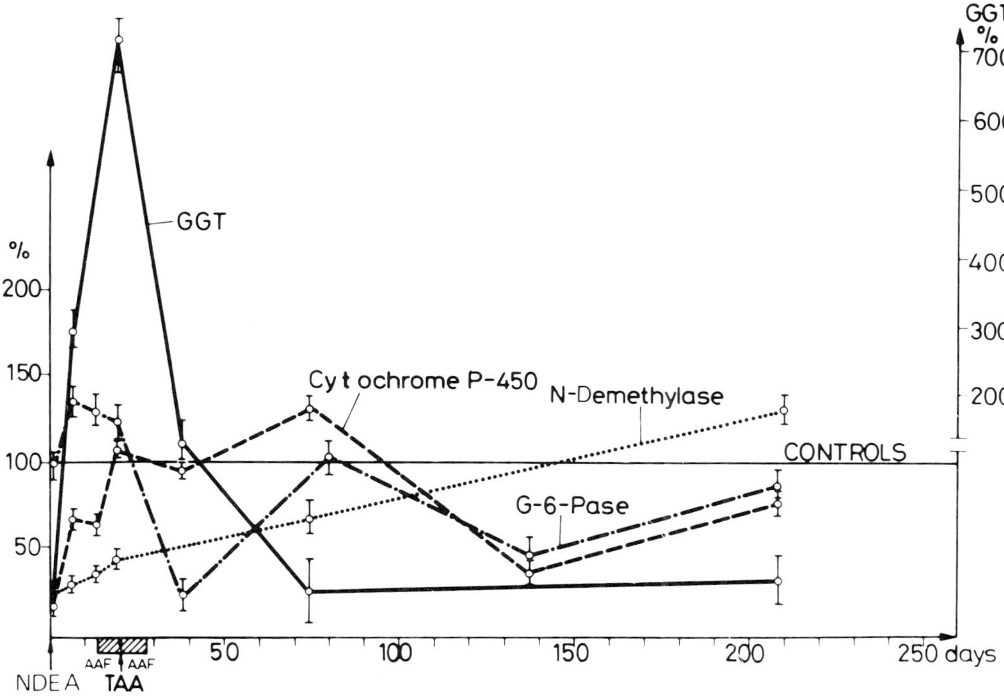


treatment with the complete hepatocarcinogen protocol (initiator + promoter) lends support to this concept. GGT has been regarded as one of the most relevant markers, because its oncofetal property has been demonstrated, and it has been detected in 90% of hepatic foci (Ogawa *et al.*, 1980; Ding *et al.*, 1982; Leonard *et al.*, 1982; Pereira *et al.*, 1983). In all the three protocols of hepatocarcinogen treatment, long-lasting, high GGT activity was observed to be correlated with the high incidence of hepatocellular carcinomas (Figs 1 and 2). Recent studies, however, queried the specificity of GGT activity as a marker of liver malignancy and gave more credit to the findings, that indicate that GGT activity is important to normal cell metabolism, including transport of neutral amino acids, glutathione conversion and detoxication of xenobiotics (Meister, 1973; Higashi *et al.*, 1976; Colombo & Colombo, 1979). GGT has been shown to be a permanent constituent of plasma membrane in liver cells, and it has been located histochemically in bile-duct cells of untreated rat liver. More importantly, the observations showed that reportedly non-carcinogenic compounds (alcohol, heroin, phenobarbital, α-naphthylisothiocyanate) also caused substantial increases of GGT activity (Colombo & Colombo, 1979; Ratanasavanh *et al.*, 1978;

Fig. 5. Alterations of chromatin proteins during hepatocarcinogenesis
1 14 days after NDEA
2 20 days after NDEA, with *N*-2-acetylaminofluorene (2-AAF) treatment during the last 6 days
3 26 days after NDEA, with 2-AAF + carbon tetrachloride treatment (model B)
4 26 days after NDEA, with 2-AAF + partial hepatectomy treatment (model A)
5 26 days after NDEA, with 2-AAF + thioacetamide treatment (model C)
6 60 days after NDEA, with 2-AAF + carbon tetrachloride treatment (model B)
7 60 days after NDEA, with 2-AAF + partial hepatctomy treatment (model A)
8 60 days after NDEA, with 2-AAF + thioacetamide treatment (model C)

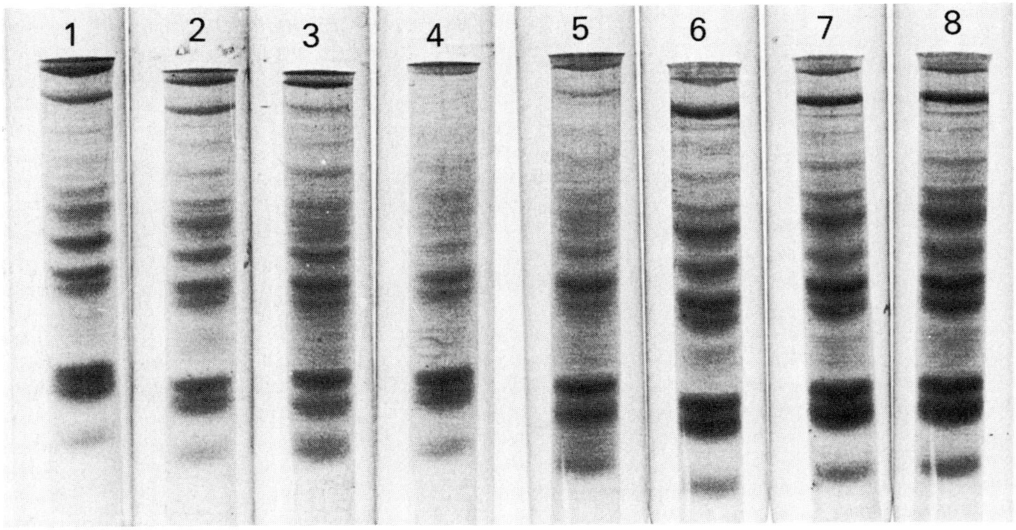


Fig. 6. Enzymatic markers in isolatec nodules and hepatocellular carcinoma (HCC)
A, Liver nodules or HCC in rats treated according to the protocol of model A; B, liver nodules or HCC in rats treated accord ng to the protocol of model B; GGT, γ-glutamyl transpeptidase

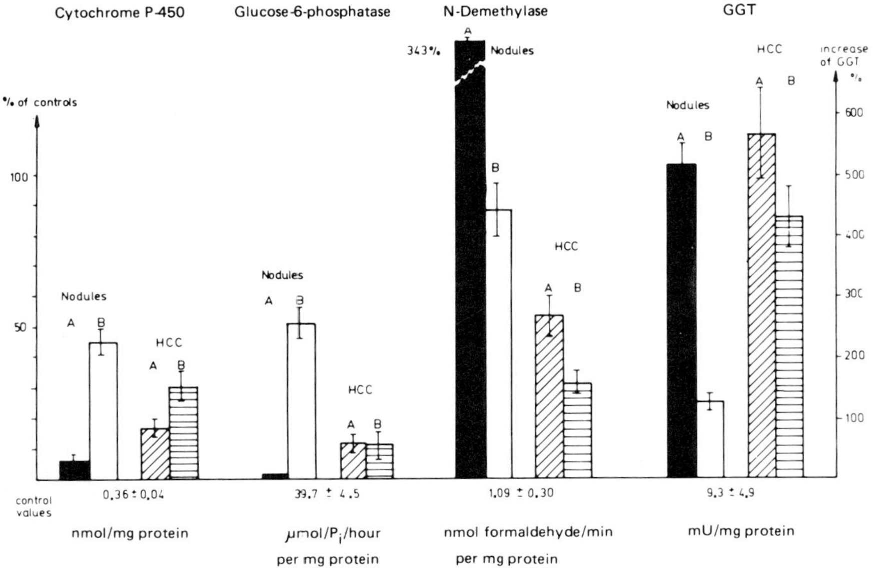

Fig. 7. Alterations of cytochrome P-450 and *N*-demethylase induced by initiator or promoters before the appearance of foci
NDEA, *N*-nitrosodiethylamine; PB, phenobarbital; AAF, *N*-2-acetylaminofluorene; PH, partial hepatectomy

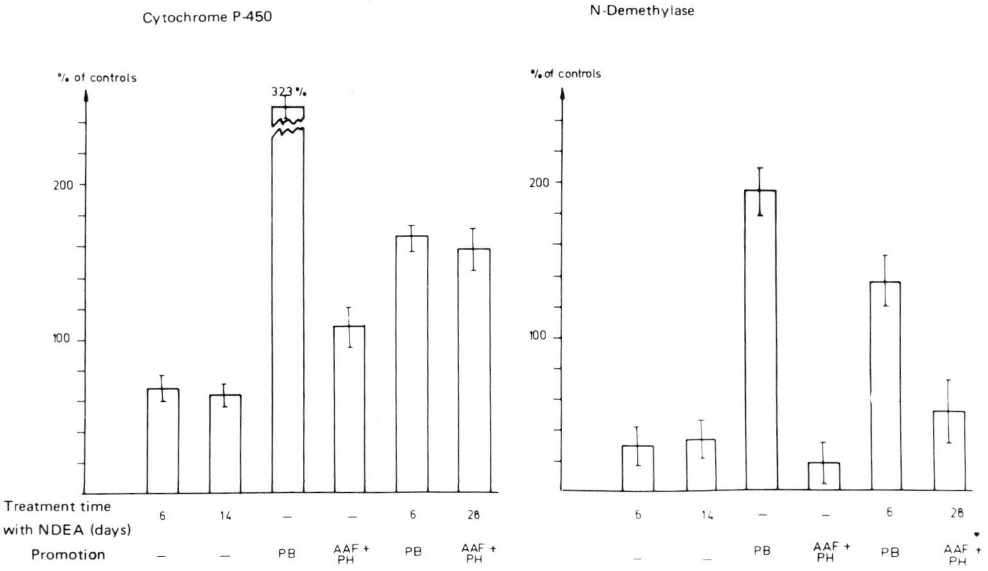


Fig. 8. Alterations of G-6-phosphatase and γ-glutamyl transferase induced by initiator or promoters before the appearance of foci
NDEA, *N*-nitrosodiethylamine; PB, phenobarbital; AAF, *N*-2-acetylaminofluorene; PH, partial hepatectomy

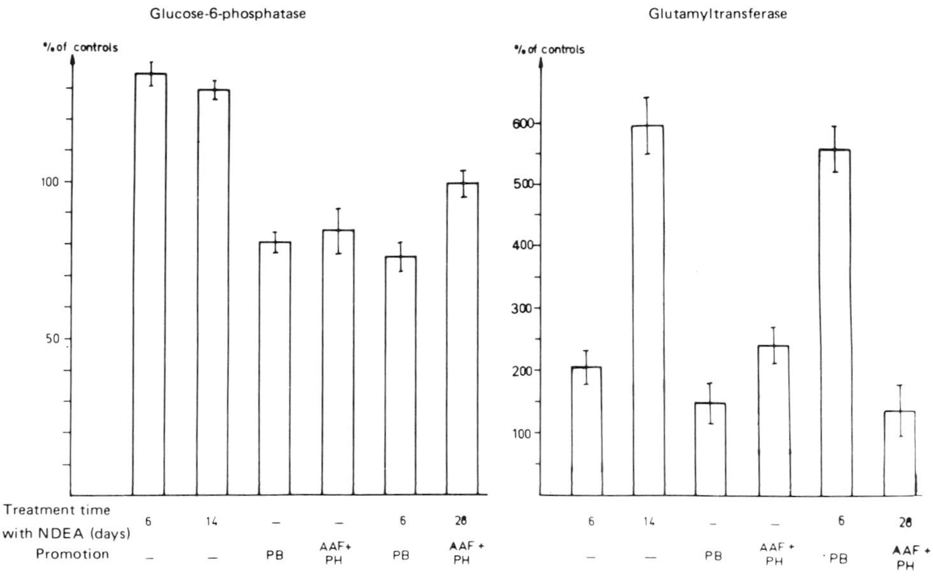

Nishimura *et al.*, 1981; Penn *et al.*, 1981; Richards *et al.*, 1982). Therefore, clarification of those enzymatic alterations regarded as specific to hepatocarcinogenesis awaits further study. Application of biochemical methods added further problems, because alterations in enzymatic activity could be demonstrated long before the appearance of foci. It may be possible, however, that these early changes have no relevance to the hepatocarcinogenic process and they represent only the toxic action of the hepatocarcinogen. Nevertheless, one should keep in mind that all metabolic processes during hepatocarcinogenesis are assumed to be directly or indirectly related to these toxic events. The data presented suggest that three stages can be distinguished in the alterations of enzyme activity during hepatocarcinogenesis.

1. An early depression that is caused by the necrogenic dose of the initiator
2. Recovery and adaptation to cellular injury. The reduced activity of some enzymes tends to return to normal, whereas the activity of others rises above the normal.
3. Long-lasting, adverse marker alterations caused by the promoter. There is a secondary depression in certain hepatic enzymes (cytochrome P-450) and an increase in others (such as GGT).

These conclusions are fully in agreement with the data of Garcea *et al.* (1982) which also showed reduction during the early period of NDEA treatment followed by a recovery. The observations of Columbano *et al.* (1981) were similar to ours. They noted differences in the action of the various types of promoters and concluded that either the mechanisms were different or the target cell populations were not the same. Farber (1980) postulated that, in these experimental models, initiation takes place as a rare event in certain cells, giving rise to foci. Conceivably, these cells have high GGT activity, are resistant to the toxic action of the initiator, and are induced to proliferate by the promoter. It seems difficult to reconcile this concept with the biochemical data presented, since induction of the enzymatic markers was demonstrated not to be an exclusive property of the initiator (Figs 7 and 8). Furthermore, the enzymatic alterations observed before the appearance of foci were too great to be attributed exclusively to these rare cells. It seems more plausible that, in our experimental model system, hepatocytes respond to the toxic action of NDEA by a higher GGT activity. An alternative mechanism might be considered which takes account of the fact that initiators – such as NDEA – induce diffuse cellular injury. However, the ensuing DNA damage and the reduction of certain enzyme activities are subjected to a repair mechanism, except in certain repair-deficient cells. The foci may be formed from these cells after the proliferative stimulation induced by the promoter. It is highly probable that the introduction of techniques for the isolation of various liver cell populations will make it possible to determine whether it is resistant cells or repair-deficient cells that give rise to foci. Furthermore, studies of the regulatory elements of gene functions – such as nuclear proteins – may contribute to the identification of the phenotypic markers in hepatocarcinogenesis. In this context, the changes in the nuclear proteins observed after promotion are noteworthy. The loss of a similar group of non-histone proteins was also observed in fibroblast culture after treatment with methylcholanthrene (Szende *et al.*, 1979).

## REFERENCES


Belmon, S. (1963) The fluorimetric determination of formaldehyde. *Anal. chim. Acta,* ***29,*** 120–126

Capouya, E.R. & Lindahl, R. (1983) Changes in the γ-glutamyltransferase activity during *N*-2-fluorenylacetamide induced rat hepatocarcinogenesis. *J. natl Cancer Inst.,* ***70,*** 359–365

Castro, I.A. & Gilette, I.R. (1967) Species and sex differences in the kinetic constant for the N-demethylation of ethyl-morphine by liver microsomes. *Biochem. biophys. Res. Commun.,* ***28,*** 426–430

Colombo, J.P. & Colombo, J. (1979) Plasma γ-glutamyltransferase in heroin addicts. *Clin. chim. Acta,* ***95,*** 483–486

Columbano, A., Rajalakshami, S. & Sarma, D.S.R. (1981) Requirement of cell proliferation for the initiation of liver carcinogenesis as assayed by three different procedures. *Cancer Res.,* ***41,*** 2079–2083

Ding, J.L., Smith, G.D. & Peters, T.J. (1982) The turnover of hepatoma cell γ-glutamyl transferase. *FEBS Lett.,* ***142,*** 207–209

Farber, E. (1980) The sequential analysis of liver cancer induction. *Biochem. biophys. Acta,* ***605,*** 149–166

Fiala, S., Fiala, A.E. & Dixon, B. (1972) Gamma-glutamyltranspeptidase in transplantable, chemically induced rat hepatomas and 'spontaneous' mouse hepatomas. *J. natl Cancer Inst.,* ***48,*** 1393–1401

Fiske, C.H. & Subbarow, Y. (1925) The colorimetric determination of phosphorus. *J. biol. Chem.,* ***66,*** 375–400

Friedrich-Freksa, A., Gossner, W. & Borner, P. (1969) Histochemische Untersuchungen der Cancerogenese in der Rattenleber nach Dauergaben von Diäthylnitrosamin. *Z. Krebsforsch.,* ***72,*** 226–241

Garcea, A.R., Cannto, R.A., Biocca, M.E., Muzio, G. & Grasso, G. (1982) Variations of cytochrome P-450 content and aminopyrene demethylase activity in rat liver microsomes during diethylnitrosamine carcinogenesis. *Cancer,* ***10,*** 703

Harper, A.E. (1963) *Glucose-6-phosphatase.* In: Bergmeyer, H.U., ed., *Methods of Enzymatic Analysis,* New York, Academic Press, pp. 788–792

Hartree, E.F. (1972) Determination of protein: a modification of the Lowry method that gives a linear photometric response. *Anal. Biochem.,* ***48,*** 422–427

Hewish, D.R. & Burgoyne, L.A. (1973) Chromatin structure. The digestion of chromatin DNA at regularly spaced sites by a nuclear deoxyribonuclease. *Biochem. biophys. Res. Commun;* ***52,*** 504–510

Higashi, T., Tateishi, N., Naruse, A. & Sakamato, Y. (1976) Decrease of glutathione and induction of γ-glutamyltransferase by dibutyryl-3′,5′-cyclic AMP in rat liver. *Biochem. biophys. Res. Commun.,* ***68,*** 1280–1286

Jeney, A., Dzurillay, É., Lapis, K. & Valkó, É. (1979) Chromatin proteins as possible target for antitumour agents: Alterations of chromatin proteins in dibromodulcitol treated Yoshida tumours. *Chem.-biol. Interact.,* ***26,*** 349–361

Lapis, K. (1982) *Morphologic expression of neoplasia in human and experimental liver tumours.* In: *Abstracts of the Proceedings of the 13th International Cancer Congress, Seattle, Washington,* p. 11

Leonard, T.B., Dent, J.G., Graichen, E., Lyght, O. & Popp, J.A. (1982) Comparison of hepatic carcinogen initiation-promotion systems. *Carcinogenesis,* ***3,*** 851–856
Meister, A. (1973) On the enzymology of amino acid transport. *Science,* ***180,*** 33–39
Nishimura, M., Stein, H., Berges, W. & Teshke, R. (1981) γ-Glutamyl-transpeptidase activity of liver plasma membrane induction following chronic alcohol consumption. *Biochem. biophys. Res. Commun.,* ***99,*** 142–148
Ogawa, K., Solt, D.B. & Farber, E. (1980) Phenotypic diversity as an early property of putative preneoplastic hepatocyte populations in liver carcinogenesis. *Cancer Res.,* ***40,*** 725–733
Omura, T. & Sato, R. (1964) The carbon monoxide-binding pigment of liver microsomes. 1. Evidence for its hemoprotein nature. *J. biol. Chem.,* ***177,*** 751–766
Penn, R., Worthington, D.J., Clarke, C.A. & Whitfield, A.G.W. (1981) γ-Glutamyltransferase and alcohol intake. *Lancet,* ***i,*** 889–890
Peraino, C., Fry, R.J.M., Staffeldt, E. & Kisielski, W.E. (1973) Effects of varying the exposure to PB on its enhancement of 2-AAF induced hepatic tumorigenesis in the rat. *Cancer Res.,* ***33,*** 2701–2705
Pereira, M.A., Lin, L.H.C. & Herren, S.L. (1983) Role of $O^6$-methylation in the initiation of GGTase positive foci. *Chem.-biol. Interact.,* ***43,*** 313–322
Pitot, H.C. & Sirica, A.E. (1980) The stages of initiation and promotion in hepatocarcinogenesis. *Biochem. biophys. Acta,* ***605,*** 191–215
Pitot, H.C., Barsness, L. & Goldsworthy, T. (1978) Biochemical characterisation of stages of hepatocarcinogenesis after a single dose of diethylnitrosamine. *Nature,* ***271,*** 456–457
Rabes, H.M., Scholze, P. & Jantsch, B. (1972) Growth kinetics of diethylnitrosamine-induced, enzyme deficient 'preneoplastic' liver cell populations in vivo and in vitro. *Cancer Res.,* ***32,*** 2577–2586
Ratanasavanh, D., Tazi, A., Galteau, M.M. & Siest, O. (1978) Localization of gamma-glutamyltransferase in subcellular fractions of rat and rabbit liver: effect of phenobarbital. *Biochem. Pharmacol.,* ***28,*** 1363–1365
Richards, W.L., Tsukada, Y. & Potter, V.R. (1982) α-Glutamyltranspeptidase and α-fetoprotein expression during α-naphthylisothiocyanate induced hepatotoxicity in rats. *Cancer Res.,* ***42,*** 5133–5138
Scherer, E. & Emmelot, P. (1975) Foci altered liver cells induced by a single dose of diethylnitrosamine and partial hepatectomy, their contribution to hepatocarcinogenesis in the rat. *Eur. J. Cancer,* ***11,*** 145–154
Solt, D. & Farber, E. (1976) New principle for analysis of chemical carcinogenesis. *Nature,* ***263,*** 701–703
Szász, G. (1969) A kinetic photometric method for serum γ-glutamyl transpeptidase. *Clin. Chem.,* ***15,*** 124–136
Szende, B., Gyapay, G., Ferenc, G., Ujhelyi, E., Lapis, K. & Jeney, A. (1979) Spontaneous and chemically induced transformation of mouse fibroblasts in culture. Biochemical aspects of the transformed cells. *Acta biol. acad. sci. hung.,* ***30,*** 309–316

# RELATIONSHIP OF HISTOCHEMICALLY DETECTABLE ALTERED HEPATOCYTE FOCI TO HEPATIC TUMORIGENESIS

C. PERAINO[1], E.F. STAFFELDT, B.A. CARNES, V.A. LUDEMAN & J.A. BLOMQUIST

*Division of Biological and Medical Research, Argonne National Laboratory, Argonne, IL 60439, USA*

S.D. VESSELINOVITCH

*Department of Radiology, The University of Chicago, Chicago, IL 60637, USA*

## SUMMARY

A new experimental system was used to examine the stages of chemically induced hepatic neoplasia in the rat. The treatment protocol involved the intraperitoneal injection of a single non-necrogenic dose of carcinogen [*N*-nitrosodiethylamine (NDEA) or benzo[*a*]pyrene (BP)] into male and female rats within one day after birth, followed by dietary exposure to promoter (0.05% phenobarbital) from weaning. Rats were killed at intervals, and their livers were examined for tumours and for histochemically detectable foci of altered hepatocytes. Six histochemical markers were used. Through serial frozen-sectioning techniques and computer-assisted image analysis, foci containing between one and six markers were identified, and their average sizes were calculated. The same complement of histochemical tests was applied to the primary hepatic tumours observed in this study.

The data showed that (1) the new treatment protocol was highly efficient in foci and tumour production; (2) growth rates and incidence levels of foci were directly related to hepatocarcinogenic effectiveness (NDEA > BP), whereas both carcinogens had similar effects on foci phenotypic properties; (3) after their formation, foci at a given level of phenotypic complexity did not become progressively more complex; (4) incidence levels of foci were sex-dependent (females > males), but growth rates of foci were the same for both sexes; (5) growth rates and growth capacities (ranges of

[1] To whom correspondence should be addressed

possible growth rates) of foci were directly related to phenotypic complexity levels of foci; (6) frequencies and phenotypic complexities of foci were inversely related; the reverse was true for tumours, although 10% of the tumours were relatively simple (three markers or fewer); (7) marker frequency distribution patterns were completely different in foci and in tumours.

From these observations, we suggest that the foci are not direct tumour progenitors but, instead, are manifestations of a mosaic of subtumorigenic effects of the carcinogenic stimulus on cellular functions associated with the control of cell division and phenotypic character. The observed foci and tumour characteristics suggest that these carcinogen-induced cellular changes define elements of the mechanism whereby a specific neoplastic transformation site is rendered more accessible to carcinogenic attack.

## INTRODUCTION

As discussed in several reviews, research in experimental hepatocarcinogenesis has been directed increasingly toward the examination of the phenotypic changes occurring in histochemically detectable foci of altered hepatocytes that invariably appear in carcinogen-treated liver prior to tumour formation (Bannasch *et al.*, 1980; Emmelot & Scherer, 1980; Farber, 1980; Pitot & Sirica, 1980; Williams, 1980; Peraino *et al.*, 1983). If, as is generally believed (preceding references), at least some of these foci are generically related to hepatic tumorigenesis, their characterization becomes important as a means of gaining insight into the elements of the neoplastic process. Moreover, in view of the responsiveness of the liver to a wide variety of tumour initiators and promoters (Peraino *et al.*, 1983), the high foci:tumour incidence ratio (Pitot *et al.*, 1978) and the relatively early appearance of foci (Peraino *et al.*, 1981), an understanding of the relationship between foci and tumours would enhance the utility of the liver tumorigenesis system as a sensitive and rapid bioassay for agents with initiating or promoting activity. Realization of these objectives, however, requires the development of simple treatment protocols that combine the maximum responsiveness to the tumorigenic effects of the administered agents with the lowest possible incidence of extraneous toxic effects that could obscure early preneoplastic changes. To this end, we have devised a treatment regimen involving the administration of a single low dose of tumour initiator, by intraperitoneal injection, to rats within one day after birth, with dietary exposure to promoter beginning at weaning (Peraino *et al.*, 1981). According to preliminary data from an experiment utilizing this procedure, initiation with *N*-nitrosodiethylamine (NDEA) or benzo[*a*]pyrene (BP) produced altered hepatocyte foci within three weeks after the rats had been weaned onto a diet containing phenobarbital as the promoter; liver tumours appeared in the NDEA- and BP-treated rats within 8 and 16 weeks after weaning, respectively (Peraino *et al.*, 1981). The present paper describes further analysis of the data obtained from that experiment after its completion. Incidences of altered hepatocyte foci and hepatic tumours were measured over an interval of 469 days after the administration of NDEA or BP to male and female rats by the procedure indicated above. Phenotypic characteristics of the foci and tumours were assessed in terms of their expression of one or more histochemically detectable changes (hereafter called 'markers'). The results suggest that the formation and characteristics of foci represent generic responses to effects of carcinogen on processes associated with the control of hepatocyte growth and phenotypic character, but that the foci themselves are probably not direct tumour progenitors.

## MATERIALS AND METHODS

### *Animal treatments*

As described previously (Peraino *et al.*, 1981), pregnant Sprague-Dawley rats (Charles River Breeding Laboratories, Wilmington, MA, USA) were obtained five days before parturition and were caged individually under constant temperature (23 °C) and a 12-h light/12-h dark illumination cycle. Water and a standard laboratory diet (Wayne Lab Blox, Allied Mills, Chicago, IL, USA) were available *ad libitum*. One day after birth, each of the offspring was injected once intraperitoneally with approximately 0.1 mL (microsyringe) of carcinogen dissolved in corn oil. NDEA was given at a dosage of 0.15 μmol/g body weight; the dosage of BP was 0.59 μmol/g body weight. Control rats were injected with corn oil alone. At 21 days of age the rats were weaned, segregated with respect to sex, and placed, three per cage, on a 30% casein diet (Teklad Test Diets, Madison, WI, USA) containing 0.05% phenobarbital (Peraino *et al.*, 1971). All groups, including the controls, were treated with phenobarbital in order to increase the responsiveness of the liver to the carcinogens. Prior investigations have demonstrated that phenobarbital enhances hepatic tumorigenesis in mice injected with NDEA at birth (Uchida & Hirona, 1979) and in rats injected with polycyclic aromatic hydrocarbons after partial hepatectomy (Hirakawa *et al.*, 1979; Pitot, 1979; Kitagawa *et al.*, 1980).

### *Histochemical analysis*

At intervals of 28, 35, 49, 77, 133, 245 and 469 days after birth, rats from each treatment group were killed and their livers were examined for the presence of histochemically detectable foci of altered hepatocytes and hepatic tumours. For the histochemical analyses, a cylindrical plug, 2 cm in diameter, was removed from the left lobe of each liver, frozen on dry ice and stored at −100 °C in a sealed, airtight container. At the time of analysis, each frozen plug was mounted in a cryostat and cut serially into 10- to 15-μm-thick frozen sections, each of which was assayed for one of the following histochemical markers in the following order; the first for increased γ-glutamyltranspeptidase (GGT), the second for increased diaphorase (D), the third for iron exclusion (Fe), the fourth for decreased glucose-6-phosphatase (G6P), the fifth for increased alkaline phosphatase (Alk), and the sixth for glycogen storage (PP, for periodic acid Schiff-positive) or glycogen depletion (PN, for periodic acid Schiff-negative). References for these assays are provided in a recent review (Peraino *et al.*, 1983). As discussed in that review, all of these histochemical markers have been used to detect putative preneoplastic hepatocyte foci in the livers of carcinogen-treated rats. For the iron exclusion assay, all rats were treated parenterally with iron dextran

(Imferon) prior to sacrifice (Hirota & Williams, 1979). Tumours were frozen and analysed histochemically as described above; sections from these tumours were also stained with haematoxylin and eosin for histopathological diagnosis.

*Quantitation of foci*

The histochemically processed sections were photographed with professional colour slide film (Kodak Ektachrome 64 professional daylight EPR-135) at 1 × magnification. The resultant photographic slides were then projected onto a sheet of vellum, in the same sequence in which they were assayed, at a magnification (approximately 178 ×) providing an image appropriate for digitizing (see below). From the projected image of each slide, the outline of the section and the foci revealed by the particular histochemical test represented by that slide were traced onto the vellum sheet, using a different colour for each tracing. As each successive image was projected, it was carefully aligned with the prior tracing. The final composite drawing consisted of the superimposed images of the six serial sections taken for each animal, representing a total tissue thickness of 60–90 μm. It should be noted that the last histochemical test in the series detected excess glycogen storage or glycogen depletion within a given focus. Each of the latter two changes was considered a separate marker but, because a single focus cannot contain both of these markers, the maximum complement of markers in a given focus is six, although the total number of markers examined is seven. (Hereafter, the complement of markers present in a given focus is termed its 'phenotype', and the number of markers per focus is considered to denote its level of 'phenotypic complexity').

Each composite drawing was digitized by means of a Hewlett-Packard 9874 A image digitizer connected to a Digital PDP11/03 computer, with the individual tracings for each composite digitized in the same sequence in which they had originally been drawn. The resultant raw data were processed to yield the number of foci of a given phenotype (i.e., showing a given complement of markers) per composite section and the maximum observed diameter for each focus (obtained from comparisons of the diameters of the sections through the focus). The latter measurement was considered to represent the closest obtainable estimation of the two-dimensional size of each focus at its equatorial plane. The processed data were then classified according to the type of carcinogen administered, the sex of the animal and the sacrifice interval at which the data were taken.

The smallest group of cells that could be reliably scored as a focus through the use of these procedures had a diameter of 50 μm, which was less than the total thickness (60–90 μm) of the superimposed serial frozen sections needed to detect foci with a phenotypic complexity level of six. Therefore, the data excluded all foci with diameters less than 90 μm.

Several different stereological methods have been developed for converting data on foci sizes and numbers obtained directly from stained liver sections to a three-dimensional base, the objective being to correct the data for inaccuracies resulting from the fact that a thin (10–15 μm) section does not pass through the equatorial planes of all the foci on the section (Pugh *et al.*, 1983). However, the existence of discrepancies between data generated by the various methods currently in use, as well as the persistence of uncertainties in estimations of foci size by the most recently devised procedure (Pugh *et al.*, 1983) suggest that none of the current stereological conversion methods provides completely reliable estimations of foci numbers and sizes. In view of the ambiguities associated with the use of these methods, we decided in the present study to address issues that depend primarily on relative responses among different experimental groups and therefore do not require knowledge of absolute numbers and sizes of foci.

## RESULTS

*Effects of carcinogen treatment and sex on incidences of tumours and foci*

Figure 1 shows the incidences of frank hepatic tumours in male and female rats treated with NDEA or BP within one day after birth and weaned onto a 0.05% phenobarbital diet. Although the administered molar dosage of NDEA was 25% that of BP, the tumour incidence rates in the NDEA-treated rats were substantially higher than those in the rats receiving BP. In both treatment groups, female rats surpassed males in tumour incidence levels, but this incremental effect of sex appeared to be

Fig. 1. Hepatic tumour incidence rates
The number next to each data point denotes the number of rats from which the data were derived. The inset shows the number of rats per data point at the three earliest sacrifice intervals (28, 35 and 49 days after birth). ●, *N*-nitrosodiethylamine (NDEA) females; ○, NDEA males; ▲, benzo[*a*]pyrene (BP) females; △, BP males

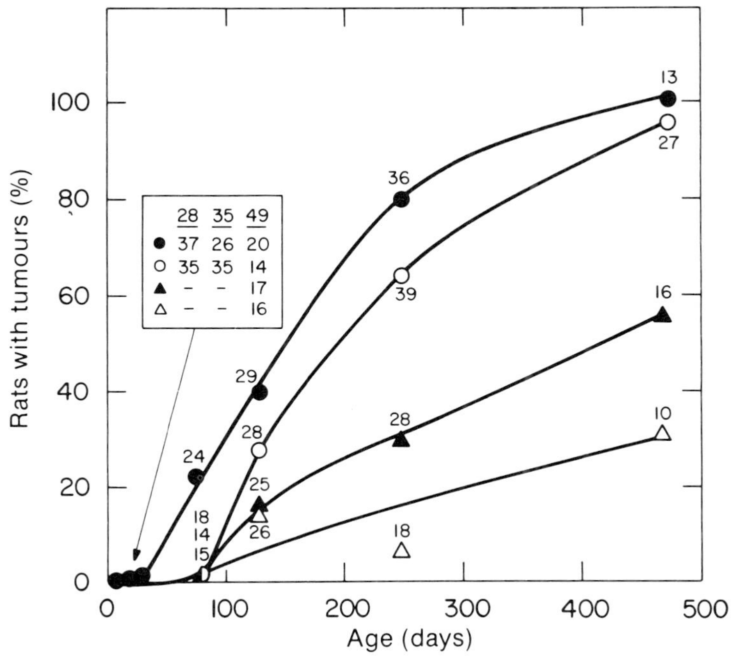

Fig. 2. Incidence rates of foci, irrespective of their phenotypes
The term 'phenotype' in this context refers to the number and types of histochemical markers seen in a given focus (see 'Methods' for further explanation). ●, *N*-nitrosodiethylamine (NDEA) females; ○, NDEA males; ▲, benzo[*a*]pyrene (BP) females; △, BP males

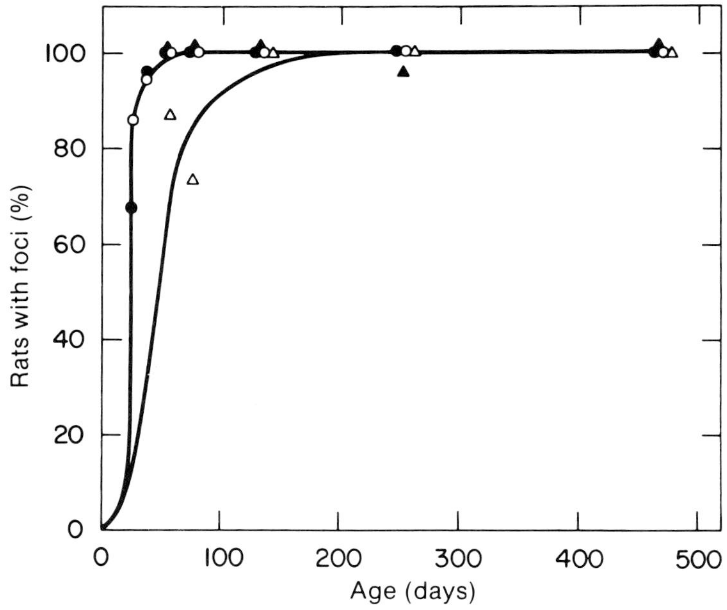


largely the result of relatively lower tumour latencies in the females, the latter phenomenon being especially evident in the NDEA-treated group. The rapidity of the tumorigenic response under these conditions is also noteworthy; despite the fact that each carcinogen was administered in a single non-necrogenic dose, the hepatic tumour incidence rates were among the highest yet achieved with these agents. As determined histologically from the haematoxylin-eosin-stained frozen sections, 2% of the tumours were frank hepatocellular carcinomas and 8% were cholangiomas, while the remainder were classified as hepatocellular adenomas by criteria used in earlier studies (Peraino *et al.*, 1980).

The data in Figure 2 represent the incidences of foci, irrespective of phenotype, in each of the experimental groups. In three of the groups, the foci incidence rates were similarly high, reaching 100% within 49 days after treatment; the BP-treated males required an additional 74 days to attain this incidence level. Comparison of Figures 1 and 2 shows that, for all groups, foci incidence rates greatly exceeded rates of tumour appearance, substantiating the utility of foci detection as a possible early indicator of carcinogen action. Comparisons of foci frequencies (pooled over time) with respect to carcinogen treatment and sex showed that rats receiving NDEA had twice the number of foci as those given BP, and foci were twice as abundant in females as in males (Table 1). These frequency differentials remained constant whether or not stereological procedures (Campbell *et al.*, 1982) were used to adjust foci numbers.

Table 1. Incidences of foci before and after stereological correction[a]

| Group | Variable | No. of foci | | No. foci per cm³ ÷ no. foci per section[b] |
|---|---|---|---|---|
| | | Per 2-cm diameter section | Per cm³ liver | |
| 1 | *N*-Nitrosodiethylamine | 35 ± 4 | 320 ± 48 | 9.7 ± 1.0 |
| 2 | Benzo[*a*]pyrene | 16 ± 3[c] | 151 ± 21[d] | 10.8 ± 0.9 |
| 3 | Females | 33 ± 4 | 311 ± 49 | 9.8 ± 1.0 |
| 4 | Males | 17 ± 3[e] | 160 ± 26[f] | 10.6 ± 0.9 |

[a] Each value is the mean ± standard error for 10 observations, each observation consisting of the mean number of foci per composite section (see 'Foci quantitation' under 'Methods') for the group of rats at each of five sacrifice intervals (when the rats were 49, 77, 133, 245 or 459 days of age – the numbers of rats are shown next to the data points in Fig. 1) in each of the four experimental groups indicated in the Table. For Groups 1 and 2, the sexes were pooled, while the carcinogen treatments were pooled for Groups 3 and 4. Student's t test for significance was used.
[b] No significant difference among the groups ($p > 0.10$)
[c] Significantly different from Group 1 ($p < 0.01$)
[d] Significantly different from Group 1 ($p < 0.002$)
[e] Significantly different from Group 3 ($p < 0.01$)
[f] Significantly different from Group 3 ($p < 0.02$)

*Effects of carcinogen treatment and sex on phenotypic complexity levels of foci*

Figure 3 shows the distribution patterns for the levels of foci phenotypic complexity (i.e., the relative frequencies of foci containing one to six markers) in rats given BP or NDEA (data pooled with respect to time and carcinogen treatment). Comparison of the data for the two carcinogens (Fig. 3) shows that, although NDEA induced higher incidences of foci and tumours than BP, the distributions of relative foci frequencies among the various phenotypic complexity levels were similar for these agents, except that the NDEA-treated rats had a somewhat higher proportion of foci with one marker. Likewise, despite the greater responsiveness of females than males in terms of foci and tumour production, foci complexity distribution patterns were similar in both sexes, except for the slightly higher proportion of foci with one marker in males (Fig. 3).

*Time-dependent changes in the phenotypic complexity of the foci population*

Figure 4 is a representation of the changing relationships among phenotype complexity levels over time in the total pooled foci population. These data show a decline in the proportion of relatively simple (single marker) foci; however, the concomitant increases in the proportions of foci with two or more marker changes were relatively evenly distributed over these higher complexity levels, i.e., the decline in the relative frequency of the simple foci did not influence preferentially the frequency of any one of the populations of higher complexity foci. An important additional feature of the relationships shown in Figure 4 is the similarity among the multiple marker foci with respect to the kinetic changes in their relative frequencies. This consistency in relationships of phenotype complexity over time suggests that the frequency of one complexity level did not change at the expense of another, i.e., once each focus had formed, its level of phenotypic complexity remained stable.

Fig. 3. Relative frequencies of foci at six levels of phenotypic complexity (number of markers expressed per focus) in rats pooled with respect to sex and given benzo[*a*]pyrene (BP) or *N*-nitrosodiethylamine (NDEA) and in male and female rats pooled with respect to carcinogen treatment
The data are expressed as a percentage of the total focus population for each experimental group. □, BP (2976 foci); ■, NDEA (8581 foci); ▨, male (4061 foci); ▧, female (7496 foci)

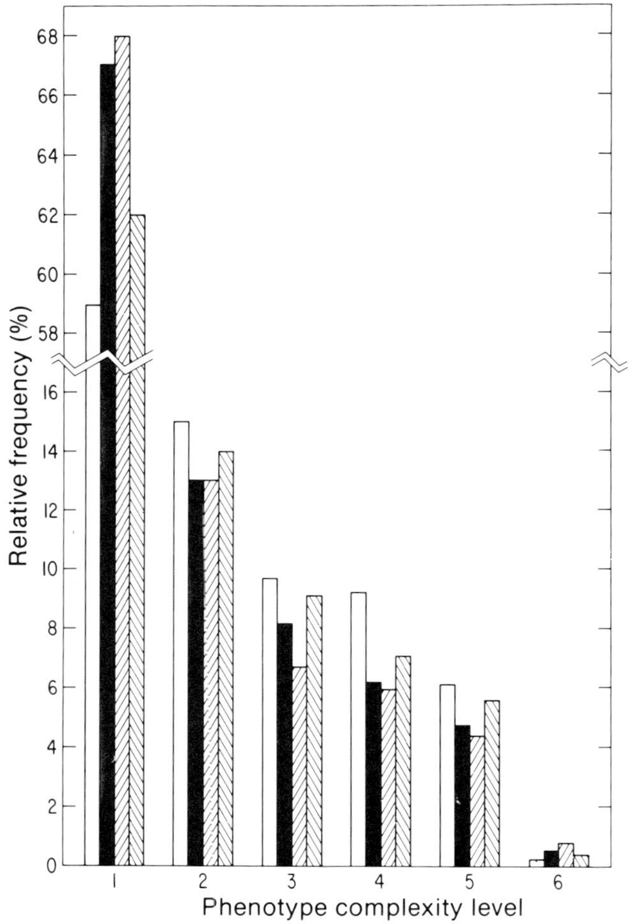


*Effects of carcinogen treatment and sex on the relative frequencies of individual markers in the foci*

Figure 5 shows the relative frequencies of each of the individual markers in the foci, irrespective of the presence or absence of other markers. The order of the markers from left to right along the abscissas in this figure reflects the descending order of marker frequencies calculated from the total pooled population of foci. For com-

Fig. 4. Time-dependent changes in the relative percentage frequencies of the six measured phenotypic complexity levels in the total pooled population of foci
□, complexity level 1; ○, complexity level 2; △, complexity level 3; +, complexity level 4; x, complexity level 5; ◇, complexity level 6

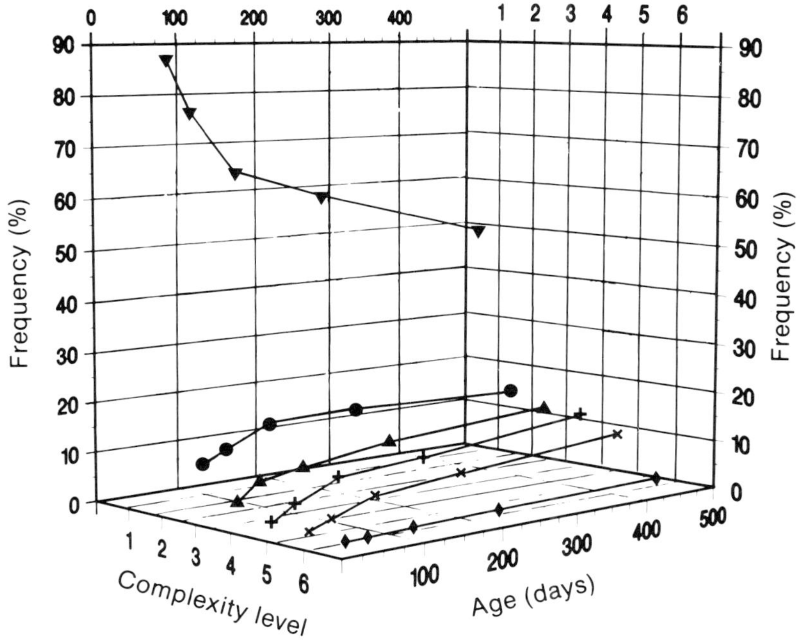


parisons of marker frequencies in rats treated with BP or NDEA, the data were pooled with respect to sex and time; for comparisons of marker frequencies in male and female rats, the data were pooled with respect to carcinogen treatment and time.

As was the case with the foci complexity patterns shown in Figure 3, BP and NDEA exerted similar effects on marker frequencies (Fig. 5). The similarity in the effects of BP and NDEA on phenotypic complexity and marker distribution suggests that individual foci phenotypes are similar in the two carcinogen treatment groups.

Comparisons of marker frequency distributions in male and female rats showed that the rank order of the diaphorase, iron exclusion and glycogen storage markers differed between the sexes (Fig. 5). Coupled with the observed similarity in the distributions of foci phenotype complexities in males and females (Fig. 3), these data suggest that the sex of the animal can influence the phenotypic composition of a given complexity level without altering the level of complexity itself.

*Relationship between phenotypic complexity levels and relative growth rates of foci*

Figure 6 depicts the relative growth rates of foci at three representative phenotypic complexity levels (1, 3 and 5) in rats given BP or NDEA; the data were pooled with respect to sex. The rates shown in Figure 6 were generated from the data in Table

Fig. 5. Relative frequencies of foci showing each marker, irrespective of the presence or absence of other markers
The remaining description is identical to that in the legend to Figure 3. GGT, γ-glutamyltranspeptidase; D, diaphorase; Fe, iron exclusion; PP, periodic acid-Schiff-positive (glycogen storage); G6P, glucose-6-phosphatase; PN, periodic acid-Schiff-negative (glycogen depletion); Alk, alkaline phosphatase. □, benzo[*a*]pyrene (2976 foci); ■, *N*-nitrosodiethylamine (8581 foci); ▨, male (4061 foci); ▧, female (7496 foci)

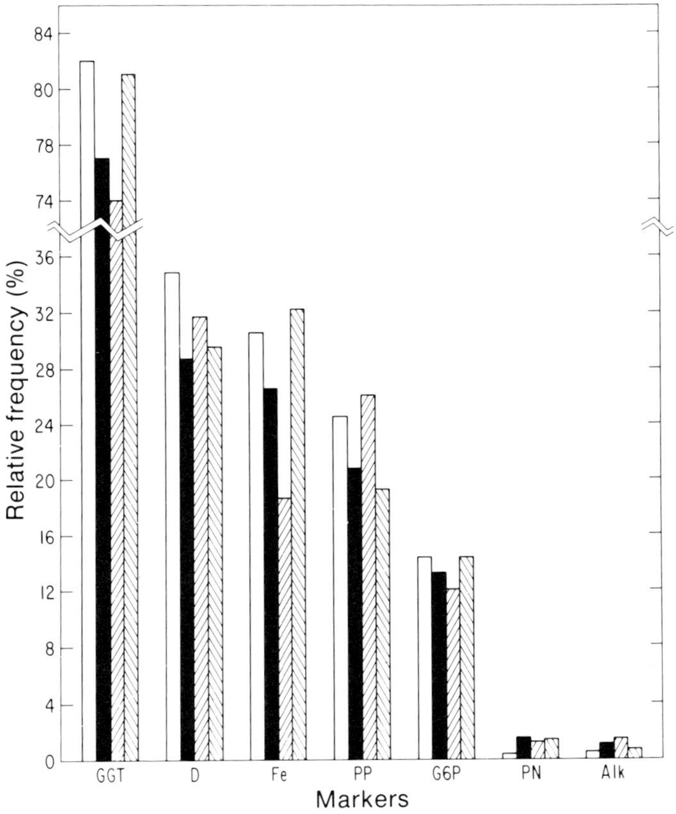


2 by means of linear regression analyses (SAS Institute Inc., 1982). Comparison of the three sets of growth rates for the three complexity levels reveals a direct relationship between phenotypic complexity and growth rate; a similar relationship was obtained when the data were expressed in terms of sex and pooled with respect to carcinogen treatment (data not shown). These observations are in accord with prior evidence (Pugh & Goldfarb, 1978) for a positive correlation between focus phenotypic complexity and labelling index.

Fig. 6. Relative growth rates of foci at phenotypic complexity levels 1, 3 and 5 (data pooled with respect to sex)

The growth rates are represented by lines generated by means of linear regression analyses of the data in Table 2. —, benzo[*a*]pyrene; ---, *N*-nitrosodiethylamine

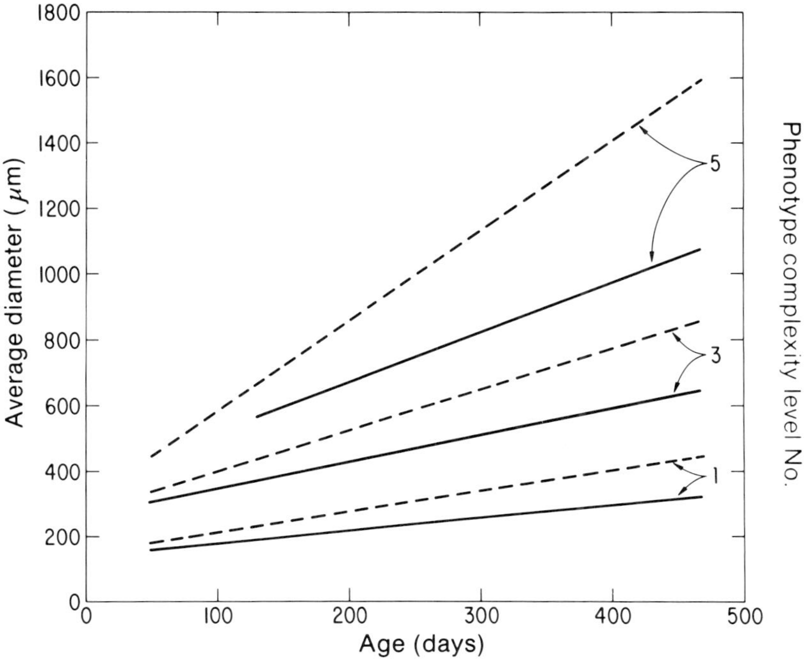


Table 2. Time-dependent changes in the sizes of foci at three levels of phenotypic complexity in rats initiated with benzo[*a*]pyrene (BP) or *N*-introsodiethylamine (NDEA) at birth

| Phenotypic complexity level | Age of rats (days) | BP | | NDEA | |
|---|---|---|---|---|---|
| | | No. of foci | Av. diameter (μm) | No. of foci | Av. diameter (μm) |
| 1 | 49 | 292 | 163 | 838 | 188 |
| | 77 | 237 | 175 | 1 257 | 199 |
| | 133 | 487 | 210 | 1 331 | 207 |
| | 245 | 404 | 235 | 1 536 | 285 |
| | 469 | 317 | 318 | 724 | 396 |
| 3 | 49 | 3 | 272 | 37 | 405 |
| | 77 | 9 | 355 | 119 | 386 |
| | 133 | 89 | 372 | 131 | 400 |
| | 245 | 77 | 453 | 255 | 568 |
| | 469 | 109 | 635 | 155 | 863 |
| 5 | 49 | – | – | 2 | 677 |
| | 77 | – | – | 40 | 521 |
| | 133 | 81 | 554 | 58 | 567 |
| | 245 | 42 | 796 | 172 | 961 |
| | 469 | 58 | 1 054 | 138 | 1 488 |

*Effects of carcinogen treatment and sex on relationship between phenotypic complexity levels and relative growth rates of foci*

Comparison of the effects of BP and NDEA on relative growth rates of foci at three representative phenotypic complexity levels (Fig. 6) showed that the NDEA-induced foci invariably grew more rapidly than those resulting from BP administration, with the incremental effects of NDEA on foci growth rates increasing in direct relation to the increases in foci complexity levels. Comparison of foci growth rates at these three complexity levels in male and female rats (data pooled with respect to carcinogen treatment) yielded identical growth rates for the two sexes (data not shown), in contrast to the differential effects of the two carcinogens on growth (Fig. 6). The latter data suggest that increases in focus phenotypic complexity levels not only engender more rapid growth, but also are associated with increases in focus growth capacities, i.e., increases in the range of possible focus growth rates.

*Comparative phenotypic complexities of foci and tumours*

Figure 7 compares the patterns of phenotypic complexity for the total pooled populations of foci and tumours. It is apparent that most foci were relatively simple (approximately 80% showing no more than two markers), whereas most tumours

Fig. 7. Comparison of the phenotypic complexity distribution patterns in the total observed populations of foci (□, 11 557) and tumours (■, 143)

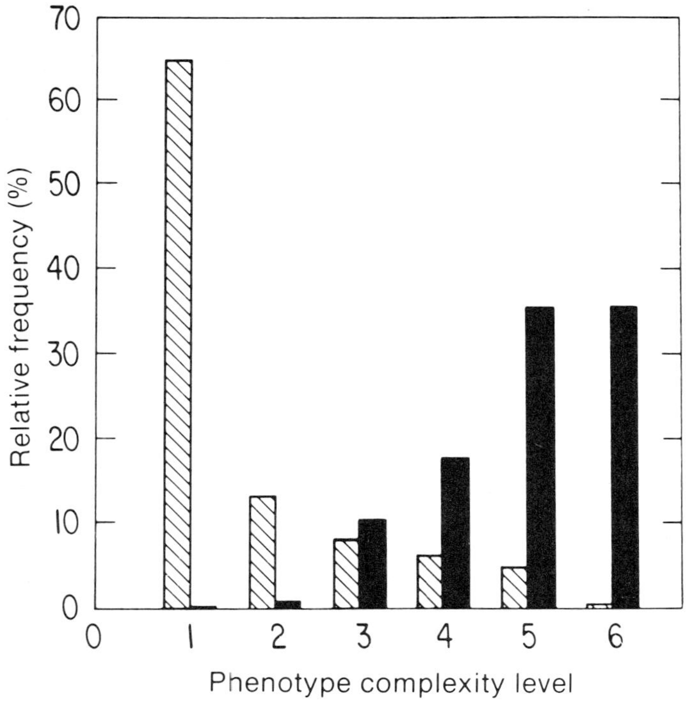

Fig. 8. Comparison of the individual marker frequency distribution patterns in the total observed populations of foci (□, 11 557) and tumours (■, 143)
GGT, γ-glutamyltranspeptidase; D, diaphorase; Fe, iron exclusion; PP, periodic acid-Schiff-positive (glycogen storage); G6P, glucose-6-phosphatase; PN, periodic acid-Schiff-negative (glycogen depletion); Alk, alkaline phosphatase

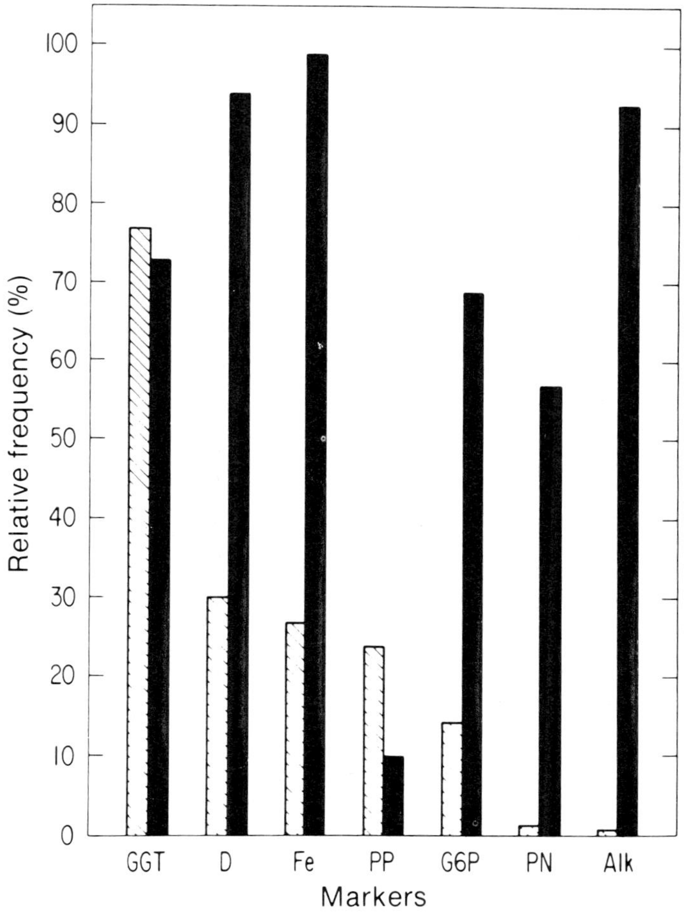


were relatively complex (approximately 75% showing five or more markers). However, the tumours did not invariably have complex phenotypes; approximately 10% showed as few as three markers. Phenotypic heterogeneity among tumours has also been observed by Goldfarb and Pugh (1981).

*Comparative frequencies of individual markers in foci and tumours*

As shown in Figure 8, the frequencies of most of the markers were substantially higher in the tumours than in the foci. This difference is in accord with the observation that most tumours were phenotypically more complex than the foci (Fig. 7). The salient aspects of the foci-tumour relationship shown in Figure 8, however, are (1) the complete absence of correspondence between the foci and tumours with respect to their marker frequency distribution patterns and (2) the observation that no single marker appeared invariably in all tumours.

## DISCUSSION

### *Effect of sex on foci and tumour production*

Our observation that, in the neonatal rat model, females were more responsive than males with respect to foci incidences (Table 1) is in accord with the results of other investigations employing initiation-promotion regimens with older rats (Deml & Oesterle, 1982; Pereira *et al.,* 1982). In those studies, the formation of foci was enhanced to a greater degree in females than in males when all rats were treated with both promoter and an initiator, whereas foci incidences were similar in both sexes when initiator alone was administered. Therefore, because all rats in the current experiment were subjected to both initiator and promoter administration, we suggest that the observed sex difference in foci production is a reflection of promoter action.

### *Dissociation of foci incidences and growth rates – relevance to tumour promotion*

The evidence that foci incidences in rats subjected to initiation and promotion were higher in females than in males, although foci relative growth rates were the same in both sexes, suggests that the rates of emergence of the foci are not necessarily related to the proliferative activities of the foci hepatocytes. This finding and the evidence that the sex differential in foci incidences in fact represents a promoter effect (Deml & Oesterle, 1982; Pereira *et al.,* 1982) suggest that the promotion mechanism does not necessarily involve stimulation of hepatic mitogenesis. Additional evidence against proliferative stimulation as the central mechanism of promotion is provided by experiments showing that (1) the promoting effect of Clophen A 50 on the production of NDEA-induced foci did not require enhanced mitogenesis (Deml & Oesterle, 1982); (2) feeding of phenobarbital enhanced the promoting effect of a choline-devoid diet but suppressed the proliferative effect of the choline deficiency (Abanobi *et al.,* 1982); and (3) a high-fat diet also enhanced the promoting effect of choline deficiency without influencing the degree of choline-deficiency-induced mitogenesis (Shinozuka *et al.,* 1982). Other studies, however, place strong emphasis on proliferative stimulation as the major promotion mechanism (Schulte-Hermann *et al.,* 1981; Barbason *et al.,* 1983). Additional discussion of the still unresolved issue of the role of mitogenic stimulation in tumour promotion is presented elsewhere (Peraino *et al.,* 1983).

### *Relationship between focus formation and hepatic neoplasia*

The observation that the phenotypic complexity levels of the foci did not increase with time (Fig. 4) suggests that the foci do not progress toward more deviated forms and are, therefore, probably not direct tumour progenitors. However, the fact that foci invariably and specifically appear in response to carcinogen administration suggests that they do represent elements of the tumorigenic process. We postulate that the foci are manifestations of a mosaic of concerted subtumorigenic effects of the carcinogenic stimulus on regulatory processes associated with the control of cell division and neoplastic transformation. The foci and tumour characteristics, as revealed by the current studies, suggest that this mosaic of effects defines the mechanism whereby the probability of a specific neoplastic event is increased. Aspects of this hypothetical mechanism, in conjunction with the empirical evidence from which they are derived, are described in the following section.

*Postulated sequence of events in the induction of foci and tumours by a chemical carcinogen*

The observation that foci growth rates are directly related to the relative hepatocarcinogenic effectiveness of NDEA and BP (Figs 1 and 6) suggests the existence of a cellular site at which the rate of mitogenesis is regulated and which has graded levels of responsiveness to carcinogenic stimuli. In conjunction with this evidence for the differential responsiveness of hepatocytes to carcinogen action, the observation that foci phenotypes are not affected by the chemical nature or tumorigenic effectiveness of the carcinogen (Figs 1, 3, and 5) suggests the existence of an additional cellular site with an all-or-none responsiveness to generic molecular properties of carcinogens that are associated with their tumorigenicity.

The observation that foci growth capacities are directly related to their levels of phenotypic complexity (Fig. 6) suggests that the processes regulating phenotype expression and growth potential are linked mechanistically; this linkage implies an integrated activation of the two regulatory sites described above. Given such integration, the indication that the weaker hepatocarcinogen, BP, is as effective as NDEA in activating one site but less effective than NDEA in activating the other suggests a hierarchical association in which the activation of the variably responsive site by carcinogen is dependent on the prior carcinogen-mediated activation of the site with the fixed level of responsiveness. Such a scheme requires that the activation of the latter site be followed by endogenously modulated carcinogen-independent events that induce a certain level of activation of the variably responsive site; the degree of this activation dictates the potential phenotypic character and associated growth characteristics that will be realized upon the subsequent interaction of this activated site with the carcinogen.

The inverse relationships of foci frequencies to their phenotypic complexity levels (Figs 3 and 7) and growth capacities (Fig. 6) suggest that the production of increasingly deviated foci (with respect to normal hepatocyte phenotypic and proliferative characteristics) involves events with progressively higher thresholds and lower probabilities. In this connection, the relatively low incidence of tumours (in comparison with foci incidences) and the preponderance of tumours with complex phenotypes (Fig. 7) suggests that the probability of tumorigenesis is increased in direct relation to the probability of complex focus formation; that is, the conditions that engender the formation of complex foci with elevated growth capacities are also most conducive to tumorigenesis.

The occurrence of a small percentage of tumours with relatively simple phenotypes (Fig. 7), the complete absence of correspondence between the distribution patterns of marker frequency in foci and tumours, and the observation that no phenotypic marker appears invariably in all tumours (Fig. 8), suggest that tumorigenesis involves a specific event that is distinct from the events responsible for the production of foci. This distinction implies the existence of a specific cellular site(s) that regulates neoplastic transformation. On the basis of the relationships described in the preceding comments, we suggest that the accessibility of this transformation site increases in direct relation to increases in the potential for the formation of phenotypically complex foci. However, rare interactions of the carcinogen with the transformation site may occur under conditions of poor site accessibility, leading to low-frequency formation of phenotypically simple tumours.

Considered collectively, the foregoing observations and interpretations lead us to postulate the following sequence of events (Fig. 9) in the interaction of a carcinogenic stimulus with the target cell. (1) The carcinogen acts on the primary site (fixed response), resulting in activation of the site and production of a secondary effector.

Fig. 9. A hypothetical sequence of events in the production of altered hepatocyte foci and tumours, as suggested by current data

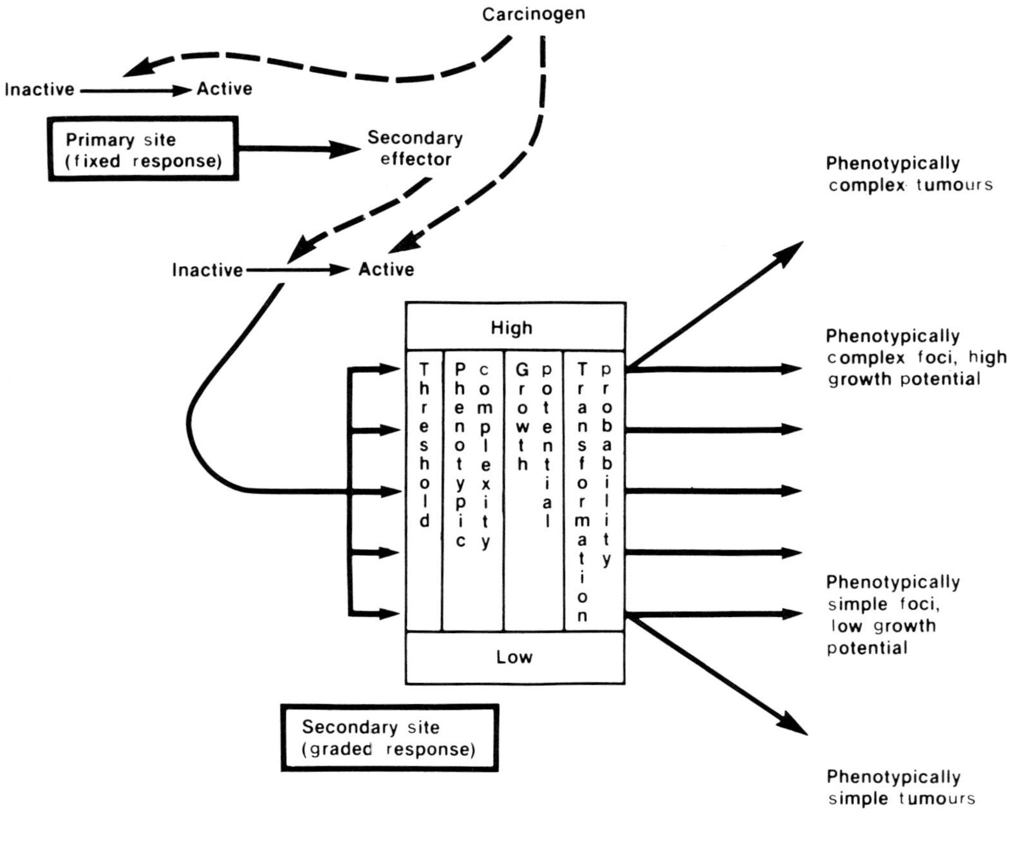

(2) The secondary effector acts on the secondary site (graded response); the efficiency of this interaction (and the consequent level of site activation) depends on intervening carcinogen-independent processes. (3) The carcinogen interacts with the activated form of the secondary site and (depending on the site activation level) produces a phenotypically simple focus with a low growth rate, a phenotypically more complex focus with a low or high growth rate (depending on the potency of the carcinogen) or a tumour. In the latter case, the probability of tumorigenesis (and the resultant tumour phenotypic complexity level) also depends on the activation level of the secondary site.

This scheme does not preclude the possibility that foci may give rise to tumours. In fact, our model predicts that the accessibility of the specific neoplastic transformation site in the hepatocytes of a focus would be enhanced in direct relation to its level of phenotypic complexity and growth capacity. This enhanced accessibility would render the hepatocytes of foci more susceptible than surrounding hepatocytes to transformation following an additional carcinogenic stimulus. The relevance of this alternative mechanism to the results of the current study appears remote, however, in view of the single carcinogen treatment used.

The tumorigenesis model described above is not presented as the definitive mechanism of chemical hepatocarcinogenesis. Instead, it represents an attempt to organize the current observations into an internally consistent pattern that defines a coherent relationship between foci and tumour production. The essence of this model, whether or not it proves to be accurate in detail, is that tumorigenesis is not simply an extension of processes that generate foci with progressively higher growth rates and greater phenotypic complexity, i.e., it is not simply the end result of an accumulation of carcinogen-induced insults. Instead, neoplastic transformation may involve a specific event, the probability of which is influenced by carcinogen-mediated events responsible for changes in hepatocyte growth control and phenotypic character associated with focus formation.

## ACKNOWLEDGEMENT

Supported by the US Department of Energy under contract No. W-31-109-ENG-38.

## REFERENCES

Abanobi, S.E., Lombardi, B. & Shinozuka, H. (1982) Stimulation of DNA synthesis and cell proliferation in the liver of rats fed a choline-devoid diet and their suppression by phenobarbital. *Cancer Res.*, ***42***, 412–415

Bannasch, P., Mayer, D. & Hacker, H.-J. (1980) Hepatocellular glycogenesis and hepatocarcinogenesis. *Biochim. biophys. Acta*, ***605***, 217–245

Barbason, H., Rassenfosse, C. & Betz, E.H. (1983) Promotion mechanism of phenobarbital and partial hepatectomy in DENA hepatocarcinogenesis cell kinetics effect. *Br. J. Cancer*, ***47***, 517–525

Campbell, H.A., Pitot, H.C., Potter, V.P. & Laishes, B.A. (1982) Application of quantitative stereology to the evaluation of enzyme-altered foci in rat liver. *Cancer Res.*, ***42***, 465–472

Deml, E. & Oesterle, D. (1982) Sex-dependent promoting effect of polychlorinated biphenyls on enzyme-altered islands induced by diethylnitrosamine in rat liver. *Carcinogenesis*, ***3***, 1449–1453

Emmelot, P. & Scherer, E. (1980) The first relevant stage in rat liver carcinogenesis. A quantitative approach. *Biochim. biophys. Acta*, ***605***, 247–304

Farber, E. (1980) The sequential analysis of liver cancer induction. *Biochim. biophys. Acta*, ***605***, 149–166

Goldfarb, S. & Pugh, T.D. (1981) Enzyme histochemical phenotypes in primary hepatocellular carcinomas. *Cancer Res.*, ***41***, 2092–2095

Hirakawa, T., Ishakawa, T., Nemoto, N., Takayama, S. & Kitagawa, T. (1979) Induction of enzyme-altered islands in rat liver by a single treatment with benzo(a)pyrene after partiel hepatectomy. *Gann*, ***70***, 393–394

Hirota, N. & Williams, G.M. (1979) The sensitivity and heterogeneity of histochemical markers for altered foci involved in liver carcinogenesis. *Am. J. Pathol.*, ***95***, 317–328

Kitagawa, T., Hirakawa, T., Ishikawa, T., Nemoto, N. & Takayama, S. (1980) Induction of hepatocellular carcinoma in rat liver by initial treatment with benzo(a)pyrene after partial hepatectomy and promotion by phenobarbital. *Toxicol. Lett.*, ***6***, 167–171

Peraino, C., Fry, R.J.M. & Staffeldt, E.F. (1971) Reduction and enhancement by phenobarbital of hepatocarcinogenesis induced in the rat by 2-acetylaminofluorene. *Cancer Res.*, ***31***, 1506–1512

Peraino, C., Staffeldt, E.F., Haugen, D.A., Lombard, L.S., Stevens, F.J. & Fry, R.J.M. (1980) Effects of varying the dietary concentration of phenobarbital on its enhancement of 2-acetylaminofluorene-induced hepatic tumorigenesis. *Cancer Res.*, ***40***, 3268–3273

Peraino, C., Staffeldt, E.F. & Ludeman, V.A. (1981) Early appearance of histochemically altered hepatocyte foci and liver tumors in female rats treated with carcinogens one day after birth. *Carcinogenesis*, ***2***, 463–465

Peraino, C., Richards, W.L. & Stevens, F.J. (1983) *Multistage hepatocarcinogenesis*. In: Slaga, T.J., ed., *Mechanisms of Tumor Promotion*, Vol. 1, *Tumor Promotion and Carcinogenesis in Internal Organs*, Boca Raton, FL, CRC Press, pp. 1–53

Pereira, M.A., Herren, S.L., Britt, A.L. & Khoury, M.M. (1982) Sex difference in enhancement of GGTase-positive foci by hexachlorobenzene and lindane in rat liver. *Cancer Lett.*, ***15***, 95–101

Pitot, H.C. (1979) *Drugs as promoters of carcinogenesis*. In: Estabrook, R.W. & Lindlaub, E., eds, *The Induction of Drug Metabolism*, New York, F.K. Schattaner-Verlag, pp. 471–483

Pitot, H.C. & Sirica, A.E. (1980) The stages of initiation and promotion in hepatocarcinogenesis. *Biochim. biophys. Acta*, ***605***, 191–215

Pitot, H.C., Barsness, L., Goldsworthy, T. & Kitagawa, T. (1978) Biochemical characterization of stages of hepatocarcinogenesis after a single dose of diethylnitrosamine. *Nature*, ***271***, 456–458

Pugh, T.D. & Goldfarb, S. (1978) Quantitative histochemical and autoradiographic studies of hepatocarcinogenesis in rats fed 2-acetylaminofluorene followed by phenobarbital. *Cancer Res.,* ***38,*** 4450–4457

Pugh, T.D., King, J.H., Koen, H., Nychka, D., Chover, J., Wahba, G., He, Y. & Goldfarb, S. (1983) Reliable stereological method for estimating the number of microscopic hepatocellular foci from their transections. *Cancer Res.,* ***43,*** 1261–1268

SAS Institute Inc. (1982) *The SAS Users Guide: Statistics,* Cory, NC

Schulte-Hermann, R., Ohde, G., Schuppler, J. & Timmermann-Trosiener, I. (1981) Enhanced proliferation of putative preneoplastic cells in rat liver following treatment with the tumor promoters phenobarbital, hexachlorocyclohexane, steroid compounds, and nafenopin. *Cancer Res.,* ***41,*** 2556–2562

Shinozuka, H., Takahashi, S., Lombardi, B. & Abanobi, S.E. (1982) Effects of varying the fat content of a choline-devoid diet on promotion of the emergence of $\gamma$-glutamyltranspeptidase positive foci in the livers of carcinogen-treated rats. *Cancer Lett.,* ***16,*** 43–50

Uchida, E. & Hirona, I. (1979) Effects of phenobarbital on induction of liver and lung tumors by diethylnitrosamine in newborn mice. *Gann,* ***70,*** 639–644

Williams, G.M. (1980) The pathogenesis of rat liver cancer caused by chemical carcinogens. *Biochem. biophys. Acta,* ***605,*** 167–190

# INITIATION-PROMOTION-INITIATION. INDUCTION OF NEOPLASTIC FOCI WITHIN ISLANDS OF PRECANCEROUS LIVER CELLS IN THE RAT

E. SCHERER[1], A.W. FERINGA & P. EMMELOT

*Division of Chemical Carcinogenesis*
*Antoni van Leeuwenhoek-Huis*
*The Netherlands Cancer Institute*
*1066 CX Amsterdam, The Netherlands*

## SUMMARY

The hypothesis that during the promotion phase of carcinogenesis a second rare event leads to a promoter-independent tumour cell was tested in an initiation-promotion-initiation type of experiment. Precancerous (island) cells induced in rat liver by 10 mg/kg *N*-nitrosodiethylamine given 24 h after partial hepatectomy were promoted by a protocol consisting of 2-acetylaminofluorene/partial hepatectomy. Administration of 25–100 mg/kg *N*-ethyl-*N*-nitrosourea served as second initiater. Microscopic foci of neoplastic cells were observed within the precancerous islands 66 days later; no such foci were noted in the appropriate controls. Deficiency of adenosine triphosphatase and glucose-6-phosphatase marker enzymes in the foci was more pronounced than in the surrounding island cells; glycogen storage was decreased and cytoplasmic basophilia slightly increased; $\gamma$-glutamyltranspeptidase staining was negative or decreased with respect to the surrounding island cells, which exhibited a partially positive reaction.

We conclude that a secondary change produced by *N*-ethyl-*N*-nitrosourea in precancerous island cells leads to focus-forming cells which grow, in the absence of promoter, into foci of neoplastic phenotype. Similar rare, initiation-like events might be involved in the process of tumour promotion in general.

[1] To whom correspondence should be addressed

## INTRODUCTION

Chemical carcinogenesis is now generally recognized as a multistage process in which the first event is initiation by a genotoxic carcinogen. A large body of evidence indicates that a rare, mutation-like event is the molecular basis of initiation. The process leading from the initiated stage to the overt cancer stage is less well understood. The operational dissection of epidermal carcinogenesis into at least two stages, i.e., initiation and promotion, and the non-carcinogenic/non-mutagenic nature of promoting agents, led to the widely-held concept that promotion is an epigenetic process leading to expression of the cancerous phenotype of initiated cells (see Scribner & Süss, 1978; Diamond *et al.*, 1980; Berenblum & Armuth, 1981). However, doubt has been expressed as to whether promotion follows solely an epigenetic pathway (Scherer & Emmelot, 1979a). Instead, it has been advocated that carcinogenesis is a multihit process (Scherer & Emmelot, 1979b), and that at least one second rare event must occur during or after the promotion phase to produce the promoter-independent, irreversibly cancerous cell. The increased proliferation of the precancerous cell population by promoter treatment should result in an increased risk that one of the precancerous cells will undergo that second, mutation-like rare event which leads to a more advanced precancerous cell or to the cancer cell (Scherer & Emmelot, 1979a). Genetic instability of precancerous cells, background carcinogenic stimuli or indirect genotoxic action of the promoter treatment could be the driving power for such mutation-like events, as long as no genotoxic substance is added deliberately. Consequently, application of an initiating carcinogen during, or at the end, of promoter treatment should strongly enhance the probability for such mutation-like events and thus lead to more and earlier tumours than the initiation-promotion protocol alone. Such an experimental design was proposed recently by Potter (1981).

To test this concept, the directly-acting carcinogen *N*-ethyl-*N*-nitrosourea (ENU) was administered to rats at the end of a 2-acetylaminofluorene (AAF)/partial hepatectomy (PH) regimen (Solt *et al.*, 1977, 1983) for promoting liver carcinogenesis initiated by a single low dose of *N*-nitrosodiethylamine (NDEA) given after PH (Scherer *et al.*, 1972). The formation of many secondary foci within the precancerous lesions is described. We conclude that the new foci represent a more advanced stage in the process of liver tumour formation, underlining the precursor function of enzyme-altered islands in hepatocarcinogenesis. Whether a similar phenotypic development occurs during liver tumour promotion generally is a matter for further study.

## MATERIALS AND METHODS

Fifty specific pathogen-free female Sprague-Dawley rats from our own inbred stock (SD-A), 130 days old and weighing 250 g at the beginning of the experiment, were divided into six groups (Fig. 1). Tap water and standard food pellets (Hope Farms, Woerden, The Netherlands) were given *ad libitum*. Experimental groups 1–4 received a single dose of 10 mg/kg NDEA (Merck, Darmstadt, Federal Republic of Germany)

Fig. 1. Schematic outline of the regimens administered to experimental (groups 1–3) and control rats (groups 4–6). Hatched area, daily applications of 15 mg/kg 2-acetylaminofluorene (AAF); PH, partial hepatectomy; NDEA, *N*-nitrosodiethylamine; ENU, *N*-ethyl-*N*-nitrosourea, +, sacrifice of animals

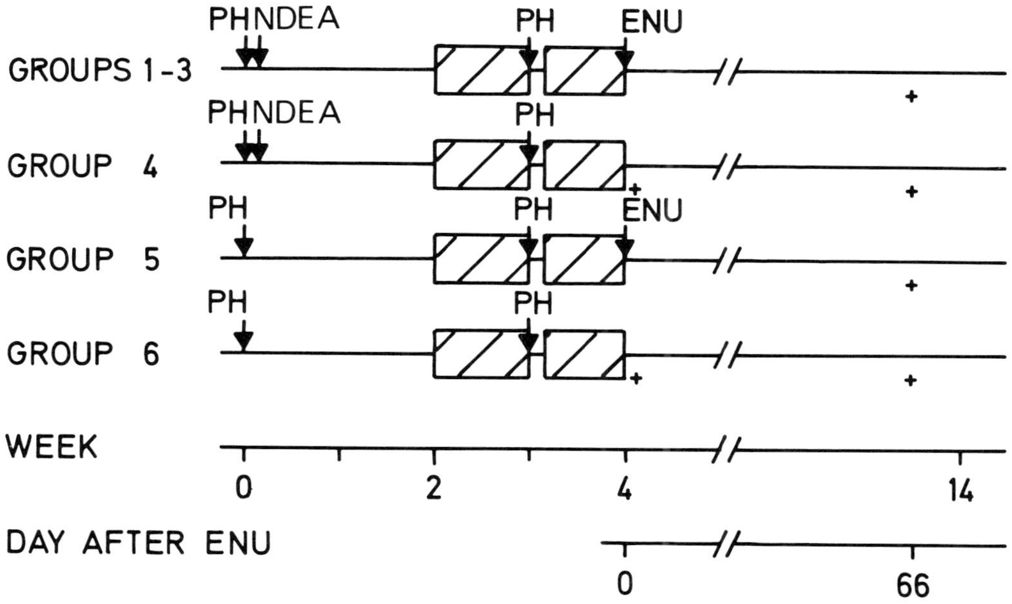


by gastric intubation 24 h after a two-thirds hepatectomy (Scherer *et al.*, 1972). After a rest period of two weeks, daily doses of AAF (Aldrich-Europe, Beerse, Belgium; 15 mg/kg dissolved in propane-1,2-diol, 7.5 mg/mL) were administered by gastric intubation for two weeks (Solt *et al.*, 1977). After one week of treatment, the anterior right sublobe of the liver was removed surgically; no AAF was given on this day. Experimental groups 1–3 received, in addition, a single gastric intubation of 100, 50 and 25 mg/kg ENU (Serva, Heidelberg, Federal Republic of Germany; 10 mg/mL in 1% acetic acid) 5 h after the last dose of AAF. Control groups 5 and 6 were not given the initiating dose of NDEA, but they received the AAF/PH regimen and (group 5) a single dose of 100 mg/kg ENU. Animals were killed 5 h after the last AAF administration, or 66 days later. The remaining animals were left for further observation. Standard pieces of the liver were combined and quickly frozen on solid carbon dioxide for the preparation of cryostat sections (10 μm; 10 series; 200 μm apart for each liver sample; section area, approximately 3 $cm^2$ each). Sections were stained for adenosine triphosphatase (ATPase) and glucose-6-phosphatase (G6Pase) by haematoxylin-eosin (HE), cresyl violet (basophilia) and the periodic acid-Schiff (PAS) reaction (Scherer *et al.*, 1972), and for γ-glutamyltranspeptidase (GGT) (Rutenburg *et al.*, 1969).

*N*(γ-L-Glutamyl)-4-methoxy-2-naphthylamide was obtained from Polysciences (Warrington, PA, USA) and Fast Blue BB salt from Serva (Heidelberg, Federal

Republic of Germany). Liver lesions were counted microscopically on the basis of decreased staining for bile canalicular and cytoplasmic ATPase. Correction of lesions/cm$^2$ to lesions/cm$^3$ liver was done by a simple computer programme (Scherer, 1981).

## RESULTS

### *Enzyme-altered islands*

Except for the loss of four animals after the first PH, no intercurrent death was noted. At autopsy, the livers were unremarkable and of normal weight. Microscopically, many small enzyme-altered islands were present at the end of the AAF treatment (Table 1, group 4). The main marker properties of these islands were ATPase deficiency and strong staining of GGT and cytoplasmic basophilia. ATPase-deficient island tissue covered 0.8% of the total liver tissue.

At the end of AAF administration, there were approximately 1000 islands/cm$^3$ liver; the number of islands was somewhat lower (500 to 900; groups 1–4) 66 days later. At day 66, strong basophilic staining was lost, and GGT staining and ATPase deficiency were less pronounced.

### *Secondary foci within islands*

In experimental groups 1–3, at day 66, multiple secondary foci were observed within islands of precancerous cells, recognizable by their more pronounced marker deficiency (ATPase, G6Pase; Fig. 2). In group 4, without ENU, such a focus was observed only once. Control groups 5 and 6 were devoid of secondary foci and contained only a few enzyme-altered islands (Table 1). Secondary foci were more or

Table 1. Number of adenosine triphosphatase (ATPase)-deficient islands and percentage of liver occupied by island tissue at the end of the selection regimen (t = 0) and 66 days later. Experimental groups as in Fig. 1, logarithmic mean

| Group | t = 0 | | | t = 66 days | | |
|---|---|---|---|---|---|---|
| | ATPase-deficient islands/cm$^3$ | | % liver occupied | ATPase deficient islands/cm$^3$ | | % liver occupied |
| 1 | | | | (2)[a] | 480 | 5.5 |
| 2 | | | | (2) | 600 | 9.1 |
| 3 | | | | (2) | 925 | 6.1 |
| 4 | (7) | 1 010<br>(450–2 300) | 0.8<br>(0.2–2.4)[b] | (2) | 540 | 4.5 |
| 5 | | | | (2) | 35 | 0.1 |
| 6 | (3) | < 25 | < 0.02 | (2) | < 20 | < 0.1 |

[a] Numbers in parentheses, number of animals
[b] Range of SD

Fig. 2. Representative secondary focus of neoplastic cells within an ATPase-deficient island. Group 2, 66 days after 50 mg/kg *N*-ethyl-*N*-nitrosourea (ENU), adenosine triphosphatase (ATPase) reaction

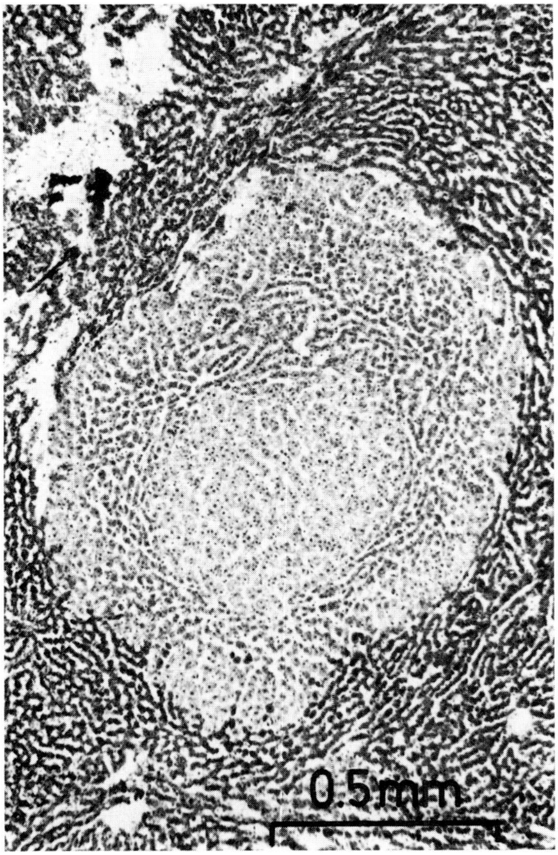


less round, exhibited plates of more than one cell thick and slightly compressed the surrounding island tissue, from which they were sharply demarcated. The plates were often discontinuous from those of the adjacent, tangentially arranged precancerous tissue. This architecture implies a centrifugal, probably clonal, growth of the secondary focus tissue. Cytoplasmic basophilia was increased, and the basophilic material was no longer present in clumps, as in normal liver and in precancerous islands, but was evenly distributed. Glycogen storage was decreased, ranging from only a few cells devoid of glycogen to its virtually complete loss in other foci.

Eosin staining of the cytoplasm was increased; GGT staining was negative or decreased as compared with the surrounding island tissue (Fig. 3).

*Quantitative aspects of secondary focus induction*

The size distribution of the secondary foci and of the ATPase-deficient islands 66 days after ENU treatment is shown in Figure 4. Most secondary foci were between 0.3 and 0.5 mm in diameter at that time. Due to the small number of animals in groups 1–3 at day 66, and the considerable variation in island numbers and in percentage of island tissue (Table 1), no dose-response data were obtained for the induction of secondary foci. If the results of the three ENU groups (groups 1–3) are combined, approximately 0.4 secondary focus was obtained per $cm^2$ of liver section. This figure corresponds to about 10 foci/$cm^3$ of liver. Therefore, in approximately one out of 50 islands, a secondary focus was present. Without ENU (group 4), less than one focus/$cm^3$ liver was obtained.

Fig. 3. Secondary focus exhibiting a negative $\gamma$-glutamyltranspeptidase (GGT) reaction (arrow) is surrounded by partially positive-staining island cells (double arrow). Group 2, GGT reaction and adenosine triphosphatase (ATPase) reaction combined

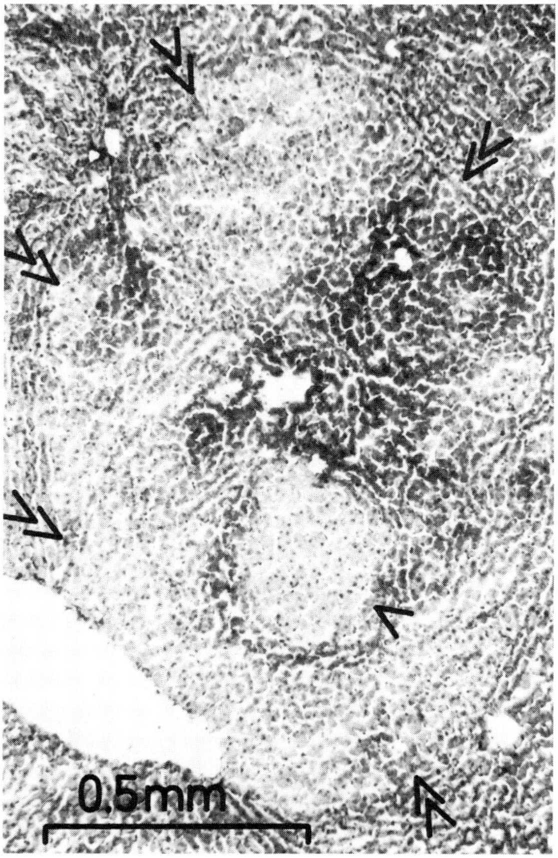

Fig. 4. Number and size of adenosine triphosphatase (ATPase)-deficient islands (groups 1–4 combined, open columns, ± SE), and of secondary foci (groups 1–3 combined, black columns) at day 66 after *N*-ethyl-*N*-nitrosourea (ENU) (see Fig. 1)

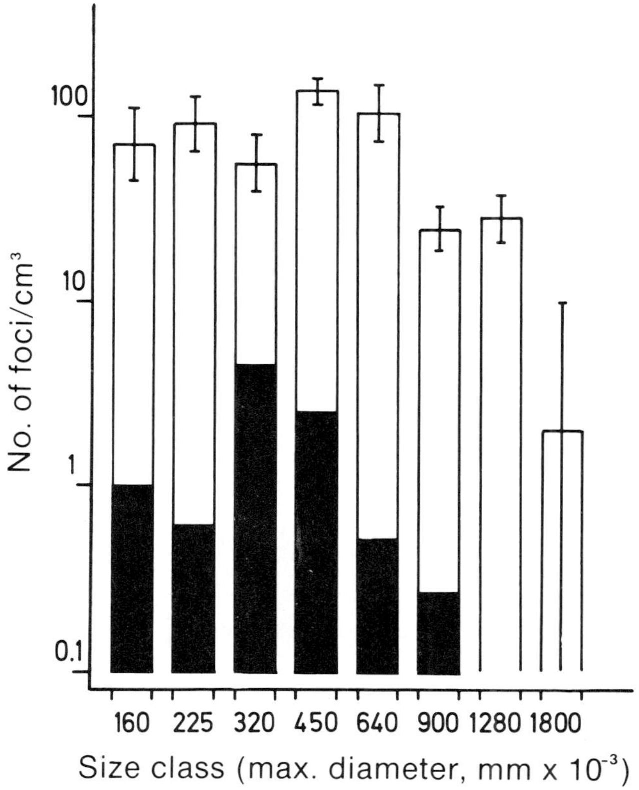


## DISCUSSION

The experiments reported here show that secondary liver cell foci can be induced within enzyme-altered islands by an initiation-promotion-initiation type of experiment. This result has been reproduced in more recent experiments (data not shown).

The secondary foci closely resemble the mixed-cell foci, as defined by Bannasch and co-workers (Bannasch *et al.*, 1980), and they qualify as neoplastic according to recommended nomenclature (Institute of Laboratory Animal Resources, 1980). Some of the secondary foci qualify as microcarcinoma since they invaded hepatic veins (compare with Koen *et al.*, 1983). The conversion of island cells into focus-forming cells is accompanied by the partial or complete loss of glycogen storage, an aspect of hepatocarcinogenesis that has been emphasized repeatedly (Bannasch *et al.*, 1980). The negative staining for GGT of the secondary foci was at variance with the concept of GGT-positive staining as the most reliable marker of precancerous and cancerous liver cell populations (Pitot *et al.*, 1978; Goldfarb & Pugh, 1981; see also Rao *et al.*, 1982).

Similar neoplastic foci within precancerous precursor tissues have been reported occasionally (Kitagawa & Sugano, 1973; Scherer & Emmelot, 1975; Solt *et al.*, 1977; Hacker *et al.*, 1982), but the study of these secondary lesions was hampered by the lack of a suitable system for reproducible induction. The present experimental system fulfills this need. In our protocol, a low dose of NDEA applied after PH serves as the first initiator; it induces a high number of enzyme-altered islands which develop slowly, in the absence of further manipulation, to nearly macroscopic size (Scherer *et al.*, 1972).

Prolonged administration of several liver cancer promoting agents, or the short-term selection regimen using AAF and a growth stimulus (Solt *et al.*, 1977), results in increased proliferation of these islands and in their progression. The short-term selection system has been chosen for the present study since it exerts the strongest proliferative stimulus (Leonard *et al.*, 1982). After 8–10 months, it leads to hepatocellular carcinoma exclusively in initiated animals, which demonstrates its strong promoting effect (Solt *et al.*, 1983). In our system, ENU was chosen as the second initiating carcinogen because of its direct alkylating activity. The relatively low liver toxicity of the doses used (similar to that of a single dose of 10 mg/kg NDEA) is not consistent with the involvement of a promoting component in its action.

After termination of the AAF/PH selection regimen, most proliferating islands reverted to less suspicious liver lesions (see also van der Heijden & Dormans, 1981; Enomoto & Farber, 1982). Most islands, however, remained detectable by at least a slight decrease in ATPase staining at their periphery. The island tissue surrounding most secondary foci exhibited the same reversion. These findings show that proliferating island cells, which later undergo phenotypic regression, can function as precursor cells for transformation into focus-forming cells.

It should be noted that a (very) small number of foci had already been obtained by the initiation-promotion protocol itself (group 4 of this study and unpublished results; Solt *et al.*, 1977, 1983; Moore *et al.*, 1983). Actually, the second initiator ENU strongly increased the occurrence of these foci. This could indicate that a common mechanism is responsible for the formation of these new cell populations due to the particular promotion stimulus alone and to the extra dose of ENU. The probability in the latter case that an island cell will be transformed into a focus-forming cell is $\sim 10^{-5}$ (assuming clonal development and one-hit kinetics: 10 foci/cm$^3$ liver develop from $0.8/100 \times 8 \times 10^7$ island cells/cm$^3$ liver serving as target cells $\rightarrow 1/6.4 \times 10^4 \sim 10^{-5}$). This probability is of the same order of magnitude as that of the first step, viz. regenerating liver cell into island-forming cell, by a similar dose (50 mg/kg) of ENU (Emmelot & Scherer, 1980; 1000 islands/cm$^3$ liver per $3 \times 10^8$ hepatocytes/cm$^3$ $\rightarrow 1/3 \times 10^{-5}$). A rare, mutation-like event may thus be involved in both the liver-island cell and island-focus cell conversions.

## REFERENCES


Bannasch, P., Mayer, D. & Hacker, H.J. (1980) Hepatocellular glycogenesis and hepatocarcinogenesis. *Biochim. biophys. Acta,* ***605,*** 217–245

Berenblum, I. & Armuth, V. (1981) Two independent aspects of tumor promotion. *Biochim. biophys. Acta,* ***651,*** 51–63

Diamond, L., O'Brien, T.G. & Baird, M. (1980) Tumor promoters and the mechanism of tumor promotion. *Adv. Cancer Res.,* ***32,*** 1–74

Emmelot, P. & Scherer, E. (1980) The first relevant cell stage in rat liver carcinogenesis. A quantitative approach. *Biochim. biophys. Acta,* ***605,*** 247–304

Enomoto, K. & Farber, E. (1982) Kinetics of phenotypic maturation of remodelling of hyperplastic nodules during liver carcinogenesis. *Cancer Res.,* ***42,*** 2330–2335

Goldfarb, S. & Pugh, T.D. (1981) Enzyme histochemical phenotypes in primary hepatocellular carcinomas. *Cancer Res.,* ***41,*** 2092–2095

Hacker, H.J., Moore, M.A., Mayer, D. & Bannasch, P. (1982) Correlative histochemistry of some enzymes of carbohydrate metabolism in preneoplastic and neoplastic lesions in the rat liver. *Carcinogenesis,* ***3,*** 1265–1272

van der Heijden, C.A. & Dormans, J.A.M.A. (1981) Short-term induction of neoplastic nodules in the rat liver. II. Study of their development and the effects of withdrawal of 2-acetylaminoflurene. *Carcinogenesis,* ***2,*** 147–156

Institute of Laboratory Animal Resources (1980) Histologic typing of liver tumors of the rat. *J. natl Cancer Inst.,* ***64,*** 178–206

Kitagawa, T. & Sugano, H. (1973) Combined enzyme histochemical and radioautographic studies on areas of hyperplasia in the liver of rats fed *N*-2-fluorenylacetamide. *Cancer Res.,* ***33,*** 2993–3001

Koen, H., Pugh, T.D., Nychka, D. & Goldfarb, S. (1983) Presence of α-fetoprotein-positive cells in hepatocellular foci and microcarcinomas induced by single injections of diethylnitrosamine in infant mice. *Cancer Res.,* ***43,*** 702–708

Leonard, T.B., Dent, J.G., Graichen, M.E., Lyght, O. & Popp, J.A. (1982) Comparison of hepatic carcinogen initiation-promotion systems. *Carcinogenesis,* ***3,*** 851–856

Moore, M.A., Hacker, H.J. & Bannasch, P. (1983) Phenotypic instability of focal and nodular lesions induced in a short term system in the rat liver. *Carcinogenesis,* ***4,*** 595–603

Pitot, H.C., Barsness, L., Goldsworthy, T. & Kitagawa, T. (1978) Biochemical characterization of stages of carcinogenesis after a single dose of diethylnitrosamine. *Nature,* ***271,*** 456–458

Potter, V.R. (1981) A new protocol and its rationale for the study of initiation and promotion of carcinogenesis in rat liver. *Carcinogenesis,* ***2,*** 1375–1379

Rao, M.S., Lalwani, N.D., Scarpelli, D.G. & Reddy, J.K. (1982) The absence of γ-glutamyl transpeptidase activity in putative preneoplastic lesions and in hepatocellular carcinomas induced in rats by the hypolipidemic peroxisome proliferator Wy-14.643. *Carcinogenesis,* ***3,*** 1231–1233

Rutenburg, A.M., Kim, H., Fischbein, J.W., Hanker, J.S., Wasserkrug, H.L. & Seligman, A.M. (1969) Histochemical and ultrastructural demonstration of γ-glutamyl transpeptidase activity. *J. Histochem. Cytochem.,* ***17,*** 517–526

Scherer, E. (1981) Use of a programmable pocket calculator for the quantitation of precancerous foci. *Carcinogenesis,* **2,** 805–807

Scherer, E. & Emmelot, P. (1975) Kinetics of induction and growth of precancerous liver-cell foci, and liver tumor formation by diethylnitrosamine in the rat. *Eur. J. Cancer,* **11,** 689–696

Scherer, E. & Emmelot, P. (1979a) *The multi-hit concept of tumor cell formation and its bearing on low dose risk assessment.* In: Emmelot, P. & Kriek, E., eds, *Environmental Carcinogenesis,* Amsterdam, Elsevier/North-Holland Biomedical Press, pp. 303–318

Scherer, E. & Emmelot, P. (1979b) *Multihit kinetics of tumor cell formation and risk assessment of low doses of carcinogen.* In: Griffin, A.C. & Shaw, C.R., eds, *Carcinogens: Identification and Mechanism of Action,* New York, Raven Press, pp. 337–364

Scherer, E., Hoffmann, M., Emmelot, P. & Friedrich-Freksa, H. (1972) Quantitative study on foci of altered liver cells induced in the rat by a single dose of diethylnitrosamine and partial hepatectomy. *J. natl Cancer Inst.,* **49,** 93–106

Scribner, J.D. & Süss, R. (1978) Tumor initiation and promotion. *Int. Res. exp. Pathol.,* **18,** 137–192

Solt, D.B., Medline, A. & Farber, E. (1977) Rapid emergence of carcinogen-induced hyperplastic lesions in a new model for the sequential analysis of liver carcinogenesis. *Am. J. Pathol.,* **88,** 595–618

Solt, D.B., Cayama, E., Tsuda, H., Enomoto, K., Lee, G. & Farber, E. (1983) Promotion of liver cancer development by brief exposure to dietary 2-acetylaminofluorene plus partial hepatectomy or carbon tetrachloride. *Cancer Res.,* **43,** 188–191

# ABERRANT EXPRESSION OF ADAPTATION TO PHENOBARBITAL MAY CAUSE SELECTIVE GROWTH OF FOCI OF ALTERED CELLS IN RAT LIVER

R. SCHULTE-HERMANN & I. TIMMERMANN-TROSIENER

*Institute of Toxicology and Pharmacology of the Phillips-University Marburg 355 Marburg a.d. Lahn, Federal Republic of Germany*

J. SCHUPPLER

*Department of Toxicology, Schering AG, Berlin (West) 65*

## SUMMARY

According to the multistage concept of carcinogenesis, promoters induce selective or preferential multiplication of initiated cells, thereby accelerating one of the rate-limiting steps in cancer formation. The driving force for this selective growth of initiated cells is not known. In normal liver, various liver tumour promoters induce expression of adaptive programmes. One such programme, induced by phenobarbital, consists of organ growth and an increase in the activity of various enzymes involved in the metabolism of lipophilic substrates. In foci of altered rat liver cells (the putative progeny of initiated cells), expression of the programme is still possible and is coupled to certain regulatory defects (excessive, unbalanced proliferation; independence from position-specific restrictions within the hepatic acinus; autonomous expression of some adaptive changes). Promoters seem to switch on this aberrant expression of the programme of adaptation, thereby leading to preferential growth of foci.

## INTRODUCTION

Current concepts of the mechanisms of tumour promotion are based mainly on studies with phorbol esters purified from croton oil (Hecker, 1978); skin was used as an in-vivo model and various types of cells as in-vitro models (Boutwell, 1974; Hecker, 1978; Weinstein *et al.*, 1979; Farber & Cameron, 1980; Hecker *et al.*, 1982). The extent to which such concepts may be valid in other organs such as the liver is not clear. This organ is particularly well suited to the study of mechanisms of promoter action. The putative progeny of the initiated cells can be discovered readily at an early stage of development in histological sections as foci or 'islands' of phenotypically altered cells (Farber & Cameron, 1980; Bannasch *et al.*, 1981), and the effects of hepatic tumour promoters on their target cells can be analysed quantitatively and qualitatively. Phenobarbital (PB), which is now widely used as a model compound to study liver tumour promotion (Peraino *et al.*, 1975), has been found to increase the number and size of foci, as well as to enhance their phenotypic deviation from the normal hepatocyte (Pitot *et al.*, 1978; Schulte-Hermann *et al.*, 1982a). These effects are consistent with the multistage concept of carcinogenesis, according to which tumour promoters cause selective or preferential multiplication of initiated cells (Farber & Cameron, 1980); however, the underlying mechanisms are not known.

A common property of PB and of most other liver tumour promoters is their ability to induce a series of adaptive responses in normal liver consisting of an increase in the activity of various drug-metabolizing enzymes and in liver growth (Schulte-Hermann, 1974, 1979). We have studied whether or not these adaptive responses also take place in preneoplastic foci identified in the liver by means of a positive $\gamma$-glutamyltransferase (GGT) reaction.

## METHODS

Young female Wistar rats (Zentralinstitut für Versuchstierzucht, Hanover, Federal Republic of Germany) received a single oral dose of 250 mg/kg body weight *N*-nitrosomorpholine (NMOR). After six weeks of recovery, PB was added to the diet at a concentration providing a daily dose of 50 mg/kg body weight. At the same time, an osmotic minipump was implanted under the dorsal skin in order to deliver $^3$H-thymidine continuously for two weeks. The animals were then killed. Serial histological sections taken from the liver were stained for GGT (Rutenberg *et al.*, 1968) and cytochrome P-450-PB by an immunoperoxidase method (Nakane & Pierce, 1967; Sternberger *et al.*, 1970). Specific antibodies were raised in rabbits against one of the major PB-inducible cytochromes P-450 that had been purified from PB-treated rat liver (Schulte-Hermann *et al.*, 1984). Autoradiography was performed on the sections, and the percentage of labelled hepatocytes (labelling index, LI) was determined.

## RESULTS AND DISCUSSION

In normal parts of the liver, cytochrome P-450-PB was detectable by immunocytochemistry only in the pericentral area; PB treatment resulted in an extension of the positive staining area, but periportal hepatocytes remained negative except for a few individual cells (Schulte-Hermann *et al.*, 1984). As in prior reports (Schulte-Hermann, 1982b, 1984), we found a number of hepatocyte foci containing the antigen in rats treated with NMOR alone or with NMOR + PB (Fig. 1). Many of these foci were also GGT positive in serial sections (Fig. 2); no focus was seen in untreated control animals of the same age. It is also noteworthy that some foci staining for cytochrome P-450-PB were located in the periportal area (Fig. 1). Apparently, expression of the antigen is less sensitive in focal cells than in normal liver to the mechanisms that restrict its presence to the centrolobular area. This finding constitutes the first regulatory defect of focal hepatocytes to be considered in this paper.

$^{3}$H-Thymidine was infused continuously during the entire period of PB treatment in an attempt to quantify the proliferative response. As indicated in Figure 3, approximately 20% of liver cells were $^{3}$H-labelled (and hence had replicated DNA) in the centrolobular area of the liver (cytochrome P-450-PB-positive). The level of DNA synthesis in the periportal area was not higher with PB treatment than without.

We showed previously that foci have higher rates of proliferation than do normal liver cells (Schulte-Hermann *et al.*, 1981, 1982a). This finding was confirmed in the present study; it was also found that the high rate of DNA synthesis was associated with the presence of cytochrome P-450-PB, with and without promoter treatment (Fig. 3). The percentage of focal cells synthesizing DNA was even higher than in normal cytochrome P-450-PB-positive hepatocytes; as shown previously, the LI in foci remains at a relatively high level for many months of PB treatment, whereas it returns to normal in the unaltered parts of the liver (Schulte-Hermann *et al.*, 1982a). This constitutes a second regulatory defect of focal hepatocytes.

Other adaptive responses to PB are also known to occur essentially in the centrolobular parts of the liver; examples are: increases in reduced glutathione transferase

Fig. 1. Immunocytochemical demonstration of cytochrome P-450-PB in rat liver pretreated with a single dose of *N*-nitrosomorpholine followed by phenobarbital
Note that, in general, periportal areas are not stained. A focus of large cytochrome P-450-positive cells is seen in the upper left corner of A and enlarged in B. Note that the focus extends into the immediate vicinity of a periportal field.

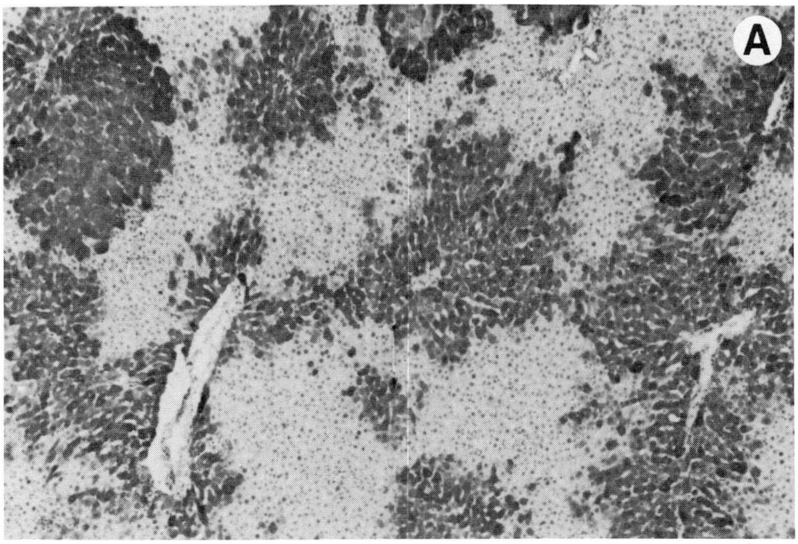

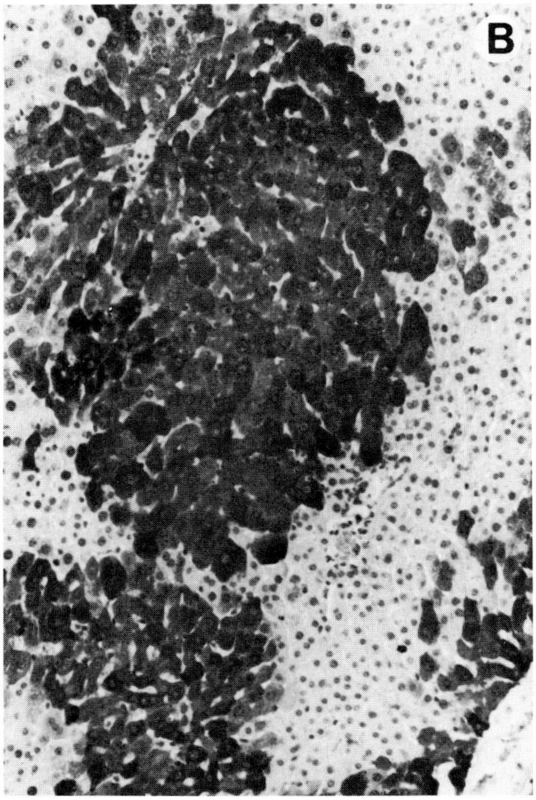


B (Kraus, Schuppler, Schulte-Hermann & Timmermann-Trosiener, unpublished data), epoxide hydratase (Bentley *et al.*, 1979) and smooth endoplasmic reticulum (Schulte-Hermann, 1974) (Fig. 4). Therefore, only a subpopulation of hepatocytes located in the central parts of the liver seem to be able to express an entire programme of adaptive responses to PB. Such a programme could also include decreases in the activities of certain enzymes; thus, glucose-6-phosphatase was found to decrease in centrolobular cells during PB treatment (Menard *et al.*, 1974).

Foci seem to express many of the responses that may be found in centrolobular cells of normal liver during PB treatment (Fig. 4). In fact, several phenotypic alterations in foci (foci 'markers') have been recognized in the last few years as adaptive responses of normal liver to PB. Some examples are listed in Figure 4, which also presents an attempt to classify and interpret the functional significance of the alterations. Several of these concern 'drug-metabolizing' enzymes, the expression of which may provide 'resistance' to cytotoxic effects of various hepatotoxins (Solt & Farber, 1976). We include GGT among these enzymes because it splits glutamine from reduced glutathione conjugates in the mercapturic acid pathway. GGT is present in normal liver and is further induced by PB; its expression in foci does not, therefore, necessarily indicate retrodifferentiation toward a foetal stage, as was assumed previously by some

Fig. 2. Cytochrome P-450-PB and $\gamma$-glutamyltransferase (GGT) in liver foci
The presence of both markers was checked in serial sections of liver tissue, and the number of foci expressing either one or both markers is expressed per cm² section area. NMOR, *N*-nitrosomorpholine; PB, phenobarbital

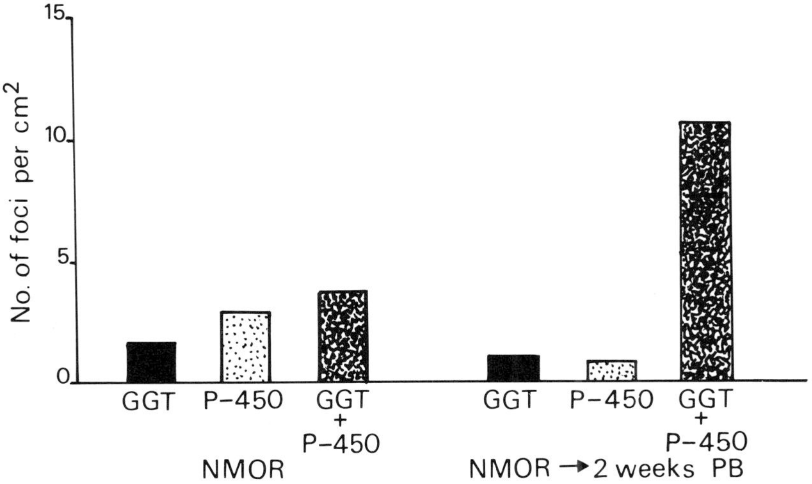


Fig. 3. Effect of phenobarbital (PB) on cytochrome P-450-PB and DNA synthesis in periportal and pericentral hepatocytes and in liver foci
DNA synthesis was measured by continuous infusion of ³H-thymidine and autoradiography, which was performed on the same sections as the immunocytochemical demonstration of cytochrome P-450. Labelling indices (LIs) of hepatocytes positive and negative for cytochrome P-450 were determined separately.

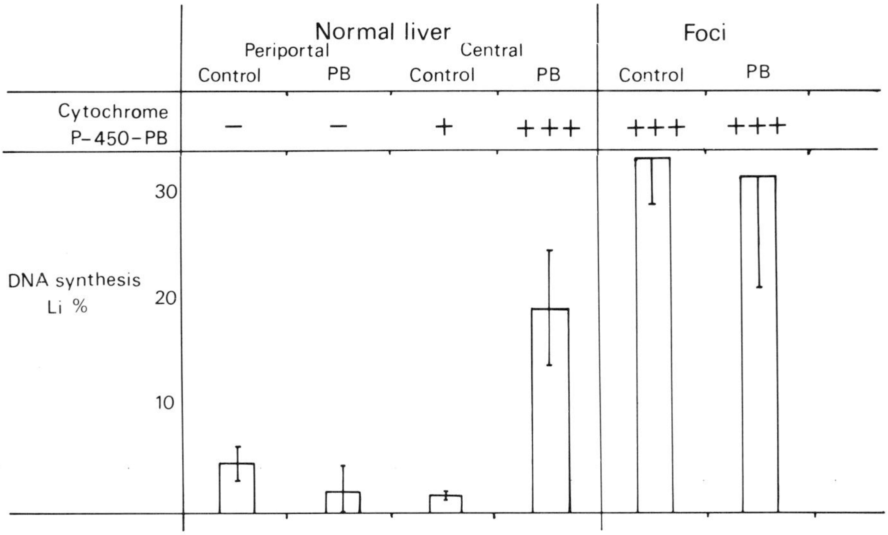

Fig. 4. Adaptive programme of normal (central hepatocytes) and of liver foci to phenobarbital (PB) (See text for explanation)

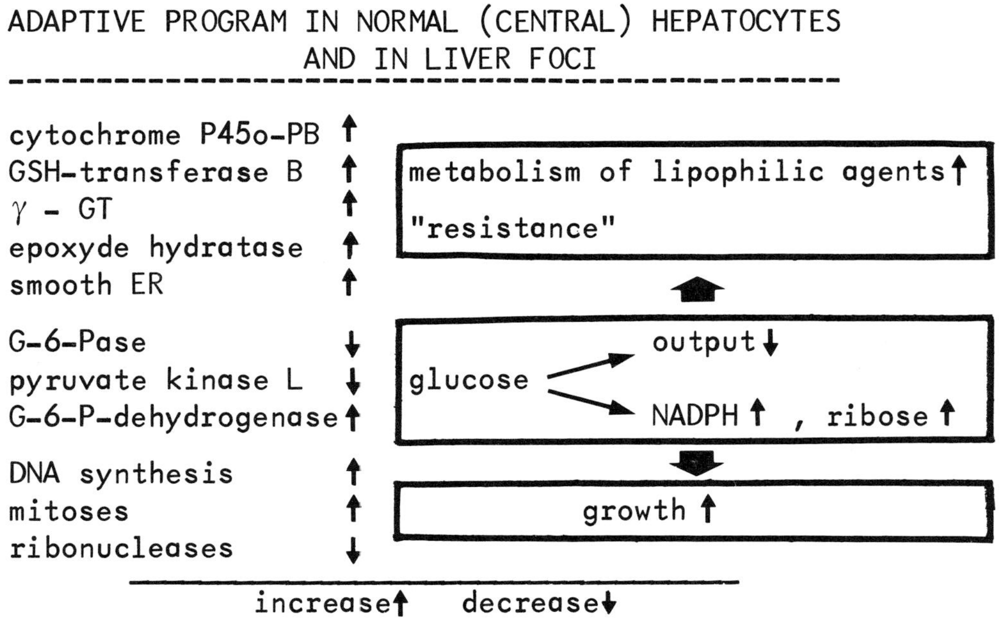


authors. A second group of enzyme changes should affect the metabolism of carbohydrates by decreasing glucose output and pyruvate formation (Reinacher *et al.* 1984), and by enhancing glucose storage and metabolism into NADPH and ribose. This shift may serve to provide substrates required for drug metabolism (monooxygenases) and nucleic acid syntheses. The third group of changes is linked more directly to cell multiplication and growth. In conclusion, we offer the hypothesis that many phenotypic alterations in foci reflect the expression of an adaptive programme, which, in normal liver, can be induced by PB and other 'inducers'.

Why should PB promote the development of the foci? As shown in Figure 2, the number and type of alterations expressed by different foci is variable; PB treatment causes a near doubling of the number of those foci detectable per $cm^2$ liver section, exclusively by increasing the number of foci that exhibit both alterations tested. Previous studies, in which several different phenotypic alterations were used to identify foci, revealed similar results (Pitot *et al.*, 1978); however, it was not clear whether such effects are due to selective growth from initiated cells of a specific subpopulation of foci (a subpopulation expressing multiple phenotypic alterations) or to expression (induction) of alterations in already existing foci. An answer to this question was provided by an experiment utilizing continuous infusion of $^3$H-thymidine. Figure 5 shows the LIs found in individual foci. If the increase in number of foci were due exclusively to selective growth of a subpopulation of initiated cells and of small foci (below the limits of detection), many foci should show LIs of 100% or

Fig. 5. DNA synthesis in individual foci
The ordinate shows the percentage of cells in γ-glutamyltransferase-positive foci that replicated DNA during two weeks of infusion of $^3$H-thymidine. NMOR, *N*-nitrosomorpholine; PB, phenobarbital

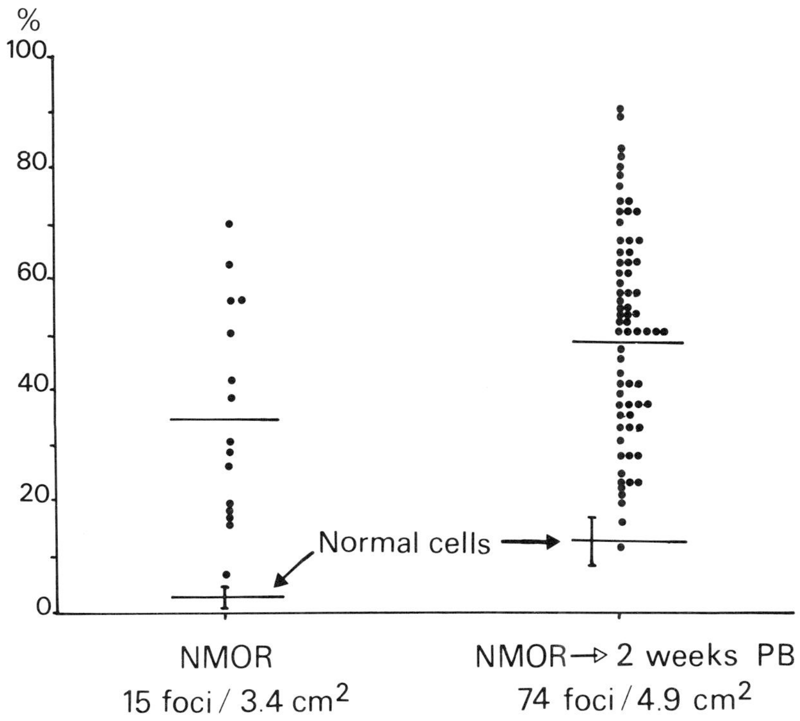


nearly 100%. This was not the case. This result strongly suggests that *induction* of GGT in preexisting but GGT-negative foci must contribute to the enhancement by PB of numbers of foci. The same conclusion was reached when cytochrome P-450-PB was used as a marker of foci. These findings indicate that foci may express some adaptive responses to PB, even in the absence of the inducer (i.e., 'autonomously'). This appears to reflect a third regulatory defect of foci. Foci still respond to PB, in that expression of the adaptive programme is enhanced and more complete after treatment with the promoter. Previous investigations by Boutwell (1974), Weinstein *et al.* (1979) and others have shown that phorbol ester tumour promoters induce qualitatively similar changes in normal and transformed cells. This phenomen also appears to be valid for PB and the liver.

The results of this study are summarized in Table 1. We believe that initiation by a (complete) carcinogen produces a cell that is 'over-specialized' in expressing a particular differentiative pathway in adult liver, that is, adaptation to lipophilic compounds such as PB. These compounds promote because they switch on or

Table 1. Excessive (facilitated) expression of the adaptive programme in liver foci

| |
|---|
| 1. Independence from local restrictions in liver lobules |
| 2. Excessive, unbalanced cell proliferation |
| 3. Expression of some adaptive changes even without inducer/promoter |
| *Foci:* 'Specialists' in expression of adaptive responses to lipophilic agents such as phenobarbital |
| *Promoters:* induce (reinforce) expression in latent foci (hormone-like); as a result, more foci exhibit unbalanced cell proliferation |

enhance the aberrant expression of the programme of adaptation in the foci. This hypothesis can easily be reconciled with current concepts of the mechanism of promoter action on other organs such as skin (Boutwell, 1974; Weinstein *et al.*, 1979; Hecker *et al.*, 1982).

## ACKNOWLEDGEMENTS

This study was supported by a grant from the BMFT/GSF-München. We are most grateful to Drs Ulrich and Graf (Homburg-Saar/Konstanz) for the generous supply of anti-cytochrome P-450 antibodies. The excellent technical assistance of J. Sprenger and G. Barthel is gratefully acknowledged.

## REFERENCES

Bannasch, P., Benner, U., Hacker, H.-J., Klimek, F., Mayer, D., Moore, M. & Zerban, H. (1981) Cytochemical and biochemical microanalysis of carcinogenesis. *Histochem. J.*, ***13***, 799–820

Bentley, P., Waechter, F., Oesch, F. & Stäubli, W. (1979) Immunochemical localization of epoxide hydratase in rat liver: Effects of 2-acetylaminofluorene. *Biochem. biophys. Res. Comm.*, ***91***, 1101–1108

Boutwell, R.K. (1974) The function and mechanism of promoters of carcinogenesis. *Crit. Rev. Toxicol.*, ***2***, 419–443

Farber, E. & Cameron, R. (1980) The sequential analysis of cancer development. *Adv. Cancer Res.*, ***31***, 125–226

Hecker, E. (1978) Co-carcinogene oder bedingt krebsauslösende Faktoren. Aktuelle neue Aspekte der Ätiologie menschlicher Tumoren und des molekularen Mechanismus der Krebsentstehung. *Naturwissenschaften*, ***65***, 640–648

Hecker, E., Fusenig, N.E., Kunz, W. Marks, F. & Thielmann, H.W., eds (1982) *Carcinogenesis*, Vol. 7, *Cocarcinogenesis and Biological Effects of Tumor Promoters*, New York, Raven Press

Menard, D., Penasse, W., Drochmans, P. & Hugon, J.S. (1974) Glucose-6-phosphatase heterogeneity within the hepatic lobule of the phenobarbital-treated rat. *Histochemistry*, ***38***, 229–239

Nakane, P.K. & Pierce, G.B. (1967) Enzyme labeled antibodies for the light and electron microscopic localization of tissue antigens. *J. Cell Biol.*, ***33***, 307–318

Peraino, C., Fry, R.J.M., Staffeldt, E. & Christopher, J.P. (1975) Comparative enhancing effects of phenobarbital, amobarbital, diphenylhydantoin, and dichlorodiphenyltrichloroethane on 2-acetylaminofluorene-induced hepatic tumorigenesis in the rat. *Cancer Res.*, ***35***, 2884–2890

Pitot, H.C., Barsness, L., Goldsworthy, T. & Kitagawa, T. (1978) Biochemical characterization of stages of hepatocarcinogenesis after a single dose of diethylnitrosamine. *Nature*, ***271***, 456–458

Reinacher, M., Eigenbrodt, E., Timmermann-Trosiener, I., Bentley, P., Waechter, F., Schoner, F. & Schulte-Hermann, R. (1984) Pyruvate kinase isoenzymes in altered foci and carcinoma of rat liver. A concept on carbohydrate metabolism during hepatocarcinogenesis. *Carcinogenesis* (in press)

Rutenberg, A.M., Kim, H., Fischbein, J., Hauker, J.S., Wasserkrug, H.C. & Seligman, R. (1968) Histochemical and ultrastructural demonstration of γ-glutamyl transpeptidase activity. *J. Histochem. Cytochem.*, ***17***, 517–526

Schulte-Hermann, R. (1974) Induction of liver growth by xenobiotic compounds and other stimuli. *Crit. Rev. Toxicol.*, ***3***, 97–158

Schulte-Hermann, R. (1979) *Reactions of the liver to injury: Adaptation.* In: Farber, E. & Fisher, M.M., eds, *Treatise on Liver, Toxic Injury of the Liver,* New York, Marcel Dekker, pp. 385–444

Schulte-Hermann, R., Ohde, G., Schuppler, J. & Timmermann-Trosiener, I. (1981) Enhanced proliferation of putative preneoplastic cells in rat liver following treatment with the tumor promoters phenobarbital, hexachlorocyclohexane, steroid compounds and nafenopin. *Cancer Res.*, ***41***, 2556–2562

Schulte-Hermann, R., Schuppler, J., Ohde, G., Bursch, W. & Timmermann-Trosiener, I. (1982a) *Phenobarbital and other liver tumor promoters.* In: Nicolini, C., ed., *Chemical Carcinogenesis,* New York, Plenum Press, pp. 231–260

Schulte-Hermann, R., Timmermann-Trosiener, I. & Schuppler, J. (1982b) Response of liver foci in rats to hepatic tumor promoters. *Toxicol. Pathol.*, ***10***, 63–68

Schulte-Hermann, R., Roome, N., Timmermann-Trosiener, I. & Schuppler, J. (1984) Immunocytochemical demonstration of a phenobarbital-inducible cytochrome $P_{450}$ in putative preneoplastic foci of rat liver. *Carcinogenesis*, ***5***, 149–153

Solt, D. & Farber, E. (1976) New principle for the analysis of chemical carcinogenesis. *Nature*, ***263***, 701–703

Sternberger, L.A., Hendy, P.H., Cuculies, I.I. & Meyer, H.G. (1970) The unlabelled antibody enzyme method of immuno-histochemistry: preparation and properties of soluble antigen-antibody complex (horse-radish peroxidase-antiperoxydase) and its use in identification of spirochaetes. *J. Histochem. Cytochem.*, ***18***, 315–333

Weinstein, B., Lee, L.-S., Fischer, P.B., Mufson, A. & Yamasaki, H. (1979) *The mechanism of action of tumor promoters and a molecular model of two stage carcinogenesis.* In: Emmelot, P. & Kriek, E., eds, *Environmental Carcinogenesis,* Amsterdam, Elsevier/North-Holland Biomedical Press, pp. 265–285

# PROMOTING EFFECT OF PHENOBARBITAL ON *N*-BIS (2-HYDROXYPROPYL)NITROSAMINE THYROID TUMORIGENESIS IN RATS. EFFECT OF VARYING DURATION OF EXPOSURE TO PHENOBARBITAL

Y. HIASA, Y. KITAHORI, N. KONISHI, N. ENOKI & T. FUJITA

*First Department of Pathology, Nara Medical University, Kashihara, Nara 634, Japan*

## SUMMARY

Male Wistar rats were injected subcutaneously with a single dose of 280 mg *N*-bis(2-hydroxypropyl)nitrosamine (DHPN) per 100 g body weight and then given a diet containing 500 mg/kg phenobarbital (PB) for 6, 12 and 19 weeks. Exposure to PB for 12 or 19 weeks enhanced the development of thyroid tumours in rats treated with DHPN. The incidences of thyroid tumours at the end of the experiment were 87% in rats given DHPN and then PB for 19 weeks, 83% in rats given DHPN and then PB for 12 weeks, 42% in rats given DHPN and then PB for 6 weeks, and 37% in rats given DHPN. The incidence of thyroid cancer was 12% in rats given DHPN and then PB for 19 weeks. The total numbers of thyroid tumours were: 241 in rats given DHPN and then PB for 19 weeks, 125 in rats given DHPN and then PB for 12 weeks, 65 in rats given DHPN and then PB for 6 weeks, and 23 in rats given DHPN alone. The total numbers of thyroid tumours were proportional to the period of exposure to PB.

## INTRODUCTION

Berenblum (1941) demonstrated that the application of multiple doses of a chemical agent to mouse skin initiated cancer induction; this effect occurred only if croton oil, 'a promoter', was subsequently applied to the treated site. Mottram (1944) described the application of a single small dose of carcinogen as 'initiation'. This two-stage concept of carcinogenesis was subsequently demonstrated in liver (Peraino *et al.*, 1971; Kitagawa *et al.*, 1979), lung (Witschi *et al.*, 1977), intestine (Narisawa *et al.*, 1974; Weisburger, 1975; Reddy *et al.*, 1977; Pollard & Luckert, 1979) and urinary bladder (Hicks *et al.*, 1973; Cohen *et al.*, 1979; Fukushima *et al.*, 1981). More recently, this action was also demonstrated in thyroid carcinogenesis (Hiasa *et al.*, 1982a,b).

The carcinogenicity of *N*-bis(2-hydroxypropyl)nitrosamine (DHPN) was reported by Mohr *et al.* (1977) and Konishi *et al.* (1978). DHPN induced tumours in the lung (100%), liver (41%), thyroid (25%), kidney (16%) and pancreas (8.1%) in rats (Mohr *et al.*, 1977). Phenobarbital (PB) (Hiasa *et al.*, 1982a) and 3-amino-1,2,4-triazole (Hiasa *et al.*, 1982b) promoted the development of thyroid tumours in rats pretreated with DHPN, although the mechanism of the action of PB is unknown.

The present paper reports studies on the effects of different periods of exposure to PB in the enhancement of thyroid tumorigenesis in male Wistar rats treated with a single dose of DHPN.

## MATERIALS AND METHODS

Two hundred six-week-old male Wistar strain rats (Kitayama Labes Animal Co., Kyoto) were given a commercial diet for one week. Then, 192 healthy rats, weighing 150–170 g, were selected and divided into eight groups.

At the beginning of the experiment, a dose of 280 mg DHPN (Nakarai Chemicals Co., Kyoto) per 100 g body weight was injected subcutaneously into rats in groups 1, 2, 3 and 4. Powdered basal diet (Oriental MF, Oriental Kobo Co., Tokyo) containing 500 mg/kg PB (Nakarai Chemicals Co., Kyoto) was given to groups 1 and 5 from week 2 to 20 (19 weeks), to groups 2 and 6 from week 2 to 13 (12 weeks) and to groups 3 and 7 from week 2 to 7 (6 weeks). Powdered basal diet without PB was given to groups 4 and 8 for 20 weeks and to the other groups at times other than those described above.

After 20 weeks of the experiment, all animals were starved for 18 h and then killed with ether. A complete autopsy, including a thorough macroscopic examination, was performed. The liver, kidneys and thyroids were then weighed and fixed in 10% buffered formalin, and the tissues were embedded in paraffin, sectioned and stained routinely with haematoxylin and eosin. Specific stains, such as periodic acid-Schiff, van Gieson and Grimelius, were employed in some cases. Thyroid tumours were counted in the largest serial sections. The morphological diagnoses of thyroid tumours were made according to the criteria of Napalkov (1958).

## RESULTS

The mean final weights of body, thyroid, liver and kidney and the effective numbers of rats in each group are shown in Table 1. No animal died before the end of the experiment. The mean final body weight in group 1 was significantly lower than those in groups 4 and 8. The mean thyroid weights in groups 1, 2 and 3 were significantly higher than those in group 8 and the weights in groups 1 and 2 were significantly higher than those in group 4. The mean liver weights in groups 1, 2 and 3 were significantly higher than those in groups 4 and 8.

Table 1. Mean (± SD) weights of body, thyroid, liver and kidney of male Wistar rats treated with *N*-bis(2-hydroxypropyl)nitrosamine (DHPN) and phenobarbital (PB)

| Experimental group (weeks of treatment) | Effective no. of rats | Final body weight (g) | Thyroid weight (mg) | Liver weight (g) | Kidney weights (g) | |
|---|---|---|---|---|---|---|
| | | | | | Left | Right |
| 1. DHPN + PB (19) | 24 | 449±39 [a,b] | 26.5±3.8 [a,b] | 14.5±2.0 [a,b] | 1.4±0.1 | 1.4±0.1 |
| 2. DHPN + PB (12) | 24 | 501±58 | 19.3±3.3 [a,b] | 13.6±1.2 [a,b] | 1.4±0.1 | 1.4±0.1 |
| 3. DHPN + PB (6) | 24 | 514±50 | 17.1±2.8 [a] | 13.1±1.7 [a,b] | 1.4±0.1 | 1.4±0.2 |
| 4. DHPN | 24 | 498±41 | 16.4±1.4 | 11.5±1.0 | 1.4±0.1 | 1.4±0.1 |
| 5. Saline + PB (19) | 24 | 497±27 | 16.9±2.7 | 13.4±1.5 [a] | 1.3±0.1 [a] | 1.3±0.1 [a] |
| 6. Saline + PB (12) | 24 | 489±35 | 15.6±3.2 | 12.5±1.5 [a] | 1.3±0.1 [a] | 1.3±0.1 [a] |
| 7. Saline + PB (6) | 24 | 502±43 | 15.4±2.4 | 11.7±1.6 | 1.4±0.1 | 1.4±0.1 |
| 8. Control | 24 | 511±21 | 15.4±2.0 | 10.7±0.4 | 1.4±0.1 | 1.4±0.1 |

[a] Significantly different from group 8 at $p < 0.05$
[b] Significantly different from group 4 at $p < 0.05$

## *Incidences of thyroid tumours*

The incidences of thyroid tumours in each group are summarized in Table 2. The incidences of adenomas were 87% in group 1, 83% in group 2, 42% in group 3 and 37% in group 4. No thyroid tumour was found in group 5, 6, 7 or 8. The incidence of cancer in group 1 was 12%.

## *Histological analysis of thyroid tumours*

The histological types of thyroid tumours in each group are also summarized in Table 2. Follicular and papillary tumours were observed, but there were no solid or C-cell tumours. The follicular adenomas were well-circumscribed and encapsulated, and their expansion caused compression and atrophy of the adjacent thyroid paren-

Table 2. Incidences of thyroid adenomas (A) and carcinomas (C) in rats treated with *N*-bis(2-hydroxypropyl)nitrosamine (DHPN) and phenobarbital (PB)

| Experimental group (weeks of treatment) | No. of rats with tumours (%) | | Total no. of tumours (per rat) | No. of tumours (No. of rats) | | | |
|---|---|---|---|---|---|---|---|
| | | | | Follicular | | Papillary | |
| | A | C | | A | C | A | C |
| 1. DHPN + PB (19) | 21 (87) [a] | 3 (12) | 241 (10.0) | 237 (21) | 3 (2) | 1 (1) | 0 |
| 2. DHPN + PB (12) | 19 (83) [a] | 0 | 125 (5.2) | 124 (18) | 0 | 1 (1) | 0 |
| 3. DHPN + PB (6) | 10 (42) | 0 | 65 (2.6) | 62 (10) | 0 | 3 (3) | 0 |
| 4. DHPN | 9 (37) | 0 | 23 (0.9) | 23 (9) | 0 | 0 | 0 |
| 5. Saline + PB (19) | 0 | 0 | 0 | 0 | 0 | 0 | 0 |
| 6. Saline + PB (12) | 0 | 0 | 0 | 0 | 0 | 0 | 0 |
| 7. Saline + PB (6) | 0 | 0 | 0 | 0 | 0 | 0 | 0 |
| 8. Control | 0 | 0 | 0 | 0 | 0 | 0 | 0 |

[a] Significantly different from group 4 at $p < 0.05$

Table 3. Histological findings in non-tumorous areas of the thyroid of rats treated with *N*-bis(2-hydroxypropyl)nitrosamine (DHPN) and phenobarbital (PB)

| Experimental group (weeks of treatment) | Hyperplasia | Colloid decrease in follicle | Size decrease of follicle |
|---|---|---|---|
| 1. DHPN + PB (19) | + + + | + + + | + + + |
| 2. DHPN + PB (12) | + + | + + | + + |
| 3. DHPN + PB (6) | + | + | + |
| 4. DHPN | + | + | + |
| 5. Saline + PB (19) | + + + | + + + | + + + |
| 6. Saline + PB (12) | − | + | + |
| 7. Saline + PB (6) | − | − | − |
| 8. Control | − | − | − |

−, none; +, slight; + +, moderate; + + +, marked

chyma. The most characteristic features of these tumours were extreme variability in size and shape of follicles. All animals in groups 1 and 2 had multiple follicular adenomas. The papillary adenomas were encapsulated, and they showed expansive and papillary growth in the follicles.

The follicular carcinomas in animals in group 1 were encapsulated and showed invasive growths into the fibrous capsule. A few mitoses were seen. No metastasis was seen in any organ.

*Histological findings in non-tumorous areas of the thyroid*

The histological findings in each group in non-tumorous areas of the thyroid are summarized in Table 3. The thyroids of rats in groups 1 and 5 showed diffuse proliferation of small follicles along with decreased colloid.

*Incidences of tumours in other organs*

The incidences of pulmonary tumours, which were well-circumscribed, encapsulated adenomas, were 12% in group 3 and 16% in group 4. The incidences of pulmonary hyperplasia were 8% in groups 3 and 4, and 4% in group 2; these areas of hyperplasia were not well-circumscribed and consisted of hyperchromatic cells. In group 3, there was an 8% incidence of renal tumours, which were well-circumscribed, encapsulated renal tubular-cell adenomas. Neither tumours nor hyperplastic nodules were found in the liver.

## DISCUSSION

We reported previously the promoting effect of PB on the development of thyroid tumours in rats given four or six subcutaneous injections of 70 mg DHPN per 100 g body weight as an initiator (Hiasa *et al.*, 1982a). The present work showed the promoting effect of PB on the development of thyroid tumours in rats given a single injection of 280 mg DHPN per 100 g body weight as an initiator.

There was a significant difference between the incidence of thyroid adenomas in rats given DHPN and then PB for 12 or 19 weeks and that of rats given DHPN and then PB for six weeks or DHPN alone. However, there was no significant difference between the incidence of thyroid adenomas in rats given DHPN and then PB for six weeks and that of rats given DHPN alone. This observation suggests that six-weeks' administration of PB has no enhancing effect on the development of thyroid adenomas in rats given DHPN, but that 12 or 19 weeks' administration does. An increase in the period of PB treatment after injection of DHPN resulted in a parallel increase in the number of thyroid tumours; that is, prolonged exposure to PB was necessary for its maximal promoting effect. These results suggest that the mechanism by which PB promotes is by increasing the probability of expression of neoplastic character by DHPN-initiated thyroid follicular cells.

Similar results have been obtained in studies of liver carcinogenesis (Peraino *et al.*, 1973): A parallel increase in the yield of hepatic tumours following an increase in the duration of PB treatment after exposure to *N*-2-acetylaminofluorene was reported (Peraino *et al.*, 1973, 1977).

Although DHPN is carcinogenic in liver (Mohr *et al.*, 1977; Konishi *et al.*, 1978) and PB has a promoting effect on liver carcinogenesis initiated by *N*-2-acetylaminofluorene (Peraino *et al.*, 1971), no liver tumour was observed in the present experiment. The promoting effect of PB on chemical carcinogenesis requires further study.

## ACKNOWLEDGEMENT

The authors thanks Ms Sachi Khono for typing the manuscript.

## REFERENCES

Berenblum, I. (1941) The carcinogenic action of croton resin. *Cancer Res.*, ***1***, 44–48

Cohen, S.M., Arai, M., Jacobs, J.B. & Friedell, G.H. (1979) Promoting effect of saccharin and DL-tryptophan in urinary bladder carcinogenesis. *Cancer Res.*, ***39***, 1207–1217

Fukushima, S., Friedell, G.H., Jacobs, J.B. & Cohen, S.H. (1981) Effect of L-tryptophan and sodium saccharin on urinary tract carcinogenesis initiated by *N*-[4-(5-nitro-2-furyl)-2-thiazolyl]formamide. *Cancer Res.*, ***41***, 3100–3103

Hiasa, Y., Kitahori, Y., Ohshima, M., Fujita, T., Yuasa, T., Konishi, N. & Miyashiro, A. (1982a) Promoting effects of phenobarbital and barbital on development of thyroid tumors in rats treated with *N*-bis(2-hydroxypropyl)nitrosamine. *Carcinogenesis*, ***3***, 1187–1190

Hiasa, Y., Ohshima, M., Kitahori, Y., Yuasa, T., Fujita, T. & Iwata, C. (1982b) Promoting effects of 3-amino-1,2,4-triazole on the development of thyroid tumors in rats treated with *N*-bis(2-hydroxypropyl)nitrosamine. *Carcinogenesis*, ***3***, 381–384

Hicks, R.M., Wakefield, J.S. & Chowaniec, J. (1973) Cocarcinogenic action of saccharin in the chemical induction of bladder cancer. *Nature*, ***243***, 347–349

Kitagawa, T., Pitot, H.C., Miller, E.C. & Miller, J.A. (1979) Promotion by dietary phenobarbital of hepatocarcinogenesis by 2-methyl-*N*,*N*-dimethyl-4-aminoazobenzene in the rat. *Cancer Res.*, ***39***, 112–115

Konishi, Y., Kondo, H., Ikeda, I., Kawabata, A., Shoji, Y. & Denda, A. (1978) Effects of dose on the carcinogenic activity of *N*-bis(2-hydroxypropyl)nitrosamine orally administered to rats. *Gann*, ***69***, 573–577

Mohr, U., Reznick, G. & Pour, P. (1977) Carcinogenic effects of diisopropanolnitrosamine in Sprague-Dawley rats. *J. natl Cancer Inst.*, ***58***, 361–366

Mottram, J.C. (1944) Developing factor in experimental blastogenesis. *J. Pathol. Bacteriol.*, ***56***, 181–187

Napalkov, N.P. (1958) Experimental tumors of thyroid gland. *Vopr. Onkol.*, ***4***, 738–750

Narisawa, T., Magadia, N.E., Weisburger, J.H. & Wynder, E.L. (1974) Promoting effect of bile acids on colon carcinogenesis after intrarectal instillation of *N*-methyl-*N'*-nitro-*N*-nitrosoguanidine in rats. *J. natl Cancer Inst.*, ***53***, 1093–1097

Peraino, C., Fry, R.J.M. & Staffeldt, E. (1971) Reduction and enhancement by phenobarbital of hepatocarcinogenesis induced in the rat by 2-acetylaminofluorene. *Cancer Res.*, ***31***, 1506–1512

Peraino, C., Fry, R.J.M., Staffeldt, E. & Kisieleski, W.E. (1973) Effects of varying the exposure to phenobarbital on its enhancement of 2-acetylaminofluorene-induced hepatic tumorigenesis in the rat. *Cancer Res.*, ***33***, 2701–2705

Peraino, C., Fry, R.J.M. & Staffeldt, E. (1977) Effects of varying the onset and duration of exposure to phenobarbital on its enhancement of 2-acetylaminofluorene-induced hepatic tumorigenesis. *Cancer Res.*, ***37***, 3623–3627

Pollard, M. & Luckert, P.H. (1979) Promotional effect of sodium barbiturate on intestinal tumors induced in rats by dimethylhydrazine. *J. natl Cancer Inst.*, ***63***, 1089–1092

Reddy, B.S., Watanabe, K. & Weisburger, J.H. (1977) Promoting effect of bile acids in colon carcinogenesis in germfree and conventional F344 rats. *Cancer Res.*, ***37***, 3238–3242

Weisburger, J.H. (1975) Large bowel cancer: Metabolic epidemiology and carcinogenesis. *Cancer*, ***36***, 2385–2386

Witschi, H., Williamson, D. & Lock, S. (1977) Enhancement of urethan tumorigenesis in mouse lung by butylated hydroxytoluene. *J. natl Cancer Inst.*, ***58***, 301–305

# THE MECHANISM OF COCARCINOGENIC ACTION OF ETHANOL IN RAT LIVER

M. SCHWARZ[1], A. BUCHMANN[1], M. MOORE[2] & W. KUNZ[1]

[1] *Institute of Biochemistry*
*and* [2] *Institute of Experimental Pathology,*
*German Cancer Research Center,*
*6900 Heidelberg, Federal Republic of Germany*

## SUMMARY

The effects of chronic alcohol consumption on nitrosamine metabolism *in vivo*, DNA synthesis and repair, and carcinogen-induced preneoplasia were studied in rat liver. Following a single injection of different doses of $^{14}$C-*N*-nitrosodimethylamine, there was no significant difference between controls and ethanol-pretreated rats in the alkylation pattern of cellular protein nor in the levels of the alkylation products 7-methylguanine and $O^6$-methylguanine isolated from liver DNA. $O^6$-Methylguanine-specific DNA repair was also unchanged. An increase in the number and size of foci staining negative for adenosine triphosphatase and/or positive for $\gamma$-glutamyltranspeptidase was observed in rats treated intermittently with ethanol and *N*-nitrosomorpholine. The numbers of clear-cell and mixed-cell foci were also increased. An ethanol-mediated enhancement of DNA synthesis, which was ascertained by different methods, may be related to this cocarcinogenic action of the alcohol. Ethanol, however, failed to demonstrate promoting activity. Long-term treatment of carcinogen pretreated rats with ethanol, according to the classical initiation-promotion protocol, had no effect on the incidence of preneoplastic foci in liver.

## INTRODUCTION

Epidemiological studies have demonstrated an association between excessive consumption of alcohol-containing beverages and an increase in cancer risk in various organs, including the liver (Tuyns, 1978). The underlying mechanism of action is not clear. Long-term animal studies with alcohol failed to demonstrate carcinogenic potential (Schmähl *et al.*, 1965; Kuratsune *et al.*, 1971). The effects of alcohol may thus result from cocarcinogenic or tumour-promoting activity.

Repeated administration of ethanol has been shown to enhance the metabolism of *N*-nitrosodimethylamine (NDMA) and other carcinogens by rat liver microsomes *in vitro* (McCoy *et al.*, 1979; Seitz *et al.*, 1979; Schwarz *et al.*, 1980; Garro *et al.*, 1981; Peng *et al.*, 1982). Inhibition of NDMA metabolism was also reported when ethanol was added *in vitro* to microsomal incubations (Schwarz *et al.*, 1980; Peng *et al.*, 1982). Pretreatment of rats with ethanol, however, did not result in any significant change in the in-vivo activation of NDMA as measured by the levels of alkylation products in liver DNA (Belinsky *et al.*, 1982; Schwarz *et al.*, 1982). An ethanol-induced increase in synthesis of liver DNA has been observed, which might be related to hepatotoxic effects of alcohol leading to an increase in cell turnover (Schwarz *et al.*, 1982). The strong influence of concomitant DNA synthesis on the carcinogenic response in liver has been well documented (Craddock, 1971; Ying *et al.*, 1981). In view of this evidence, we have investigated the effect of intermittent and sequential ethanol treatment on nitrosamine-induced hepatocarcinogenesis. Various preneoplastic markers were analysed in order to make this study.

## MATERIALS AND METHODS

The analytical procedures for the determination of specific radioactivity of liver protein and of DNA alkylation and repair in $^{14}$C-NDMA-injected rats, as well as those for the measurement of incorporation of $^{3}$H-thymidine into liver DNA of controls and ethanol-pretreated animals were described recently (Schwarz *et al.*, 1982).

The influence of ethanol on the extent of carcinogen-induced enzyme-altered foci was studied in female Wistar rats weighing an average of 65 g at start of the experiment. *N*-Nitrosomorpholine (NMOR; a kind gift of Professor Preussmann, this centre) was administered in the drinking-water (40 mg/L) on four consecutive days in every week for 15 weeks. Ethanol (10% in the drinking-water, three days per week) was given intermittently with the carcinogen; the interval between both treatments was always 12 h, to avoid the presence of alcohol during activation metabolism of the carcinogen.

The effects of ethanol post-treatment were studied in rats weighing an average of 200 g. Animals were treated with *N*-nitrosodiethylamine (NDEA) by stomach tube, 3 mg/kg body weight, three times per week for nine weeks. Ethanol (10% in the drinking-water) was administered subsequently for 16 weeks.

The rats were killed 14 days after the end of treatments. Serial 10-μm frozen sections were prepared from each rat liver and stained enzyme-histochemically for ATPase (Wachstein & Meisel, 1957) and γ-glutamyl transpeptidase (GGT) (Lojda *et al.*, 1976) activity. Clear-cell and mixed-cell foci (for classification, see Bannasch, 1976) were analysed in haematoxylin and eosin-stained sections prepared from formalin-fixed parts of each liver. The number of foci per cm$^3$ was calculated according to the method of Campbell *et al.* (1982). Intergroup differences were analysed by the Wilcoxon rank sum test.

## RESULTS AND DISCUSSION

Carcinogenic nitrosamines are activated, yielding highly reactive intermediates which may bind covalently to nucleophilic centres in cellular macromolecules. Using $^{14}$C-NDMA, the radioactively-labelled reaction products, 7-methylguanine and $O^6$-methylguanine – among others – can be quantitated in DNA; the level of these products relates indirectly to the activation of the carcinogen. 7-Methylguanine and $O^6$-methylguanine formation in rat liver DNA from controls and from ethanol pretreated animals is shown in Table 1. There was no significant difference between alcohol-treated and non-treated rats at the different NDMA dose levels. Similar results were obtained with respect to specific radioactivity levels of liver-cell protein: These were even slightly decreased in ethanol pretreated rats (Table 1). The results obtained are in agreement with data in the literature (Belinsky *et al.*, 1982), but they contrast sharply with those observed *in vitro*, where incubation of liver microsomes obtained from ethanol pretreated rats resulted in a strong increase in NDMA metabolism (Schwarz *et al.*, 1980; Garro *et al.*, 1981; Peng *et al.*, 1982). The reason for this difference is unknown.

DNA repair was analysed by determining the ratio of $O^6$- to 7-methylguanine. Ethanol pretreatment did not change these ratios (Table 1). These data, therefore, fail to support the concept that the increase in liver cancer risk observed in human alcoholics is due to an effect on activation pathways of environmental carcinogens or on DNA repair capacity.

Table 1. Effect of ethanol on *N*-nitrosodimethylamine (NDMA)-mediated alkylation of liver macromolecules and on metabolite incorporation into guanine isolated from liver DNA[a]

| Dose of NDMA (mg/kg body weight) | Ethanol pre-treatment | Specific radioactivity of protein (dpm/mg) | 7-Methyl-guanine: guanine × $10^6$ | $O^6$-Methyl-guanine: guanine × $10^6$ | $O^6$-Methyl-guanine × $10^3$: 7-methylguanine | Incorporation into guanine (dpm/μmol guanine) |
|---|---|---|---|---|---|---|
| 0.25 | − | 427 | 63.2 | 0.54 | 8.5 | 195 |
| | + | 406 | 73.7 | ND | ND | 628 |
| 0.5 | − | 858 | 117.1 | 1.34 | 11.4 | 354 |
| | + | 819 | 128.6 | 2.85 | 22.2 | 1 377 |
| 1 | − | 1 802 | 223.8 | 6.69 | 29.9 | 695 |
| | + | 1 351 | 231.9 | 7.74 | 33.4 | 2 428 |
| 2 | − | 3 162 | 507.9 | 32.5 | 64.0 | 1 147 |
| | + | 2 664 | 562.0 | 28.8 | 51.2 | 4 605 |
| 5 | − | 8 249 | 1 304.1 | 109.3 | 83.8 | 1 172 |
| | + | 6 837 | 1 221.3 | 94.1 | 77.1 | 3 798 |
| 10 | − | 18 282 | 2 416.0 | 232.1 | 96.1 | 1 315 |
| | + | 13 035 | 2 537.0 | 223.5 | 88.1 | 4 854 |
| 20 | − | 26 420 | 5 071.6 | 481.0 | 94.8 | 1 440 |
| | + | 24 468 | 4 811.3 | 416.5 | 86.6 | 9 956 |

[a] From Schwarz *et al.* (1982). Various doses of $^{14}$C-NDMA were injected intraperitoneally into rats, which were killed 4 h later. DNA was isolated, hydrolysed and base analysis performed by ion-exchange chromatography. Ethanol (20% w/v) was administered *via* the drinking-water for 14 days and was omitted 24 h before NDMA treatment. Each value represents the mean of estimations from two individual animals.
ND, not determined

Formaldehyde is a primary reaction product of oxidative demethylation of $^{14}C$-NDMA during carcinogen activation. This radioactive product can be incorporated into purine bases *via* the $C_1$ pool. During DNA synthesis, such labelled bases are incorporated into the nucleic acid, and they may be used as an indirect parameter of prior DNA synthesis in liver. At all of the NDMA dose levels used, a strong increase in radioactivity in guanine was seen in liver DNA of rats pretreated with ethanol (Table 1), suggesting enhancement of DNA synthesis. These preliminary results were further confirmed by the analysis of incorporation of tritium-labelled thymidine in DNA. Measurement of specific radioactivity levels in liver DNA from controls resulted in values of 792 ± 402 dpm/mg (mean ± SD, n = 5), while 2 899 ± 420 (n =

Fig. 1. Effect of ethanol on the number of enzyme-altered foci induced in rat liver by *N*-nitrosomorpholine (NMOR)
Ethanol (10% in drinking-water, 3 days/week) was given intermittently with NMOR (40 mg/L in drinking-water, 4 days/week) for 15 weeks. Enzyme-altered foci were demonstrated histochemically in serial liver sections. Means ± SD of 9 rats/group; *, $p < 0.05$; **, $p < 0.01$; ***, $p < 0.001$; *versus* controls. ▨, NMOR; □, NMOR plus ethanol; GGT, γ-glutamyl transpeptidase

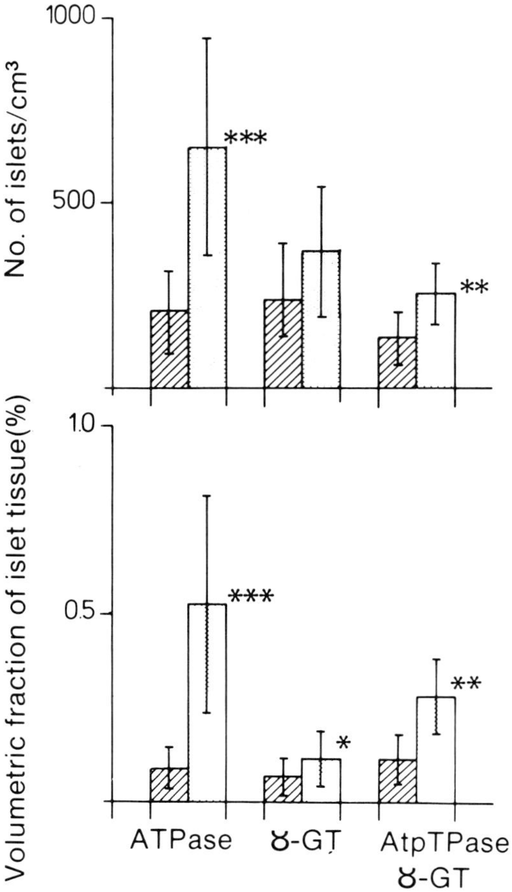

4) and 5 185 ± 1 551 (n = 4) dpm/mg were found in rats pretreated for 14 days with 5% or 10% ethanol, respectively, in the drinking-water.

The response of chemically induced tumours in liver is strongly influenced by concomitant DNA synthesis. Partial hepatectomy, for example, enhances tumour formation when performed shortly before or shortly after carcinogen administration, but not at prolonged time intervals after carcinogen treatment (Rajewsky *et al.*, 1966; Emmelot & Scherer, 1980; Ishikawa *et al.*, 1980). Therefore, liver regeneration seems to affect tumour initiation rather than subsequent stages of carcinogenesis. For this reason, we assessed the effect on hepatocarcinogenesis of ethanol given simultaneously or sequentially with the carcinogen.

Fig. 2. Effect of ethanol on the number of clear-cell and mixed-cell foci induced by *N*-nitrosomorpholine (NMOR)
For experimental details, see footnote to Figure 1. Means ± SD; *, $p < 0.05$; **, $p < 0.01$; *versus* controls. ▨, NMOR; □, NMOR plus ethanol

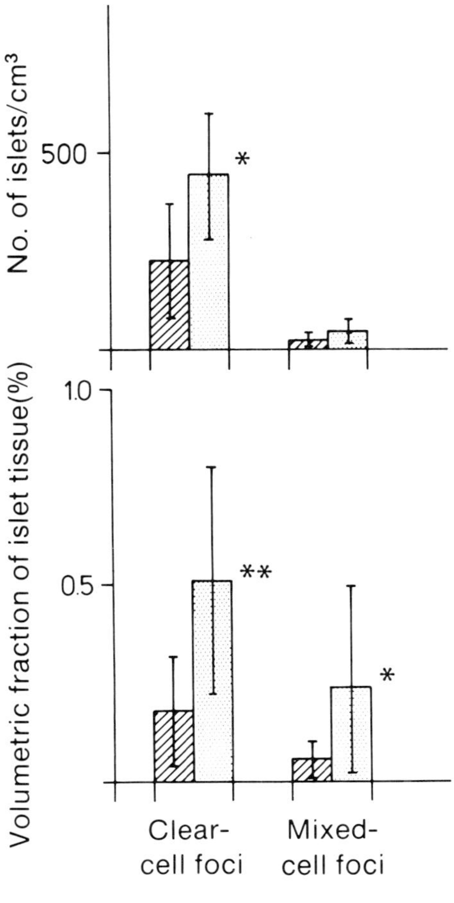

Fig. 3. Effect of ethanol on the number of ATPase-deficient foci when given after cessation of *N*-nitrosodiethylamine (NDEA) treatment
Rats were treated with NDEA (3 mg/kg) three times per week for 9 weeks. Ethanol (10% in the drinking-water) was administered after the end of carcinogen treatment for an additional 16 weeks. Means ± SD of 9 rats/group.

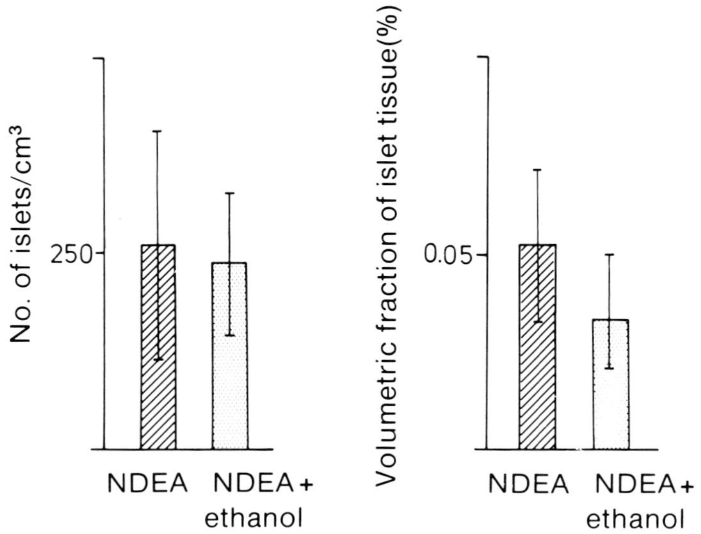


The extent of preneoplastic foci in liver was quantitated as a parameter of carcinogenic effectiveness. The following markers were used: (1) ATPase-deficient and/or GGT-positive foci, as demonstrated enzyme-histochemically; (2) focal lesions, characterized histologically as clear-cell foci with glycogen storage or mixed-cell populations, which may contain more progressed basophilic cells.

The effect of ethanol on liver carcinogenesis induced by NMOR is shown in Figure 1. One group of rats received carcinogen only, whereas a second group was subjected to intermittent treatment with carcinogen and ethanol. Intermittent ethanol/carcinogen treatment resulted in a strong increase in both the number and total volume of ATPase-negative foci. More moderate effects were seen with islets staining positive for GGT and with those showing both of these enzyme-histochemical markers. Similar findings were obtained with regard to the extent of clear-cell and mixed-cell foci (Fig. 2). Opposite results have also been reported, showing a decrease in liver tumour incidence in rats treated with NDEA and ethanol (Habs & Schmähl, 1981). Differences in feeding schedule and the higher ethanol dose used in the present study may explain this discrepancy.

The enhancement of total islet volume was due predominantly to an increase in foci with larger diameters. Analyses of islet size distributions observed in rats treated under various experimental conditions showed an ethanol-mediated increase in the number of very large foci of presumably progressed neoplastic character (data not shown). Such enhancement seems to be restricted, however, to a feeding protocol in which the alcohol is given during the period of carcinogen administration. Long-term treatment of carcinogen-pretreated animals with ethanol, according to the classical initiation-promotion protocol, had no effect on the number of preneoplastic foci in liver (Fig. 3). Ethanol itself failed to induce any enzyme-altered foci (data not shown).

In conclusion, ethanol exhibits neither carcinogenic nor tumour-promoting activity in liver. The observed cocarcinogenicity of this compound appears to be related to its hepatotoxicity, which may lead to chronic liver regeneration. The effects of ethanol are, therefore, entirely opposite to those seen with classical tumour promoters such as phenobarbital, which are effective only when given after the initiating insult of a carcinogen, but which inhibit tumour formation when given simultaneously with the carcinogen.

## ACKNOWLEDGEMENTS

The authors thank Ms J. Hummel, Mrs G. Robinson, Mr M. Maor and Mr R. Schmidt for excellent technical assistance and helpful discussions.

## REFERENCES

Bannasch, P. (1976) Cytology and cytogenesis of neoplastic (hyperplastic) hepatic nodules. *Cancer Res.*, ***36***, 2555–2562

Belinsky, S.A., Bedell, M.A. & Swenberg, J.A. (1982) Effect of chronic ethanol diet on the replication, alkylation and repair of DNA from hepatocytes and nonparenchymal cells following dimethylnitrosamine administration. *Carcinogenesis*, ***3***, 1293–1297

Campbell, H.A., Pitot, H.C., Potter, V.R. & Laishes, B.A. (1982) Application of quantitative stereology to the evaluation of enzyme-altered foci in rat liver. *Cancer Res.*, ***42***, 465–472

Craddock, V.M. (1971) Liver carcinomas induced in rats by single administration of dimethylnitrosamine after partial hepatectomy. *J. natl Cancer Inst.*, ***47***, 899–907

Emmelot, P. & Scherer, E. (1980) The first relevant cell stage in rat liver carcinogenesis: A quantitative approach. *Biochem. biophys. Acta*, ***605***, 247–304

Garro, A.J., Seitz, H.K. & Lieber, C.S. (1981) Enhancement of dimethylnitrosamine metabolism and activation to a mutagen following chronic alcohol consumption. *Cancer Res.*, ***41***, 120–124

Habs, M. & Schmähl, D. (1981) Inhibition of the hepatocarcinogenic activity of diethylnitrosamine (DENA) by ethanol in rats. *Hepato-gastroenterology*, ***28***, 242–244

Ishikawa, T., Takayama, S. & Kitagawa, T. (1980) Correlation between time of partial hepatectomy after a single treatment with diethylnitrosamine and induction of adenosinetriphosphatase-deficient islands in rat liver. *Cancer Res.*, ***40***, 4261–4264

Kuratsune, M., Kohchi, S., Horie, A. & Nishizumi, M. (1971) Test of alcohol beverages and ethanol solutions for carcinogenicity and tumor-promoting activity. *Gann*, ***62***, 395–405

Lojda, Z., Gossrau, R. & Schiebler, T.H. (1976) *Enzymhistochemische Methoden,* Heidelberg, Springer, pp. 182–184

McCoy, G.D., Chen, C.B., Hecht, S.S. & McCoy, E.C. (1979) Enhanced metabolism and mutagenicity of nitrosopyrrolidine in liver fractions isolated from chronic ethanol-consuming hamsters. *Cancer Res.,* ***39,*** 793–796

Peng, R., Tu, Y.Y. & Yang, C.S. (1982) The induction and competitive inhibition of a high affinity microsomal nitrosodimethylamine demethylase by ethanol. *Carcinogenesis,* ***3,*** 1457–1461

Rajewsky, M.F., Dauber, W. & Frankenberg, H. (1966) Liver carcinogenesis by diethylnitrosamine in the rat. *Science,* ***152,*** 83–85

Schmähl, D., Thomas, C., Sattler, W. & Scheld, G. (1965) Experimentelle Untersuchungen zur Syncarcinogenese. 3. Mitteilung: Versuche zur Krebserzeugung bei Ratten bei gleichzeitiger Gabe von Diäthylnitrosamine und Tetrachlorkohlenstoff bzw. Äthylalkohol, zugleich ein experimenteller Beitrag zur Frage der 'Alkoholcirrhose'. *Z. Krebsforsch.,* ***66,*** 526–532

Schwarz, M., Appel, K.E., Schrenk D. & Kunz W. (1980) Effect of ethanol on microsomal metabolism of dimethylnitrosamine. *J. Cancer Res. clin. Oncol.,* ***97,*** 233–240

Schwarz, M., Wiesbeck, G., Hummel, J. & Kunz, W. (1982) Effect of ethanol on dimethylnitrosamine activation and DNA synthesis in rat liver. *Carcinogenesis,* ***3,*** 1071–1075

Seitz, H.K., Garro, A.J. & Lieber, C.S. (1979) Increased activation of procarcinogens after ethanol. *Fed. Proc.,* ***38,*** 1404

Tuyns, A. (1978) *Alcool et Cancer (IARC Scientific Publications, Monographie hors série),* Lyon, International Agency for Research on Cancer

Wachstein, M. & Meisel, E. (1957) Histochemistry of hepatic phosphatases at a physiological pH. *Am. J. clin. Pathol.,* ***27,*** 13–23

Ying, T.S., Sarma, D.S.R. & Farber, E. (1981) Role of acute hepatic necrosis in the induction of early steps in liver carcinogenesis by diethylnitrosamine. *Cancer Res.,* ***41,*** 2096–2102

# TUMOUR PROMOTION
# IN OTHER ORGANS

# URINARY BLADDER CARCINOGENESIS

S.M. COHEN, R. HASEGAWA, R.E. GREENFIELD & L.B. ELLWEIN

*Department of Pathology & Laboratory Medicine and The Eppley Institute for Research in Cancer, University of Nebraska Medical Center, Omaha, NE, USA*

## INTRODUCTION

Cancer of the lower urinary tract has been associated etiologically with chemicals since the observation by Rehn in 1895 that workers in the German aniline dye industry developed a high incidence of the disease. Subsequently, numerous chemicals have been identified as human bladder carcinogens, including 2-naphthylamine, benzidine, 4-aminobiphenyl and cyclophosphamide (Price, 1971). In addition, models have been developed in rodents and dogs using chemicals that are specific for the lower urinary tract. The models most commonly used today include those in which *N*-butyl-*N*-(4-hydroxybutyl)-nitrosamine (BBN) is administered in the drinking-water or subcutaneously (Druckrey *et al.*, 1964), *N*-[4-(5-nitro-2-furyl)-2-thiazolyl]formamide (FANFT) administered in the diet (Erturk *et al.*, 1967), or *N*-methyl-*N*-nitrosourea (MNU) administered by intravesicalar instillation (Hicks & Wakefield, 1972).

Although exposure of animals or man specifically to one of these agents results in an increased incidence of bladder cancer, the more common situation with regard to humans is exposure to numerous chemicals that may act in an enhancing or inhibitory fashion. Ito and his colleagues in Japan demonstrated that the simultaneous administration of low doses of four bladder carcinogens—BBN, FANFT, 2-acetylaminofluorene (AAF) and 3,3′-dichlorobenzidine (DCB)—to rats for short periods of time resulted in the induction of bladder cancer, whereas administration of the chemicals individually to the rats did not induce tumours over the period of the experiment (Tsuda *et al.*, 1977); administration of higher doses or of low doses for longer periods of time, however, induces bladder cancer in animals (Price, 1971). Tatematsu *et al.* (1977) demonstrated further that the administration of these four compounds sequentially rather than simultaneously also resulted in the induction of bladder cancer.

## INITIATION AND PROMOTION IN BLADDER CARCINOGENESIS

The first indication that the two-stage model of carcinogenesis – initially demonstrated in the mouse skin model and stated to consist of initiation and promotion (Boutwell, 1964; Scribner & Suss, 1978) – might be applicable to the urinary bladder came from studies in the 1960s utilizing the pellet implantation technique. Bryan and Springberg (1966) showed that administration of the 8-methyl ether of xanthurenic acid (XAE) in a cholesterol pellet implanted into the mouse urinary bladder induced an increased incidence of bladder tumours compared with that produced by the cholesterol pellet alone. In addition, they showed that administration of XAE by subcutaneous injection followed by implantation into the bladder of a cholesterol pellet (without XAE) resulted in a similar increase in the incidence of bladder tumours. A comparable sequence was demonstrated by Clayson *et al.* (1967) with the compound 2-aminodiphenylene oxide administered either in a paraffin pellet or by oral administration in the diet before implantation of a paraffin pellet. Although these experiments are suggestive of a two-stage model of carcinogenesis, they have been difficult to interpret because of the use of the pellet implantation technique (Jull, 1975).

A more classical model of initiation and promotion in the urinary bladder was reported by Hicks and her colleagues in the UK in the 1970s; they used a 'subcarcinogenic' dose of MNU followed by oral administration of either sodium saccharin or sodium cyclamate (Hicks *et al.*, 1973, 1975; Hicks & Chowaniec, 1977). This sequence resulted in a markedly increased incidence of bladder tumours compared with that in animals receiving either sodium saccharin or sodium cyclamate without previous instillation of MNU. In this model, cyclophosphamide was not a promoting agent.

At the same time, we were developing a similar model, based on the use of FANFT as the initiating chemical (Cohen *et al.*, 1979). Six weeks' administration of 0.2% FANFT in the diet was used as the initiating dose, and 5% sodium saccharin or 2% DL-tryptophan was used as the promoting agent (Table 1). The promoting agents were administered either immediately after initiation or after a six-week delay, during which time the animals were fed control diet. This delay was instituted (1) to allow for regression of the mild hyperplasia present after six weeks' administration of FANFT (so that the bladder epithelium appeared normal histologically and ultrastructurally at the time the promoting agent was given), (2) to allow adequate time for FANFT to be excreted from the animal before administering the promoting agent, and (3) to get an indication of the potential irreversibility of the initiating event, as in the mouse skin model. Appropriate control groups received FANFT only for six weeks, the promoting agents alone, no agent or long-term administration of FANFT (as a positive control). As expected, long-term administration of FANFT induced a 100% incidence of bladder tumours, and administration of either of the promoting agents or of control diet alone did not result in bladder tumours. Administration of FANFT followed by sodium saccharin or DL-tryptophan, either immediately after FANFT or after a six-week delay, resulted in an increased incidence of bladder tumours compared with that seen after six weeks of FANFT followed by control diet. There was essentially no difference in the results if the promoting agent was adminis-

Table 1. Lesions of the urinary bladder induced after 6 weeks' administration of *N*-[4-(5-nitro-2-furyl)-2-thiazolyl]formamide (FANFT) as initiator and administration of sodium saccharin or DL-tryptophan as promoter[a]

| Treatment group | Effective no. of rats | Urinary bladder lesion | | | | |
|---|---|---|---|---|---|---|
| | | Normal | Simple hyperplasia | Nodular or papillary hyperplasia | Papilloma | Cancer |
| FANFT → saccharin | 19 | 0 | 0 | 1 | 0 | 18 |
| FANFT → control → saccharin | 18 | 0 | 1 | 4 | 0 | 13 |
| Control → saccharin | 20 | 18 | 2 | 0 | 0 | 0 |
| FANFT → tryptophan | 19 | 0 | 5 | 3 | 1 | 10 |
| FANFT → control → tryptophan | 20 | 0 | 3 | 3 | 4 | 10 |
| Control → tryptophan | 19 | 16 | 3 | 0 | 0 | 0 |
| Control | 42 | 37 | 4 | 1 | 0 | 0 |
| FANFT → control | 20 | 5 | 9 | 1 | 1 | 4 |
| FANFT → control → FANFT → control | 16 | 0 | 0 | 0 | 0 | 16 |
| Control → FANFT → control | 19 | 0 | 0 | 0 | 0 | 19 |
| FANFT | 40 | 0 | 0 | 0 | 0 | 40 |

[a] From Cohen *et al.* (1979)

tered immediately after the initiating agent or six weeks later. It should be noted that administration of sodium saccharin was discontinued after 83 weeks of the experiment, because many of the animals already had bladder tumours. Since most of the animals had bladder tumours even at the end of the experiment at 104 weeks (21 weeks after saccharin administration was discontinued), it would appear that the tumours induced by this regimen were irreversible.

The results of these experiments were similar to those of Hicks using the MNU model and were consistent with a two-stage model of carcinogenesis in the urinary bladder. Similar results have been obtained by Ito and his colleagues (Nakanishi *et al.*, 1980a,b), using BBN as the initiating agent and sodium saccharin as the promoting agent. However, no experiment in which the sequence of administration is reversed (giving the promoting agent first, followed by the initiating agent) has yet been reported.

Since six weeks' administration of FANFT in our first experiment resulted in a low but significant incidence of bladder tumours, we repeated the experiment giving FANFT for four weeks as the initiator and either sodium saccharin or L-tryptophan as the promoter (Fukushima *et al.*, 1981a; Table 2). No tumour was induced after four weeks' administration of FANFT alone, but a significant incidence of tumours was induced in the group administered sodium saccharin after FANFT. The incidence was increased with L-tryptophan, but not significantly.

In our laboratory and those of others, other chemicals have been shown to have promoting activity for the urinary bladder; L-tryptophan has promoting activity not only in our rat model but also in mice (Matsushima, 1977) and in dogs (Radomski

Table 2. Lesions of the urinary bladder induced after 4 weeks' administration of *N*-[4-(5-nitro-2-furyl)-2-thiazolyl]formamide (FANFT) as initiator and administration of sodium saccharin or L-tryptophan as promoter[a]

| Treatment group | Effective no. of rats | Urinary bladder lesion | | | | |
|---|---|---|---|---|---|---|
| | | Normal | Simple hyperplasia | Nodular or papillary hyperplasia | Papilloma | Carcinoma |
| 1. FANFT → saccharin | 26 | 14 | 4 | 1 | 2 | 5[b, c] |
| 2. Control → saccharin | 26 | 21 | 5 | 0 | 0 | 0 |
| 3. FANFT → tryptophan | 26 | 14 | 5 | 2 | 3 | 2[d] |
| 4. Control → tryptophan | 26 | 24 | 2 | 0 | 0 | 0 |
| 5. FANFT → control | 25 | 22 | 2 | 0 | 1 | 0 |
| 6. FANFT | 8 | 0 | 0 | 0 | 0 | 8[e] |
| 7. Control | 27 | 25 | 2 | 0 | 0 | 0 |

[a]From Fukushima *et al.* (1981a)
[b]One had metastases to lymph nodes and mesenteric fat
[c]Compared to Group 5, $p < 0.03$ for incidences of carcinoma and for incidences of papilloma plus carcinoma
[d]Compared to Group 5, $p > 0.1$ for incidences of carcinoma, but $p < 0.03$ for incidences of papilloma plus carcinoma, plus nodular or papillary hyperplasia
[e]Four showed invasion: two into submucosa; one into muscle; and one through the serosa

*et al.,* 1977); more recently, Ito and his colleagues have provided evidence that phenacetin (Nakanishi *et al.,* 1978) and sodium ascorbate (Fukushima *et al.,* 1983) have promoting activity when administered after initiation by BBN.

## PROPERTIES OF PROMOTERS

Sodium saccharin and L-tryptophan have many of the properties that have become associated with promoting agents in various tissue systems. For example, sodium saccharin appears not to be active in various in-vitro mutagenic assays, including the Ames assay (Fukushima *et al.,* 1981a), but appears to have chromosome altering properties at high doses in various assays (Moore & Schmick, 1979) and has effects on intercellular communication *in vitro* (Trosko *et al.,* 1980). One characteristic of promoting agents is that they induce hyperplasia in a target tissue without prior initiation (Boutwell, 1964; Scribner & Suss, 1978). Initial reports of experiments with sodium saccharin indicated that hyperplasia is rarely observed (Hicks *et al.,* 1973; Cohen *et al.,* 1979; Arnold *et al.,* 1980); but the sensitive techniques of scanning electron microscopy and autoradiography made it possible for us to demonstrate that a slight, multifocal hyperplasia does occur (Fukushima & Cohen, 1980). The labelling index rose within one week after administration of sodium saccharin in the diet, and that index and changes seen in scanning electron microscopy showed an essentially linear dose-response curve (Murasaki & Cohen, 1981). The induction by sodium saccharin of hyperplasia in various strains of rats has now also been demonstrated by others (Chowaniec & Hicks, 1979), and a dose-response similar to that observed in our experiment was observed by Nakanishi *et al.* (1980a).

## EFFECT OF REGENERATIVE HYPERPLASIA

A perplexing problem encountered with the FANFT and BBN models of two-stage carcinogenesis has been the fact that relatively large doses and long periods of administration of these compounds are necessary to effect initiation. It is well known from studies in other in-vitro and in-vivo models that a cycle of cell division is required for initiation to occur and to be fixed irreversibly (Scribner & Suss, 1978). One possible reason that initiation is relatively difficult to institute in the bladder model (as in the liver model) is that the bladder mucosa is normally mitotically quiescent; it has a turnover rate of approximately 100–200 days (Tiltman & Friedell, 1972; Murasaki & Cohen, 1983a). To test this hypothesis, we (Cohen *et al.*, 1982) administered FANFT in the diet for two weeks immediately following ulceration by

Fig. 1. Experimental design to test the effect of bladder ulceration on the carcinogenicity of *N*-[4-(5-nitro-2-furyl)-2-thiazolyl]formamide (FANFT) and sodium saccharin (From Cohen *et al.*, 1982); ■, 0.2% FANFT; ▨, 5.0% saccharin; □, control; v, freeze ulceration; ▼, i.p. injection of 100 mg/kg bw cytoxan

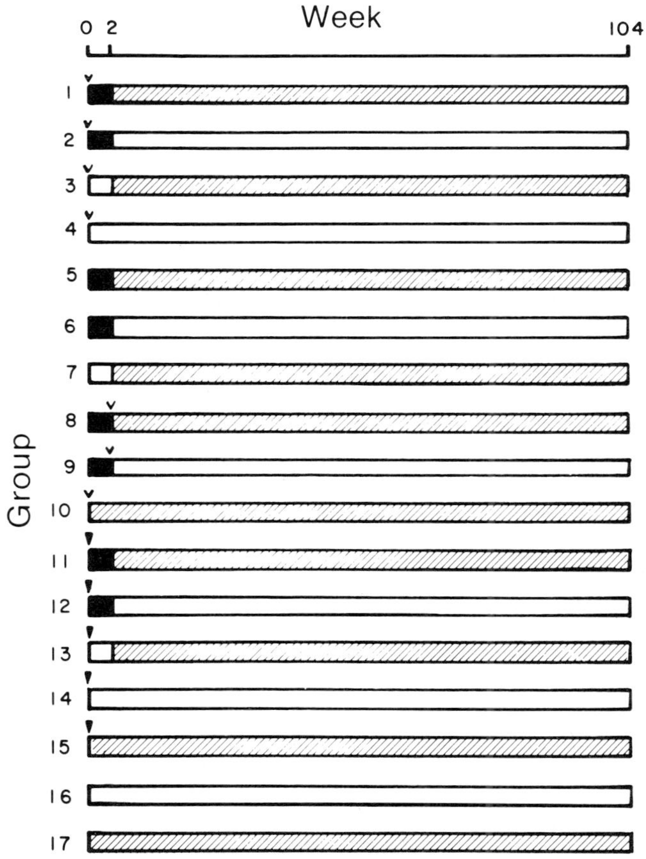

Table 3. Urinary bladder lesions induced in a study evaluating the effect of ulceration and regenerative hyperplasia on the carcinogenicity of *N*-[4-(5-nitro-2-furyl)-2-thiazolyl]formamide (FANFT) and sodium saccharin[a]

| Treatment group[b] | Effective no. of rats | Lesions of the urinary bladder[c] | | | | | | | | | | |
|---|---|---|---|---|---|---|---|---|---|---|---|---|
| | | Simple hyper-plasia | Nodular or papillary hyper-plasia | Papilloma | Carcinoma | | | | | Calcifi-cation in muscle layer | Scar in sub-mucosa | Calculus |
| | | | | | Total | Non-invasive | Invasive | | | | | |
| | | | | | | | Stalk | Sub-mucosa | Muscle | | | |
| 1 Ul → F → S | 23 | 5 (22) | 8 (35) | 0 – | 4 (17)[d] | 2 | 2 | 0 | 0 | 3 | 1 | 1 |
| 2 Ul → F | 22 | 7 (32) | 1 (5) | 0 – | 0 – | | | | | 5 | 0 | 0 |
| 3 Ul → Cont → S | 20 | 7 (35) | 2 (10) | 1 (5) | 5 (25)[d,e] | 2 | 0 | 2 | 1 | 0 | 0 | 1 |
| 4 Ul | 23 | 4 (17) | 1 (4) | 0 – | 0 – | | | | | 2 | 2 | 0 |
| 5 F → S | 21 | 10 (48) | 0 – | 0 – | 1 (5) | 1 | 0 | 0 | 0 | 0 | 0 | 0 |
| 6 F | 19 | 2 (11) | 0 – | 0 – | 0 – | | | | | 0 | 0 | 0 |
| 7 S | 17 | 7 (41) | 1 (6) | 0 – | 0 – | | | | | 0 | 0 | 0 |
| 8 F → Ul → S | 22 | 5 (23) | 4 (18) | 1 (5) | 8 (36)[d,e] | 4 | 3[f] | 0 | 1[g] | 6 | 6 | 0 |
| 9 F → Ul | 21 | 5 (24) | 2 (10) | 0 – | 2 (10) | 0 | 1 | 0 | 1 | 2 | 2 | 0 |
| 10 Ul → S | 21 | 4 (19) | 2 (10) | 2 (10) | 2 (10)[d] | 1 | 1 | 0 | 0 | 3 | 3 | 0 |
| 11 Cp → F → S | 22 | 11 (50) | 2 (9) | 3 (14) | 4 (18) | 1 | 2 | 1 | 0 | 0 | 0 | 1 |
| 12 Cp → F | 9 | 2 (22) | 0 – | 0 – | 0 – | | | | | 0 | 0 | 0 |
| 13 Cp → Cont → S | 17 | 2 (12) | 4 (24) | 2 (12) | 3 (18)[d,e] | 2 | 1 | 0 | 0 | 0 | 0 | 0 |
| 14 Cp | 7 | 0 – | 0 – | 1 (14) | 0 – | | | | | 0 | 0 | 0 |
| 15 Cp → S | 17 | 4 (24) | 2 (12) | 3 (18) | 3 (18)[d,e] | 2 | 0 | 1 | 0 | 0 | 0 | 0 |
| 16 Cont | 32 | 0 – | 0 – | 0 – | 0 – | | | | | 0 | 0 | 0 |
| 17 S | 20 | 6 (30) | 0 – | 0 – | 0 – | | | | | 0 | 0 | 0 |

[a] From Cohen *et al.* (1982)
[b] Ul = ulcer; F = FANFT; S = sodium saccharin; Cont = control diet; Cp = cyclophosphamide
[c] Each rat is tabulated in the column of the most advanced lesions present in the urinary bladder; numbers in parentheses are percentages of effective number of rats in the group
[d] $p < 0.05$ for incidence of carcinoma and incidence of carcinoma plus papilloma compared to Group 16
[e] $p < 0.05$ for incidence of carcinoma plus papilloma compared to Group 5
[f] One had squamous-cell metaplasia
[g] Poorly differentiated transitional-cell carcinoma

either freezing or intraperitoneal injection of cyclophosphamide (Fukushima *et al.*, 1981b) (Fig. 1). Following ulceration by either of these techniques, there is marked regenerative hyperplasia, and nodular, and papillary hyperplastic lesions are induced. The hyperplasia regresses and is repaired within three to four weeks, and the bladder epithelium returns to normal microscopically and ultrastructurally and remains so for the lifetime of the rat (Fukushima *et al.*, 1981b,c). The groups receiving the various other combinations of these agents or each agent alone were the appropriate controls for this experiment (Table 3). As predicted, the groups (1 and 11) administered FANFT after ulceration and then promoted with sodium saccharin developed bladder tumours. If our hypothesis had been correct, the other groups should not have developed tumours. It can be seen that this did not occur! To summarize, it would appear that sodium saccharin administered after ulceration, either immediately or after a two-week delay, induces bladder tumours whether FANFT is present or not. It must be noted that in this protocol, administration of sodium saccharin immediately after freeze ulceration or after administration of cyclophosphamide or two weeks later took place at a time when the urinary bladder epithelium was markedly hyperplastic. The presence of FANFT, which produces mutagenic urine when administered in the diet (Klemencic & Wang, 1978), did not enhance the incidence of tumours, and

Fig. 2. Sequential incidences of nodular and papillary hyperplasia in rat bladder at different times after freeze ulceration and/or feeding of sodium saccharin
– –, ulceration → saccharin; ---, ulceration → 2 weeks' control → saccharin; –·–·, saccharin; —, ulceration → control

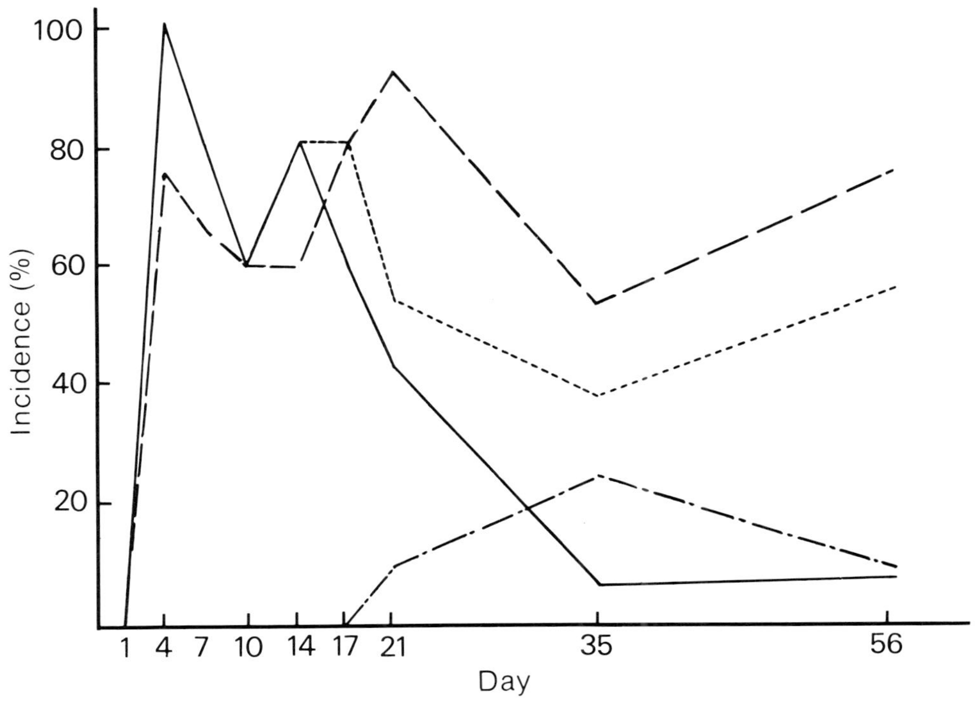

Fig. 3. Labelling index in rat bladder mucosa at different times after freeze ulceration and/or feeding of sodium saccharin
– –, ulceration → saccharin; —-, ulceration → 2 weeks' control → saccharin; –·–·–, saccharin; —, ulceration → control; –··–··–, control, as observed by autoradiography

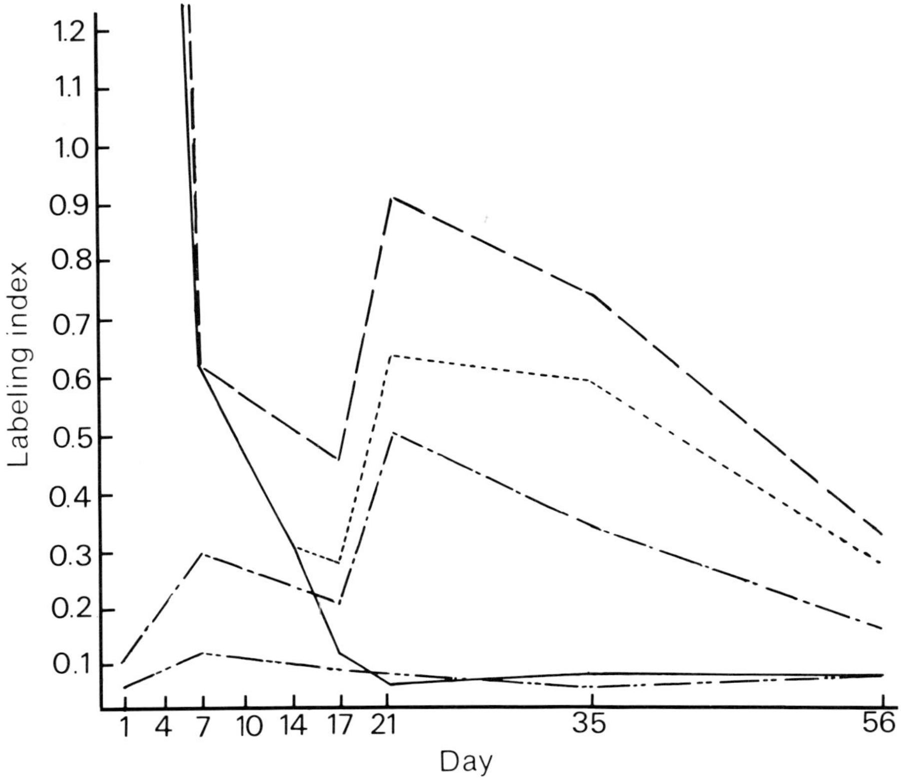


induction of ulceration with cyclophosphamide as opposed to freezing did not increase the incidence of bladder tumours. Cyclophosphamide also produces a mutagen in the urine (Mohn & Ellenberger, 1976).

These data would suggest that the carcinogenic process proceeded without the presence of a typical mutagenic initiating agent in the regimen. The results are similar in many respects to those of previous studies in which only sodium saccharin was administered in a two-generation experiment (Arnold *et al.*, 1980) and in pellet implantation studies (Bryan *et al.*, 1970). In all three circumstances, sodium saccharin was administered during a period of marked hyperplasia of the bladder. In the ulceration experiments that we have reported (Cohen *et al.*, 1982), hyperplasia is induced by either freezing or cyclophosphamide administration. In the two-generation study, a marked proliferative state of the bladder epithelium is normally present in fetuses (Clayson & Cooper, 1970). In the pellet implantation technique, hyperplasia is induced by the surgical procedure for implanting the pellet and by the presence of the pellet itself. The surgical procedure for pellet implantation results in a hyperplastic response in which the tissue kinetics are similar to those following freeze ulceration (Fukushima *et al.*, 1981b).

The mechanism by which sodium saccharin induces bladder tumours under these circumstances is not known. However, we have demonstrated that neither nitrosamines nor mutagens (detectable by the Ames assay) are generated by freeze ulceration with or without sodium saccharin (S.M. Cohen *et al.*, unpublished data). Bacterial contamination does not occur. However, we have demonstrated recently that one characteristic of this regimen is that the hyperplasia induced by the ulceration technique (Fig. 2) is maintained if sodium saccharin is administered sometime during the hyperplastic phase of regeneration and repair (Murasaki & Cohen, 1983a). In addition, the marked increase in labelling index in the bladder mucosa during regeneration is maintained by subsequent administration of sodium saccharin (Fig. 3).

## COCARCINOGENESIS

These studies and others provide considerable evidence that the initiation and promotion model can be applied to the urinary bladder and that it is reasonable to use sodium saccharin as a promoting agent in these studies. Another type of experimental protocol, for the evaluation of more than one compound, is the model of cocarcinogenesis (Scribner & Suss, 1978). This model infers the administration of two or more agents simultaneously rather than sequentially. We have demonstrated

Table 4. Incidence of bladder lesions in a study evaluating the cocarcinogenicity of sodium saccharin with other agents[a]

| Treatment group[b] | Effective no. of rats | Urinary bladder lesion | | | | | |
|---|---|---|---|---|---|---|---|
| | | Normal (%) | Hyperplasia | | Tumour | | |
| | | | Simple | Nodular and papillary | Papilloma | Cancer | Total (%) |
| Sac + L–Trp | 13 | 13 (100) | 0 | 0 | 0 | 0 | 0 |
| Sac + FANFT | 16 | 2 (13)[c] | 4 | 5 | 3 | 2[d] | 5 (31)[e] |
| Sac | 20 | 16 (80) | 4 | 0 | 0 | 0 | 0 |
| L–Trp | 16 | 16 (100) | 0 | 0 | 0 | 0 | 0 |
| FANFT | 11 | 9 (82) | 0 | 2 | 0 | 0 | 0 |
| Control | 23 | 23 (100) | 0 | 0 | 0 | 0 | 0 |

[a] From Murasaki & Cohen (1983b)
[b] Sac, 5% sodium saccharin; L–Trp, 2% L-tryptophan; FANFT, 0.005% *N*-[4-(5-nitro-2-furyl)-2-thiazolyl]formamide; Control, control diet only
[c] Group 2 compared with Group 5, $p < 0.001$
[d] Transitional-cell carcinoma, non-invasive
[e] Group 2 compared with Group 5, $p < 0.06$

recently that sodium saccharin is not only a promoting agent for the urinary bladder but also has cocarcinogenic activity with FANFT (Murasaki & Cohen, 1983b). FANFT, administered at a dose of 0.005% of the diet, did not induce bladder tumours over a two-year period, but if it was combined with 5% sodium saccharin in the diet there was an increased incidence of bladder tumours (Table 4). No tumour was found after administration of sodium saccharin alone or with L-tryptophan or after L-tryptophan alone.

The mechanism by which this effect occurs is not known, but at least two possibilities exist. One is that sodium saccharin modifies the metabolism of FANFT such that an increased amount of the activated form of FANFT reaches the bladder epithelium. In collaboration with Dr Craig Schnell (C. Schnell *et al.*, unpublished data), we have demonstrated that there is no increase in liver enzymes in the microsomal drug metabolizing system following administration of sodium saccharin. This does not exclude the possibility that other enzymes might be involved in the activation of FANFT (Cohen *et al.*, 1981). Another alternative is that sodium saccharin increases the mitotic rate and cell number in the bladder epithelium (Murasaki & Cohen, 1981), resulting in the availability of an increased number of target cells for the action of FANFT.

## THE ROLE OF URINE IN BLADDER CARCINOGENESIS

The experiments described above involved the administration of exogenous chemicals; the role of endogenous factors must also be considered. It has been known for several decades that exogenously administered carcinogens act on the urinary bladder primarily by excretion and concentration in the urine. However, beginning with experiments reported by Chapman *et al.* (1973), evidence has accumulated that urine, or substances in urine, might play a more direct role in bladder carcinogenesis than merely transporting carcinogens. Those authors showed that when the urinary bladder was divided in half and a pellet inserted into each half, only the half exposed to urine developed tumours.

More direct evidence for the role of urine in bladder carcinogenesis has been provided by a series of experiments by Oyasu and colleagues (Oyasu *et al.*, 1981; Izumi *et al.*, 1981; Babaya *et al.*, 1983) and Rowland *et al.* (1980). Administration of FANFT to male Fischer rats for 14 weeks followed by control diet resulted in the induction of bladder tumours by 30 weeks. However, if at 14 weeks when FANFT administration was discontinued the rats underwent bilateral ureterosigmoidostomy, effectively diverting the flow of urine away from the bladder to the colon, a markedly decreased incidence of bladder tumours resulted. Thus, even though a supposedly carcinogenic dose of FANFT had been administered, it was necessary for urine to be present for expression of these tumours. Similarly, by using the heterotopic bladder model (Oyasu *et al.*, 1981; Babaya *et al.*, 1983) and an in-vitro assay for mitogenesis and ornithine decarboxylase induction (Izumi *et al.*, 1981; Babaya *et al.*, 1983), a direct action of urine has been demonstrated: at least two active fractions have been identified, with approximate molecular weights of 37 000 and 4 300 Daltons. It would appear that each acts as a growth stimulating factor in urinary bladder carcinogenesis.

## A PROBABILISTIC MODEL OF CARCINOGENESIS

The above experiments and others provide support for the hypothesis that carcinogenesis occurs in two steps. Because of their complexity, the interrelationships of the biological events are difficult to evaluate by use of in-vivo models. Solutions to some of these questions can be obtained from experiments involving tissue cultures, but these systems have certain limitations that have been well documented in the literature. Another approach is to utilize a computer-based model that can analyse the interrelationships in mathematical terms and thus aid in identifying critical experiments necessary for furthering our understanding of carcinogenesis.

On the basis of data from the urinary bladder carcinogenesis experiments described above and others, we have devised a probabilistic model of two-stage carcinogenesis which may be applicable to other tumour systems (Greenfield *et al.,* 1984). Several assumptions have been made concerning the carcinogenic process: the first is that carcinogenesis requires two specific events, each of which is irreversible. Secondly, these critical events can occur only during cell replication; they cannot occur when the cell is at rest. Thirdly, the critical events occur only in stem cells in the urinary bladder (there could be stem cell equivalents in other tissues). Our model is probabilistic; under normal circumstances, each event is obviously rare.

The various possible cellular transitions are depicted in Figure 4. The critical transitions for carcinogenesis are from normal to initiated to transformed stem cell. The probability that a single normal cell will become initiated during cell replication is given as $p_{1,2}$, and the probability that an individual initiated stem cell will become

Fig. 4. Possible cellular transition
(Downward arrows represent cell death)

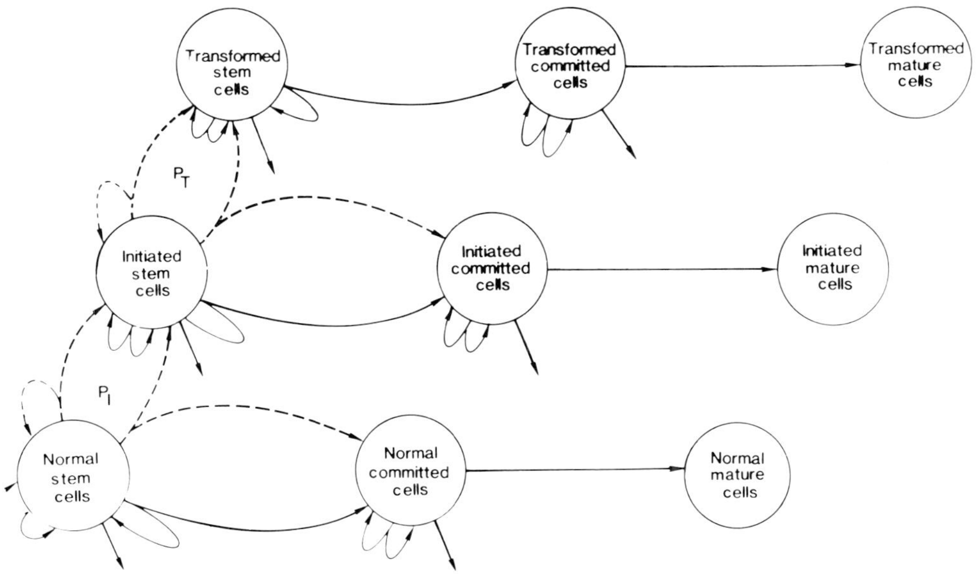

a transformed stem cell is given as $p_{2,3}$. There are approximately $10^6$ cells in the urinary bladder of the rat, and we estimate that approximately $10^5$ of these are stem cells. The likelihood of developing a tumour within a specific period of time is thus a function of: the number of cells in each of the stem-cell populations, the number of mitotic events in each stem-cell population during that period, and the probabilities $p_{1,2}$ and $p_{2,3}$. The number of cells can be estimated by histopathological examination of the urinary bladder at different periods following the administration of various stimuli, such as FANFT or sodium saccharin, and the mitotic rate can be determined experimentally by autoradiography. Obviously, estimates must be made of the transition probabilities, $p_{1,2}$ and $p_{2,3}$. It should be recognized that the stimulus can cause any of the above parameters to change in value as a function of time.

Using the FANFT Fischer rat model, it has been shown that hyperplasia (an increase in the number of cells) appears rapidly and increases gradually with time of administration of the chemical (Erturk *et al.*, 1969; Tiltman & Friedell, 1971). In addition, the mitotic rate increases (Tiltman & Friedell, 1972). If FANFT is withdrawn from the diet, the hyperplasia decreases (Jacobs *et al.*, 1977). The computer-based model reflects these changes over time on the basis of one-day increments. By using data from the above experiments, predictions can be made of the rate of tumour formation and growth. On the basis of this model, we can show that $p_{1,2}$ must increase dramatically over background levels during FANFT administration, but that the transition probability, $p_{2,3}$, does not change from the background. In fact, $p_{2,3}$ must remain at background levels for the model to replicate empirically observed tumour incidences. Sodium saccharin was shown by the computer model to alter neither $p_{1,2}$ nor $p_{2,3}$; the entire effect of sodium saccharin can be explained by increased cell numbers (hyperplasia) and increased mitotic rate, which have been demonstrated experimentally.

Although this model involves two events in carcinogenesis, it is a more general formulation than the classical initiation and promotion concept described originally in mouse skin. Thus, an increase in tumour incidence occurs after application of any agent that increases one or more of the critical variables: number of normal stem cells, mitotic rate of normal stem cells, probability of transition from normal to initiated stem cell ($p_{1,2}$), number of initiated stem cells, mitotic rate of initiated stem cells, and probability of transition from initiated stem cell to transformed stem cell ($p_{2,3}$). Using such a model, it can also be demonstrated that the critical factors in most promotion experiments, including those in mouse skin with phorbol esters, are an increase in the stem-cell population and an increased mitotic rate rather than an actual change in $p_{2,3}$. The properties of the classical initiation and promotion experiments (Boutwell, 1964; Scribner & Suss, 1978), such as irreversibility of initiation, importance of sequence of administration and even the subdivision of promotion into various stages (Slaga *et al.*, 1980), can readily be explained by such a model. The importance of changes in the size of the stem-cell population and mitotic rates appears to have been underestimated. It is also essential to distinguish between the proliferation of stem cells and the proliferation of non-stem cells in relating hyperplasia to the carcinogenic process.

We believe that synthesis of data from various animal studies through computer-based modelling is a valuable, relatively cheap and rapid approach towards furthering the understanding of the complex interrelationships between multiple exposures to exogenous or endogenous agents and the development of tumours. The availability of a model that is applicable to animals and to man may also assist in the extrapolation of data from animal experiments to human problems.

## ACKNOWLEDGEMENTS

We gratefully acknowledge the advice and comments of Dr Gilbert H. Friedell and the work of numerous colleagues in our laboratories. We also thank Jan Leemkuil and Margaret St John for preparing this manuscript. Work reported in this manuscript from our laboratories was supported in part by USPHS Grants CA32513, CA28874 and CA32313 from the National Cancer Institute, the former two through the National Bladder Cancer Project.

## REFERENCES

Arnold, D.L., Moodie, C.A., Grice, H.C., Charbonneau, S.M., Stavric, B., Collins, B.T., McGuire, P.F., Zawidzka, Z.Z. & Munro, I.C. (1980) Long-term toxicity of ortho-toluene sulfonamide and sodium saccharin in the rat. *Toxicol. appl. Pharmacol.*, ***52***, 113–152

Babaya, K., Izumi, K., Ozono, S., Miyata, Y., Morikawa, A., Chmiel, J.S. & Oyasu, R. (1983) Capability of urinary components to enhance ornithine decarboxylase activity and promote urothelial tumorigenicity. *Cancer Res.*, ***43***, 1774–1782

Boutwell, R.K. (1964) Some biological aspects of skin carcinogenesis. *Prog. exp. Tumor Res.*, ***4***, 207–250

Bryan, G.T. & Springberg, P.D. (1966) Role of the vehicle in the genesis of bladder carcinomas in mice by the pellet implantation technic. *Cancer Res.*, ***26***, 105–109

Bryan, G.T., Erturk, E. & Yoshida, O. (1970) Production of urinary bladder carcinomas in mice by sodium saccharin. *Science*, ***168***, 1238–1240

Chapman, W.H., Kirchkin, D. & McRoberts, J.W. (1973) Effect of the urine and calculus formation in the incidence of bladder tumors in rats implanted with paraffin wax pellets. *Cancer Res.*, ***33***, 1225–1229

Chowaniec, J. & Hicks, R.M. (1979) Response of the rat to saccharin with particular reference to the urinary bladder. *Br. J. Cancer*, ***39***, 355–375

Clayson, D.B. & Cooper, E.H. (1970) Cancer of the urinary tract. *Adv. Cancer Res.*, ***13***, 271–381

Clayson, D.B., Lawson, T.A. & Pringle, J.A.S. (1967) The carcinogenic action of 2-aminodiphenylene oxide and 4-aminodiphenyl on the bladder and liver of the $C_{57} \times$ IF mouse. *Br. J. Cancer*, ***21***, 755–762

Cohen, S.M., Arai, M., Jacobs, J.B. & Friedell, G.H. (1979) Promoting effect of saccharin and D,L-tryptophan in urinary bladder carcinogenesis. *Cancer Res.*, ***39***, 1207–1217

Cohen, S.M., Zenser, T.V., Murasaki, G., Fukushima, S., Mattammal, M.B., Rapp, N.S. & Davis, B.B. (1981) Aspirin inhibition of *N*-[4-(5-nitro-2-furyl)-2-thiazolyl]-formamide-induced lesions of the urinary bladder correlated with inhibition of metabolism by bladder prostaglandin endoperoxide synthetase. *Cancer Res.*, ***41***, 3355–3359

Cohen, S.M., Murasaki, G., Fukushima, S. & Greenfield, R.E. (1982) Effect of regenerative hyperplasia on the urinary bladder: Carcinogenicity of sodium saccharin and *N*-[4-(5-nitro-2-furyl)-2-thiazolyl]formamide. *Cancer Res.*, ***42***, 65–71

Druckrey, H., Preussmann, R., Ivankovic, S. & Schmidt, C.H. (1964) Selective induction of bladder cancer in rats by dibutyl- and *N*-butyl-*N*-butanol-(4)-nitrosamine. *Z. Krebsforsch.*, ***66***, 280–290

Erturk, E., Price, J.M., Morris, J.E., Cohen, S., Leith, R.S., VonEsch, A.M. & Crovetti, A.J. (1967) The production of carcinoma of the urinary bladder in rats by feeding *N*-[4-(5-nitro-2-furyl)-2-thiazolyl]formamide. *Cancer Res.*, ***27***, 1998–2002

Erturk, E., Cohen, S.M., Price, J.M. & Bryan, G.T. (1969) Pathogenesis, histogenesis, histology and transplantability of urinary bladder carcinomas induce in albino rats by oral administration of *N*-[4-(5-nitro-2-furyl)-2-thiazolyl]formamide. *Cancer Res.*, ***29***, 2219–2228

Fukushima, S. & Cohen, S.M. (1980) Saccharin-induced hyperplasia of the rat urinary bladder. *Cancer Res.*, ***40***, 734–736

Fukushima, S., Friedell, G.H., Jacobs, J.B. & Cohen, S.M. (1981a) Effect of L-tryptophan and sodium saccharin on urinary tract carcinogenesis initiated by *N*-[4-(5-nitro-2-furyl)-2-thiazolyl]formamide. *Cancer Res.*, ***41***, 3100–3103

Fukushima, S., Cohen, S.M., Arai, M., Jacobs, J.B. & Friedell, G.H. (1981b) Scanning electron microscopic examination of reversible hyperplasia of the rat urinary bladder. *Am. J. Pathol.*, ***102***, 373–380

Fukushima, S., Arai, M., Cohen, S.M., Jacobs, J.B. & Friedell, G.H. (1981c) Scanning electron microscopy of cyclophosphamide-induced hyperplasia of the rat urinary bladder. *Lab. Invest.*, ***44***, 89–96

Fukushima, S., Imaida, K., Sakata, T., Okamura, T., Shibata, M. & Ito, N. (1983) Promoting effects of sodium L-ascorbate on 2-stage urinary bladder carcinogenesis in rats. *Cancer Res.*, ***43***, 4454–4457

Greenfield, R.E., Ellwein, L.B. & Cohen, S.M. (1984) A general probabilistic model of carcinogenesis: Analysis of experimental urinary bladder cancer. *Carcinogenesis*, ***5***, 437–445

Hicks, R.M. & Chowaniec, J. (1977) The importance of synergy between weak carcinogens in the induction of bladder cancer in experimental animals and humans. *Cancer Res.*, ***37***, 2943–2949

Hicks, R.M. & Wakefield, J.St J. (1972) Rapid induction of bladder cancer in rats with *N*-methyl-*N*-nitrosourea. I. Histology. *Chem.-biol. Interact.*, ***5***, 139–152

Hicks, R.M., Wakefield, J.St J. & Chowaniec, J. (1973) Co-carcinogenic action of saccharin in the chemical induction of bladder cancer. *Nature*, ***243***, 347–349

Hicks, R.M., Wakefield, J.St J. & Chowaniec, J. (1975) Evaluation of a new model to detect bladder carcinogens or co-carcinogens; Results obtained with saccharin, cyclamate and cyclophosphamide. *Chem.-biol. Interact.*, ***11***, 225–233

Izumi, K., Hirao, Y., Hopp, L. & Oyasu, R. (1981) In vitro induction of ornithine decarboxylase in urinary bladder carcinoma cells. *Cancer Res.*, ***41***, 405–409

Jacobs, J.B., Arai, M., Cohen, S.M. & Friedell, G.H. (1977) A long-term study of reversible and progressive urinary bladder cancer lesions in rats fed *N*-[4-(5-nitro-2-furyl)-2-thiazolyl]formamide. *Cancer Res.*, ***37***, 2817–2821

Jull, J.W. (1975) Carcinogenesis by chemicals implanted into the bladder: An evaluation. *Gann Monogr.*, ***17***, 383–392

Klemencic, J.M. & Wang, C.Y. (1978) *Mutagenicity of nitrofurans*. In: Bryan, G.T., ed., *Carcinogenesis. A Comprehensive Survey*, Vol. 4, New York, Raven Press, pp. 99–130

Matsushima, M. (1977) The role of the promoter L-tryptophan on tumorigenesis in the urinary bladder. 2. Urinary bladder carcinogenicity of FANFT (initiating factor) in mice. *Jpn. J. Urol.*, ***68***, 731–736

Mohn, G.R. & Ellenberger, J. (1976) Genetic effects of cyclophosphamide, ifosfamide and trafosfamide. *Mutat. Res.*, ***32***, 331–360

Moore, C.W. & Schmick, A. (1979) Genetic effects of impure and pure saccharin in yeast. *Science*, ***205***, 1007–1010

Murasaki, G. & Cohen, S.M. (1981) Effect of dose of sodium saccharin on the induction of rat urinary bladder proliferation. *Cancer Res.*, ***41***, 942–944

Murasaki, G. & Cohen, S.M. (1983a) Effect of sodium saccharin on urinary bladder epithelial regenerative hyperplasia following freeze ulceration. *Cancer Res.*, ***43***, 182–187

Murasaki, G. & Cohen, S.M. (1983b) Co-carcinogenicity of sodium saccharin and *N*-[4-(5-nitro-2-furyl)-2-thiazolyl]formamide for the urinary bladder. *Carcinogenesis*, ***4***, 97–99

Nakanishi, K., Fukushima, S., Shibata, M., Shirai, T., Ogiso, T. & Ito, N. (1978) Effect of phenacetin and caffeine on the urinary bladder of rats treated with *N*-butyl-*N*-(4-hydroxybutyl)nitrosamine. *Gann*, ***69***, 395–400

Nakanishi, K., Hagiwara, A., Shibata, M., Imaida, K., Tatematsu, M. & Ito, N. (1980a) Dose response of saccharin in induction of urinary bladder hyperplasias in Fischer 344 rats pretreated with *N*-butyl-*N*-(4-hydroxybutyl)nitrosamine. *J. natl Cancer Inst.*, ***65***, 1005–1010

Nakanishi, K., Hirose, M., Ogiso, T., Hasegawa, R., Arai, M. & Ito, N. (1980b) Effects of sodium saccharin and caffeine on the urinary bladder of rats treated with *N*-butyl-*N*-(4-hydroxybutyl)nitrosamine. *Gann*, ***71***, 490–500

Oyasu, R., Hirao, Y. & Izumi, K. (1981) Enhancement by urine of urinary bladder carcinogenesis. *Cancer Res.*, ***41***, 478–481

Price, J. M. (1971) *Etiology of bladder cancer*. In: Maltry, E., ed, *Benign and Malignant Tumors of the Urinary Bladder*, New York, Medical Examination Publication Co., pp. 189–251

Radomski, J.L., Radomski, T. & MacDonald, W.E. (1977) Cocarcinogenic interaction between D,L-tryptophan and 4-aminobiphenyl or 2-naphthylamine in dogs. *J. natl Cancer Inst.*, ***58***, 1831–1834

Rowland, R.G., Henneberry, M.O., Oyasu, R. & Grayhack, J.T. (1980) Effects of urine and continued exposure to carcinogen on progression of early neoplastic urinary bladder lesions. *Cancer Res.*, ***40***, 4524–4527

Scribner, J.D. & Suss, R. (1978) Tumor initiation and promotion. *Int. Rev. exp. Pathol.*, ***18***, 137–198

Slaga, T.J., Fischer, S.M., Nelson, K. & Gleason, G.L. (1980) Studies on the mechanism of skin tumor promotion: Evidence for several stages in promotion. *Proc. natl Acad. Sci. USA*, ***77***, 3659–3663

Tatematsu, M., Miyata, Y., Mizutani, M., Hananouchi, M., Hirose, M. & Ito, N. (1977) Summation effect of *N*-butyl-*N*-(4-hydroxybutyl)nitrosamine, *N*-[4-(5-nitro-2-furyl)-2-thiazolyl]formamide, *N*-2-fluorenylacetamide, and 3,3′-dichlorobenzidine on urinary bladder carcinogenesis in rats. *Gann*, ***68***, 193–202

Tiltman, A.J. & Friedell, G.H. (1971) The histogenesis of experimental bladder cancer. *Invest. Urol.*, ***9***, 218–226

Tiltman, A.J. & Friedell, G.H. (1972) Effect of feeding *N*-[4-(5-nitro-2-furyl)-2-thiazolyl]formamide on mitotic activity of rat urinary-bladder epithelium. *J. natl Cancer Inst.*, ***48***, 125–129

Trosko, J.E., Dawson, B., Yotti, L.P. & Chang, C.C. (1980) Saccharin may act as a tumour promoter by inhibiting metabolic cooperation between cells. *Nature*, ***285***, 109

Tsuda, H., Miyata, Y., Murasaki, G., Kinoshita, H., Fukushima, S. & Ito, N. (1977) Synergistic effect of urinary bladder carcinogenesis in rats treated with *N*-butyl-*N*-(4-hydroxybutyl)nitrosamine, *N*-[4-(5-nitro-2-furyl)-2-thiazolyl]formamide, *N*-2-fluorenylacetamide, and 3,3′-dichlorobenzidine. *Gann*, ***68***, 183–192

# STUDIES ON THE ACTION OF TUMOUR PROMOTERS AND ANTIPROMOTERS ON RESPIRATORY-TRACT EPITHELIUM

P. NETTESHEIM, J.C. BARRETT, M.J. MASS, V.E. STEELE & T.E. GRAY

*National Institute of Environmental Health Sciences, Laboratory of Pulmonary Function and Toxicology, Research Triangle Park, NC 27709, USA*

## SUMMARY

Studies were carried out to examine the susceptibility of normal and initiated tracheal epithelial cells of rats to known tumour-promoting agents. The ability of normal rat tracheal epithelial cells to form colonies in cultures was enhanced markedly by addition of known tumour promoters to the medium. Several retinoids were shown to reduce the ability of these cells to form colonies in culture and to inhibit this effect of 12-*O*-tetradecanoylphorbol-13-acetate (TPA).

A transformation assay of tracheal epithelial cells was used to study promotional effects of TPA in cultures initiated with *N*-methyl-*N'*-nitro-*N*-nitrosoguanidine. In this assay, four stages of transformation are recognized. TPA did not affect measurably the first two transformation stages, i.e., the development of transformed colonies (enhanced growth variants) and the 'immortalization' of enhanced growth variant-derived subcultures. However, treatment of cultures with TPA during the early post-initiation period resulted in a marked enhancement of the appearance of the third transformed phenotype, which is characterized by anchorage independence of growth. The findings of these in-vitro initiation-promotion studies paralleled, in all major respects, the results obtained in in-vivo – in-vitro studies. Tracheas exposed *in vivo* to initiator and promoter were shown to develop the same transformants observed in the in-vitro assay. TPA affected primarily the late anchorage-independence phenotype. Parallel tumour induction studies showed that TPA increased markedly the incidence of tracheal carcinomas following initiation with a low dose of 7,12-dimethylbenz[*a*]anthracene. The studies thus demonstrate that TPA is an effective tumour promoter for rat tracheal epithelium, causing an increase in tracheal carcinomas. They further suggest that the action of TPA on an early transformed cellular phenotype enhances the development of later phenotypes, including neoplastic cell variants.

## INTRODUCTION

One of the major sites of cancer development in humans is the lung. The epidemiological studies that have been conducted over the last three decades leave little doubt that tobacco smoke is the most important agent involved in the etiology of lung cancer (Hammond, 1966; Wynder *et al.*, 1970). Numerous chemical and biological investigations have been carried out to identify the essential carcinogenic agents in tobacco smoke. These studies have led to the widely accepted conclusion that its carcinogenicity is due to the presence of tumour-initiating as well as tumour-promoting agents (Hoffmann & Wynder, 1971; Van Duuren & Goldschmidt, 1976).

Although the potential role of tumour promoters in the carcinogenicity of tobacco smoke has been recognized, few investigations have been conducted to determine the response of airway epithelium to tumour promoters. One study has shown that, in mice, butylated hydroxytoluene promotes the development of pulmonary adenomas induced by urethane (Witschi *et al.*, 1977). Most investigations performed to identify tobacco smoke carcinogens and promoters have been conducted with the mouse skin tumour assay.

In our laboratory, a number of experiments were carried out during the last few years with rat tracheal epithelium, using either the heterotopic tracheal transplant system or an organ culture system to determine the effects of promoters on airway epithelium. These investigations indicated that the mouse skin tumour promoter 12-*O*-tetradecanoylphorbol-13-acetate (TPA) (Pal *et al.*, 1978; Steele *et al.*, 1980; Topping & Nettesheim, 1980a; Steele & Nettesheim, 1983), as well as asbestos (Topping & Nettesheim, 1980b), can enhance neoplastic development in airway epithelium in two-stage carcinogenesis experiments.

In the present communication, we discuss more recent studies on the effect of tumour promoters on airway epithelium, in which a quantitative epithelial cell transformation system was used. The purpose of these studies was: (1) to examine the effects of known promoting agents on normal airway epithelium cells in primary culture; (2) to determine the effects of promoters on transformed cells; and (3) to elucidate the cellular mechanism of promotion during different stages of neoplastic development.

## EFFECTS OF KNOWN TUMOUR PROMOTERS AND ANTIPROMOTERS ON THE COLONY-FORMING EFFICIENCY OF PRIMARY RAT TRACHEAL EPITHELIAL CELLS

TPA and its active analogues are known to be mitogenic agents, causing hyperplastic responses in a variety of tissues. It was, therefore, important to determine whether these agents have a similar effect on tracheal cells in culture, and, if so, to quantitate its magnitude (Mass *et al.*, in preparation). Rat tracheal epithelial (RTE) cells harvested by proteolytic procedures were seeded into culture dishes which were either coated with collagen or contained lethally irradiated 3T3 feeder layers. Methods for culturing RTE cells have been established previously by our laboratory (Wu *et al.*, 1982; Pai *et al.*, 1983; Gray *et al.*, 1983). The effects on the colony-forming efficiency (CFE) of

RTE cells of phorbol ester derivatives and a variety of other agents with known hyperplasiogenic and/or promoting effects in mouse skin were examined. Figure 1 shows the marked concentration-dependent increase in CFE induced by TPA and phorbol dibutyrate. Phorbol, the parent alcohol, lacked this activity. The maximum stimulation achieved with tracheal cells grown on 3T3 feeder layers raised the CFE from 3% to nearly 30%. There was little or no effect on the size of the day-8 colonies, suggesting that the effect of the promoting agents was limited to triggering colony formation but that it did not significantly affect the subsequent rate of cell replication. (It was noted, however, that when RTE cells were grown under suboptimal culture conditions, TPA increased colony size markedly.) Other phorbol esters found to be active, in order of decreasing effectiveness, were: mezerein, phorbol didecanoate, phorbol dibenzoate, 4-*O*-methyl TPA and phorbol diacetate. Teleocidin was another promoting agent that caused a marked stimulation of CFE and, on a molar basis, was the most potent of all the chemicals examined, its activity being more than ten-fold greater than that of TPA. Benzoylperoxide, anthralin, calcium ionophore A23187 and

Fig. 1. Enhancement of colony-forming efficiency (CFE) of rat tracheal epithelial (RTE) cells by tumour promoters
Freshly harvested RTE cells were plated onto lethally irradiated 3T3 feeder layers in media containing different phorbol esters. CFE was determined on day 7 of culture. ▲, 12-*O*-tetradecanoylphorbol-13-acetate; ●, phorboldibutyrate; □, phorbol; ○, controls (Mass *et al.*, unpublished data)

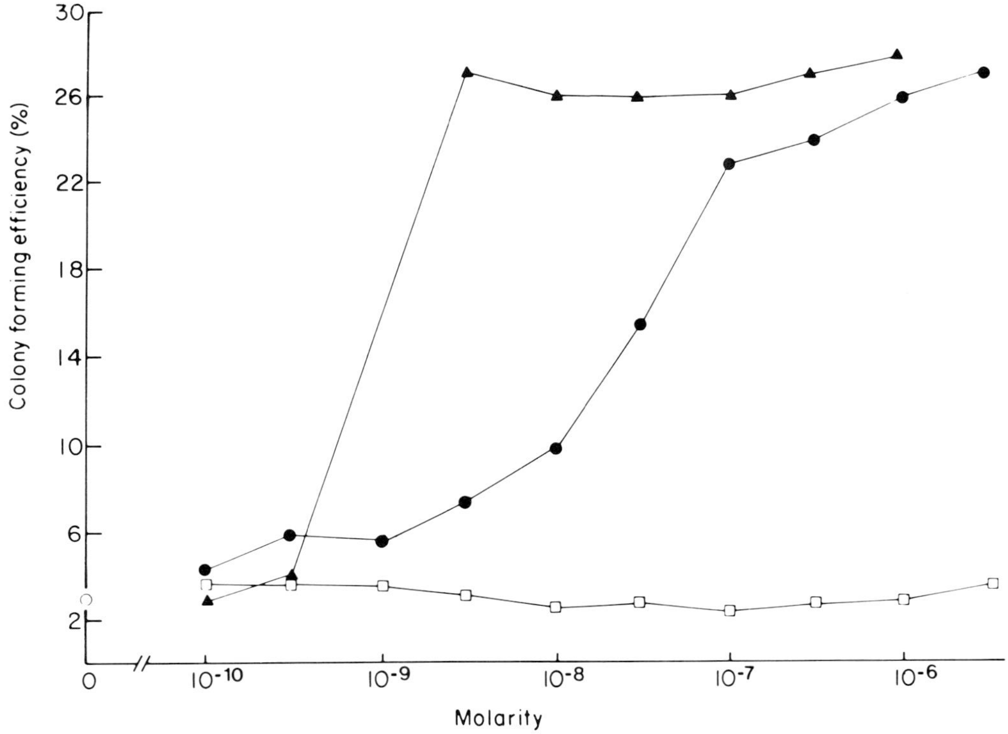

Table 1. Effect of retinoids on colony-forming efficiency (CFE) of rat tracheal epithelial (RTE) cells in primary cultures

| Retinoids | Inhibition of CFE (%)[a] |
|---|---|
| Retinylacetate | 40 |
| Retinol | 85 |
| Retinal | 90 |
| All-*trans*-retinoic acid | 99 |

[a]Freshly harvested RTE cells were plated in media containing various concentrations of retinoids. Maximum inhibition of CFE, obtained with concentrations of 0.2–0.5 mg/mL, is given (Mass *et al.*, unpublished data).

phenobarbital caused little or no increase in CFE at the concentrations tested. Only agents that show substantial affinity for the phorbol dibutyrate receptor (Blumberg, 1981) were capable of enhancing growth of RTE cells.

Certain retinoids have proved to be powerful antipromoting agents *in vivo*. In addition, they are known to have profound effects on the control of cell proliferation and on cell replication in a variety of cell systems, including epithelial cells of the conducting airways (for reviews, see Nettesheim, 1980; Sporn & Roberts, 1983). Retinoids have also been shown to modulate the sensitivity of airway epithelium to carcinogenic insults (Nettesheim & Williams, 1976; Nettesheim *et al.*, 1979). It was thus of considerable interest to examine the effects of retinoids on the CFE of normal as well as TPA-stimulated tracheal cells. Four retinoids were tested (see Table 1) at concentrations ranging from 0.01–0.5 μg/ml. All of them reduced the CFE of normal RTE cells in a concentration-dependent manner (Mass *et al.*, in preparation). Furthermore all-*trans*-retinoic acid (RA) inhibited the stimulation of CFE by TPA. The degree of inhibition was dependent on the amount of TPA used to stimulate the RTE cells. At a concentration of 1 ng/mL TPA, which caused a seven-fold increase in CFE, simultaneous treatment with 0.05 μg/mL RA reduced the number of colony-forming cells by approximately 60%. However, with 10- or 50-fold higher concentrations of TPA, the inhibition of CFE by RA was only marginal, even when RA concentrations were increased to 0.5 mg/mL. Higher RA concentrations were cytotoxic.

We concluded from these studies that RTE cells in culture are sensitive to a variety of tumour promoters and retinoids (antipromoters), which stimulate and inhibit, respectively, their CFE. Apparently, these agents modulate the ability of the colony formers among the RTE cells to enter the cell cycle and divide in culture.

## RAT TRACHEAL CELL TRANSFORMATION SYSTEM

Over the last several years, we have used the RTE cell system to study neoplastic transformation of cells exposed to carcinogenic agents *in vivo* (Terzaghi & Nettesheim, 1979; Terzaghi *et al.*, 1981; Pai *et al.*, 1982; Terzaghi *et al.*, 1982, 1983;

Fig. 2. Effect of exposure to *N*-methyl-*N'*-nitro-*N*-nitrosoguanidine (MNNG) on the growth of primary tracheal cell cultures
○, Cultures treated with 0.2% dimethylsulfoxide; ▲, cultures exposed to 0.1 µg/mL MNNG. Mean number of cells per dish ± SD; 3 dishes per point (modified from Pai *et al.*, 1983)

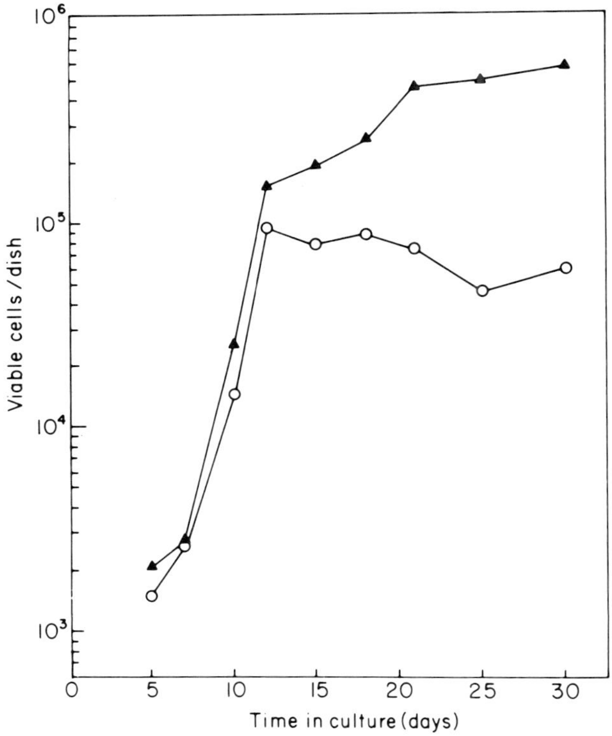


Terzaghi & Nettesheim, 1983) and *in vitro* (Nettesheim *et al.*, 1982; Nettesheim & Barrett, 1984; Pai *et al.*, 1983; Thomassen *et al.*, 1983). Since RTE cells can be grown at clonal densities, this transformation system can be readily quantitated in terms of the number of transformants per surviving colony-forming cell, by correcting for the cytotoxicity of the transforming agent.

The presence of transformed cells in RTE cell cultures became apparent in two ways. Normal RTE cell cultures characteristically ceased to grow after about 10–12 days of rapid replication (Fig. 2). At this time, some signal was generated, switching off growth in the cultures. However, following carcinogen treatment, some cells in the cultures continued to grow for at least several more weeks. Thus, either the growth-arresting signal was not generated or some cells in the culture had become insensitive to such a signal. Besides this characteristic difference in the growth curves of normal and carcinogen-treated cultures, a morphological change became apparent as a result of carcinogen exposure: densely packed, expanding colonies developed that were composed of small, highly refractile, dividing cells, characterized by high nuclear-

Fig. 3. Enhanced growth (EG) variant
A. Tissue culture dish showing an EG variant 6 weeks after exposure to *N*-methyl-*N'*-nitro-*N*-nitrosoguanidine (MNNG)
B. Part of an EG variant colony showing closely-packed, small, refractile cells 6 weeks after exposure to MNNG. Only a few large, flat epithelial cells are found in control dishes at 6 weeks (Thomassen *et al.*, 1983)

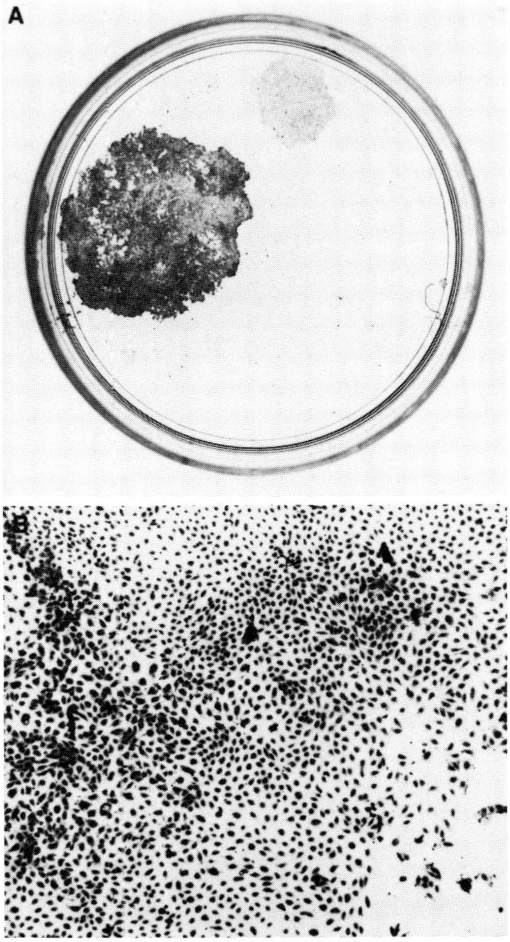

cytoplasmic ratios (Fig. 3). These transformed colonies were named 'enhanced growth (EG) variants', because they exhibit an enhanced capacity to grow continuously, which is entirely atypical of normal RTE cell cultures. They were scored between four and six weeks after exposure. Control cultures at this time only rarely showed continuously expanding colonies and, instead, contained scattered patches of large, spread-out epithelial cells, the remnants of the early colonies, scored on day 8 during the logarithmic growth phase of the cultures. The EG variant was the first

Fig. 4. Frequency of transformants (enhanced growth variants) per colony-forming cell in primary rat tracheal epithelium cell cultures as a function of dose of *N*-methyl-*N′*-nitro-*N*-nitrosoguanidine (MNNG) (from Thomassen *et al.*, 1983)

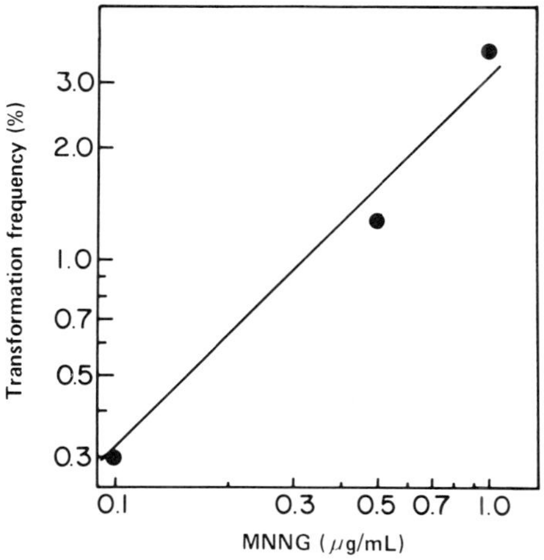


Fig. 5. Diagram of phenotypic changes during neoplastic progression of rat tracheal epithelium (RTE) cells (from Nettesheim & Barrett, 1984)
EG, enhanced growth

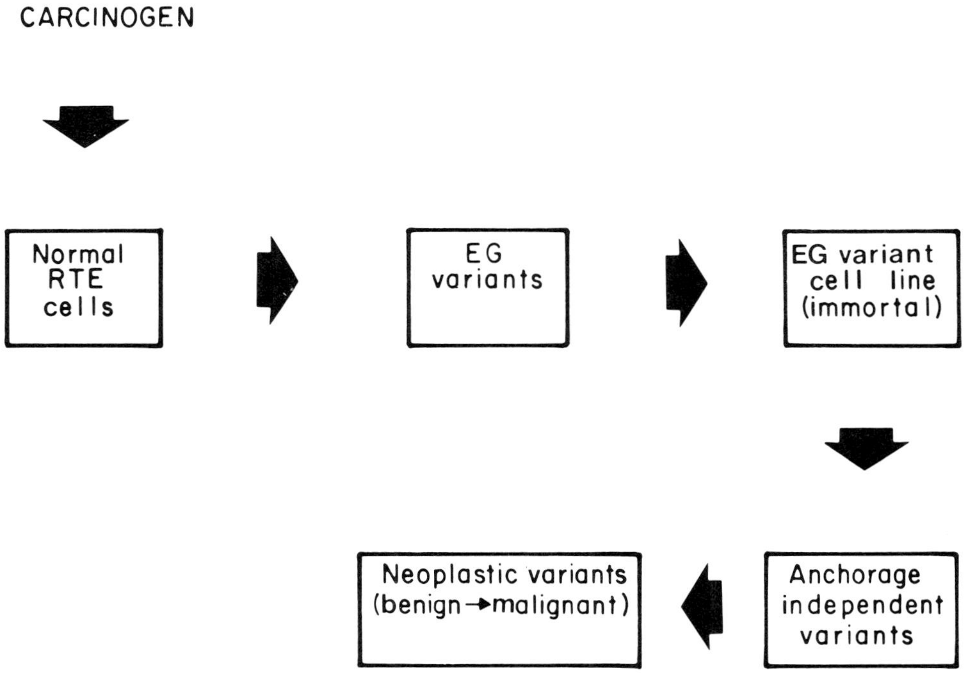

observable transformed phenotype induced in primary RTE cell cultures by a variety of carcinogens. Besides the directly-acting carcinogen *N*-methyl-*N*′-nitro-*N*-nitrosoguanidine (MNNG), which was shown to produce a dose-dependent EG variant response (Fig. 4), benzo[*a*]pyrene, nickel salts, arsenicals and γ-radiation were also found to be effective transforming agents (Nettesheim & Barrett, 1984).

The EG capacity of these transformed cultures became even more apparent when four- to six-week-old primary cultures were subcultured on plastic. At this time, cells obtained from control cultures had very low replating efficiency: only one control culture out of ten formed colonies upon replating ($10^4$ cells seeded). In marked contrast, eight out of ten MNNG-treated cultures produced colonies upon replating on plastic. Many of these cultures could be subcultured repeatedly, and a large proportion became 'immortal', i.e., they could be subcultured indefinitely and thus became stable cell lines. We presently consider the attainment of 'cell line status' as the second stage of transformation (see Fig. 5). However, we are not as yet certain whether the first stage (EG variant) and the second stage ('immortalization') are truly biologically distinct stages or whether they are merely operationally separate. Following these two types of early transformants, two later phenotypic alterations—anchorage-independent growth ($AG^+$) and neoplastic growth—were acquired by many of the carcinogen-treated cultures. Thus, the RTE cell transformation system differs from most other cell transformation systems in that four sequential stages of transformation are recognized. Whether or not all four stages constitute obligatory steps of neoplastic progression is presently under investigation.

## INITIATION-PROMOTION STUDIES IN RAT TRACHEAL EPITHELIAL CELL CULTURES

In viewing this model of neoplastic development (see Fig. 5), a number of important questions emerge: (1) What factors govern the rates of transition from one stage to another? (2) Can tumour promoters affect transition rates? (3) At which stages are tumour promoters effective?

Experiments were designed to determine whether the induction of the first transformant, the EG variant, is influenced by the tumour promoter TPA. Following treatment with MNNG, RTE cell cultures were exposed to various concentrations of TPA, using a variety of different exposure regimens (Table 2). The cultures were exposed to MNNG on day 1 for four hours at concentrations ranging from levels that do not induce transformation above background to concentrations that induce a near maximal frequency of early transformants. In no instance did TPA increase the number of MNNG-induced EG variants scored at 5–6 weeks after MNNG exposure. This suggests that the processes leading to development of early variants in the transformation of RTE cells were insensitive to the promoting effects of TPA. However, other studies indicated that treatment of transformed cultures with TPA may cause qualitative changes in the exposed cell population (Steele *et al.*, unpublished data). Multiple TPA exposures of carcinogen-treated cultures (10 pg/mL TPA, two times per week between days 6–40) resulted in significant enhancement of the replating efficiency of

Table 2. Experimental designs of promotion experiments

| | |
|---|---|
| *N*-Methyl-*N'*-nitro-*N*-nitrosoguanidine concentrations tested: | 0.01, 0.1, 0.3, 0.5 μg/mL |
| 12-*O*-Tetradecanoylphorbol-13-acetate (TPA) concentrations tested: | 0.1, 0.01 μg/mL |
| TPA exposure schemes: | |
| continuous exposure | day 2 through day 7 |
| | day 2 through day 40 |
| 1-hour pulses | day 2 and day 7 |
| biweekly 1-hour pulses | day 4 through day 40 |
| | day 14 through day 40 |

Table 3. Effects of 12-*O*-tetradecanoylphorbol-13-acetate (TPA) on replating efficiency of late primary cultures transformed with *N*-methyl-*N'*-nitro-*N*-nitrosoguanidine (MNNG)

| Treatment[a] | CFE of replated cultures (%)[b] |
|---|---|
| – | 0.1 |
| TPA | 0.4 |
| MNNG | 0.6 |
| MNNG followed by TPA | 1.8 |

[a] Primary RTE cell cultures were either exposed repeatedly to TPA (10 pg/mL, 1 h, 2× per week, days 6–30 of culture) or to MNNG (0.1 μg/mL, 1 h on day 1 of culture) or to MNNG on day 1 and to TPA 2× per week from day 6 to day 30. Control cultures received solvent treatment.

[b] On day 40 the primary cultures were dissociated and the colony-forming efficiency (CFE) was determined by reseeding the cells from each culture at various cell densities into plastic tissue culture dishes and scoring the resulting colonies 7 days later (Steele *et al.*, unpublished data).

such cultures determined on day 40, i.e., the time at which the EG variants were normally scored (Table 3). Thus, in cultures treated with initiator as well as promoter, the growth fraction in the transformed cell population (as measured by the colony-forming assay) was larger than in cultures treated with initiator only or with promoter only. Although this difference was not large, it might be biologically very important since the expansion of transformed colony formers is presumably an important factor in progression to neoplastic transformation *in vitro*.

Treatment of initiated primary cultures with TPA also led to other changes, which became apparent after the cultures had been passaged several times. As can be seen in Table 4, the $AG^+$ phenotype developed in a large proportion of the cultures treated with MNNG and TPA, but it was rare in cultures treated with only one of the two agents. Thus, TPA treatment soon after carcinogen exposure appeared to promote development of the late-appearing $AG^+$ phenotype (see Fig. 5). This development may have been the result of either an increase in the frequency of conversion to $AG^+$ phenotype or of selection for cells with this phenotype.

Another manifestation of promoter-induced changes in transformed cultures became evident even before the appearance of the $AG^+$ phenotype (Vanderlaan *et al.*,

Table 4. Effect of treatment of initiated rat tracheal epithelial (RTE) cell cultures with 12-*O*-tetradecanoylphorbol-13-acetate (TPA) on the induction of the anchorage-independent growth ($AG^+$)-phenotype[a]

| *N*-Methyl-*N'*-nitro-*N*-nitrosoguanidine (MNNG) (μg/mL) | Time after start of culture[b] | | | |
|---|---|---|---|---|
| | Day 60 | | Day 120 | |
| | No TPA | TPA | No TPA | TPA |
| 0 | 0/7 | 1/15 | 0/1 | 2/11 |
| 0.1 | 0/11 | 7/13 | 1/9 | 7/12 |

[a] RTE cell cultures were treated with MNNG and/or TPA (10 pg/mL), see Table 3; at day 40 of primary culture, they were dissociated and (when possible) passaged serially; at day 60 and day 120 (total time in culture), the cultures were tested for anchorage independence of growth.
[b] Data are expressed as number of cultures showing anchorage independence of growth ($AG^+$) per number of cultures tested (same experiment as in Table 3). The number of cultures tested in each group (and time point) varies because subculturability depends on treatment; only a few control cultures survive beyond the fifth passage (Steele *et al.*, unpublished data).

1983). Measurements of cellular DNA content by flow cytometry showed very heterogeneous DNA profiles, particularly in cultures treated with MNNG plus TPA (Fig. 6), which suggests the presence of multiple cell populations with different modal DNA values. We assume that this is an indication of polyploidy and heteroploidy of the MNNG-induced transformants, which seems to be further exaggerated by repeated TPA exposure.

*Analysis of cellular events during in-vivo tumour promotion*

Over the last five years, many investigators have examined the cellular and biochemical effects of tumour promoters in cell cultures (e.g., Blumberg, 1981). These investigations have produced a wealth of information and have revealed an enormous diversity of effects of the TPA-related phorbol esters, involving virtually all levels of cellular and subcellular organization. Despite this rapid expansion of knowledge, the basic phenomenon of tumour promotion in the skin as well as in other organ systems remains largely unexplained. The pleiotropy of the phorbol ester effects makes it difficult to determine which of the effects relate to tumour promotion. On the one hand, information obtained with in-vivo tumour promotion systems is generally difficult to analyse mechanistically, while, on the other hand, uncertainty exists regarding the relevance to tumour promotion of many of the phenomena produced by promoting chemicals in cell culture. A major problem of interpreting initiation-promotion studies carried out in cell culture systems stems from the fact that homeostatic mechanisms operating *in vivo,* which control the proliferative steady state of the tissue, are either non-existent or in only rudimentary form in most cell culture systems. The disruption of this tissue homeostasis may indeed be one of the essential elements of tumour promotion (for review, see Horowitz & Weinstein, 1983).

It seemed to us that one useful approach to the study of mechanisms of tumour promotion might be to allow initiation and promotion to occur *in vivo* in intact tissue and to analyse periodically the resulting cellular changes in the target tissue using a

Fig. 6. Changes in DNA content of 60-day-old primary rat tracheal epithelium (RTE) cell cultures following exposure to *N*-methyl-*N'*-nitro-*N*-nitrosoguanidine (MNNG) and 12-*O*-tetradecanoylphorbol-13-acetate (TPA)
(Data obtained from experiment summarized in Tables 3 and 4)
A. Control culture exposed between days 6 and 30 to dimethylsulfoxide only; note $G_1$ peak at channel 76 (DNA value of diploid control cells) and unusually high $G_2$ peak near channel 150; B. Culture exposed seven times to 10 pg/mL TPA between days 6 and 30 shows near-normal $G_1$ and $G_2$ peak; C. Culture exposed to 0.1 µg/mL MNNG on day 1: besides the normal $G_1$ peak, several other peaks have appeared; D. Culture exposed to 0.1 µg/mL MNNG on day 1 and between days 6 and 30 to 10 pg/mL TPA; note multiple DNA peaks, consistent with presence of multiple, probably aneuploid as well as polyploid cell populations. (Modified from Vanderlaan *et al.*, 1983)

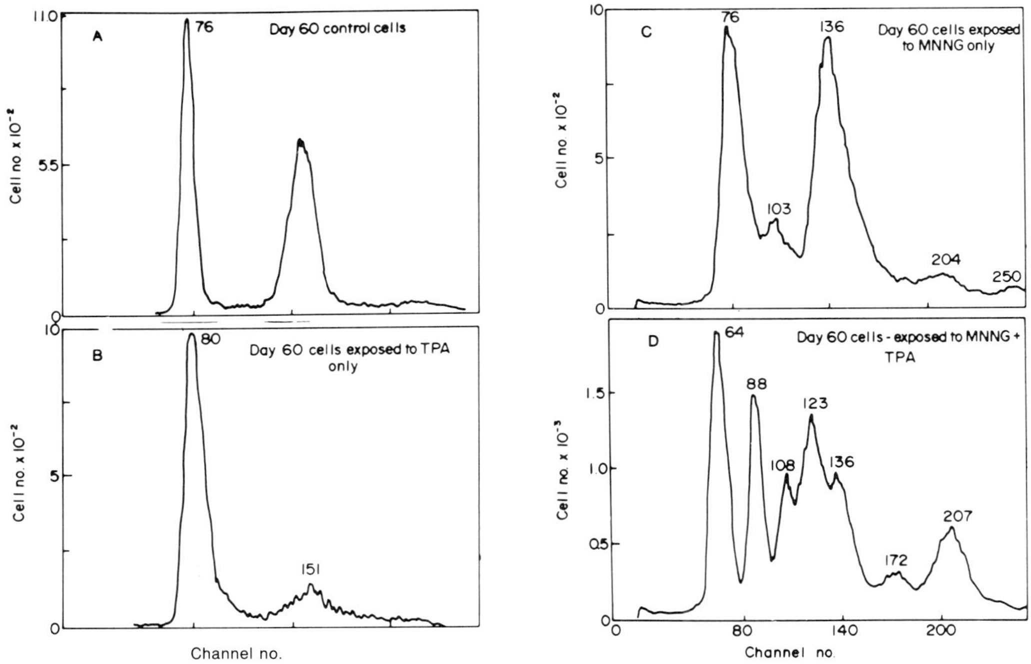


cell culture assay with which it is possible to discern different classes of cell transformants (Terzaghi & Nettesheim, 1979; Terzaghi *et al.*, 1982). This approach would allow us to monitor the cell population submitted to initiator and promoter effects *in vivo* and to measure the qualitative and quantitative changes in the target cell population evolving during the course of tumour promotion. The utility of such an in-vivo/in-vitro approach for analysing the progression of neoplastic disease as a function of time after carcinogen exposure has been reported previously (Pai *et al.*, 1982; Terzaghi & Nettesheim, 1979, 1983; Terzaghi *et al.*, 1981, 1982, 1983). The same phenotypic changes and markers of transformation described for the in-vitro transformation studies (see Fig. 5) are observed when epithelial cells obtained from carcinogen-exposed tracheas are placed in culture. We previously reported that the number of transformed foci (called 'epithelial foci', EF, in the in-vivo/in-vitro studies, equivalent to the EG variants in the in-vitro transformation studies) did not change markedly either with time after exposure or with dose of carcinogen administered *in vivo*. However, the frequency of 'immortalized' and even more so of $AG^+$-transformants increased as a function of time after exposure and of carcinogen dose. The early increase in $AG^+$-transformants observed following high doses of carcinogen was particularly striking (Terzaghi *et al.*, 1982). It was thus of interest to determine how treatment of initiated tracheal epithelium with the tumour promoter TPA would affect the dynamics of the evolution of the various transformed phenotypes.

A tracheal tumour induction study was performed simultaneously with the in-vivo/in-vitro experiments to determine the effect of TPA treatment on 7,12-dimethylbenz[*a*]anthracene (DMBA)-exposed tracheas. An earlier study (Topping & Nettesheim, 1980a) suggested that TPA might indeed enhance the induction of tracheal carcinomas. Heterotopic tracheal transplants were exposed to low doses of DMBA for two weeks and subsequently to TPA for four to six months (for details of procedures employed, see Nettesheim *et al.*, 1977 and Terzaghi *et al.*, 1983). Only a very low carcinoma incidence was observed in the tracheas exposed to DMBA alone (Fig. 7), while a 30% carcinoma incidence occurred in the initiated and promoted tracheas. It is noteworthy that this promotion effect became apparent quite late, namely at about 15 months after the start of exposure.

Fig. 7. Tumour promotion in rat tracheas initiated with 7,12-dimethylbenz[*a*]anthracene (DMBA) and promoted with 12-*O*-tetradecanoylphorbol-13-acetate (TPA)
Heterotopic tracheal transplants were exposed for 2 weeks to pellets containing 35 μg DMBA and subsequently to 100 μg TPA released from intraluminal pellets over a period of approximately 4–6 months. Carcinoma incidence in tracheas exposed to DMBA only (●) and to DMBA followed by TPA (▲) (From Terzaghi *et al.*, 1983)

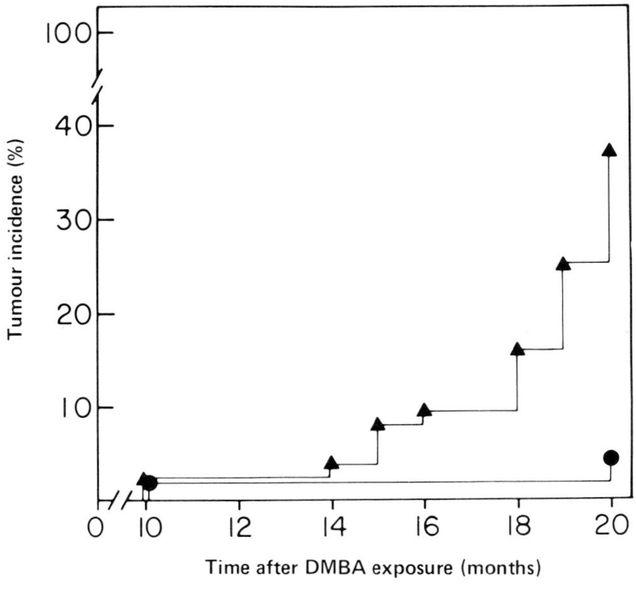

Fig. 8. Cellular analysis of in-vivo tumour promotion in rat tracheas
Heterotopic tracheal transplants were exposed to 7,12-dimethylbenz[*a*]anthracene (DMBA) and subsequently to 12-*O*-tetradecanoylphorbol-13-acetate (TPA), as described in the legend to Fig. 7. At the end of DMBA exposure, and also 3, 12 and 18 months later, tracheas were removed, the epithelium was dissociated enzymatically, and the resulting single-cell suspensions were plated in culture to determine the number of transformants per $10^5$ tracheal cells. Three types of transformant were recognized: those forming late proliferating epithelial foci (EF); those forming EF with subculturable offspring ($EF_s$); and those with subculturable and anchorage-independent offspring ($EF_sAG^+$). ○, results obtained with cells recovered from DMBA-exposed tracheas; ●, results obtained with cells recovered from DMBA- and TPA-exposed tracheas. Control tracheas (including controls exposed only to TPA) yielded <1 EF/$10^4$ cells. (Modified from Terzaghi *et al.*, 1983)

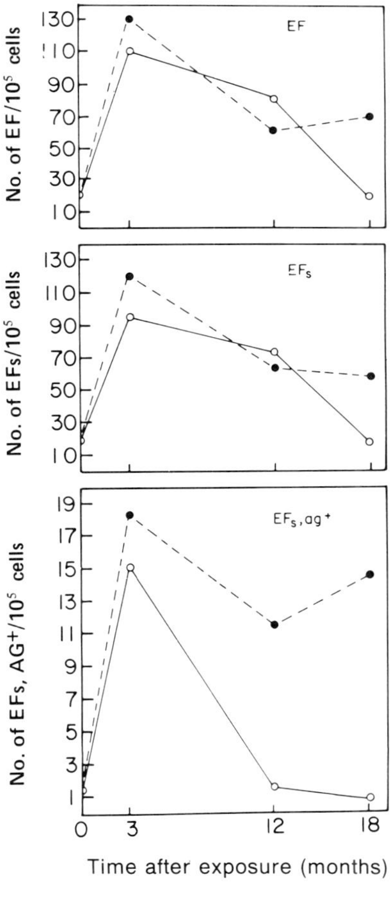


In order to study the cellular evolution of neoplasia in initiated and promoted tracheal epithelium, similarly treated tracheas were harvested periodically, and epithelial cells collected from the tracheas were cultured and assayed for the presence or absence of transformed cells. Several interesting observations were made (Fig. 8): (1) With exposure to DMBA only, the peak number of all three types of transformants was observed at three months; a roughly ten-fold reduction in two of the variants, namely the EF and its subculturable descendents ($EF_s$), occurred over the subsequent 15 months. Such a reduction in transformants has not been observed in previous studies in which much higher doses of DMBA were used (Terzaghi *et al.*, 1982), and it might be a highly significant temporal effect related to 'reversion' or loss of transformants induced by low doses of carcinogen. (2) Promotion of DMBA-initiated tracheas with TPA did *not* increase the number of any of the three types of transformants over and above the peak value observed at three months (TPA alone did not induce a significant number of transformants). TPA did not affect the frequency of EF or $EF_s$ transformants at any time. (3) However, TPA treatment of DMBA-initiated tracheas almost completely prevented the reduction in the $AG^+$-transformants (designated $EF_s$ $AG^+$), observed between three and twelve months after exposure to DMBA only (see bottom panel of Fig. 8). Thus, both the tumour induction study and the in-vivo/in-vitro cell transformation study suggest that the effect of TPA treatment during the first few months after initiation manifests itself *late* during neoplastic transformation of rat tracheal epithelium. This finding is, indeed, reminiscent of the in-vitro promotion effects. In these studies, TPA treatment during the first four weeks after initiation also failed to affect the appearance of the early phenotype but, instead, affected the late $AG^+$-transformant (see Table 4).

## DISCUSSION AND CONCLUSION

Our studies demonstrate clearly that rat tracheal epithelium, which is used as a model for the epithelium of various types of conducting airways, is responsive to TPA and to other known mouse skin tumour promoters. The investigations produced three important findings: (1) TPA and other promoters markedly stimulate normal tracheal cells to proliferate; (2) TPA does not enhance the frequency of early RTE cell transformants; but (3) TPA enhances progression of the early transformants to more advanced phenotypes which appear during the late stages of neoplastic development.

Culturing normal tracheal cells in medium containing TPA resulted in marked stimulation of epithelial cell colony-forming efficiency, i.e., the promoting agent triggered into cell cycle those cells that would not have proliferated otherwise. Presumably, the cells that were stimulated belong to the 'reserve' cell population, since their proliferative capacity appeared to be considerable (it takes about 10 cell divisions to produce an average colony as measured in the colony-forming assay). A maximum of about 30% of the cells seeded could be stimulated to replicate by various promoting agents. This might suggest that the so-called 'basal cells', which are presumed to be the 'reserve' cells of the tracheobronchial epithelium and which are responsible for its normal cellular regeneration, were selectively triggered into cell cycle. About one-third of the cells harvested from normal rat tracheas can be identified ultrastructurally as basal cells (Wu *et al.*, 1982), the other two major cell types being mucous and ciliated. However, further studies will be needed to determine unequivocally which cell type or cell types are stimulated to divide by tumour promoters.

The stimulation of colony formation by TPA was inhibited significantly by retinoids. Neither TPA nor the retinoids affected colony size (provided the culture conditions used were 'optimal' for growth). Thus, these agents seemed primarily to activate or to inactivate the colony-forming cells present in the tracheal cell population rather than to modify generally the rate of cell replication in the epithelial colonies.

The second important finding was that TPA treatment of MNNG-initiated RTE cell cultures did *not* increase the number of transformants (EG variants). These results were supported by virtually identical findings made in the in-vivo/in-vitro studies in which treatment with initiator and promoter was carried out in structurally intact tracheas and in which the number of transformants was subsequently determined with a cell culture assay. These negative findings may be surprising, since other investigators (Mondal & Heidelberger, 1976; Mondal *et al.*, 1976; Kennedy *et al.*, 1978; Popescu *et al.*, 1980; Frazelle *et al.*, 1983), using the C3H 10T½ mouse embryo fibroblast transformation system, have reported that TPA enhances transformation in cell culture.

In discussing cell-culture studies of initiation and promotion, one faces several difficulties. One problem is due to uncertainties in interpreting the phenomena of the mouse skin assay itself. For example, it is not known whether the papilloma that arises from initiation and promotion of mouse skin is simply a clone of initiated cells or whether papilloma cells differ qualitatively from the initiated cells from which they arose. TPA has been reported to induce chromosomal aneuploidy and aberrations as well as sister chromatid exchanges (Emeritt & Cerutti, 1981; Nagasawa & Little, 1981; Parry *et al.*, 1981; Kinsella *et al.*, 1983). This raises the possibility that TPA might be able to confer qualitative changes on initiated cells. Another difficulty stems from the fact that we do not know whether the cell culture phenomena and the observed in-vivo phenomena have a common biological basis. Yet, the definitions of initiation and promotion are based on observations of mouse skin tumour induction. Are the transformants scored in various cell culture transformation systems 'initiated' cells or do they represent a different, possibly more advanced stage in the evolution of neoplastic cells? The situation becomes further complicated when one tries to compare findings made in different transformation systems. We do not know whether the transformants scored in the C3H 10T½ system and in the RTE cell system are equivalent stages in neoplastic development. In spite of the obvious risk of misinterpretation, we believe that it is important to view results from in-vitro transformation studies in the context of in-vivo carcinogenesis. Without an implicit or explicit reference to cancer development as it occurs *in vivo,* much of the cell culture transformation work would be without genuine objective.

Our interpretation of the RTE cell initiation-promotion studies is as follows. Diploid epithelial cells are initiated either *in vivo* or *in vitro* by exposure to a low dose of carcinogen. Subsequently, the initiated cells undergo extensive proliferation due to the fact that the dissociated epithelial cells are cultured at low cell density. Disruption of cell-cell contact and rapid cell proliferation may constitute a promotional stimulus inherent in the RTE cell culture system that is similar in its effects to TPA exposure on mouse skin. The carcinogen-exposed RTE cell population contains initiated as well as uninitiated cells. The latter also respond to the replicative stimulus, but they cease to divide after eight to ten rounds of replication and appear to differentiate. At that point, the expanding clones of initiated cells (EG variants) emerge, since they continue to replicate. The EG variant, and the skin papilloma, may both result from clonal expansion of an initiated cell. If this interpretation is correct, it should not be surprising that addition of the promoter TPA did not increase the frequency of transformed clones, since in the RTE cell cultures the initiated cells are presumably already subjected to the culture-inherent promotional factors. This analogy between papilloma and EG variant is made even more attractive because of a recent finding that indicates that retinoids suppress the development of EG variants (Mass *et al.*, in preparation). Inhibition of promotion in the mouse skin tumour assay by retinoids has been amply documented (e.g., Verma *et al.*, 1979).

Several lines of evidence indicate that TPA administered during the early post-initiation period, although it does not enhance the number of EG variants, nevertheless affects the cells of the EGV colonies and also has an effect on later stages of transformation. This was manifested in several ways. (1) Initiated and TPA-treated primary RTE cell cultures contained increased numbers of colony-forming cells compared with cultures treated only with MNNG or only with TPA, suggesting preferential stimulation of initiated colony-forming cells. This stimulation may subsequently influence the likelihood of progression. (2) Initiated cultures treated with promoter showed evidence of enhanced heteroploidy, as suggested by the complexity of the DNA profiles measured by flow cytometry. (3) TPA enhanced the development of the $AG^+$ phenotype, which is considered to be a marker for a late stage of RTE cell transformation. Thus, early TPA treatment—during the formation of the EG variant colonies in the primary cultures—resulted in enhancement of the late $AG^+$ phenotype in the subcultures (see Fig. 5). Preliminary experiments indicate that TPA exposure during the stage of cell line formation can also result in increased conversion of the $AG^-$ to the $AG^+$ phenotype.

One of the advantages of the RTE cell transformation system is that it has an in-vivo counterpart which can be used to study tracheal tumour formation (e.g., Nettesheim *et al.*, 1977; Topping & Nettesheim, 1980a) and to analyse the evolution *in vivo* of preneoplastic and neoplastic tracheal cell populations (e.g., Terzaghi & Nettesheim, 1979; Terzaghi *et al.*, 1982). This provides us with the opportunity to compare the effects of TPA *in vitro* and *in vivo*. In a tracheal tumour promotion study, TPA markedly increased the incidence of carcinomas in DMBA-initiated tracheas: the tumours appeared eight to ten months after TPA exposure had ceased. Analysis of the evolution of transformed cellular phenotypes in these tracheas showed that TPA, as in the in-vitro promotional studies, had no effect on the incidence of early transformants. However, it had an effect on the $AG^+$-transformants, causing the number of DMBA-induced $AG^+$ variants to remain at high levels for many months; without TPA treatment, these cell variants as well as their precursors decreased with time after DMBA exposure. If the $AG^+$ transformant is, as we are assuming, a close precursor of the neoplastic variant, then it seems reasonable to expect that persistence of this preneoplastic phenotype in large numbers would increase the probability of neoplastic conversion. These findings seem to be consistent with those recently reported by Hennings *et al.* (1983), who showed that TPA, although it does not convert skin papillomas directly into carcinomas, nevertheless plays a crucial role in the induction of carcinomas, which continued to develop for 40 weeks after cessation of TPA treatment. In the tracheal initiation-promotion studies, the effects of TPA treatment during early phases of neoplastic development become manifest only during the evolution of late preneoplastic and neoplastic phenotypes. It is presently uncertain whether the TPA effects are exclusively a result of expansion of the initiated cell pool, thus increasing the probability of malignant conversion. TPA might have other effects (e.g., chromosomal effects) which could be important in the progression of premalignant to malignant cell variants. Further studies are needed to resolve this problem.

## ACKNOWLEDGEMENTS

The authors wish to thank Ms Diane Beeman for her excellent technical assistance and Ms Alma Gonzalez for preparing the manuscript.

## REFERENCES

Blumberg, P.M. (1981) *In vitro* studies on the model of the phorbol esters, potent tumor promoters. *Crit. Rev. Toxicol.*, ***8***, 179–234

Emeritt, J. & Cerutti, P.A. (1981) Tumor promoter phorbol-12-myristate-13-acetate induces chromosomal damage via indirect action. *Nature*, ***293***, 144–146

Frazelle, J.H., Abernethy, D.J. & Boreiko, C.J. (1983) Factors influencing the promotion of transformation in chemically-initiated C3H 10T½ Cl8 mouse embryo fibroblasts. *Carcinogenesis*, ***4***, 709–715

Gray, T.E., Thomassen, D.G., Mass, M.J. & Barrett, J.C. (1983) Quantitation of cell proliferation, colony formation and carcinogen induced cytotoxicity of rat tracheal epithelial cells grown in culture on 3T3 feeder layers. *In Vitro*, ***19***, 559–570

Hammond, E.C. (1966) Smoking in relation to the death rates of one million men and women. *Natl Cancer Inst. Monogr.*, ***19***, 127–204

Hennings, H., Shores, R., Wenk, M.L., Spangler, E.F., Tarone, R. & Yuspa, S.H. (1983) Malignant conversion of mouse skin tumors is increased by tumor initiators and unaffected by tumor promoters. *Nature*, ***304***, 67–69

Hoffmann, D. & Wynder, E.L. (1971) Tobacco carcinogenesis. XI. Tumor initiators, tumor accelerators and tumor promoting activity of condensate fractions. *Cancer*, ***27***, 848–864

Horowitz, A.D. & Weinstein, J.B. (1983) *Tumor promoters and their relevance to endogenous growth factors*. In: Garoff, G., ed., *Growth and Maturation Factors*, Vol. 1, New York, John Wiley & Sons, pp. 155–191

Kennedy, A.R., Mondal, S., Heidelberger, C. & Little, J.B. (1978) Enhancement of X-ray transformation by 12-*O*-tetradecanoylphorbol-13-acetate in a clonal line of C3H mouse embryo cells. *Cancer Res.*, ***38***, 439–443

Kinsella, A.R., Gainer, H.St C. & Butler, J. (1983) Investigation of a possible role of superoxide-ion production in tumor promotion. *Carcinogenesis*, ***4***, 717–719

Mondal, S. & Heidelberger, C. (1976) Transformation of C3H 10T½ Cl8 mouse embryo fibroblasts by ultraviolet radiation and a phorbol ester. *Nature*, ***260***, 710–711

Mondal, S., Brankow, D.W. & Heidelberger, C. (1976) Two-stage chemical oncogenesis in cultures of C3H 10T½-cells. *Cancer Res.*, ***36***, 2254–2260

Nagasawa, H. & Little, J.B. (1981) Factors influencing the induction of sister chromatid exchanges in mammalian cells by 12-*O*-tetradecanoylphorbol-13-acetate. *Carcinogenesis*, ***2***, 601–607

Nettesheim, P. (1980) Inhibition of carcinogenesis by retinoids. *Can. med. Assoc. J.*, ***122***, 757–765

Nettesheim, P. & Barrett, J.C. (1984) Tracheal epithelial cell transformation: A model system for studies on neoplastic progression. *Crit. Rev. Toxicol.*, ***12***, 215–239

Nettesheim, P. & Williams, M.L. (1976) The influence of vitamin A on the susceptibility of the rat lung to 3-methylcholanthrene. *Int. J. Cancer*, ***17***, 351–357

Nettesheim, P., Griesemer, R.A., Martin, D.H. & Caton, J.E. (1977) Induction of preneoplastic and neoplastic lesions in grafted rat tracheas continuously exposed to benzo(a)pyrene. *Cancer Res.*, ***37***, 1271–1278

Nettesheim, P., Snyder, C. & Kim, J.C.S. (1979) Vitamin A and the susceptibility of respiratory tract tissues to carcinogenic insults. *Environ. Health Perspect.*, ***29***, 89–93

Nettesheim, P., Pai, S.B., Steele, V.E. & Wu, R. (1982) *In vitro* studies of normal airway epithelium and of its neoplastic transformation. *Cancer Forum*, ***6***, 130–148

Pai, S.B., Steele, V.E. & Nettesheim, P. (1982) Identification of early carcinogen induced changes in nutritional and substrate requirements in cultured tracheal epithelial cells. *Carcinogenesis*, ***3***, 1201–1206

Pai, S.B., Steele, V.E. & Nettesheim, P. (1983) Neoplastic transformation of primary tracheal epithelial cell cultures. *Carcinogenesis*, ***4***, 369–374

Pal, B.C., Topping, D.C., Griesemer, R.A., Nelson, F.R. & Nettesheim, P. (1978) Development of a system for controlled release of benzo(a)pyrene, 7,12-dimethylbenz(a)anthracene and phorbol ester for tumor induction in heterotopic tracheal grafts. *Cancer Res.*, ***38***, 1376–1383

Parry, J.M., Parry, E.M. & Barrett, J.C. (1981) Tumor promoters induce mitotic aneuploidy in yeast. *Nature*, ***294***, 263–265

Popescu, N.C., Amsbaugh, S.C. & DiPaolo, J.A. (1980) Enhancement of *N*-methyl-*N′*-nitro-*N*-nitrosoguanidine transformation of Syrian hamster embryo cells by a phorbol diester is independent of sister chromatid exchanges and chromosome aberrations. *Proc. natl Acad. Sci. USA*, ***77***, 7282–7286

Sporn, M.B. & Roberts, A.B. (1983) Role of retinoids in differentiation and carcinogenesis. *Cancer Res.*, ***43***, 3034–3040

Steele, V.E. & Nettesheim, P. (1983) *Tumor promotion in respiratory tract carcinogenesis.* In: Slaga, T.J., ed., *Mechanisms of Tumor Promotion*, Vol. 2, *Tumor Promotion and Carcinogenesis in Internal Organs*, Boca Raton, FL, CRC Press, pp. 91–105

Steele, V.E., Marchok, A.C. & Nettesheim, P. (1980) Enhancement of carcinogenesis in cultured respiratory tract epithelium by 12-*O*-tetradecanoylphorbol-13-acetate. *Int. J. Cancer*, ***26***, 343–348

Terzaghi, M. & Nettesheim, P. (1979) Dynamics of neoplastic development in carcinogen exposed tracheal mucosa. *Cancer Res.,* ***39,*** 4003–4010

Terzaghi, M. & Nettesheim, P. (1983) *Combined* in vivo – in vitro *studies of neoplastic development in rat respiratory tissues.* In: Reznik-Schuller, H.M., ed., *Comparative Respiratory Tract Carcinogenesis,* Vol. 2, Boca Raton, FL, CRC Press, pp. 189–197

Terzaghi, M., Nettesheim, P., Yarita, T. & Williams, M.L. (1981) Epithelial focus assay for early detection of carcinogen-altered cells in various organs of rats exposed in situ to *N*-nitrosoheptamethyleneimine. *J. natl Cancer Inst.,* ***67,*** 1057–1062

Terzaghi, M., Nettesheim, P. & Riester, L. (1982) Effect of carcinogen dose on the dynamics of neoplastic development in rat tracheal epithelium. *Cancer Res.,* ***42,*** 4511–4518

Terzaghi, M., Klein-Szanto, A.J.P. & Nettesheim, P. (1983) Effect of the promoter TPA on the evolution of 'carcinogen altered' cell population in tracheas initiated with DMBA. *Cancer Res.,* ***43,*** 1461–1466

Thomassen, D.G., Gray, T.E., Mass, M.J. & Barrett, J.C. (1983) High frequency of carcinogen-induced early, preneoplastic changes in rat tracheal epithelial cells in culture. *Cancer Res.,* ***43,*** 5956–5963

Topping, D.C. & Nettesheim, P. (1980a) Promotion-like enhancement of tracheal carcinogenesis in rats by 12-*O*-tetradecanoyl-phorbol-13-acetate. *Cancer Res.,* ***40,*** 4352–4355

Topping, D.C. & Nettesheim, P. (1980b) Two-stage carcinogenesis studies with asbestos in Fischer 344 rats. *J. natl Cancer Inst.,* ***65,*** 627–630

Vanderlaan, V., Steele, V.E. & Nettesheim, P. (1983) Increased DNA content as an early marker of transformation in carcinogen-exposed rat tracheal cell cultures. *Carcinogenesis,* ***4,*** 721–727

Van Duuren, B.L. & Goldschmidt, B.M. (1976) Cocarcinogenic and tumor promoting agents in tobacco carcinogenesis. *J. natl Cancer Inst.,* ***56,*** 1237–1242

Verma, A.K., Shapas, B.G., Rice, H.M. & Boutwell, R.K. (1979) Correlation of the inhibition of retinoids on tumor promotion-induced mouse epidermal ornithine decarboxylase activity and of skin tumor promotion. *Cancer Res.,* ***39,*** 419–425

Witschi, H.P., Williamson, D. & Lock, S. (1977) Enhancement of urethan tumorigenesis in mouse lung by butylated hydroxytoluene. *J. natl Cancer Inst.,* ***58,*** 301–305

Wu, R., Groelke, J.W., Chang, L.Y., Porter, M.E., Smith, D. & Nettesheim, P. (1982) *Effects of hormones on the multiplication and differentiation of tracheal epithelial cells in culture.* In: Sirbasku, D., Sato, G.H. & Pardee, A.B., eds, *Growth of Cells in Hormonally Defined Media (Cold Spring Harbor Conferences on Cell Proliferation, Vol. 9),* Cold Spring Harbor, NY, Cold Spring Harbor Laboratory, pp. 641–656

Wynder, E.L., Mabuchi, E.L. & Beattie, E.J. (1970) The epidemiology of lung cancer. Recent trends. *J. Am. med. Assoc.,* ***213,*** 2221–2228

# THE EFFECT OF PROMOTERS ON 1,2-DIMETHYL-HYDRAZINE-INDUCED COLON CARCINOGENESIS

O. CSUKA, Z. SZENTIRMAY & J. SUGÁR

*National Institute of Oncology,*
*Research Institute of Oncopathology,*
*1122 Budapest, Hungary*

## SUMMARY

The influence of 12-*O*-tetradecanoylphorbol 13-acetate (TPA) and vincristine (VCR) on the development of colon carcinoma induced by 1,2-dimethylhydrazine (DMH) has been studied by light and electron microscopy. The ability of TPA to induce the appearance of cells with a heterogeneous genotype has been investigated by cytophotometric evaluation of DNA content. The TPA-induced phenotypic alterations have been studied by quantitative histochemistry. The influence of promoters on the outcome of DMH-induced carcinogenesis has been investigated in DMH-resistant C57 Black mice. Aneuploid DNA populations were detected in hyperplasias induced by DMH or TPA; in carcinomas, the percentage of hyperdiploid cell populations was further increased. DNA aneuploidy is defined as the genetic instability of cells that can be induced by TPA treatment alone. TPA can induce dedifferentiation of hyperplastic cells, as demonstrated by quantitative histochemistry of the intestinal mucins. TPA increased the colon tumour incidence in DMH-resistant C57 Black mice. A promoter-like action of VCR could also be observed.

## INTRODUCTION

12-*O*-Tetradecanoylphorbol 13-acetate (TPA) has been shown recently to induce hyperplasia and carcinoma of the forestomach in mice pretreated with carcinogens (Goerttler *et al.*, 1979) and to affect cell morphology and the proliferative capacity of primary cultures of human premalignant colonic epithelial cells (Friedman, 1981). These data imply that TPA can act as a promoting agent on gastrointestinal epithelium. The two-stage mechanism of 1,2-dimethylhydrazine (DMH)-induced, TPA-promoted carcinogenesis has not been studied because DMH alone is a powerful carcinogen with a high propensity for cancer production in the large intestine. However, in some mouse strains, for example in C57 Black mice, DMH has been proven to be a weak carcinogen (Evans *et al.*, 1974; Corbett *et al.*, 1975). The present investigation deals with the effect of the tumour promoter TPA on DMH-induced colon carcinogenesis in C57 Black mice.

The structural and differential unit in the colonic epithelium of mammals is the crypt of Lieberkühn, and there is evidence that colonic tumours develop in a single crypt (Chang, 1978). Any disturbance in the proliferative capacity of cells in Lieberkühn's crypt might influence the maturation and differentiation of colonic epithelium and result in the development of carcinomas. Keeping this in mind, we studied the effect of the well-known mitotic inhibitor, vincristine, on DMH-induced colon carcinogenesis.

Tumour promoters can block terminal differentiation of various cells (Diamond *et al.*, 1980). The differentiated function of colonic epithelial cells is the production of mucins. In order to detect dedifferentiation and phenotypic alterations, changes in the mucin pattern of colonic epithelium have been investigated in mice treated with TPA and/or DMH.

Genomic effects due to TPA have also been proposed. A TPA-induced aneuploidy concomitant with the expression of neoantigens (Kopelovich *et al.*, 1979) and selective gene amplification have also been reported (Varshavsky, 1981). The consequence of this DNA rearrangement within the genome might be genetic instability of the tumour cells and the occurrence of cells with heterogeneous genotype. Computer-controlled cytophotometric analysis revealed the ability of TPA to induce the appearance of cells with aneuploid DNA content.

## MATERIALS AND METHODS

### *Animals and treatments*

Outbred Swiss male mice and inbred C57 Black female mice were treated with DMH for 8–20 weeks, either with DMH alone or with DMH followed by TPA. DMH (Aldrich, Beerse, Belgium) was dissolved in 0.001 mol/L ethylenediamine tetraacetic acid (EDTA) and adjusted to pH 6.5 with sodium bicarbonate. DMH was administered subcutaneously once a week at a dose of of 20 mg/kg body weight. TPA (Sigma, St Louis, MO, USA) was given at a concentration of 100 ng/ml in drinking-water available *ad libitum* during a period of three months. VCR (Richter, Budapest, Hungary) was given intraperitoneally weekly at a dose of 0.1 mg/kg body weight for two months. The experimental groups, of ten mice each, were as follows: (1) normal controls; (2–4) 10, 15 and 20 weeks of DMH treatment; (5–7) carcinogen treatment followed by TPA administration; (8–10) carcinogen treatment followed by VCR administration; (11–12) promoter treatment alone. The mice were killed between one and thirty weeks after treatment.

### *Tissue preparation, histochemistry*

The colon tissue was fixed in 4% formaldehyde for light microscopy and in 2.5% glutaraldehyde for electron microscopy. The periodic acid-Schiff reaction was used to detect neutral mucin. Alcian blue staining at pH 1 (Lev & Spicer, 1964) and the HID reaction (Spicer, 1965) were used to detect sulfomucin. $C_{7-8}$-*O*-Acyl-substituted sialomucins were detected according to the method of Culling *et al.*, (1976). The non-substituted sialomucins in the colonic epithelium were investigated by staining with the cationic carbocyanine dye, 'stains all' (Green, 1978).

*Cytophotometry*

The DNA content of Feulgen's stained cells was determined under a Carl Zeiss type 1K Scanning microscope photometer interfaced with a Hewlett Packard 9825 B type computer. The data were collected and processed by an APAMOS 3 T programme. Spectral analysis of birefrigency in 'stains-all' stained specimens (Taylor *et al.*, 1974) was carried out using crossed Nicol prisms and a grating emission monochromator. The mathematical analysis used in the present study was developed by Szentirmay *et al.* (unpublished data).

## RESULTS

The most characteristic action of the tumour promoter TPA is the induction of colonic hyperplasia. TPA also increased the number of hyperplasias induced by low doses of DMH (Fig. 1), and TPA was found to induce glandular hyperplasia in the pyloric region of the stomach. Histochemical analysis of epithelial mucins in TPA- and DMH-induced hyperplasias and in DMH-induced colonic lesions shows a de-

Fig. 1. Effect of 12-O-tetradecanoylphorbol-13-acetate (TPA) on the induction of hyperplasias of the colon
1,2-Dimethylhydrazine (DMH) was administered for 10 weeks and TPA for 16 weeks

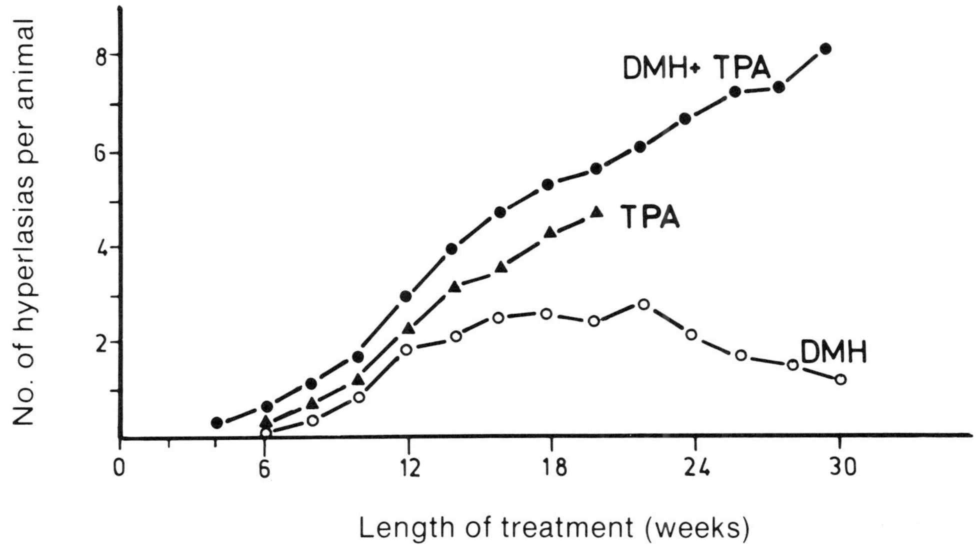

Fig. 2. Spectral transmittance ($T = \frac{I}{I_o}$) of anizotropic 'stains-all' stained mucins in the large bowel 1, embryonic colon; 2, intact adult colon; 3, hyperplasia

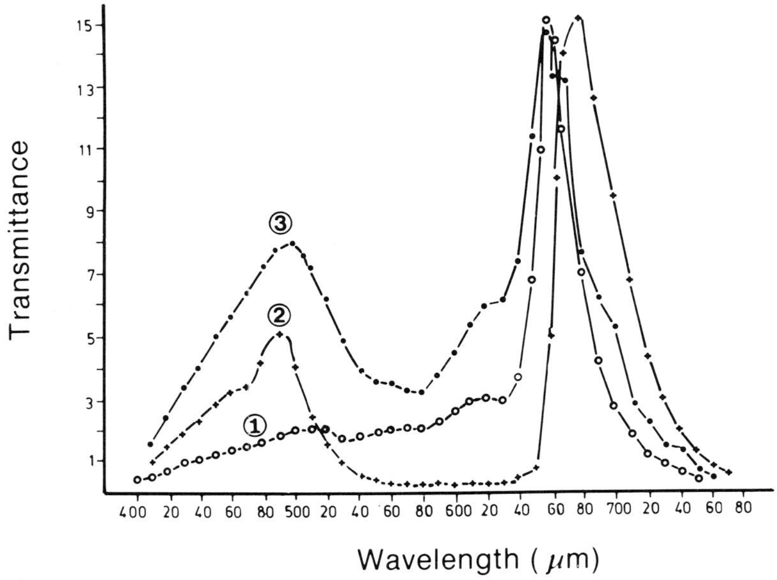


Table 1. Spectral transmittance analysis of birefrigency in the 'stains-all' stained mucins of the large bowel; DMH, 1,2-dimethylhydrazine; TPA, 12-*O*-tetradecanoylphorbol-13-acetate

| Tissue | First maximum (μm) | Second maximum (μm) |
|---|---|---|
| Embryonic large bowel | 500 ± 0.6 | 662.0 ± 0.7 |
| Adult large bowel | 492.5 ± 4.2 | 674.3 ± 2.9 |
| DMH-induced hyperplasia | 491.9 ± 12.8 | 670.1 ± 6.7 |
| TPA-induced hyperplasia | 500.7 ± 5.9 | 664.7 ± 3.6 |
| DMA-induced carcinoma | 497.7 ± 6.4 | 664.8 ± 3.1 |

crease in sulfomucins and in the *O*-acyl-substituted sialomucin content of dysplasias, adenomas and carcinomas. The detectability of non-substituted sialomucins did not change in DMH-induced carcinogenesis or in TPA- and DMH-induced hyperplasias.

Changes in the structure or in the composition of these sialomucins can be observed by quantitative histochemistry and spectral analysis of transmitted light of birefrigency in 'stains-all' stained specimens. Two peaks of transmitted light were observed in embryonic, adult and hyperplastic colonic mucosa (Fig. 2). The values of light transmitted from DMH-induced hyperplasia also differ from those transmitted from intact epithelium and carcinoma; however, the values of the peaks in TPA-induced hyperplasia, embryonic colon and carcinomas are quite similar (Table 1). Phorbol ester-induced dedifferentiation and decreased intercellular communication were detected by electron microscopy. The intercellular gaps are dilated, and dividing cells can be observed at the upper part of the crypt in TPA-treated animals. VCR treatment arrests cells in metaphase, and these cells can move to the surface of the

Fig. 3. Metaphase-arrested cells (→) induced by treatment with vincristine observed in the colon of Swiss mice

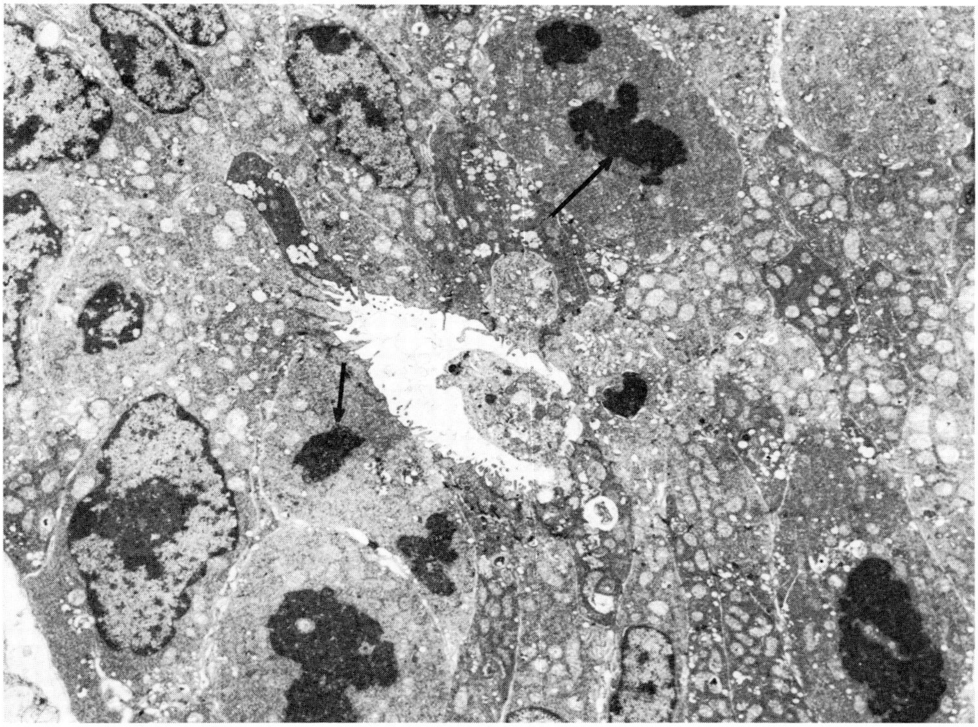

Table 2. DNA distribution in different lesions of the large bowel; TPA, 12-*O*-tetradecanoylphorbol-13-acetate; DMH, 1,2-dimethylhydrazine

| Tissue | Subpopulations with different DNA ploidy | Relative frequency of subpopulations | Mean cell number of subpopulations (%) |
|---|---|---|---|
| Intact mucosa | Diploid | 1.00 | 100 |
| DMH-induced | Diploid | 1.00 | 88.7 ± 10.69 |
| hyperplasia | Hyperdiploid aneuploid | 0.60 | 11.3 ± 2.37 |
| TPA-induced | Diploid | 1.00 | 77.4 ± 12.83 |
| hyperplasia | Hyperdiploid aneuploid | 0.80 | 22.6 ± 3.26 |
| DMH-induced | Diploid | 0.67 | 31.1 ± 4.92 |
| carcinoma | Hyperdiploid aneuploid | 0.87 | 38.9 ± 6.8 |
| | Near triploid aneuploid | 0.67 | 29.9 ± 5.2 |

Table 3. Cell cycle distribution of cells in colonic mucosa treated with 1,2-dimethylhydrazine (DMH) and 12-*O*-tetradecanoylphorbol-13-acetate (TPA)

| Sample | No. of cases | Mean number cells in | | |
|---|---|---|---|---|
| | | $G_1$ region (%) | S region (%) | $G_2$ region (%) |
| Intact mucosa | 5 | $96.1 \pm 2.25$ | $2.4 \pm 1.26$ | $1.5 \pm 1.28$ |
| DMH-induced hyperplasia | 4 | $87.3 \pm 5.65$ | $7.6 \pm 2.0$ | $4.7 \pm 2.06$ |
| TPA-induced hyperplasia | 8 | $71.6 \pm 6.12$ | $16.1 \pm 4.43$ | $12.1 \pm 4.77$ |
| DMH-induced carcinoma | 6 | $71.2 \pm 7.83$ | $20.1 \pm 3.41$ | $9.6 \pm 5.15$ |

colonic epithelium (Fig. 3) and complete their division, which results in the appearance of surface dysplasias. VCR treatment also increased the incidence of DMH-induced perianal tumours in Swiss mice from 18% to 34%. TPA alone increased the colonic tumour incidence in DMH-resistant C57 Black mice from 13% to 42%.

Cytophotometric analysis of cellular DNA content revealed a hyperdiploid cell population in 22.6% of TPA-induced and in 11.3% of DMH-induced hyperplasias and carcinomas. The hyperdiploid cell population in DMH-induced carcinomas was increased to 38.9%, and a near-triploid cell population (29.9%) was also detected (Table 2). A high percentage of cells in S phase in TPA-induced hyperplasia and in DMH-induced carcinoma, reflecting the presence of a large proportion of proliferating cells, was observed (Table 3).

## DISCUSSION

That TPA can induce hyperplasias in skin has been known for many years (Berenblum, 1954; Boutwell, 1969); however, TPA-induced glandular hyperplasia of the stomach has not been reported previously. Hyperplasias caused by TPA are thought to be reversible and not related to the specific promoter action of that compound. Our studies show that TPA-induced hyperplasia is accompanied by a structural change in non-substituted sialomucins, resembling embryonic mucins. This finding is in accordance with the ability of TPA to induce dedifferentiation of cells (Diamond *et al.*, 1980) and might indicate that hyperplasias should not be considered simple outgrowths of tissues. The appearance of a cell population with an aneuploid DNA content in TPA-induced hyperplasias could be related to the genomic effect of TPA. This is plausible, because TPA has been reported to facilitate sister chromatid exchange (Kinsella & Radman, 1978) and to enhance the frequency of specific locus mutations (Trosko *et al.*, 1977). The occurrence of cells with polyploid DNA content in DMH-induced tumours agrees with previous data indicating the presence of polyploid populations in different tumours (Böhm & Sandritter, 1975; Szentirmay *et al.*, 1982; Wolley *et al.*, 1982).

The promoter action of TPA in DMH-induced carcinogenesis has been verified in C57 Black mice. VCR treatment increased the incidence of perianal tumours in DMH-treated Swiss mice but not in C57 Black mice. This promoter action might be attributed to the reversible mitotic block induced by VCR, resulting in the appearance of dysplasias on the mucosal surface. Surface dysplasias have been shown to be significant in the development of colon carcinomas (Chang, 1978). Some data in the literature lend further support to a promoter-like action of VCR, e.g., the induction of chromosomal aberrations (Degraeve, 1978) and of an increase in ornithine decarboxylase activity (Rumsby & Puck, 1982). Further investigation is needed to clarify this point.

## REFERENCES

Berenblum, I. (1954) A speculative review: The probable nature of promoting action and its significance in the understanding of the mechanisms of carcinogenesis. *Cancer Res.*, ***14***, 471–477

Böhm, N. & Sandritter, W. (1975) DNA in human tumors: A cytophotometric study. *Curr. Topics Pathol.*, ***60***, 151–219

Boutwell, R.K. (1969) The functions and mechanism of promoters of carcinogenesis. *CRC crit. Rev. Toxicol.*, ***2***, 419–443

Chang, W.W.L. (1978) Histogenesis of symmetrical 1,2-dimethylhydrazine-induced neoplasms of the colon in the mouse. *J. natl Cancer Inst.*, ***60***, 1405–1412

Corbett, T.H., Griswold, P.P., Jr, Roberts, B.J., Peckham, J.C. & Schabel, F.M., Jr (1975) Tumor induction relationships in development of transplantable cancers of the colon in mice for chemotherapy assays, with a note on carcinogen structure. *Cancer Res.*, ***35***, 2434–2439

Culling, C.F.A., Reid, P.E. & Dunn, W.L. (1976) A new histochemical method for the identification and visualization of both side chain acylated and nonacylated sialic acids. *J. Histochem. Cytochem.*, ***24***, 1225–1230

Degraeve, N. (1978) Genetic and related effects of *Vinca rosea* alkaloids. *Mutat. Res.*, ***55***, 31–42

Diamond, L., O'Brien, T.G. & Baird, W. (1980) Tumor promoters and the mechanism of tumor promotion. *Adv. Cancer Res.*, ***32***, 1–74

Evans, J.T., Hauschka, T.S. & Mittelman, A. (1974) Brief communication: differential susceptibility of four mouse strains to induction of multiple large-bowel neoplasms by 1,2-dimethylhydrazine. *J. natl Cancer Inst.*, ***52***, 999–1000

Friedman, E.A. (1981) Differential response of premalignant epithelial cell classes to phorbol ester tumour promoters and to deoxycholic acid. *Cancer Res.*, ***35***, 4588–4599

Goerttler, K., Loehrke, H., Schweizer, J. & Hesse, B. (1979) Systemic two-stage carcinogenesis in the epithelium of the forestomach of mice using 7,12-dimethylbenz(a)anthracene as initiator and the phorbol ester 12-O-tetradecanoylphorbol-13-acetate as promoter. *Cancer Res.*, ***39***, 1293–1297

Green, M.R. (1978) Simultaneous differential staining of phosphoproteins, sialoglycoproteins, hyaluronic acid, sulfated glycosaminoglycans, proteins and nucleic acids in human breast tissue with a cationic carbocyanine dye. *J. natl Cancer Inst.*, ***61***, 951–960

Kinsella, A.R. & Radman, M. (1978) Tumor promoter induces sister chromatid exchanges: relevance to mechanisms of carcinogenesis. *Proc. natl Acad. Sci. USA*, ***75***, 6149–6153

Kopelovich, L., Bias, N. & Helson, L. (1979) Tumour promoter alone induces neoplastic transformation of fibroblasts from humans genetically predisposed to cancer. *Nature*, ***282***, 619–661

Lev, R. & Spicer, S.S. (1964) Specific staining of sulphate groups with alcian blue at low pH. *J. Histochem. Cytochem.*, ***12***, 309–310

Rumsby, G. & Puck, T.T. (1982) Ornithine decarboxylase induction and the cytoskeleton in normal and transformed cells. *J. Cell Physiol.*, ***111***, 133–139

Spicer, S.S. (1965) Diamine methods for differentiating mucosubstances histochemically. *J. Histochem. Cytochem.*, ***13***, 211–234

Szentirmay, Z., Sugar, J. & Kralovanszky, J. (1982) Early detection of human gastric cancer based on morphologic and enzymologic studies. *Cancer Detect. Prev.*, ***5***, 185–194

Taylor, D.L., Allen, R.D. & Benditt, E.P. (1974) Determination of the polarisation optical properties of the amyloid-congo red complex by phase modulation microspectrophotometry. *J. Histochem. Cytochem.*, ***22***, 1105–1112

Trosko, J.E., Chang, C.C., Yotti, L.P. & Chu, E.H.Y. (1977) Effect of phorbol myristate acetate on the recovery of spontaneous and ultraviolet light-induced 6-thioguanine and ouabain-resistant Chinese hamster cells. *Cancer Res.*, ***37***, 188–193

Varshavsky, A. (1981) Phorbol ester dramatically increases incidence of methotrexate-resistant mouse cells: possible mechanisms and relevance to tumor promotions. *Cell*, ***25***, 561–572

Wolley, R.C., Schreiber, K., Koss, L.G., Kavas, M. & Sherman, A. (1982) DNA distribution in human colon carcinomas and its relationship to clinical behavior. *J. natl Cancer Inst.*, ***69***, 15–22

# MEMBRANE INTERACTION OF TUMOUR-PROMOTING AGENTS

# ANALYSIS OF MEMBRANE AND CYTOSOLIC PHORBOL ESTER RECEPTORS

P.M. BLUMBERG[1], B. KÖNIG, N.A. SHARKEY, K.L. LEACH, S. JAKEN & A.Y. JENG

*Molecular Mechanisms of Tumour Promotion Section, Laboratory of Cellular Carcinogenesis and Tumor Promotion, National Cancer Institute, Bethesda, MD 20205, USA*

## SUMMARY

Specific phorbol ester receptors are found in the particulate fraction of cells. In addition, cytosol contains a phorbol ester apo-receptor, which requires phospholipids for reconstitution. The apo-receptor corresponds to protein kinase C, and the quantitatively major membrane receptor appears to be a protein kinase C-phospholipid complex. The ability to reconstitute the phorbol ester apo-receptor into different lipid domains now makes it possible to begin elucidation of the role of the lipid domain in phorbol ester action. Studies reviewed here indicate that diglycerides competitively inhibit phorbol ester binding, consistent with their being the postulated endogenous phorbol ester analogues. Highly lipophilic phorbol esters inhibit effectively only if they are incorporated into the lipid phase, indicating that it is the membrane-dissolved form of the ligand which is recognized. The binding affinity of $^3$H-phorbol 12,13-dibutyrate for holo-receptor depends markedly ($>$20-fold range) on the phospholipid environment, and heterogeneous phorbol ester binding (i.e., curved Scatchard plots) can be generated by use of heterogeneous lipid environments in the reconstitution. The possible existence of other phorbol ester receptors in addition to protein kinase C-phospholipid complexes remains to be resolved.

## INTRODUCTION

The rationale for studying the mechanism of action of the phorbol ester tumour promoters is that the phorbol esters are the most potent class of tumour promoters for mouse skin; therefore, it should be easier to distinguish specific from non-specific

[1] To whom correspondence should be addressed.

effects of these compounds than with less specific agents such as iodoacetic acid or phenol. A second rationale is that the phorbol esters have profound effects on a variety of biological systems (Blumberg, 1980; Diamond *et al.*, 1980; Hecker *et al.*, 1982). These effects include (1) potentiation of other cellular effectors, e.g., epidermal growth factor, (2) inhibition and/or induction of cellular differentiation and differentiated cell functions, (3) modulation of membrane activities, and (4) (reversible) induction in normal cells of a partially transformed phenotype. Understanding the mechanism of action of the phorbol esters may help to clarify the mechanisms of control of these other biological processes as well.

Efforts in this laboratory have focused on defining the initial events in the interaction of the phorbol esters with cells. Identification of such events should highlight critical biochemical processes causally involved in tumour promotion. Such processes may provide useful points for intervention or for monitoring.

We and subsequently others have demonstrated that the phorbol esters bind specifically to cells and to tissue preparations (Blumberg *et al.*, 1982, 1983a,b, 1984, and references cited therein). Binding analysis was made possible by our introduction of the phorbol ester derivative $^3$H-phorbol 12,13-dibutyrate (PDBu), a ligand which, although less potent than phorbol 12-myristate 13-acetate (PMA),[1] the standard phorbol derivative used in promotion studies, has a more favourable ratio of specific to non-specific binding. Quantitative structure-activity analysis strongly argues that these binding sites mediate phorbol ester responses, that is, that these binding sites function as phorbol ester receptors. The properties of these receptors have been characterized in detail and the results reviewed elsewhere (Blumberg *et al.*, 1984).

One approach taken to identify the biochemical function of the phorbol ester receptors was by direct purification. An alternative approach was suggested by the observation that the level of receptors in brain, 30 pmol/mg of protein, corresponded to the receptor constituting approximately 1/500 of the total brain protein (Dunphy *et al.*, 1980). Therefore, it seemed possible that the receptor might have been already isolated by workers studying it because of some other function which it possessed. In fact, comparison of the properties of the phorbol ester receptors with those of the calcium phospholipid-dependent protein kinase (see Takai *et al.*, 1982, for review), also known as 'protein kinase C', revealed striking similarities (Table 1).

It was therefore a source of considerable excitement that Castagna, Nishizuka and co-workers were able to demonstrate direct activation of protein kinase C by nanomolar concentrations of phorbol esters under appropriate in-vitro conditions (Castagna *et al.*, 1982). This finding was particularly cogent since, in contrast to the wide range of phorbol ester responses observed in intact cells, only one other report of an

Table 1. Similarities between the phorbol ester receptor and protein kinase C

| |
|---|
| 1. Tissue distribution |
| 2. Absolute level in brain |
| 3. Evolutionary conservation |
| 4. High sensitivity to calcium ion |
| 5. Phospholipid association |

[1] Identical to 12-*O*-tetradecanoyl phorbol-13-acetate (TPA).

effect of the phorbol esters at nanomolar concentrations in a broken cell preparation had been reported (Puszkin & Zucker, 1973). Direct confirmation of the relationship between phorbol ester binding and protein kinase C has been obtained by both this laboratory (Leach *et al.*, 1983) and a number of others (Ashendel *et al.*, 1983; Niedel *et al.*, 1983; Sando & Young, 1983), showing that the two activities co-fractionate during purification.

Protein kinase C itself is an apo-enzyme that has an absolute requirement for acidic phospholipids to achieve reconstitution. A critical concept, therefore, which is perhaps emphasized inadequately, is that the functional entity – the holo-receptor or holo-enzyme – is thus not simply the protein moiety but is rather a lipid-protein complex. The ability to manipulate the lipid domain separately from the apo-protein has made possible the exploration of a number of previously inaccessible questions.

## RELATION OF CYTOSOLIC AND MEMBRANE BINDING ACTIVITIES

Although many of the properties of protein kinase C resembled those of the phorbol ester receptors, the observed subcellular localizations were strikingly different. Whereas protein kinase C was found largely in the cytosolic fraction, the phorbol ester binding activity in brain was found to be particulate (Dunphy *et al.*, 1981). The explanation is that complete binding activity was being compared to that of the apo-enzyme. When binding was assayed in the cytosol under conditions permitting protein kinase C reconstitution, cytosolic phorbol ester binding could be recovered (Leach *et al.*, 1983; Niedel *et al.*, 1983; Sando & Young, 1983). Since the cytosolic binding activity requires phospholipid for reconstitution, we refer to it as a 'phorbol ester apo-receptor'.[1] Assays used to measure cytosolic binding include gel filtration (Niedel *et al.*, 1983), precipitation with cold acetone (Ashendel *et al.*, 1983) and precipitation with polyethylene glycol (Leach *et al.*, 1983; Sando & Young, 1983).

Although the relationship of the cytosolic apo-receptor to the previously characterized membrane receptor remains to be determined conclusively, the two activities probably represent different states of the same protein. We have found that in rat pituitary cells, the distribution of cellular binding recovered in the membrane fraction as compared to the cytosolic fraction depends on the lysis conditions (manuscript in preparation). More cellular binding is associated with the membranes in the presence of calcium; and more is found in the cytosol if the cells are lysed in the presence of EGTA. Under both conditions, total activity recovered in lysates is similar to that of the intact cells. A shift of phorbol ester binding and of protein kinase C activity (Kikkawa *et al.*, 1982; Niedel *et al.*, 1983) between cytosol and membranes as a function of free calcium ion has also been observed in rat brain. These observations help explain the similarity in tissue distribution between cytosolic protein kinase C activity and membrane phorbol ester binding activity. The former analyses were carried out routinely in the presence of EGTA, the latter in the absence of chelators.

A second treatment leading to a shift in distribution (as determined in cells lysed in the presence of EGTA) is exposure of cells to phorbol esters. Such treatment of

[1] The term 'phorbol ester apo-receptor' is used to describe activity characterized operationally by binding, whereas the term 'protein kinase C' is used for activity characterized by enzymatic assay.

Table 2. Binding affinities of phorbol esters for mouse brain membranes and cytosol[a]

| Compound | $K_i$ (nM) | |
|---|---|---|
| | Membrane | Cytosol |
| Phorbol 12-myristate 13-acetate (PMA) | 0.066 | 0.041 |
| Phorbol 12,13-didecanoate | <2.8 | <7.7 |
| Phorbol 12,13-dibutyrate | 7.4 | 1.3 |
| Phorbol 12,13-diacetate | 560 | 440 |
| 4-*O*-Methyl PMA | ND | 510 |

[a] From Leach *et al.* (1983)
ND, not determined

intact EL4 mouse thymoma and parietal yolk sac cells causes virtually complete transfer of protein kinase C to the particulate fraction (Kraft *et al.*, 1982; Kraft & Anderson, 1983). In rat pituitary cells, transfer, measured for $^3$H-PDBu binding, still occurs but is less complete (manuscript in preparation).

It should be noted that the current data do not distinguish between some and all of the phorbol ester receptors in the membranes being related to protein kinase C.

We have carried out limited structure-activity comparison between mouse brain cytosolic apo-receptor reconstituted into phosphatidylserine (PS) and the membrane receptor (Leach *et al.*, 1983). Affinities for the apo-receptor among active derivatives ranged from 0.04 nM for PMA to 440 nM for phorbol 12,13-diacetate (Table 2). These values were all within a factor of three of those determined previously for the membrane receptor. Our measured affinity for PMA is approximately 30-fold higher than that reported by Castagna *et al.* (1982) for activation of protein kinase C. This discrepancy may reflect the conditions under which the enzyme was assayed by these workers (e.g., an enzyme concentration greater than the equilibrium dissociation constant ($K_d$) for PMA. In the $GH_4C_1$ rat pituitary cell system, we find good agreement between the $K_d$ for PDBu binding to the apo-receptor and for protein kinase C activation.

## LIPID DEPENDENCE OF BINDING

Different phospholipids varied in their ability to reconstitute specific $^3$H-PDBu binding activity (Leach *et al.*, 1983; and manuscript in preparation). Using partially purified apo-receptor to reduce contamination by lipids retained in the cytosol fraction (which otherwise give partial reconstitution in the absence of added phospholipid) and maintaining chelator excess, we found that PS was most effective at reconstitution, with a half-maximally effective dose ($ED_{50}$) of 7 μg/ml. The negatively charged phospholipids phosphatidylinositol (PI) and phosphatidic acid (PA) were also active, with similar $ED_{50}$ values, whereas the uncharged phospholipids phosphatidylethanolamine (PE) and phosphatidylcholine (PC) failed to reconstitute activity if added alone. The inability of PE to reconstitute binding may reflect, in part, its inability to form liposomes in the absence of other phospholipids. A 1:1 mixture of PE and PC gave partial reconstitution, although only at high concentrations (approximately 1 mg/ml).

Reconstitution was achieved with mixtures of PS and either PE or PC. The dose-response curves were shifted to higher phospholipid concentrations, however. For example, a 1:2 PS:PC mixture yielded an $ED_{50}$ for reconstitution of approximately 40 μg/ml. Reconstitution into a phospholipid mixture resembling that of the human red blood cell (PC:PE:PS:SM:PI:DPG, 30:30:13:25:1:1, mole ratio) yielded an $ED_{50}$ of 80 μg/ml.

The dose-response curves for reconstitution of binding by phospholipid depend on the calcium ion concentration. In the presence of excess calcium ion over chelator, the $ED_{50}$ for PS, for example, is reduced to less than 1μg/ml.

Sphingomyelin (SM) differs from the glycerolphospholipids in its behaviour in the apo-receptor reconstitution system. At high concentrations, it gives apparent specific binding, as measured by a difference in the amount of $^3$H-PDBu bound in the presence and absence of 30 μM non-radioactive PDBu. However, identical results are obtained in the absence of apo-receptor, indicating that the SM itself was responsible for the binding rather than acting to reconstitute the apo-receptor. Scatchard analysis yielded a $K_d$ of $>> 200$ nM, consistent with a low-affinity interaction. $^3$H-PMA has also been reported to show 'specific binding' to SM (Esumi & Fujiki, 1983). Low affinity, competing interactions between ligands and secondary binding sites are not unusual. The opiates, for example, have been reported to bind to glass fibre filters and to cerebrosides (Snyder *et al.*, 1975). In the case of the phorbol esters, there is no evidence that such low-affinity interactions are biologically significant. Whether SM could account for the low (μM)-affinity binding sites reported by Horowitz *et al.* (1981) remains to be determined.

The phospholipids used for the reconstitution not only determine whether the apo-receptor can bind $^3$H-PDBu but also help to determine the binding affinity. Under assay conditions in which the $K_d$ of $^3$H-PDBu for the apo-receptor reconstituted into PS is 0.8 nM, reconstitution into dioleoyl phosphatidic acid or into the human red blood cell phospholipid mixture yields a $K_d$ of approximately 20 nM. These values are in the range observed typically for $^3$H-PDBu binding to intact cells, whereas the $K_d$ for apo-receptor reconstituted into PS is of higher affinity than is usually observed. These results clearly emphasize that the holo-receptor is the lipid-protein complex rather than the protein alone.

Implications of these findings are, first, that different measured receptor affinities in intact cells or membrane preparations may reflect different lipid domains for the same apo-receptor rather than different proteins. Secondly, the agreement in absolute affinities between the apo-receptor reconstituted into PS and the brain membrane receptor described above may be, in part, the fortuitous result of the choice of reconstitution conditions. Since different receptor sub-classes may show different structure-activity relations for phorbol esters as well as different absolute affinities for $^3$H-PDBu, we predict and are currently trying to verify that the lipid component of the holo-receptor may affect differentially the affinity for different phorbol esters.

Previous analysis of the thermodynamics of $^3$H-PDBu binding to the phorbol ester receptor in brain membranes had indicated that the binding was entropy driven, consistent with the binding largely resulting from hydrophobic interactions (Dunphy *et al.*, 1981). Insertion of the phorbol ester side chains into the phospholipid bilayer could represent part of this interaction.

## A PHOTOACTIVATABLE PHORBOL ESTER AS A PROBE OF THE LIPID ENVIRONMENT OF THE MEMBRANE RECEPTOR

Reconstitution experiments provide information about the influence of different lipids on the properties of the lipid-apo-receptor complex. The photoactivatable phorbol ester derivative phorbol 12-*p*-azidobenzoate 13-benzoate (PaBB), which we synthesized, provides a probe for the actual micro-environment of the binding site for the membrane receptor (Delclos *et al.*, 1983). In studies carried out with the brain membrane receptor before identification of the cytoplasmic apo-receptor and demonstration of the relationship between protein kinase C and the phorbol ester receptor, we showed that incubation with PaBB followed by ultraviolet irradiation induced specific, irreversible labelling by the ligand. Although the specific, irreversible binding was protease sensitive, consistent with a protein component to the binding site, analysis of the specific adducts formed indicated that they were phorbol ester-phospholipid conjugates. Fractionation by thin-layer chromatography (TLC) yielded two peaks. Both peaks were degraded by phospholipase $A_2$, which shifted their mobilities to a position near the solvent front, consistent with attachment of the phorbol ester to the side chains released from position 2 of phospholipids by the enzyme. The lower mobility peak was identified as a phorbol ester-PS adduct on the basis of its susceptibility to degradation by the specific enzyme phosphatidylserine decarboxylase (Fig. 1). The resulting product, a phorbol ester-PE adduct, co-chromatographed with the second peak.

Brain contains a significant amount of alk-1-enyl 2-acyl phosphoglycerides (plasmalogens), particularly in the PE fraction. These are not distinguishable from the corresponding diacyl phosphoglycerides by their mobility on TLC, but they can be identified by their sensitivities to mercuric chloride. Treatment with mercuric chloride degraded the putative phorbol ester-PE adduct by 60%, which corresponds to the proportion of plasmalogen in brain PE.

The lipid profile suggests that the apo-receptor in brain membranes is, in fact, associated with those lipids that are effective in in-vitro reconstitution of protein kinase C activity. PS is very efficient at reconstitution of the kinase (Takai *et al.*, 1982), and PE further enhances reconstitution of the enzymatic activity although not that of the binding activity. Whether the phorbol esters influence the lipid domain into which the apo-receptor is inserted remains to be determined.

There are two possible explanations for the selective reaction of PaBB with lipids rather than with the protein portion of the receptor. One is based on the location of the reactive nitrene generated from the aryl azide on the PaBB at the far end of the side chain from the phorbol moiety. If the terminus of the phorbol ester side chain were buried entirely in the lipid bilayer rather than bound in a hydrophobic pocket formed by both protein and phospholipid, it might not be in close enough proximity to react with the protein. An alternative explanation may be that although it is in adequate proximity to both protein and lipid, the nitrene reacts selectively. Such

Fig. 1. Treatment of the putative $^3$H-phorbol 12-*p*-azidobenzoate 13-benzoate-phosphatidylserine ($^3$HPaBB-PS) adduct with serine decarboxylase
A. Adduct incubated with enzyme (---); adduct incubated without enzyme (——)
B. Putative $^3$H-PaBB-phosphatidylethanolamine (PE) adduct incubated without enzyme. The samples in both panels were subjected to thin-layer chromatography using a solvent system of chloroform : methanol : water, 70 : 30 : 4 (vol/vol). From Delclos *et al.* (1983)

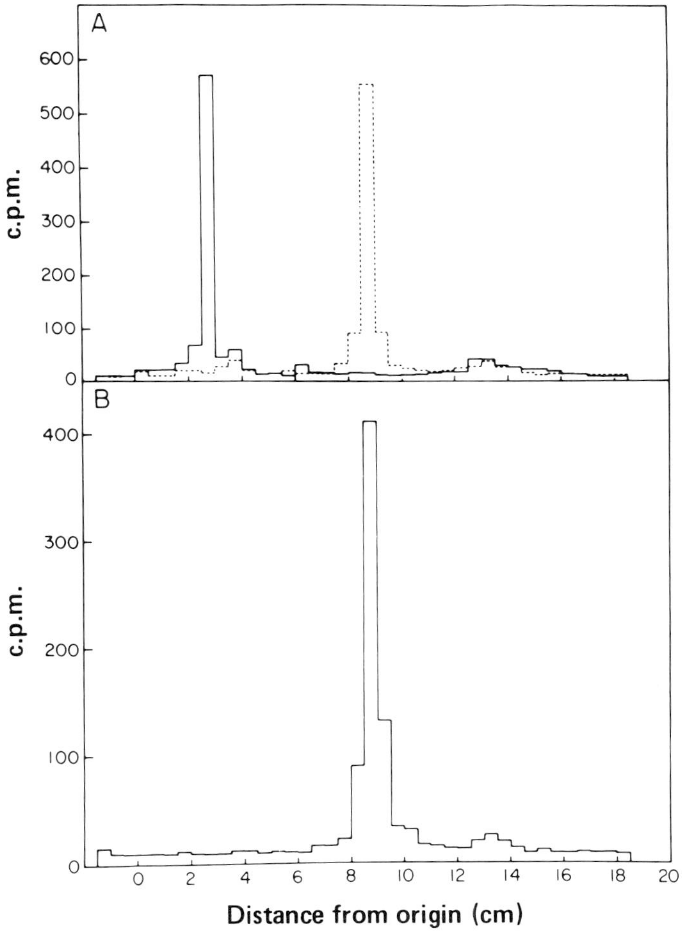


behaviour has been observed in some (Quay *et al.*, 1981) but not in other (Brunner & Richards, 1980) systems with nitrene-generating phospholipid derivatives.

## DIACYLGLYCEROL AS AN ENDOGENOUS PHORBOL ESTER ANALOGUE

The phorbol ester receptor has been highly conserved over evolution. Both the number of binding sites and the $^3$H-PDBu binding affinity for sea urchins, fruit flies and nematodes fall within the range observed for vertebrate systems (Blumberg *et al.*, 1984). In the case of the nematode, moreover, the structure-activity relations for binding have been characterized and found to resemble closely those for mouse skin. In analogy with evolutionarily-conserved binding sites for other exogenous ligands such as the opiates, the existence of an endogenous ligand that could exert a constraint on the divergence of the binding site over the course of evolution seemed probable. Although initial efforts to identify endogenous, *competitive* inhibitors of $^3$H-PDBu binding in tissue extracts were unsuccessful (see Blumberg *et al.*, 1984, for review), the screening assays were carried out under conditions that would have failed to detect the activity of transient or highly lipophilic compounds.

The similarity in the activation of protein kinase C by diacylglycerol and by phorbol esters suggested that diacylglycerol was a possible candidate for the predicted endogenous analogue of the phorbol esters. To test this hypothesis, we examined the ability of the diacylglycerol derivative diolein to inhibit $^3$H-PDBu binding to the mouse brain apo-receptor reconstituted into PS (Sharkey *et al.*, 1984). Diolein inhibited binding by more than 90%. Scatchard analysis indicated that the decreased binding reflected an altered affinity for $^3$H-PDBu rather than a change in maximal binding (Fig. 2). The change in binding affinity could reflect either a general perturbation of the phospholipid environment into which the apo-receptor was reconstituted or specific competition at the binding site itself. For a competitive inhibitor, the change in apparent $^3$H-PDBu binding affinity as a function of diolein concentration should fit the relationship $K_a = K_d (1 + I/K_I)$, where $K_a$ is the apparent dissociation constant for $^3$H-PDBu in the presence of diolein, $K_d$ is the dissociation constant for $^3$H-PDBu in the absence of diolein, I is the concentration of diolein, and $K_I$ is the apparent dissociation constant for diolein. This relationship was, in fact, found, yielding values for $K_d$ and $K_I$ of 3.7 nM and 3.5 µg/ml, respectively. These values agree well with the $K_d$ of 3.1 nM for $^3$H-PDBu, determined by Scatchard analysis, and with the $K_I$ of 3.6 µg/ml, determined by competition at a fixed $^3$H-PDBu concentration, under these assay conditions. Further testable predictions are that diolein should interact stoichiometrically with the receptor and that it should bind at the same site on the protein as does PDBu.

The $K_I$ for diolein could represent either its concentration in aqueous solution or its concentration in the PS lipid phase into which the apo-receptor is reconstituted. The latter result is predicted, since diolein should be insoluble in aqueous solution and should thus be present in solution in the PS. To distinguish the two possibilities experimentally, the $K_I$ for diolein was determined as a function of the amount of PS used for reconstitution of the apo-receptor. Over a 400-fold range in PS concentration, the $K_I$ for diolein showed little variation in relation to PS (0.35–1.1% of the phospholipid) and a corresponding, marked variation in relation to volume (6.9–0.05 µg/ml). For $^3$H-PDBu, in contrast, the $K_I$ in relation to its aqueous concentration showed little variation with PS concentration, which is again the expected result, since only a few percent of this more hydrophilic ligand partition into the liposomes under these conditions (the concentration of $^3$H-PDBu in the liposomes is also essentially independent of the amount of PS under these conditions).

We compared a series of different diacylglycerol derivatives to determine which structural features were required for inhibition of $^3$H-PDBu binding. In addition to

Fig. 2. Scatchard analysis of specific $^3$H-phorbol 12,13-dibutyrate (PDBu) binding as a function of diolein concentration
Specific binding was measured in the presence of 960 μg/ml of phosphatidylserine (PS) and of diolein at ○, 0 μg/ml; ●, 1.5 μg/ml; ■, 3.0 μg/ml; and ▲, 12 μg/ml. From Sharkey *et al.* (1984)

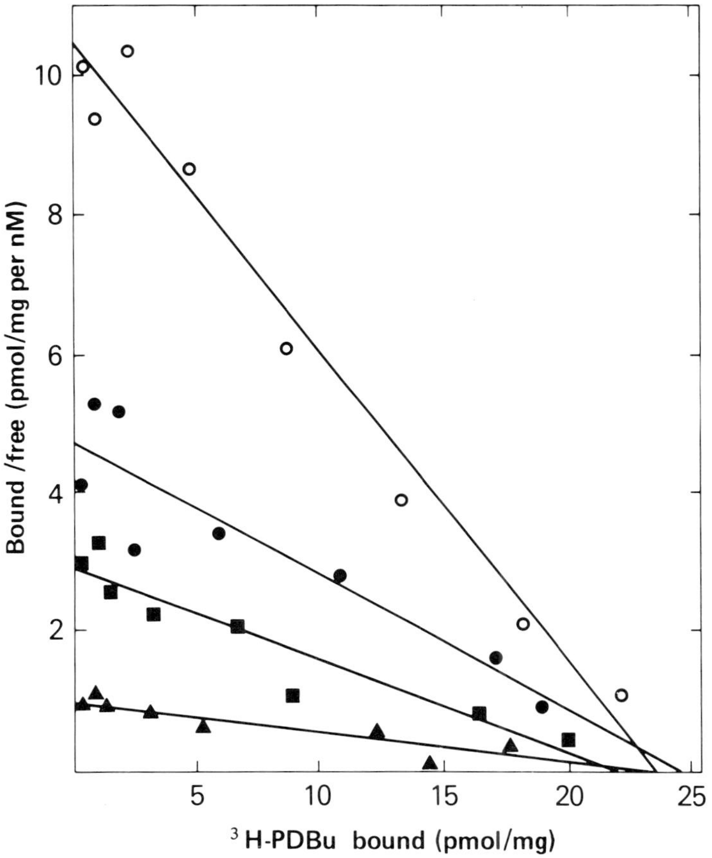


diolein, the symmetrically substituted glycerol derivatives with short, saturated fatty acid side chains (dicaproin, dicaprylin and dilaurin) were also active, whereas those with longer saturated side chains were not (Fig. 3). We interpret these findings as an indication that side chains in a disordered or fluid state at 37 °C may be required for maximal activity of the compounds.

Although diolein acts as a competitive inhibitor of $^3$H-PDBu binding, it is much less potent. If the $K_d$ for $^3$H-PDBu is expressed in terms of its actual concentration in the liposomes, a difference in affinities of $6 \times 10^4$ is obtained. For the homologous pair of compounds, phorbol 12,13-dilaurate and 1,2-glycerol-dilaurate, the difference is substantially smaller: $K_i$ values of 17 nM and 300 nM were obtained, respectively, using both ligands incorporated into mixed liposomes (see below). Whether both ligands incorporate with equal effectiveness is not known, however. Despite their

Fig. 3. Inhibition of specific $^3$H-phorbol 12,13-dibutyrate (PDBu) binding by glycerol derivatives Specific binding of $^3$H-PDBu was measured in the presence of 960 μ g/ml of phosphatidylserine (PS) and 160 μg/ml of the indicated derivatives. Adapted from Sharkey *et al.* (1984)

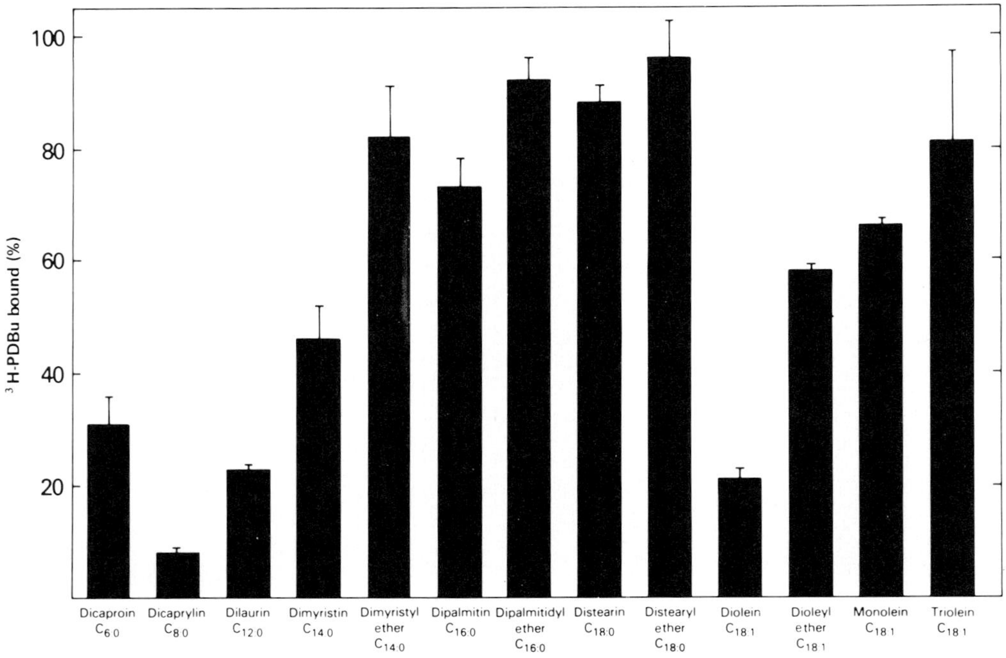


lower absolute potency, the effective concentrations of diacylglycerols do not appear to be unphysiological. Evidence, at least in the platelet system as described by Nishizuka and co-workers, suggests that diacylglycerols play a functional role as endogenous activators of protein kinase C (Kawahara *et al.,* 1980; Kaibuchi *et al.,* 1983; Sano *et al.,* 1983).

## ACTIVITY OF HIGHLY INSOLUBLE PHORBOL ESTERS

A continuing uncertainty in the analysis of phorbol ester structure-activity relations has been whether the receptor recognizes those phorbol ester molecules that are dissolved in the lipid bilayer or those that are free in aqueous solution. The indirect evidence so far available has provided some support for both viewpoints. On the one hand, derivatives more lipophilic than PMA, e.g., phorbol 12,13-didecanoate, are less potent, although they should partition more strongly into the membranes. On the other hand, since diacylglycerols, which are insoluble, compete for phorbol ester binding, the simplest model would be that the phorbol esters are also recognized after they dissolve in the lipid bilayer.

An experimental approach to this question was to synthesize a series of highly lipophilic phorbol derivatives—phorbol 12,13-dimyristate, phorbol 12,13-distearate and phorbol 12,13-dioleate. On the basis of aqueous solubilities of $2 \times 10^{-6}$ and $5 \times 10^{-8}$ M for PMA and phorbol 12,13-didecanoate, respectively, these derivatives would be expected to show aqueous solubilities too low to achieve an effective inhibitory concentration. Like diolein, however, these derivatives can be mixed in organic solvents with PS and be incorporated directly into the liposomes used to reconstitute the apo-receptor. The results obtained with all three derivatives were similar (Sharkey & Blumberg, 1984). When incorporated directly into the liposomes, they displayed apparent $K_d$ values of between 5 and 35 nM. When added to the aqueous phase of the binding assay, they only inhibited with apparent $K_d$ values of 3 to $>20$ μM. In contrast, for the more soluble phorbol 12,13-didecanoate, identical values were obtained by either route of addition.

The low activity of the highly hydrophilic phorbol esters when added to the aqueous phase presumably reflects their slow rate of transfer from phorbol ester micelles to the PS liposomes. Addition of low concentrations of detergent would be expected to accelerate the rate of transfer. In fact, incubation with 0.03% Triton X-100 overnight reduced the $K_i$ for phorbol 12,13-distearate (i.e., increased its apparent affinity) to 12.5 nM. In analogy with phospholipid exchange proteins, the phorbol ester binding protein from serum described by Shoyab and Todaro (1982) may be able to function similarly to promote equilibration.

The phorbol esters cause an apparent transfer of protein kinase C from the cytosolic to the membrane fraction. Recognition by the receptor of phorbol ester dissolved in the membranes suggests that the 'cytosolic receptor' is either loosely or transiently membrane-associated.

## HETEROGENEITY OF PHORBOL-ESTER BINDING AND ITS RELATION TO THE APO-RECEPTOR

Biological evidence for heterogeneity of phorbol ester receptors is suggested by different dose-response curves and structure-activity requirements for different biological responses, at least in certain systems. The subdivision of tumour promotion into first and second stages is a particularly cogent example. Additional examples are cited by Blumberg *et al.* (1983a). Direct evidence for heterogeneity of high-affinity phorbol ester binding has been obtained for mouse skin particulate preparations (Dunn & Blumberg, 1983), for NRK cells (unpublished observations) and, in unconfirmed studies, for myeloid cells (Colburn *et al.*, 1983). Preliminary reports also suggest the possible existence of distinct nuclear binding activity (Perella *et al.*, 1982).

The origin of the heterogeneity in phorbol ester binding remains to be determined. It could reflect multiple targets for the phorbol esters in addition to protein kinase C. Alternatively, it could reflect differential modification of protein kinase C, by proteolysis, phosphorylation or different lipid environments. Modulation of receptor affinity by variation of the phospholipid composition or the diacylglycerol content in the phospholipids has been described above. By maintaining heterogeneity of the lipid environment used for reconstitution, curved Scatchard plots can be obtained. For example, Scatchard plots of $^3$H-PDBu binding data for receptors reconstituted into liposomes of PS, 1.8% diolein in PS or a 1:1 mixture of the two types of liposomes were determined. The 1:1 mixture yielded a curved Scatchard plot fitting that predicted for reconstitution into the two distinct liposome populations. Similarly, addition of small amounts of PS (0.05 μg/ml) to the cytosol fraction from brain (which contains small amounts of phospholipid if not further fractionated) yielded a biphasic Scatchard plot, whereas an excess of PS yielded a linear plot.

A crucial unresolved issue is whether the heterogeneity in structure-activity relations which has been observed, and not simply the heterogeneity in $^3$H-PDBu binding affinity, can be generated from the apo-receptor in the presence of the appropriate lipid domain. A second issue is whether heterogeneity in lipid domain does in fact occur in particulate preparations or intact cells. The availability of photoaffinity ligands such as PaBB, described above, should provide a means of probing this microenvironment.

## GENERAL DISCUSSION

The convergence on two independent lines of research, analysis of phorbol ester binding and of protein kinase C, promises to foster rapid progress in understanding the initial events in the mechanism of action of the phorbol esters. The two approaches are complementary. On the one hand, the enzymatic studies permit characterization of the subsequent steps in the phorbol ester response pathway. On the other hand, the phorbol ester binding provides the best evidence for the functional role of protein kinase C in most systems and the best means for analysing the membrane-bound form of the enzyme.

As described above, an important unresolved issue is whether protein kinase C is the sole, functional phorbol ester apo-receptor or whether it is simply the quantitatively major form in the tissues examined. The antibiotic penicillin, for example, interacts specifically with half a dozen different, related proteins in bacteria (Blumberg & Strominger, 1974). For several of these proteins, penicillin binding leads independently to cell killing, and one such binding protein in *Escherichia coli* accounts for only 0.75% of the total penicillin bound (Spratt, 1977). Comparable, quantitatively minor phorbol ester binding activities would not have been detected. Indeed, for the special case of the resiniferonol derivative resiniferatoxin, the pharmacological evidence that it acts through a different receptor, albeit indirect, is quite compelling (Driedger & Blumberg, 1980).

Although the phorbol esters appear to be diacylglycerol analogues, it does not follow that the two classes of compound should function identically. First, whereas the phorbol esters are relatively stable, diacylglycerols are metabolized rapidly. The phorbol esters should, therefore, lead to abnormal, chronic stimulation of protein kinase C. Secondly, the hormonally-activated turnover of PI should generate diacylglycerol at the plasma membrane. The phorbol esters, in contrast, should be able to equilibrate with internal membranes in the cell. They may, therefore, cause an abnormal distribution of activated kinase; the altered distribution of kinase may result, in turn, in an altered pattern of phosphorylation. Thirdly, the endogenous generation of diacylglycerol is associated with an elevation of intracellular calcium ion, which can activate enzymes in addition to protein kinase C, e.g., myosin light-chain kinase. The phorbol esters do not elevate intracellular calcium ion (Tsien *et al.*, 1982). Fourthly, protein kinase C can be cleaved proteolytically to a 51 000 molecular weight active fragment which no longer requires phospholipids, calcium ion or diacylglycerols for activation and which no longer binds to membranes (Kishimoto *et al.*, 1983). The susceptibility to cleavage of protein kinase C is enhanced when the enzyme is in the activated state (Kishimoto *et al.*, 1983). Chronic activation of kinase C by phorbol esters may, therefore, lead to enhanced conversion to the constitutive, cytosolic form and again lead to an altered pattern of phosphorylation. This process, incidentally, could be involved in the reported anti-promoting affects of protease inhibitors.

The ability of the phospholipid component of the holo-receptor to regulate its binding affinity for the phorbol ester highlights another important difference between an exogenous and an endogenous ligand. A shift in $K_d$ for the phorbol esters simply means that a higher concentration of the phorbol ester must be added to achieve maximal stimulation. In contrast, for diacylglycerol generated in response to an external stimulus, a shift in binding affinity will result in a shift in the absolute level of activation of protein kinase C. A change in lipid environment could, therefore, regulate the coupling between external stimulus and cellular response.

Hecker (1968) reported that phorbol 12-acyl 13-acetate derivatives showed progressive loss of promoting activity for fatty acids longer than myristic acid. Similarly, Thielmann and Hecker (1969) observed decreased inflammatory and promoting activities for symmetrically substituted phorbol diesters with side chains longer than octanoic acid. On the basis of differences in the relative inflammatory and promoting activities of phorbol 12,13-dibutyrate as compared to phorbol 12,13-dimyristate, Scribner and Boutwell (1972) argued that these two responses were mediated through different mechanisms.

Results obtained with the highly lipophilic phorbol esters help to clarify these findings. Firstly, the lack of activity of highly lipophilic phorbol esters probably represents in part a pharmacological artefact, *viz*. that the lipophilic derivatives have failed to equilibrate over the time course of the assays. Secondly, even when the lipophilic derivatives are already incorporated into the lipid phase, they appear to be intrinsically less potent. The equivalent $K_d$ value for PDBu, were it to partition entirely into the lipid phase, would be 0.02 nM under the conditions in which phorbol 12,13-distearate (incorporated into the liposomes) yielded a $K_d$ of 9 nM.

The slow equilibration of lipophilic phorbol esters suggests a potential kinetic mechanism by which different phorbol esters could lead to different biological outcomes. Although the mechanism is speculative and may well be wrong, it is presented here in the hope of stimulating other groups to be alert to results related to its predictions.

*In vitro*, the phorbol esters induce association of protein kinase C with PS liposomes. In intact cells, likewise, phorbol esters cause the transfer of cytosolic protein kinase C to the particulate fraction. As we have suggested above, phorbol esters equilibrated with internal membranes of the cell such as those of the mitochondria or nucleus may cause the ectopic localization of protein kinase C to those sites. If the pattern of phosphorylation reflects the subcellular localization of the membrane-associated kinase, then different subcellular distributions of phorbol ester would lead to different phosphorylation profiles. Highly lipophilic phorbol esters might be expected to show not only a slower rate of transfer from phorbol-ester micelles to phospholipid bilayers but also a slower rate of transfer between bilayers. At early stages, therefore, they might show preferential localization in the plasma membrane as compared to internal membranes, relative to less lipophilic derivatives. In this context, it is perhaps worth noting that phorbol 12-retinoate 13-acetate, one of the paradigms for a second-stage tumour promoter, is among the most lipophilic of the commonly studied phorbol derivatives.

For the pharmacologist, a striking feature of the tumour promotion process is that it does not reflect simple equilibrium occupancy of a static receptor. Although PMA functions as a promoter when administered only once or twice a week, in experiments in which inhibitors are added together with PMA, the timing of the additions is important. For example, in experiments of Verma *et al.* (1979), addition of retinoic acid 24 hours after each PMA application caused no reduction in the incidence of papillomas, whereas administration one hour before each PMA application led to an 84% reduction. It would thus appear that processes are activated which reach a refractory stage fairly rapidly. The stimulation of ornithine decarboxylase by PMA may be a good example: it peaks at six to eight hours after PMA addition and is no longer inhibited by indomethacin added more than two hours after PMA application (Verma *et al.,* 1980). The relative rates at which processes are activated over a relatively short time scale may, therefore, be important.

A further argument for their potential importance is evidence, albeit limited, that some responses induced by the phorbol esters may be mutually antagonistic. In several systems, phorbol esters yield bell-shaped dose-response curves (Yamamoto & zur Hausen, 1979; Kopelovich & Bias, 1980). In two studies, simultaneous addition of PMA together with a second phorbol ester gave a reduced tumour yield compared to addition of PMA alone (e.g., Schmidt & Hecker, 1982). In macrophages, chemotaxis in response to PMA was blocked by addition of phorbol 12,13-diacetate, which by itself could not induce chemotaxis (Sturm *et al.,* 1983).

## ACKNOWLEDGEMENT

The work of K.L.L. was supported in part by Public Health Service Grant CA 07054, awarded by the National Cancer Institute.

## REFERENCES

Ashendel, C.L., Staller, J.M. & Boutwell, R.K. (1983) Protein kinase activity associated with a phorbol ester receptor purified from mouse brain. *Cancer Res.*, ***43***, 4333–4337

Blumberg, P.M. (1980) In vitro studies on the mode of action of the phorbol esters, potent tumour promoters. *Crit. Rev. Toxicol.*, ***8***, 153–234

Blumberg, P.M. & Strominger, J.L. (1974) Interaction of penicillin with the bacterial cell: penicillin-binding proteins and penicillin-sensitive enzymes. *Bacteriol. Rev.*, ***38***, 291–335

Blumberg, P.M., Delclos, K.B., Dunphy, W.G. & Jaken, S. (1982) *Specific binding of phorbol ester tumour promoters to mouse tissues and cultured cells.* In: Hecker, E., Fusenig, N.E., Kunz, W., Marks, F. & Thielmann, H.W., eds, *Carcinogenesis,* Vol. 7, *Cocarcinogenesis and Biological Effects of Tumour Promoters,* New York, Raven Press, pp. 519–535

Blumberg, P.M., Delclos, K.B., Dunn, J.A., Jaken, S., Leach, K.L. & Yeh, E. (1983a) Phorbol ester receptors and the *in vitro* effects of tumour promoters. *Ann. N.Y. Acad. Sci.*, ***407***, 303–315

Blumberg, P.M., Delclos, K.B. & Jaken, S. (1983b) *Tissue and species specificity for phorbol ester receptors.* In: Langenbach, R., Nesnow, S. & Rice, J.M., eds, *Organ and Species Specificity in Chemical Carcinogenesis,* New York, Plenum, pp. 201–229

Blumberg, P.M., Dunn, J.A., Jaken, S., Jeng, A.Y., Leach, K.L., Sharkey, N.A. & Yeh, E. (1984) *Specific receptors for phorbol ester tumour promoters and their involvement in biological responses.* In: Slaga, T.J., ed., *Mechanisms of Tumor Promotion,* Vol. 3, *Tumor Promotion and Cocarcinogenesis in Vitro,* Boca Raton FL, CRC Press, pp. 143–184

Brunner, J. & Richards, F.M. (1980) Analysis of membranes photolabeled with lipid analogs. *J. biol. Chem.*, ***255***, 3319–3329

Castagna, M., Takai, Y., Kaibuchi, K., Sano, K., Kikkawa, U. & Nishizuka, Y. (1982) Direct activation of calcium-activated, phospholipid-dependent protein kinase by tumour promoting phorbol esters. *J. biol. Chem.*, ***257***, 7847–7851

Colburn, N.H., Gindhart, T.D., Dalal, B. & Hegamyer, G.A. (1983) *The role of phorbol ester receptor binding in responses to promoters by mouse and human cells.* In: Langenbach, R., Nesnow, S. & Rice, J.M., eds, *Organ and Species Specificity in Chemical Carcinogenesis,* New York, Plenum, pp. 189–200

Delclos, K.B., Yeh, E. & Blumberg, P.M. (1983) Specific labeling of mouse brain membrane phospholipids with [20-$^3$H]phorbol 12-*p*-azidobenzoate 13-benzoate, a photolabile phorbol ester. *Proc. natl Acad. Sci. USA*, ***80***, 3054–3058

Diamond, L., O'Brien, T.G. & Baird, W.M. (1980) Tumor promoters and the mechanism of tumor promotion. *Adv. Cancer Res.*, ***32***, 1–74

Driedger, P.E. & Blumberg, P.M. (1980) Different biological targets for resiniferatoxin and phorbol 12-myristate 13-acetate. *Cancer Res.*, ***40***, 1400–1404

Dunn, J.A. & Blumberg, P.M. (1983) Specific binding of [20-$^3$H] 12-deoxyphorbol 13-isobutyrate to phorbol ester receptor subclasses in mouse skin particulate preparations. *Cancer Res.*, ***43***, 4632–4637

Dunphy, W.G., Delclos, K.B. & Blumberg, P.M. (1980) Characterization of specific binding of [$^3$H]phorbol 12,13-dibutyrate and [$^3$H]phorbol 12-myristate 13-acetate to mouse brain. *Cancer Res.*, ***40***, 3635–3641

Dunphy, W.G., Kochenburger, R.J., Castagna, M. & Blumberg, P.M. (1981) Kinetics and subcellular localization of specific [$^3$H]phorbol 12,13-dibutyrate binding by mouse brain. *Cancer Res.*, ***41***, 2640–2647

Esumi, M. & Fujiki, H. (1983) Sphingomyelin is a possible constituent of binding sites for the tumor promoters phorbol ester, indole alkaloids, and polyacetates. *Biochem. biophys. Res. Commun.*, ***112***, 709–716

Hecker, E. (1968) Cocarcinogenic principles from the seed oil of *Croton tiglium* and from other Euphorbiaceae. *Cancer Res.*, ***28***, 2338–2349

Hecker, E., Fusenig, N.E., Kunz, W., Marks, F. & Thielmann, H.W., eds (1982) *Carcinogenesis—A Comprehensive Survey,* Vol. 7, *Cocarcinogenesis and Biological Effects of Tumor Promoters,* New York, Raven Press

Horowitz, A.D., Greenebaum, E. & Weinstein, I.B. (1981) Identification of receptors for phorbol ester tumor promoters in intact mammalian cells and of an inhibitor of receptor binding in biological fluids. *Proc. natl Acad. Sci. USA*, ***78***, 2315–2319

Kaibuchi, K., Takai, Y., Sawamura, M., Hoshijima, M., Fujikara, T. & Nishizuka, Y. (1983) Synergistic functions of protein phosphorylation and calcium mobilization in platelet activation. *J. biol. Chem.*, ***258***, 6701–6704

Kawahara, Y., Takai, Y., Minakuchi, R., Sano, K. & Nishizuka, Y. (1980) Phospholipid turnover as a possible transmembrane signal for protein phosphorylation during human platelet activation by thrombin. *Biochem. biophys. Res. Commun.*, ***97***, 309–317

Kikkawa, U., Takai, Y., Minakuchi, R., Inohara, S. & Nishizuka, Y. (1982) Calcium-activated, phospholipid dependent protein kinase from rat brain. Subcellular distribution, purification, and properties. *J. biol. Chem.*, ***257***, 13341–13348

Kishimoto, A., Kajikawa, N., Shiota, M. & Nishizuka, Y. (1983) Proteolytic activation of calcium-activated, phospholipid-dependent protein kinase by calcium-dependent neutral protease. *J. biol. Chem.*, ***258***, 1156–1164

Kopelovich, L. & Bias, N.E. (1980) Tumor promoter induces loss of anchorage dependence in human skin fibroblasts from individuals genetically predisposed to cancer. *Exp. Cell Res.*, ***48***, 207–217

Kraft, A.S. & Anderson, W.B. (1983) Phorbol esters increase the amount of $Ca^{++}$, phospholipid-dependent protein kinase associated with plasma membrane. *Nature*, ***301***, 621–623

Kraft, A.S., Anderson, W.B., Cooper, H.L. & Sando, J.J. (1982) Decrease in cytosolic calcium/phospholipid-dependent protein kinase activity following phorbol ester treatment of EL4 thymoma cells. *J. biol. Chem.*, ***257***, 13193–13196

Leach, K.L., James, M.L. & Blumberg, P.M. (1983) Characterization of a specific phorbol ester aporeceptor in mouse brain cytosol. *Proc. natl Acad. Sci. USA*, ***80***, 4208–4212

Niedel, J.E., Kuhn, L.J. & Vandenbark, G.R. (1983) Phorbol diester receptor copurifies with protein kinase C. *Proc. natl Acad. Sci. USA*, ***80***, 36–40

Perella, F.W., Ashendel, C.L. & Boutwell, R.K. (1982) Specific high affinity binding of the phorbol ester tumor promoter 12-*O*-tetradecanoyl-phorbol-13-acetate to isolated nuclei and nuclear macromolecules in mouse epidermis. *Cancer Res.*, ***42***, 3496–3501

Puszkin, E.G. & Zucker, M.B. (1973) Enhancement of platelet and muscle actomyosin ATPase activity and superprecipitation by the tumor promoter 12-*O*-tetradecanoyl-phorbol-13-acetate (PMA). *Nature-New Biol.*, ***245***, 277–280

Quay, S.C., Radhakrishnan, R. & Khorana, H.G. (1981) Incorporation of photosensitive fatty acids into phospholipids of *Escherichia coli* and irradiation-dependent cross-linking of phospholipids to membrane proteins. *J. biol. Chem.*, ***256***, 4444–4449

Sando, J.J. & Young, M.C. (1983) Identification of high-affinity phorbol ester receptor in cytosol of EL4 thymoma cells: requirement for calcium, magnesium, and phospholipids. *Proc. natl Acad. Sci. USA*, ***80***, 2642–2646

Sano, K., Takai, Y., Yamanishi, J. & Nishizuka, Y. (1983) A role of calcium-activated phospholipid-dependent protein kinase in human platelet activation. Comparison of thrombin and collagen actions. *J. biol. Chem.*, ***258***, 2010–2013

Schmidt, R. & Hecker, E. (1982) *Simple phorbol esters as inhibitors of tumor promotion by TPA in mouse skin.* In: Hecker, E., Fusenig, N.E., Kunz, W., Marks, F. & Thielmann, H.W., eds, *Carcinogenesis,* Vol. 7, *Cocarcinogenesis and Biological Effects of Tumor Promoters,* New York, Raven Press, pp. 57–63

Scribner, J.D. & Boutwell, R.K. (1972) Inflammation and tumor promotion: selective protein induction in mouse skin by tumor promoters. *Eur. J. Cancer*, ***8***, 617–621

Sharkey, N.A. & Blumberg, P.M. (1984) Highly lipophilic phorbol esters as inhibitors of specific [$^{3}$H]phorbol 12,13-dibutyrate binding. *Cancer Res.* (in press)

Sharkey, N.A., Leach, K.L. & Blumberg, P.M. (1984) Competitive inhibition by diacylglycerol of specific phorbol ester binding. *Proc. natl Acad. Sci. USA*, ***81***, 607–610

Shoyab, M. & Todaro, G.J. (1982) Partial purification and characterization of a binding protein for biologically active phorbol and ingenol esters from murine sera. *J. biol. Chem.*, ***257***, 439–445

Snyder, S.H., Pasternak, G.W. & Pert, C.B. (1975) *Opiate receptor mechanisms.* In: Iverson, L.L., Iverson, S.D. & Snyder, S.H., eds, *Handbook of Psychopharmacology,* Vol. 5, New York, Plenum, pp. 329–360

Spratt, B.G. (1977) Properties of the penicillin-binding proteins of *Escherichia coli K12*. *Eur. J. Biochem.*, ***72***, 341–352

Sturm, R.J., Smith, B.M., Lane, R.W., Laskin, D.L., Harris, L.S. & Carchman, R.A. (1983) Antagonist of phorbol ester receptor-mediated chemotaxis in mouse peritoneal macrophages. *Cancer Res.*, ***43***, 4552–4556

Takai, Y., Kishimoto, A. & Nishizuka, Y. (1982) *Calcium and phospholipid turnover as transmembrane signaling for protein phosphorylation.* In: Cheung, W.Y., ed., *Calcium and Cell Function,* Vol. 2, New York, Academic Press, pp. 385–412

Thielmann, H.W. & Hecker, E. (1969) *Beziehungen zwischen der Struktur von Phorbolderivaten und ihren entzündlichen und tumorpromovierenden Eigenschaften.* In: Schmidt, C.G., ed., *Fortschritte der Krebsforschung,* Stuttgart-New York, Schattauer, pp. 171–179

Tsien, R.Y., Pozzan, T. & Rink, T.J. (1982) T-cell mitogens cause early changes in cytoplasmic free $Ca^{++}$ and membrane potential in lymphocytes. *Nature*, ***295***, 68–70

Verma, A.K., Shapas, B.G., Rice, H.M. & Boutwell, R.K. (1979) Correlation of the inhibition by retinoids of tumor promoter-induced mouse epidermal ornithine decarboxylase activity and of skin tumor promotion. *Cancer Res.*, ***39***, 419–425

Verma, A.K., Ashendel, C.L. & Boutwell, R.K. (1980) Inhibition by prostaglandin synthesis inhibitors of the induction of epidermal ornithine decarboxylase activity, the accumulation of prostaglandins, and the tumor promotion caused by 12-*O*-tetradecanoylphorbol-13-acetate. *Cancer Res.*, ***40***, 308–315

Yamamoto, N. & zur Hausen, H. (1979) Tumor promoter TPA enhances transformation of human leukocytes by Epstein-Barr virus. *Nature*, ***280***, 244–245

# A PHORBOL ESTER-BINDING INHIBITORY FACTOR FROM HUMAN PLACENTA. PARTIAL PURIFICATION, CHARACTERIZATION AND BIOLOGICAL EFFECTS

E. HAMEL & H. YAMASAKI

*International Agency for Research on Cancer, 69372 Lyon Cedex 08, France*

J.L. TAYOT

*Institut Merieux, Marcy-l'Etoile, France*

## SUMMARY

A factor which inhibits the binding of $^{3}$H-phorbol-12,13-dibutyrate (PDBu) on different types of cells has been partially purified from human placenta. This factor, phorbol ester binding inhibitory factor (PEBIF), is sensitive to pepsin, but resistant to trypsin, heat and acid (pH 3) treatments and can be precipitated by 80% ethanol with no loss of activity. Inhibition occurs both at 37 °C and 4 °C and is rapid and reversible. Inhibition on human epithelial cells (FL), on mouse erythroleukaemia cells (FELC clone 19-10) and on rat liver cells (IAR clone 6-1 and clone 20) is non-competitive, whereas on IAR clone 6 and clone 6-7 it is competitive. Differentiation of FELC induced by hexamethylene bisacetamide (HMBA) can be inhibited by 12-*O*-tetradecanoyl phorbol-13-acetate (TPA) only if TPA-sensitive cells are used, and no inhibition was observed with TPA-resistant cells. PEBIF can also inhibit the differentiation induced by HMBA of TPA-sensitive cells and has no effect on the differentiation of TPA-resistant cells. The extent of inhibition of PDBu binding by PEBIF was similar in these two clones. Like TPA, PEBIF can increase 2-deoxyglucose uptake in mouse fibroblasts (BALB/3T3 cells). Thus, TPA and PEBIF share two biological responses; however, PEBIF failed to mimic other TPA effects, such as induction of Epstein-Barr virus from Raji cells, inhibition of intercellular communication and induction of differentiation of human promyelocytic leukaemia cells (HL-60).

These data suggest that this factor may play a role in the regulation of cell differentiation and/or in the modulation of carcinogenesis.

## INTRODUCTION

In-vitro studies on the mechanism of action of tumour-promoting phorbol esters have suggested that these compounds interact with a variety of cells at specific binding sites (Weinstein *et al.*, 1979). Recently, the existence of high-affinity, specific receptors for biologically active phorbol esters in a variety of tissue culture cells and in animal tissues using $^{3}$H-phorbol-12,13-dibutyrate ($^{3}$H-PDBu) as a ligand has been reported (Shoyab & Todaro, 1981; Blumberg *et al.*, 1982). Further characterization of the binding sites revealed that the phorbol ester receptors copurify with the phospholipid-sensitive calcium ion-dependent protein kinase (Ashendel *et al.*, 1983; Niedel *et al.*, 1983), and 12-*O*-tetradecanoyl phorbol 13-acetate (TPA), the most potent tumour promoter, and related tumour promoters have been shown to activate this enzyme in the presence of calcium and phospholipid (Castagna *et al.*, 1982). Thus, it has been suggested that protein kinase C is the phorbol ester receptor (Ashendel *et al.*, 1983).

Since the interaction of phorbol esters with the cellular membrane is an important determinant of their subsequent action in the cells, we tried to find a physiological factor that modulates the binding of phorbol esters to the receptors and influences the biological effects of phorbol esters. We chose human placenta as a source and report here the partial purification, the characterization and some biological effects of a placental factor that can inhibit $^{3}$H-PDBu binding on different types of cell.

## MATERIALS AND METHODS

### *Chemicals*

TPA and PDBu were purchased from Chemicals for Cancer Research (Eden Prairie, MN, USA). $^{3}$H-PDBu (13–17 Ci/mmol), [2-$^{3}$H]-deoxy-D-glucose (8.2 Ci/mmol) and $^{32}$P-adenosine triphosphate (8–10 Ci/mmol) were purchased from New England Nuclear Corp. (Boston, MA, USA). CM Sephadex and G100 Sephadex were obtained from Pharmacia Fine Chemicals; Con A Sepharose, phosphatidylserine, diolein and histone from Sigma Chemical Co (St Louis, MO, USA). Hexamethylene bisacetamide (HMBA) was synthesized by Dr K. Shibata of Osaka City University, Osaka, Japan.

### *PDBu binding assay*

Binding of $^{3}$H-PDBu to intact FL, BALB 3T3 and rat liver epithelial cells was assayed directly in Linbro culture plates (Blumberg *et al.*, 1982). Specific binding of $^{3}$H-PDBu to Friend erythroleukaemia cells (FELC) was measured by the filtration assay method, as described previously (Yamasaki *et al.*, 1982).

### *Measurement of cell differentiation*

In order to determine differentiation of FELC, $10^5$ cells were inoculated into the well of a Linbro tissue culture plate containing 1 mL of culture medium in the presence of 4 mM HMBA, and the percentage of haemoglobin-containing cells was determined by benzidine reaction after four and five days, as described previously (Yamasaki *et al.*, 1982).

### *Measurement of 2-deoxy-D-glucose uptake*

2-Deoxy-D-glucose uptake by BALB 3T3 cells was assayed directly in 60-mm Petri dishes. Cells in confluency were washed twice with glucose-free Hank's solution pre-warmed to the assay temperature and then incubated at 37 °C for 10 min with the same solution containing 0.5 μCi/mL of $^3$H-2-deoxy-D-glucose. The cells were then washed three times with ice-cold Hank's solution, drained and taken up directly into 1.0 mL trichloroacetic acid (5%). The radioactivity was counted in a liquid scintillation counter.

## RESULTS

### *Purification and characterization of phorbol ester binding inhibitory factor (PEBIF)*

Purification of PEBIF from α, β and γ globulin- and haemoglobin-deprived human placental blood fraction (Tayot *et al.*, 1981) is summarized in Table 1. The detailed procedure of purification is reported elsewhere (Hamel *et al.*, 1984). Each purification step was followed by measurement of $ID_{50}$, defined as the concentration of protein per mL required to produce 50% binding of $^3$H-PDBu to FL cells. We obtained a 133-fold purification of PEBIF with an $ID_{50}$ of 0.2 mg protein/mL, as compared with 26.7 mg protein/mL for the supernatant after removal of γ globulin, haemoglobin and α and β globulin.

PEBIF is stable at pH 3 and is not inactivated by heating in boiling water for 20 min. Thus, it differs from the heat- and acid-labile binding protein for biologically

Table 1. Purification of PEBIF from human placenta extract

| Step | | $ID_{50}$ [a] (mg protein/ml) | Purification −fold |
|---|---|---|---|
| I | Supernatant after removal of γ globulin, haemoglobin and α and β globulin | 26.7 | 1 |
| II | Alcohol, 75%, pH 3 | 2.3 | 12 |
| III | CM Sephadex | 1 | 27 |
| IV | Con-A Sepharose | 0.3 | 90 |
| V | Sephadex G 100 | 0.2 | 133 |

[a] Concentration of protein/mL required to produce 50% binding of $^3$H-PDBu to FL cells

Fig. 1. A. Time course of $^3$H-PDBu binding to FL cells (●) and inhibition by PEBIF (□) (7.8 mg protein/mL, step II concentrated by 80% ethanol) added 30 min and 120 min after $^3$H-PDBu incubation for the indicated period.
B. Time course of PEBIF inhibition (●) (3.4 mg protein/mL, step II) of $^3$H-PDBu binding to FL cells and reversibility of inhibition. At 120 min, PEBIF was removed and the binding assay was carried out at different times (□).

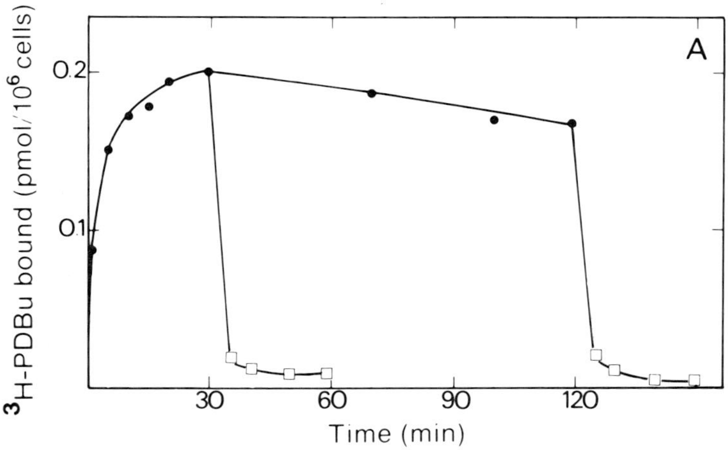


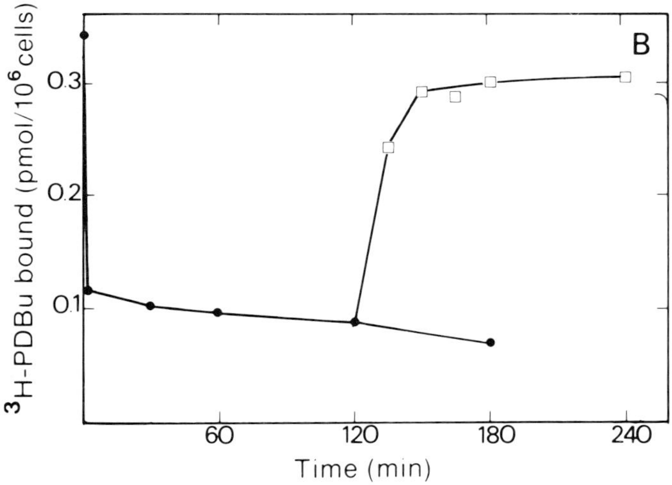


active phorbol esters reported by Shoyab and Todaro (1981) and from the heat-labile factor purified by Horowitz *et al.* (1981). Its molecular weight, determined by gel filtration (Sephadex G75), is 52 000 daltons.

## *Nature of $^3$H-PDBu binding inhibition by PEBIF*

PEBIF can interfere with the process of $^3$H-PDBu binding to its receptors and/or replace already bound $^3$H-PDBu molecules, depending on whether it is added before or after incubation (data not shown). When it was added to a culture in which the

PDBu binding was at equilibrium, there was rapid removal of PDBu from FL cells, both at 37 °C (Fig. 1A) and at 4 °C (data not shown). The inhibition was readily reversible when the cells were washed to remove PEBIF (Fig. 1B). PEBIF can also inhibit PDBu binding to a particulate membranous fraction and to glutaraldehyde-fixed FL cells to the same extent as in native FL cells (data not shown).

*Kinetics of PEBIF action on $^3$H-PDBu binding*

Kinetic studies of FL cells have shown a reduction in the number of available binding sites from $4 \times 10^5$ per cell in the control to $2.4 \times 10^5$ per cell and to $1.5 \times 10^5$ per cell in the presence of 0.9 mg protein/mL and 2.6 mg protein/mL of PEBIF (step

Fig. 2. Effect of phorbol-12,13-dibutyrate (PDBu) concentration on the binding of PDBu on FL cells (A) or on IAR 6 cells (B) in the presence or absence of phorbol ester binding inhibitory factor (PEBIF) (Scatchard analysis)
A. (□) No PEBIF; (●) 0.8 mg protein/mL PEBIF; (△) 2.2 mg protein/mL PEBIF
B. (□) No PEBIF; (●) 0.9 mg protein/mL PEBIF; (△) 2.6 mg protein/mL PEBIF. PEBIF used was from purification step II.

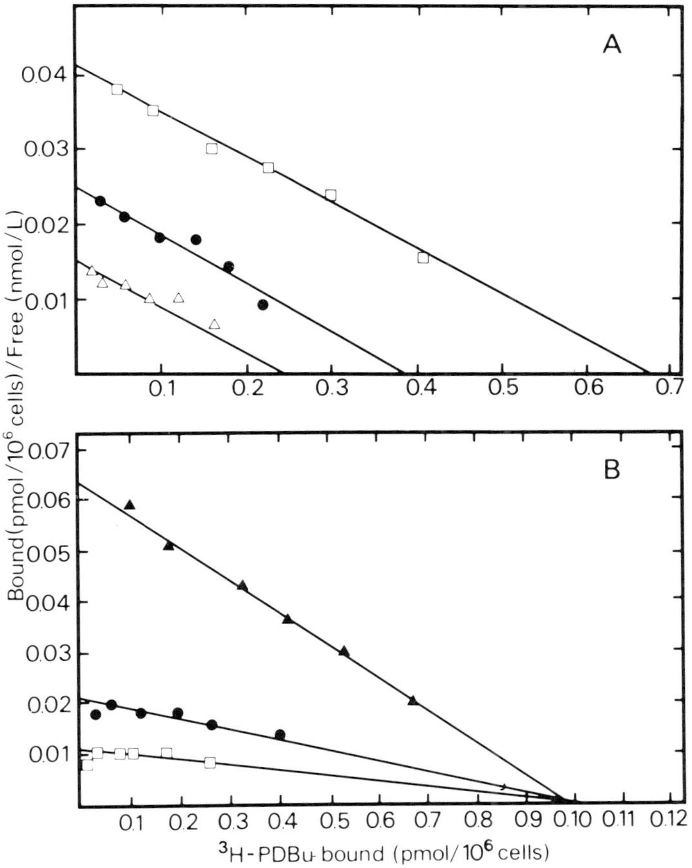

II), respectively. In all three cases, the dissociation constants (Kd) were in the vicinity of 16 nM (Fig. 2A). Similar kinetics have been observed for FELC clone 19-10 with a similar extent of inhibition by PEBIF (data not shown).

Kinetic studies on rat liver cell lines established by Dr Montesano (IARC), IAR 6-1 and IAR 20, also indicate non-competitive inhibition by PEBIF (data not shown), whereas kinetics of clones 6 and 6–7 show a decrease of the affinity of receptors from 14.4 nM in the control to 40 nM and 88 nM for IAR 6 cells (Fig. 2B) and from 11.1 nM in the control to 25.4 nM and 73 nM for IAR 6-7 cells with 0.8 mg protein/mL and 2.2 mg protein/mL of PEBIF (step II), respectively, with a constant number of available binding sites ($5.6 \times 10^5$ sites/IAR 6 cells and $2.9 \times 10^5$ sites/IAR 6-7 cells). These results are characteristic of competitive inhibition of binding.

## *Effect of PEBIF fraction on FELC differentiation*

In order to determine whether PEBIF acts as an endogenous agonist with properties similar to those of the biologically active phorbol esters, we studied its effects on

Fig. 3. Effect of 12-*O*-tetradecanoylphorbol 13-acetate (TPA) and phorbol ester binding inhibitory factor (PEBIF) on differentiation and $^3$H-phorbol-12,13-dibutyrate ($^3$H-PDBu) binding of Friend erythroleukaemia (FELC) cells
FELC ($10^5$ cells/mL) (clone TS 19-10, ●; clone TR 19-9, □) were cultured with 4 mM hexamethylene bisacetamide for 4 days, and cell differentiation was scored by benzidine positivity (B+). The indicated amounts of PEBIF (Step III) (A) or TPA (B) were added at the same time as hexamethylene bisacetamide. The binding assay on FELC cells ($10^6$ cells/mL) was carried out by the filtration method in the presence of different amounts of PEBIF (step III) and % inhibition of specific PDBu binding was calculated (C). Symbols are the same as those for A and B.

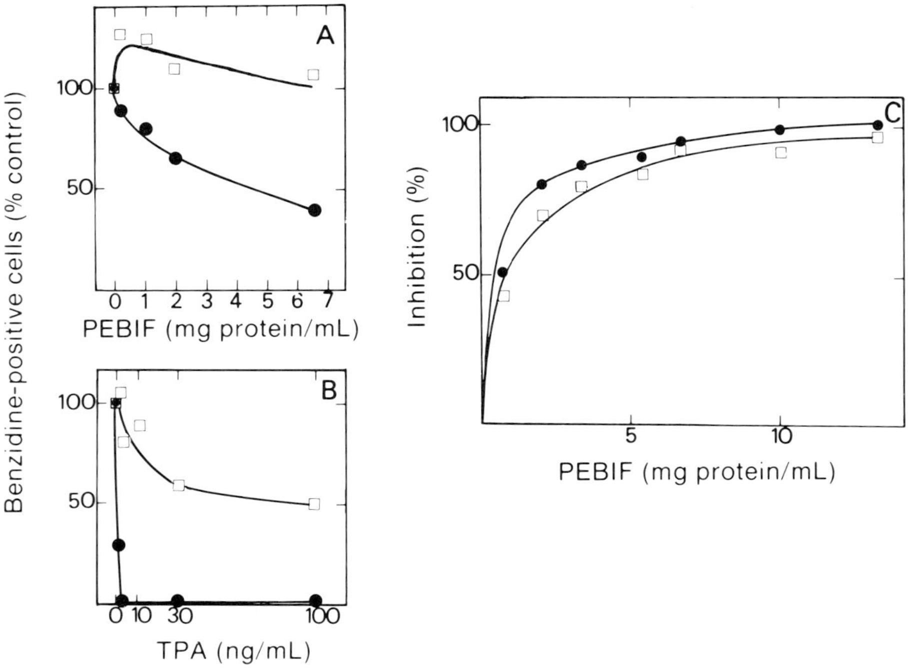

inhibition of the induced differentiation of mouse erythroleukaemia cells (FELC), TPA-sensitive clone 19-10, and on TPA-resistant cells, clone 19-9. Differentiation of FELC induced by HMBA can be inhibited by TPA only if TPA-sensitive cells are used with 3 ng TPA, whereas much less inhibition is observed with TPA-resistant cells with 100 ng TPA. Partially purified PEBIF (step III) also inhibits the differentiation induced by HMBA of TPA-sensitive cells and has no effect on the differentiation of TPA-resistant cells (Fig. 3A, B).

Since these two clones have about the same number of phorbol ester receptors, with no difference in their affinity, we suggested that the mechanism of TPA resistance lies at a point beyond the binding of phorbol esters (Yamasaki *et al.*, 1982). The extent of inhibition of $^{3}$H-PDBu binding by PEBIF was similar in TPA-sensitive and -resistant FELC (Fig. 3C), again suggesting that TPA resistance is determined after direct membrane interactions.

*Effect of PEBIF fraction on 2-deoxy-D-glucose uptake*

TPA (100 ng) induced four-fold stimulation of 2-deoxy-D-glucose uptake, while partially purified PEBIF (step III, 3 mg protein) stimulated the uptake by seven to eight fold in confluent cultures of mouse fibroblast BALB 3T3 cells.

## DISCUSSION

We used human placenta from which to purify (by 133-fold) a ‘phorbol ester binding inhibitory factor’, since many growth factors are known to be present in that tissue. Heat and acid stability make this factor different from the heat- and acid-labile binding protein for biologically active phorbol esters reported by Shoyab and Todaro (1981) and from the heat-labile factor purified by Horowitz *et al.* (1981). The inhibition observed with PEBIF of $^{3}$H-PDBu binding on FL cells is rapid, temperature-independent and reversible, indicating that PEBIF exerts its inhibitory effect without cellular metabolism, receptor destruction, complex alterations in membrane structure or alteration in macromolecular synthesis. The same degree of inhibition of binding on native FL cells, on FL cells fixed with glutaraldehyde and on particulate membrane fraction from FL cells indicates that neither intact cells nor cellular metabolism nor intact membrane fluidity nor a change in the membrane protein micro-environment of PDBu receptors is required for the action of PEBIF. Kinetic studies show that PEBIF does not act like a binding protein for PDBu, which would compete with inhibition of PDBu binding to cells; however, competitive inhibition of binding on IAR 6 and 6-7 cells suggests a possible direct interaction with at least one class of phorbol ester receptors. In the biological model of FELC differentiation, PEBIF acts in the same way as TPA, although the non-competitive nature of PEBIF inhibition of $^{3}$H-PDBu binding indicates an indirect interaction of PEBIF with phorbol ester receptors. It is known that the effect of TPA on FELC differentiation is not mediated by cytotoxicity, and it remains to be determined whether the PEBIF fraction exerts its inhibitory effect through cytotoxicity, through more specific modulation of gene expression (like TPA), or through another, unknown mechanism. A further similarity between the PEBIF fraction and TPA is that both can stimulate 2-deoxyglucose uptake by rat embryo fibroblast BALB 3T3 cells.

Recent results show that the calcium-activated phospholipid-dependent protein kinase can be co-purified with the phorbol ester receptors, and that tumour-promoting phorbol esters bind to a homogeneous preparation of protein kinase C (Ashendel *et al.,* 1983; Niedel *et al.,* 1983) and directly activate this kinase in the presence of calcium and phospholipid (Castagna *et al.,* 1982). We are investigating whether the PEBIF fraction can interact with this enzyme: preliminary results show that the fraction can modulate the kinase C activity from mouse brain. Further studies are needed to elucidate that interaction and should help to determine its physiological significance, if any.

## REFERENCES

Ashendel, C.L., Staller, J.M. & Boutwell, R.K. (1983) Identification of a calcium- and phospholipid-dependent phorbol ester binding activity in the soluble fraction of mouse tissues. *Biochem. biophys. Res. Commun.,* ***111,*** 340–345

Blumberg, P.M., Delclos, K.B., Dunphy, W.G. & Jaken, S. (1982) *Specific binding of phorbol ester tumor promoters to mouse tissue and cultured cells.* In: Hecker, E., Fusening, N.E., Kunz, W., Marks, F. & Thielmann, H.W., eds, *Carcinogenesis,* Vol. 7, *Cocarcinogenesis and Biological Effects of Tumor Promoters,* New York, Raven Press, pp. 519–535

Castagna, M., Takai, Y., Kaibuchi, K., Sanom, K., Kikkawa, U. & Nishizuka, Y. (1982) Direct activation of calcium-activated phospholipid-dependent protein kinase by tumor promoting phorbol esters. *J. biol. Chem.,* ***257,*** 7847–7851

Hamel, E., Martel, N., Tayot, J.L. & Yamasaki, H. (1984) Characterization of a human placental factor which inhibits specific binding of phorbol esters to cultured cells. *Carcinogenesis* ***5,*** 15–21

Horowitz, A.D., Greenebaum, E. & Weinstein, I.B. (1981) Identification of receptors for phorbol ester tumor-promoters in intact mammalian cells and of an inhibitor of receptor binding in biologic fluids. *Proc. natl Acad. Sci. USA,* ***78,*** 2315–2319

Niedel, J.E., Kuhn, L.J. & Vandenbark, G.R. (1983) Phorbol diester receptor copurifies with protein kinase C. *Proc. natl Acad. Sci. USA,* ***80,*** 36–40

Shoyab, M. & Todaro, G.J. (1981) Partial purification and characterization of a binding protein for biologically active phorbol and ingenol esters from murine sera. *J. biol. Chem.,* ***257,*** 439–445

Tayot, J.L., Grandgeorge, M., Blanc, P., Gattel, P., Tardy, M., Paturel, J., Pla, J., Debrus, A., Liautaud, J., Plan, R. & Peyron, L. (1981) *Chromatographie industrielle, production et qualité de l'albumine humaine d'origine placentaire.* In: Fondation Merieux, ed., *Cooperation internationale et derives sanguins,* Talloires/Lyon

Weinstein, I.B., Lee, L.S., Fisher, P.B., Mufson, R.A. & Yamasaki, H. (1979) Action of phorbol esters in culture: Mimicry of transformation altered differentiation and effects on cell membranes. *J. supramol. Struct.,* ***12,*** 195–208

Yamasaki, H., Drevon, C. & Martel, N. (1982) Specific binding of phorbol esters to Friend erythroleukemia cells. General properties, down regulation and relationship to cell differentiation. *Carcinogenesis,* ***3,*** 905–910

# SPECIFIC LIPID COMPONENTS IN MEMBRANE RECEPTORS OF 12-*O*-TETRADECANOYLPHORBOL-13-ACETATE AS REVEALED BY DIRECT PHOTOAFFINITY LABELLING

M. HERGENHAHN & E. HECKER

*Institute of Biochemistry, German Cancer Research Center*
*6900 Heidelberg, Federal Republic of Germany*

## SUMMARY

The use of [20-$^{3}$H]-12-*O*-tetradecanoylphorbol-13-acetate ($^{3}$H-TPA) as a direct photoaffinity probe of receptors was investigated. When membrane receptors in a particulate fraction from mouse brain were loaded with the high-affinity agonist $^{3}$H-TPA, irradiation of such preparations with ultraviolet (UV) light resulted in specific irreversible binding of the label to the membrane lipids phosphatidylethanolamine (PE) and phosphatidylserine (PS); evidence for labelling of proteins was lacking. The labelled lipids were tentatively identified by co-chromatography; they corresponded to selected reference lipids obtained by photoaffinity labelling. When a variety of natural and synthetic reference lipids was irradiated in the presence of $^{3}$H-TPA, photoadducts were obtained primarily from natural lipids containing unsaturated acyl chains in position 2. The synthetic 1,2-dipalmitoyl derivatives of phosphatidylcholine (PC), PE and phosphatidyl glycerol were refractory. When the photoadducts from PC and PE were treated with phospholipases $A_2$ and C, the chromatographic pattern of cleavage products obtained was in accordance with that of phospholipids carrying the $^{3}$H-TPA label on the acyl moiety in the 2-position. Since previous evidence had suggested that a lipid-protein complex was the phorbol ester receptor, it may, therefore, be concluded that the receptor(s) contain PE and PS in specific interaction with protein(s). Accordingly, PE- and PS-dependent enzymes (or other proteins) are considered prime candidates for phorbol ester receptors.

## INTRODUCTION

Diterpenes of the phorbol ester type are the most active initiation promoters presently known. Moreover, as inducers or modulators, they may influence many important cellular functions (for overviews see Hecker *et al.*, 1982). Considerable efforts are directed to the isolation and characterization of phorbol ester receptors, which were described first by Driedger and Blumberg (1980). Subsequent studies have demonstrated sensitivity of the receptors to heat and papain (Dunphy *et al.*, 1980; Schmidt & Hecker, 1982), to trypsin (Hergenhahn & Hecker, 1982; Schmidt & Hecker, 1982), to sulfhydryl reagents (Schmidt & Hecker, 1982), to phospholipase $A_2$ (Dunphy *et al.*, 1980; Hergenhahn & Hecker, 1982; Schmidt & Hecker, 1982) and to phospholipase C (Hergenhahn & Hecker, 1982; Schmidt & Hecker, 1982; Jones & Murray, 1983). Evidence for degradation of receptors in parallel with lipid peroxidation was also presented (Delclos & Blumberg, 1982). This body of evidence seems to suggest that phorbol ester receptor(s) are proteinaceous and dependent on a lipid environment.

Photoaffinity labelling is a powerful approach to characterization of receptor components (Bailey & Knowles, 1977). Consequently, we have investigated methods of labelling receptors irreversibly with appropriate phorbol esters.

An obvious group of compounds to be tested is the phorbol esters with a photoactivatable group in one or both of the acyl chains. However, there is evidence that suggests 'anchoring' of phorbol esters in the lipid bilayer of membranes *via* the 12-*O*-acyl chain of the phorbol moiety (Pečar *et al.*, 1982; Hergenhahn *et al.*, 1983). Furthermore, degradation studies of the phorbol ester receptors using hydrophilic agents support the notion that part of the receptor is exposed to a hydrophilic environment or is sensitive to changes in the hydrophilic area of the membrane. Thus, a photoreactive group in the more hydrophilic phorbol moiety of the esters may be expected to label preferentially accessible protein structures in its vicinity. The $\alpha,\beta$-unsaturated keto function in the five-membered ring, which is present inherently in every phorbol ester, may be considered such a group. Photoactivation of these chromophores (Bailey & Knowles, 1977) in phorbol esters at about 300–330 nm would lead to an excited $n \rightarrow \pi^*$ state, which might form covalent bonds with appropriate groups in close proximity.

Since high-affinity, specific binding of [20-$^3$H]-12-*O*-tetradecanoylphorbol-13-acetate ($^3$H-TPA) to membranes from mouse brain was demonstrated (Dunphy *et al.*, 1980; Hergenhahn & Hecker, 1981), $^3$H-TPA itself was selected as the photoaffinity probe of choice.

We report here on direct photoaffinity labelling of membranes from mouse brain using $^3$H-TPA. A short account of this work has been given elsewhere (Hergenhahn *et al.*, 1983).

## MATERIALS AND METHODS

The particulate fraction from mouse brain was prepared as described previously (Hergenhahn & Hecker, 1981). A fraction enriched in receptors was obtained by separating the particulate fraction on a Percoll gradient. To this end, 3 mL of the particulate fraction plus 5 mL Percoll/saline plus 12 mL of $T_{50}$ buffer (50 mmol/L Tris·hydrochloric acid, pH 7.4) were mixed and spun for 25 min at 36 500 × *g* in a Beckman 50.2 Ti rotor, at 2 °C. The second, voluminous band from the top was removed by aspiration, diluted five fold with $T_{50}$, and pelleted at 100 000 × g for 30 min at 2 °C. The pellet was resuspended in $T_{50}$ at a concentration of about 10 mg protein/mL and stored at −70 °C. For photoaffinity labelling of a membrane suspension, the membrane fraction was thawed and diluted to 1 mg/mL in buffer; 5 μL $^{3}$H-TPA in ethanol containing about 25 pmol were added to either 100 μg of membrane protein in 100 μL (final concentration of $^{3}$H-TPA, 250 nmol/L), or to 400 μg of protein in 1 mL (final concentration, 25 nmol/L). After vortexing, the membrane suspensions were incubated for 20 min at 37 °C followed by chilling to 0 °C for 30 min. Irradiation was performed in one or four Pyrex tubes (Sorvall, Bad Nauheim, Federal Republic of Germany), respectively, in a photoreactor emitting UV light at about 320 nm, at 2 × 200 mA (Graentzel, Karlsruhe, Federal Republic of Germany), for 20 min at room temperature. (The tubes were kept at room temperature by directing an intense stream of air at them.) The lipids were extracted with either 150 μL or 750 μL chloroform:methanol (2:1) in each Pyrex tube by vigorous vortexing; separation of the layers was achieved by brief centrifugation in Eppendorf vials (Eppendorf, Hamburg, Federal Republic of Germany). The lipid extracts were concentrated by rotatory evaporation, and taken up in 100 or 400 μL chloroform:methanol (2:1), respectively. Volumes of 100 μL (Fig. 1, A, C) or 100 μL plus 100 μL of a mixture of the reference lipids plus photoadducts (B) were chromatographed on silica gel plates.

For irradiation of membranes on filters, 200 μg of membrane protein in 1 mL were incubated with 5 μL $^{3}$H-TPA in ethanol (final concentration, 12.5 nmol/L) plus either 5 μL of ethanol, or 5 μL of nonradioactive TPA in ethanol (final concentration, $10^{-6}$ mol/L) to determine non-specific binding. After incubation for 20 min at 37 °C, the suspensions were filtered over Whatman GF/C filters and washed rapidly with 2 × 1 mL acetone at −20 °C (Hergenhahn & Hecker, 1981) followed by 1 mL buffer at 0 °C. The wet filters were irradiated in Pyrex tubes as above; lipids were extracted twice with 3 mL chloroform:methanol and filtered over a cotton-wool plug; the organic extracts were concentrated on a rotatory evaporator. After addition of 250 μL chloroform:methanol (2:1), the fluid phases were transfered to an Eppendorf vial, where the phases were separated by brief centrifugation. The lower phase was taken for chromatography. For preparation of lipid adducts, the lipids were dispersed in $T_{50}$ at 1 mg/mL by either vigorous vortexing or brief sonification at 0 °C of a lipid film obtained by evaporation of chloroform:methanol solutions. Then, 5 μL $^{3}$H-TPA containing 25 pmol in ethanol were added to 100 μL lipid suspension, which was incubated briefly at 37 °C, cooled to 0 °C and irradiated in Pyrex tubes, as above. After extraction with 150 μL chloroform:methanol (2:1), the lower phase was used for chromatography. For degradation of the phosphatidylcholine (PC) and phosphatidylethanolamine (PE) adducts, respectively, with phospholipases, 200 μL PC or PE (from bovine brain) were irradiated with 10 μL $^{3}$H-TPA, as above; however, no extraction was performed. Instead, 60 μL each of the irradiated suspensions were incubated with 100 μL of a phospholipase $A_2$ solution (1 mg/mL in $T_{50}$), plus 16 μL of 20 mmol/L calcium chloride, or 100 μL phospholipase C (1 mg/mL in $T_{50}$), or

Fig. 1. Irreversible binding of [20-$^3$H]-12-*O*-tetradecanoylphorbol-13-acetate ($^3$H-TPA) to membrane lipids induced by ultraviolet irradiation. Typical experiment out of three

After incubation of brain membranes with $^3$H-TPA (see Materials and Methods), the membrane suspensions were irradiated at 320 nm. Buffered aqueous suspensions of reference lipids were processed under the same conditions. Extracts (with chloroform:methanol, 2:1) of the irradiated membrane and lipid suspensions, respectively, were chromatographed on silica gel plates with chloroform:methanol:ammonia, 65:35:4; the plates were scanned for radioactivity as described. Arrows indicate origin (left) and front (right). TPA chromatographs where indicated.

1, Extract of membranes, irradiated at a final concentration of $^3$H-TPA: 25 nmol/L (saturating level

2, Extract of membranes, irradiated at a final concentration of $^3$H-TPA: 250 nmol/L. For identification of the peaks, reference lipids, phosphatidylethanolamine (PE), phosphatidylcholine (PC), phosphatidylserine (PS), plus their photoadducts were added to one-quarter of the membrane extract.

3, Same as 2, without reference lipids and their photoadducts

4, PE plus $^3$H-TPA, extract after irradiation; PI, phosphatidylinositol

5, PC plus $^3$H-TPA, extract after irradiation

6, PS plus $^3$H-TPA, extract after irradiation

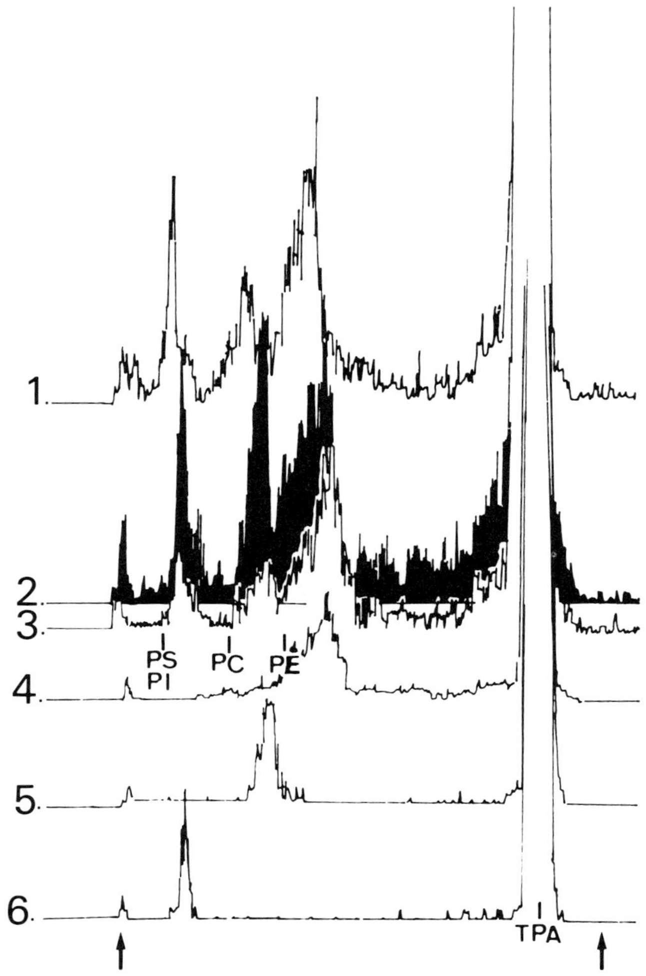

100 μL of a solution containing 100 μg bovine serum albumin, overnight at 37 °C. Subsequently, the aqueous phases were extracted with 200 μL chloroform:methanol (2:1), and the lower phases were used.

For thin-layer chromatography, glass-backed silica gel plates (E. Merck, Darmstadt, Federal Republic of Germany), were used. Lipids were visualized with iodine vapour; radioactivity on the plates was scanned with a Linear II scanner equipped with a multichannel analyser (Berthold, Wildbad, Federal Republic of Germany). Lipids and phospholipases were from Sigma (Munich), while $^3$H-TPA (specific activity, 20 Ci/mmol) was from NEN (Dreieich). Percoll was provided by Pharmacia (Freiburg). Protein was estimated by the Lowry method using bovine serum albumin as a standard.

## RESULTS

Several pilot experiments had shown that optimal amounts of photoproducts were obtained from membrane/$^3$H-TPA complexes after irradiation for 20 min at room temperature; therefore, this time period was used in the experiments.

When a particulate fraction from mouse brain was incubated with $^3$H-TPA at 25 nmol/L (close to the saturation level) or at a higher concentration followed by irradiation at 320 nm (Fig. 1), no significant binding to proteins was observed since (1) most of the radioactivity could be extracted into the organic phase, (2) when aliquots of irradiated membrane/$^3$H-TPA suspensions were applied to thin-layer chromatographic plates and chromatographed after drying on the plate, radioactivity at the origin was very low (data not shown). In contrast, lipid extracts of the membranes were shown to display three major radioactive peaks, in addition to some minor peaks (Fig. 1). The major peaks co-chromatographed with those from lipid extracts obtained after irradiation of $^3$H-TPA in the presence of the reference lipids PE, PC and phosphatidylserine (PS), respectively. At saturating conditions, the yields of photoproducts of the major phospholipids were in the range of 3–10%, with some variation (Fig. 1).

Specific and irreversible binding of $^3$H-TPA to PE and PS was demonstrated by another approach (Fig. 2): after binding of $^3$H-TPA to membranes, specific *versus* non-specific binding was increased dramatically by washing the membranes with cold acetone on a filter support (Ashendel & Boutwell, 1981; Hergenhahn & Hecker, 1981). Following irradiation of washed membranes on filters, extraction of lipid-$^3$H-TPA adducts was possible in yields of $\leq$ 1%. As shown by co-chromatography with photoproducts obtained from reference lipids, the products may be derived from PE and PS. The same peaks were reduced considerably if $^3$H-TPA was displaced competitively from membrane receptors by inclusion of an excess of nonradioactive TPA in the assay (Fig. 2A). The thin-layer chromatographic system used in Figure 2A, however, does not separate phosphatidylinositol (PI), PS and their TPA photoadducts; such a separation is possible in a system of chloroform:methanol:acetic acid:water, 65:45:3:1 (R. Schmidt, personal communication) (Fig. 2B). When lipid extracts from irradiated filters carrying washed membranes were chromatographed in this system, two major photoadducts were seen, which

Fig. 2. Specific irreversible binding of [20-$^3$H]-12-*O*-tetradecanoylphorbol-13-acetate ($^3$H-TPA) to lipids from brain membranes. Representative experiment out of four

A, Membranes were incubated with $^3$H-TPA (final concentration, 12.5 nmol/L), subsequently washed with cold acetone and buffer (see Materials and Methods). To determine nonspecific binding of $^3$H-TPA to the membranes, an excess of nonradioactive TPA (final concentration, 1 μmol/L) was included in parallel incubations; nine samples were used in each case.
After ultraviolet irradiation, the filters were extracted with chloroform:methanol, 2:1; the extracts were chromatographed on silica gel with chloroform:methanol:ammonia, 65:35:4, and scanned as above. Arrows indicate origin (left) and front (right). TPA chromatographs where indicated.
1, Extract of incubation with $^3$H-TPA; the positions of major lipids are indicated.
2, Extract of incubation with $^3$H-TPA plus an excess of nonradioactive TPA. Sensitivity of the scan was increased 2.5 fold with respect to 1.
For generation of reference photoadducts, suspensions of phosphatidylethanolamine (PE), phosphatidylcholine (PC) and phosphatidylserine (PS) were each irradiated with $^3$H-TPA (see legend to Fig. 1). Aliquots of extracts were chromatographed together on lane 3.
3, Combined photoadducts of PE, PC and PS. Note that the positions of the lipids and lipid adducts in lane 3 were shifted consistently to the right. PI, phosphatidylinositol

B, Incubation of membranes and preparation of photoadducts as in A. Chromatography on silica gel with the alternative solvent system chloroform:methanol:acetic acid:water, 65:45:3:1.
1, Extract of incubation with $^3$H-TPA
2, PE plus $^3$H-TPA, extract after irradiation
3, PI plus $^3$H-TPA, extract after irradiation
4, PS plus $^3$H-TPA, extract after irradiation
5, PC plus $^3$H-TPA, extract after irradiation

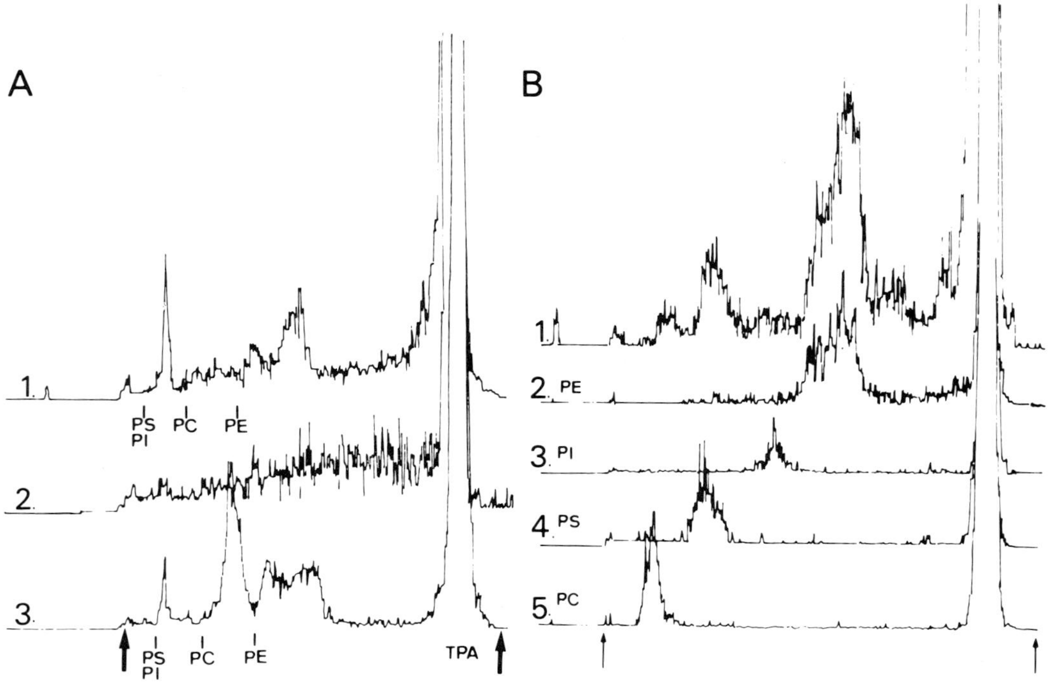

cochromatographed with the adducts from PE and PS; minor peaks seemed to coincide with the adducts of PC and PI.

In order to locate the site of photolabelling of lipids by $^3$H-TPA, aqueous suspensions of natural or synthetic lipids carrying unsaturated or saturated acyl chains were reacted with $^3$H-TPA by irradiation. The pattern shown in Table 1 was obtained.

When a new radioactive peak was obtained, it migrated in a manner similar to that of the phospholipid from which it was derived. In the case of the synthetic dipalmitoylphosphatidylethanolamine (DPPE), only a shoulder on the left-hand side of the $^3$H-TPA peak was observed consistently.

The site of the radioactive probe in the adducts was further addressed in experiments involving phospholipases (Fig. 3): PC incubated with phospholipase $A_2$ from bee venom produces lysophosphatidylcholine plus an (unsaturated) acid, and phospholipase C from *Clostridium perfringens* gives rise to the diacylglycerol derivative plus phosphocholine. In actual experiments, the photoadduct was cleaved with either phospholipase $A_2$ or C. Alternatively, PC was exposed first to the phospholipases, followed by irradiation of the cleavage products in the presence of $^3$H-TPA. Organic extracts of the suspensions gave the pattern shown in Figure 3A.

Similarly, the PE adduct was treated with phospholipases $A_2$ (from bee venom) and C (from *Clostridium perfringens* or *Bacillus cereus*). It was noted that, of the two phospholipases C, only that from *B. cereus* was capable of degrading the PE-TPA photoadduct. The following pattern (Fig. 3B) was obtained: after treatment with phospholipase $A_2$, which resulted in partial degradation, more radioactivity was associated with the region migrating further than the peak of the photoadduct, while the peak of the PE-TPA photoadduct was reduced considerably. Degradation by phospholipase C resulted in a new product, which migrated ahead of $^3$H-TPA.

Table 1. Photoproducts after irradiation of suspensions of natural and synthetic reference lipids in the presence of [20-$^3$H]-12-*O*-tetradecanoylphorbol-13-acetate ($^3$H-TPA)

| Lipid | | Photoproduct on radioactive thin-layer chromatography |
|---|---|---|
| Phosphatidylcholine | (natural) | + |
| Phosphatidylethanolamine | (natural) | + |
| Phosphatidylserine | (natural) | + |
| Phosphatidylinositol | (natural) | + |
| Sphingomyelin | (natural) | + |
| Dipalmitoylphosphatidylcholine | (synthetic) | − |
| Dipalmitoylphosphatidylethanolamine | (synthetic) | ? |
| Lysophosphatidylcholine | (natural) | − |
| Lysophosphatidylethanolamine | (natural) | (+) |
| Diolein | (synthetic) | + |
| Dipalmitin | (synthetic) | − |
| Oleic acid | (natural) | + |

Lipid suspensions were prepared and photolabelled as described in the legend to Figure 1. The photoproducts migrated slightly ahead of the particular phospholipid used, while diolein and oleic acid migrated in front of the photoproducts (compare with Fig. 3). The table is a compilation of several experiments using different solvent systems.

Fig. 3. Degradation of [20-$^3$H]-12-*O*-tetradecanoylphorbol-13-acetate ($^3$H-TPA) adducts with phosphatidylcholine (PC) (A) and phosphatidylethanolamine (PE) (B) by phospholipases $A_2$ and C. One of two similar experiments is shown.

A, A suspension of PC was irradiated in the presence of $^3$H-TPA, as above (Fig. 1); aliquots were treated overnight at 37 °C with phospholipase $A_2$ (bee venom), with phospholipase C *(Clostridium perfringens)* or with bovine serum albumin as control. Alternatively, PC was degraded first by treatment with the phospholipases, the mixtures were incubated with $^3$H-TPA, and irradiated; all preparations were extracted with chloroform:methanol, 2:1. Suspensions of diolein and lysophosphatidylcholine were irradiated with $^3$H-TPA and extracted as above. The extracts were chromatographed on silica gel, first with chloroform:methanol: ammonia, 65:35:4, to a height of 9.5 cm (front indicated by CMA), then with cyclohexane: acetone, 4:1, to 17 cm (front indicated by CA). Arrows indicate origin (left) and fronts (right).

1, Extract of PC-$^3$H-TPA adduct, control (incubation with bovine serum albumin)
2, Extract of adduct after phospholipase $A_2$ treatment, FA, mixture of fatty acids
3, Extract of adduct after phospholipase C treatment; DG, diacylglycerol(1,2-diolein plus traces of the 1,3-isomer in lane 7); adduct peak (black) disappears, new peaks (black) appear
4, Extract when PC was degraded first with phopholipase C
5, Extract when PC was degraded first with phopholipase $A_2$; LPC, lysophosphatidylcholine
6, Extract of irradiated lysophosphatidylcholine/$^3$H-TPA suspension
7, Extract of irradiated diolein/$^3$H-TPA suspension

B, The phospholipid adduct of PE was obtained by irradiation in the presence of $^3$H-TPA, as above (Fig. 1); aliquots were treated overnight at 37 °C with phospholipase $A_2$ (bee venom), with phospholipase C *(Bacillus cereus)* or with bovine serum albumin as control. Suspensions of diolein and oleic acid were also irradiated in the presence of $^3$H-TPA. Extraction and chromatography were performed as in A.

1, Extract of PE-$^3$H-TPA adduct in bovine serum albumin (control)
2, Extract of adduct after phospholipase $A_2$ treatment
3, Extract of adduct after phospholipase C treatment
4, Diolein plus $^3$H-TPA, extract after irradiation
5, Oleic acid plus $^3$H-TPA, extract after irradiation

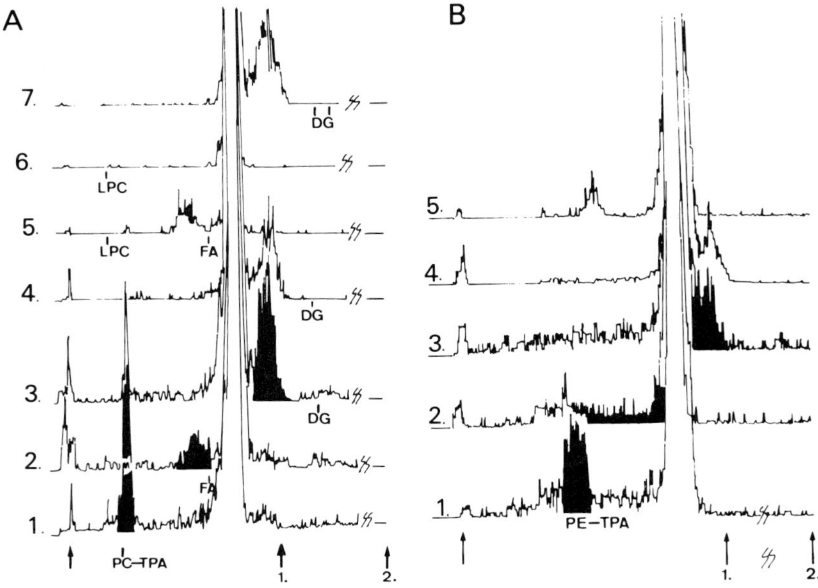

## DISCUSSION

In contrast to initial expectations, the use of $^3$H-TPA as a direct photoaffinity label induced formation of photoadducts of specific membrane phospholipids, instead of membrane proteins. This conclusion is warranted by (1) the absence of these products when UV irradiation of the membrane/$^3$H-TPA complex is omitted; (2) lack of evidence for notable UV-induced TPA degradation or hydrolysis in the presence of membranes (data not shown ); (3) dependence of formation of photoadducts on the presence of particular lipids (Table 1, Figs 1–3); and (4) degradation of phospholipid adducts by phospholipases $A_2$ and C, respectively (Fig. 3). Only limited amounts of the photoadducts were produced, presumably due to the low energy yield of the reaction.

When nonspecific binding in relation to specific (reversible) binding in the membranes was high, the major photoadducts were derived from PE and PS, in addition to PC, as suggested by cochromatography of the products with those obtained from reference lipids. After reduction of nonspecific binding to $\leq$ 10% of total binding by the cold acetone-filter assay (Ashendel & Boutwell, 1981; Hergenhahn & Hecker, 1981), however, UV irradiation induced photoadducts of PE and PS, in addition to some minor products. The specificity of $^3$H-TPA binding to PE and PS was indicated by the much lower level and more uniform distribution of the radioactivity when radioactive TPA was in competition with an excess of non-radioactive TPA (Fig. 2A). Some indication of the attachment site of the radioactive probe in the photoadducts was obtained in experiments involving the use of phospholipases. When the PC-TPA adduct was degraded by phospholipases $A_2$ or C, or when PC was degraded first, followed by photolabelling of the mixtures of products with $^3$H-TPA, the results were in accordance with covalent binding of the TPA to (unsaturated) acyl chains in position 2 of the phospholipid (Fig. 3A). Since radioactive products were also observed after photolabelling of diolein or oleic acid with $^3$H-TPA (Fig. 3, Table 1), a single unsaturated carbon-carbon bond in an acyl chain may be sufficient for photoadduct formation. This conclusion was supported by the failure to induce, under similar conditions, products with the synthetic dipalmitoyl-phosphatidylcholine and DPPE (Table 1). However, a radioactive shoulder on the $^3$H-TPA peak was observed consistently with DPPE, indicating either formation of an adduct with the head group or facilitation of degradation of $^3$H-TPA (data not shown). Evidence was obtained that the PE-TPA adduct can also be degraded by phospholipases $A_2$ from bee venom and C from *B. cereus* (Fig. 3B). In analogy, it may be assumed that $^3$H-TPA reacts preferentially with unsaturated acyl chains in position 2 of other phospholipids. Thus, the preferential labelling of PE and PS in a situation in which most receptors were occupied by $^3$H-TPA and nonspecific binding was low may indicate that these two phospholipids were primarily involved in binding sites of phorbol ester receptors.

Similar conclusions were advanced in very recent reports from Blumberg's and from this laboratory. The two groups have used binding of different phorbol esters carrying a photoactive group in one of the acyl moieties to receptors in either a particulate fraction from mouse brain (Delclos *et al.*, 1983) or a particulate fraction from mouse epidermis (Schmidt *et al.*, 1983, and unpublished data). On the basis of the similar results of this study, using direct photoaffinity binding to the phorbol moiety, we tend to conclude that, in addition to the acyl residue(s), the phorbol moiety of TPA is also located in a position favourable to binding of specific phospholipids. Remarkably, none of the two photoaffinity labelling approaches has produced evidence for labelling of proteins, which may indicate topological limitations of the phorbol ester-receptor interaction and/or restricted reactivity of the various photoreactive groups used.

The importance of phospholipids in phorbol ester binding to specific receptors in membranes is also supported by (1) the studies cited in the introduction to this report, (2) the large change in entropy observed on binding of a phorbol ester to receptors, which is typical of a strong hydrophobic interaction (Dunphy *et al.*, 1980); (3) the induction of specific phorbol ester receptors in cytosol from various organs (Leach *et al.*, 1982; Ashendel *et al.*, 1983) and in a solubilized fraction from mouse epidermis (Schmidt & Hecker, 1982) by addition of PS; and (4) the requirement of PS for both phorbol ester binding and protein kinase activity of a phospholipid/calcium ion-dependent protein kinase C (Castagna *et al.*, 1982; Niedel *et al.*, 1983). Thus, the specific binding of phorbol esters to receptors may involve modification of specific phospholipid-protein interactions, with subsequent activation of specific enzymatic reactions. Although there is considerable evidence that protein kinase C is a prime candidate for a receptor, there may be other specific associations of PE and PS with proteins, which also display properties of functional phorbol ester receptors.

## ACKNOWLEDGEMENT

The valuable technical assistance of Ms U. Stanior and Ms I. Thome is gratefully acknowledged.

## REFERENCES

Ashendel, C.L. & Boutwell, R.K. (1981) Direct measurement of specific binding of highly lipophilic phorbol diester to mouse epidermal membranes using cold acetone. *Biochem. biophys. Res. Commun.*, ***99***, 543–549

Ashendel, C.L., Staller, J.M. & Boutwell, R.K. (1983) Identification of a calcium- and phospholipid-dependent phorbol ester binding activity in the soluble fraction of mouse tissues. *Biochem. biophys. Res. Commun.*, ***111***, 340–345

Bailey, H. & Knowles, J.R. (1977) Photoaffinity labeling. *Meth. Enzymol.*, ***46***, 69–114

Castagna, M., Takai, Y., Kaibuchi, K., Sano, K., Kikkawa, U. & Nishizuka, Y. (1982) Direct activation of calcium-activated, phospholipid-dependent protein kinase by tumor-promoting phorbol esters. *J. biol. Chem.*, ***257***, 7847–7851

Delclos, K.B. & Blumberg, P.M. (1982) Identification of ascorbic acid as the heat-stable factor from brain which inactivates the phorbol ester receptor. *Cancer Res.*, ***42***, 1227–1232

Delclos, K.B., Yeh, E. & Blumberg, P.M. (1983) Specific labeling of mouse brain membrane phospholipids with (20-$^3$H)phorbol 12-p-azidobenzoate 13-benzoate, a photolabile phorbol ester. *Proc. natl Acad. Sci. USA*, ***80***, 3054–3058

Driedger, P.E. & Blumberg, P.M. (1980) Specific binding of phorbol ester tumor promoters. *Proc. natl Acad. Sci. USA, 77*, 567–571

Dunphy, W.G., Delclos, K.B. & Blumberg, P.M. (1980) Characterization of specific binding of ($^3$H)phorbol 12,13-dibutyrate and ($^3$H)phorbol 12-myristate 13-acetate to mouse brain. *Cancer Res.*, ***40***, 3635–3641

Hecker, E., Fusenig, N.E., Kunz, W., Marks, F. & Thielmann, H.W., eds (1982) *Carcinogenesis – A Comprehensive Survey*, Vol. 7, *Cocarcinogenesis and Biological Effects of Tumor Promoters*, New York, Raven Press

Hergenhahn, M. & Hecker, E. (1981) Specific binding of the tumor promoter TPA in various mouse organs as measured by a 'cold acetone-filter assay'. *Carcinogenesis*, ***2***, 1277–1281

Hergenhahn, M. & Hecker, E. (1982) Specific binding sites for the tumor promoter TPA – studies on distribution, specificity and nature of the sites. *Periodicum biol.*, ***85***, Suppl. 2, 143–145

Hergenhahn, M., Marston, A. & Hecker, E. (1983) Lipids in a cellular TPA recognition site – studies using amino acyl esters of phorbol, enzyme degradation of membrane phospholipids, and photoaffinity labeling. *J. Cancer Res. clin. Oncol.*, ***105***, CH 17 (Abstract)

Jones, M.D. & Murray, A.W. (1983) Decreased (20-$^3$H)phorbol-12,13-dibutyrate binding to phospholipase C pretreated epidermal cells. *Cancer Lett.*, ***19***, 91–95

Leach, K.L., James, M.L. & Blumberg, P.M. (1982) Specific apo-binding activity for phorbol ester tumor promoters in mouse brain cytosol. *J. Cell Biol.*, ***95***, 431a (Abstract)

Niedel, J.E., Kuhn, L.J. & Vandenbark, G.R. (1983) Phorbol diester receptor copurifies with protein kinase C. *Proc. natl Acad. Sci. USA*, ***80***, 36–40

Pečar, S., Šentjurc, M., Schara, M., Nemec, M., Sorg, B. & Hecker, E. (1982) *Spin-labeled phorbol esters and their interaction with cellular membranes*. In: Hecker, E., Fusenig, N.E., Kunz, W., Marks, F. & Thielmann, H.W., eds, *Carcinogenesis – A Comprehensive Survey*, Vol. 7, *Cocarcinogenesis and Biological Effects of Tumor Promoters*, New York, Raven Press, pp. 1–553

Schmidt, R. & Hecker, E. (1982) Characterization of particulate and solubilized binding sites for $^3$H-phorbol-12,13-dipropionate of mouse skin epidermis. *Periodicum biol.*, ***85***, Suppl. 2, 155–157

Schmidt, R., Sorg, B., Marston, A. & Hecker, E. (1983) Bivalent and photoaffinity-labeled ligands to study specific binding sites of phorbol esters in mouse epidermis. *J. Cancer Res. clin. Oncol.*, ***105***, CH 45 (Abstract)

# MEMBRANE-MEDIATED RESPONSES TO 12-*O*-TETRADECANOYLPHORBOL-13-ACETATE IN HUMAN SKIN FIBROBLASTS

A.R. KINSELLA, A.D. WHETTON, E. DE WYNTER & G.W. BAZILL

*Paterson Laboratories, Christie Hospital and Holt Radium Institute, Manchester M20 9BX, UK*

C.M. HEYWORTH & M.D. HOUSLAY

*Department of Biochemistry and Molecular Biology, University of Manchester Institute of Science and Technology, Manchester M60 1QD, UK*

## SUMMARY

The effects on primary human skin fibroblasts of the structurally unrelated tumour promoters 12-*O*-tetradecanoylphorbol-13-acetate (TPA) and teleocidin B were compared with those of epidermal growth factor and the non-promoting derivative 4-*O*-methyl TPA by means of two-dimensional gel electrophoresis. Both TPA and teleocidin B caused a marked increase in the synthesis of two polypeptides of molecular weights 44 kilodaltons (P44) and 55 kilodaltons (P55). P55 was complexed in cell lysates by antiactin antibody and was shown to be a component of the cytoskeleton. P44 migrated very near to actin, but it was shown not to be a variant form of actin. No such specific increase in polypeptide synthesis was observed following treatment with either epidermal growth factor or 4-*O*-methyl TPA. TPA inhibited the β-adrenergic hormone response in the same human skin fibroblasts.

## INTRODUCTION

It has been speculated that 12-*O*-tetradecanoylphorbol-13-acetate (TPA) and the phorbol esters might exert their effects on the cell by usurping or disturbing cellular receptor response pathways, thereby eliciting a variety of effects leading to transformation (Lee & Weinstein, 1978a). The earliest changes that occur in response to TPA *in vitro* occur at the cell membrane within minutes, in the absence of RNA and protein synthesis. These changes include increased 2-deoxyglucose uptake, altered cell adhesion and morphology, increased release of arachidonic acid from membrane phospholipids and inhibition of epidermal growth factor (EGF) binding to its cellular receptor. In fact, TPA and the phorbol esters share many of the characteristics of hormonal agents, in that many of their effects are mediated at nanomolar concentrations *via* highly specific phorbol ester receptors, and culminate in the induction of highly pleiotropic and reversible effects (Weinstein *et al.*, 1979).

In addition to this ability to modulate growth factor binding (Brown *et al.*, 1979; Shoyab *et al.*, 1979), TPA is also known to modulate or uncouple β-adrenergic hormone receptor interactions (Garte & Belman, 1980) and modulate or perturb gene expression. Evidence for the modulation of gene expression in response to TPA includes the induction of plasminogen activator (Wigler & Weinstein, 1976) and ornithine decarboxylase activities (O'Brien *et al.*, 1975), depression of histidase activity (Colburn *et al.*, 1975), induction of viral genes (zur Hausen *et al.*, 1978; Amtmann & Sauer, 1982), and a possible influence on gene amplification (Varshavsky, 1981; Bojan *et al.*, 1983, and this volume p. 265). Thus, it seemed pertinent to the assessment of the nature of the changes induced by TPA and by tumour promoters to investigate both the extent of the changes in gene expression induced by these agents and the ability of TPA to modulate normal hormonal responses in the same in-vitro system. To these ends, we have employed two-dimensional gel electrophoresis to compare the effects of TPA, EGF, teleocidin B and the non-promoting derivative of TPA, 4-*O*-methyl TPA (4-*O*-MeTPA) on gene expression in human skin fibroblasts. We also investigated the influence of TPA on β-adrenergic hormone-stimulated cyclic AMP accumulation.

## MATERIALS AND METHODS

Skin fibroblast cultures were established from freshly isolated skin biopsies from (1) a 10–12-week-old fetus (FSII), (2) an eight-year-old male donor (FF1) and (3) a 51-year-old female donor. All cultures were maintained routinely in Dulbecco's modification of Eagle's minimal essential medium (Flow Laboratories Ltd, Irvine, UK) (DMEM) supplemented with penicillin (100 U/mL) streptomycin (50 μg/mL) and 10% fetal bovine serum (DMEM 10%) and placed in a humidified gas incubator at 37° C with 5% carbon dioxide in air gas phase.

### *Labelling of cells with $^{35}$S-methionine*

For exposure to TPA, teleocidin B, EGF and 4-*O*-MeTPA, $2 \times 10^5$ cells were plated per 16-mm well and allowed to attach prior to treatment for 12–15 h with 0.1 μg/mL of the appropriate test agent. The medium was then removed and the cells washed once with methionine-free minimal essential medium containing 10% fetal bovine serum (MEM 10%). The cells were pre-incubated for 20 min in MEM 10% containing 0.1 μg/mL of test agent, when appropriate. This medium was then replaced by 0.21 mL of MEM 10% containing, in addition, 1.0 μg/mL methionine and 330 μCi/mL $^{35}$S-methionine. The cells were incubated for four hours at 37 °C. The radioactive medium was then removed, the cells washed twice with 1.0 mL phosphate buffered saline (PBS) and then lysed *in situ* by the addition of 0.1 mL of O'Farrell lysis buffer (O'Farrell, 1975).

*Electrophoresis*

The procedure followed was essentially that described by O'Farrell *et al.* (1977) for non-equilibrium pH gradient gel electrophoresis (NEPHGE), using LKB ampholines in the range 3.5–10.0. Focusing was carried out for 2 000 volt-hours. Lysate equivalent to 2 × 10$^5$ cpm was applied to the focusing gel. In the second dimension, gels were run at pH 8.3 at 20 mA per gel with voltage limited to 200 V. Autoradiographs were made on Kodak NS2T X-ray film.

*Peptide mapping by digestion with Staphylococcal V8 protease*

The method employed was essentially that described by Cleveland *et al.* (1977). Three stained and dried gels bearing TPA-stimulated polypeptides were selected, and the actin spot and the area containing the polypeptide of molecular weight 44 kilodaltons (P44) were cut out. The paper backing was removed and the gel fragments rehydrated in a solution containing 0.1 M Tris-hydrochloric acid, pH 6.89, 0.1% SDS and 1 mM ethylenediaminetetraacetic acid (EDTA). The gel fragments were transferred to sample wells and digested during electrophoresis with 0.25 μg *Staphylococcal* V8 protease (Sigma).

*Test for cross-reaction with anti-actin antibody*

FF1 cells (2 × 10$^5$) growing on 3-cm plastic petri dishes were treated with 0.1 μg/mL TPA for 18 h in parallel with untreated controls. The medium was then removed and the cells were washed with PBS, pre-incubated in MEM containing 1.0 μg/mL methionine for 30 min and labelled in 0.5 mL medium containing 300 μCi/mL $^{35}$S-methionine, as described above. After 5 h incubation, the cells were washed, then lysed in 0.5 mL of a solution containing 1% Nonidet NP40, 5 mM ethylenediaminetetraacetic acid, 50 mM Tris-hydrochloric acid pH 6.8 and 0.25 mM phenyl methyl sulfonyl fluoride. A portion of each lysate (50 μL) was kept as a control to make sure that TPA had stimulated the synthesis of P44 and the polypeptide of molecular weight 55 kilodaltons (P55), as in previous experiments. To the remainder was added 20 μL (approximately 20 μg protein) of antiactin antibody, and the mixture was kept overnight at 4 °C. Approximately 0.3 mL of washed protein A sepharose (Sigma) was added. The suspension was maintained at room temperature for two hours and then stored overnight at 4 °C. The sepharose beads were washed five times by centrifugation in 5 mL PBS. Finally, the buffer was removed, and 0.2 mL lysis buffer

(O'Farrell, 1975) was added to the beads. Protein equivalent to about 50 000 cpm was analysed by NEPHGE, as described previously. The gels were dehydrated and impregnated with 2,5-diphenyloxazole by the procedure of Laskey and Mills (1975). Fluorograms were exposed at –70 °C.

*Measurement of the intact cell response to isoproterenol*

FF1 cells were plated at a density of $4 \times 10^4$ cells, in a 2-mL volume of DMEM 10% in standard glass scintillation vials. Twenty-four hours prior to determination of the cyclic AMP (cAMP) response, TPA was added to give a final concentration of 0.1 μg/mL in 3 mL DMEM 10%, and the vials incubated at 37° C. Immediately prior to the determination of the cAMP response, the cell sheets were washed three times and 0.5 mL of serum-free medium plus the phosphodiesterase inhibitor isobutyl methyl xanthine (IBMX; 1.0 nM) added. The cells were pre-incubated at 37° C for 15 min. All incubations ± the various agonists were carried out for 10 min, and they were terminated by boiling. The vials were then cooled and the contents sonicated for 10 sec to rupture the cells. After sonication, the samples were transferred to 1-mL microfuge tubes, and the protein deposit was removed by centrifugation at 12 000 × *g* for one minute. The resulting supernatants were assayed for cAMP using a competitive binding assay (Houslay *et al.*, 1976).

## RESULTS

Investigation of promoter-induced alterations in gene expression induced by 0.1 μg/mL TPA and 0.1 μg/mL teleocidin B showed a manifold increase in the intensity of two spots corresponding to polypeptides of molecular weights 44 and 55 kilodaltons (P44 and P55), in three independent human fibroblast cultures established from donors of different ages (Fig. 1; data for FS11 cells only). Neither polypeptide was induced following treatment with either 0.1 μg/mL 4-*O*-MeTPA or EGF (Fig. 2). To establish whether or not P44, which migrated close to actin (Fig. 1, b & c), was a modified form of actin, the proteins in the P44 gel fragment were digested with *Staphylococcal* V8 protease (Cleveland *et al.*, 1977), and the resulting peptides compared with those of actin (Fig. 3). The fluorograms (Fig. 3) show that P44 is not a modified form of actin. This was confirmed when anti-actin antibody was added to FF1 cell lysates: The antibody-bound proteins were run under NEPHGE conditions (O'Farrell *et al.*, 1977) in the second dimension, and fluorograms of these gels (Fig. 4) show P44 to be absent from both the control and TPA-treated cell lysates, although actin (marked A) is clearly visible. One spot that was present on the 'TPA-treated' autoradiograph (Fig. 4b) but absent from the control (Fig. 4a) corresponded exactly to the position of P55. Consistent with this finding was the observation that P44 was absent from cytoskeletal preparations of teleocidin B-treated cells, while P55 was clearly visible (data not shown).

Analysis of the β-adrenergic response of the FF1 cells showed that a 24-h pre-incubation with TPA inhibits isoproterenol-stimulated cAMP accumulation almost completely (Fig. 5).

Fig. 1. Two-dimensional gel electrophoresis of $^{35}$S-methionine-labelled polypeptides from: a, untreated 10–12-week-old fetus (FSII) skin fibroblasts; b, FSII cells treated with 0.1 μg/mL 12-*O*-tetradecanoylphorbol-13-acetate; c, FSII cells treated with 0.1 μg/mL teleocidin B

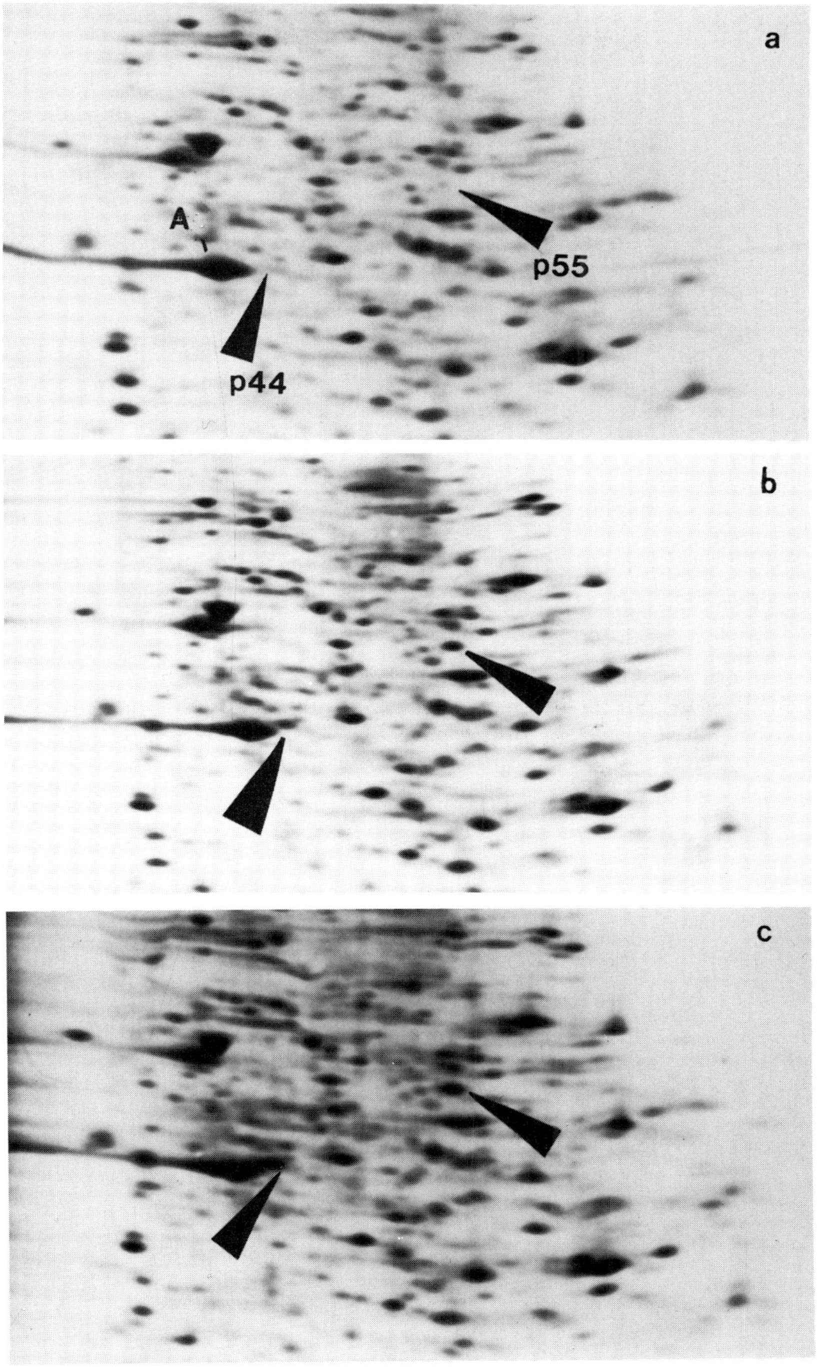

Fig. 2. Two-dimensional gel electrophoresis of $^{35}$S-methionine-labelled polypeptides from: a, untreated 10–12-week-old fetus (FSII) cells; b, FSII cells treated with 0.1 g/mL 4-*O*-methyl-12-*O*-tetradecanoylphorbol-13-acetate; c, FSII cells treated with 0.1 μg/mL epidermal growth factor

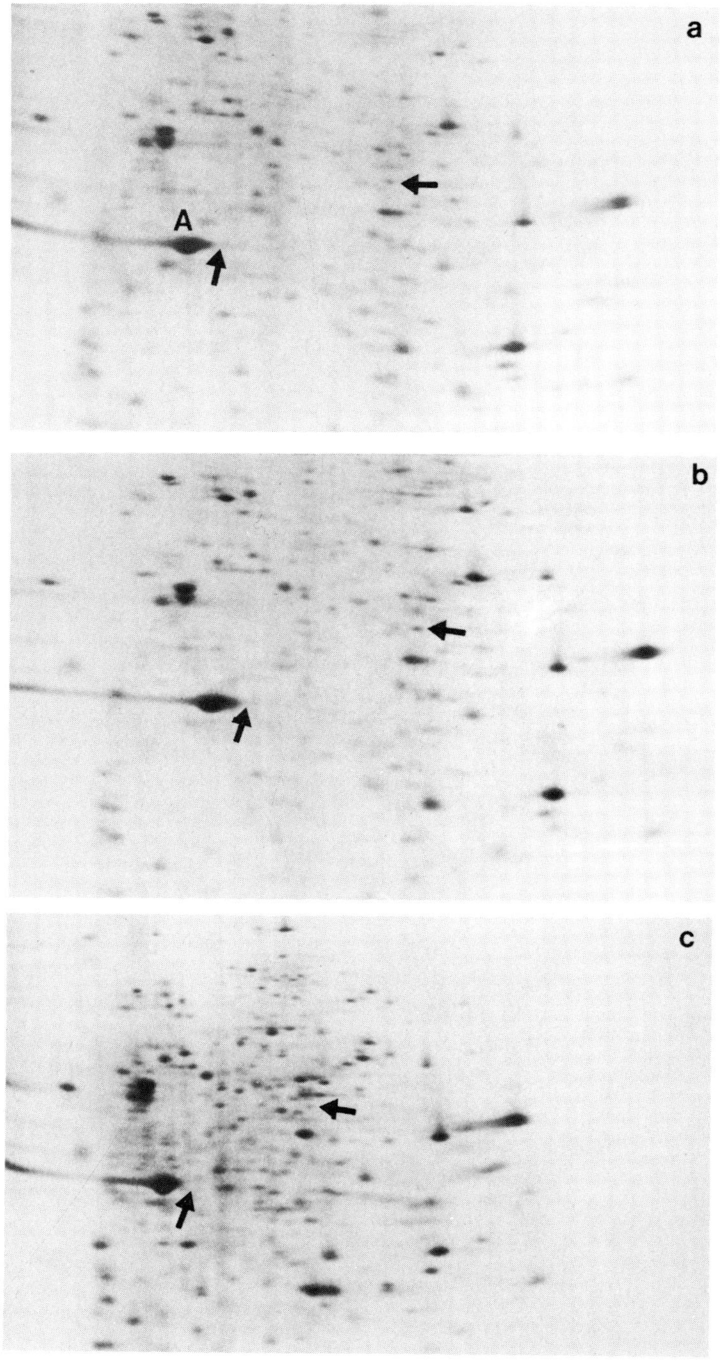

Fig. 3. One-dimensional gel electrophoresis of the peptides generated by *Staphylococcal* V8 protease treatment of: a, actin; b, polypeptide molecular weight 44 kilodaltons; and c, actin

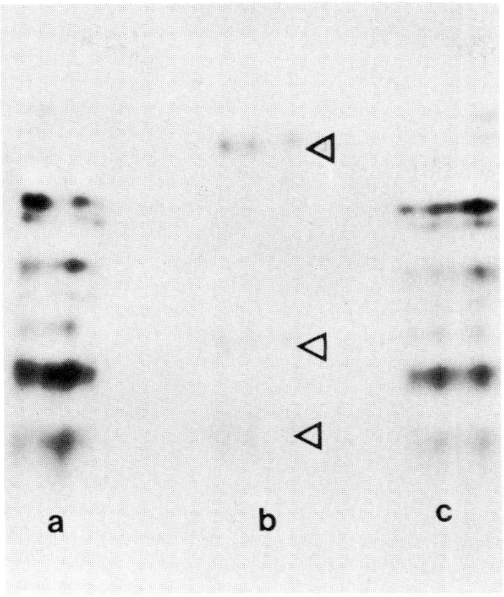


## DISCUSSION

Our data demonstrate the ability of two structurally unrelated promoters, TPA and teleocidin B (Fujiki *et al.*, 1979, 1981) to bring about the same specific changes in protein synthesis in three different human skin fibroblast cells lines. Although the identities of these promoter-induced polypeptides are not known, we have confirmed that P44, which migrates close to actin, is not a modified form of actin. Modified forms of actin have been reported previously in a chemically-transformed human fibroblast cell line (Leavitt & Kakunaga, 1980) and in a sarcoma cell line (Bravo *et al.*, 1981). In fact, analysis of the protein bound by anti-actin antibody (Fig. 4) showed P55, and not P44, to be one of a small group of proteins bound selectively by anti-actin antibody. However, it is unlikely that these polypeptides are all modified forms of actin and, in all probability, they are merely 'actin-associated' cytoskeletal proteins. No such specific change was observed with either the non-promoting derivative of TPA, 4-*O*-MeTPA (Marks, 1976) or EGF, which shares a number of biological effects with TPA and teleocidin B (Rose *et al.*, 1976; DiPasquale *et al.*, 1978; Lee & Weinstein, 1978b; Fisher *et al.*, 1981).

Thus, the specificity of the response to TPA and teleocidin B is consistent with the view that the pleiotropic effects of these agents are the result of binding to either a specific receptor or to different receptors with a common effector mechanism. Also, although both TPA and teleocidin B inhibit EGF binding to its cellular receptor (Lee & Weinstein, 1978a; Umezawa *et al.*, 1981) and EGF has been reported to enhance tumour formation (Rose *et al.*, 1976) and in-vitro cellular transformation (Fisher *et*

Fig. 4. Autoradiographs of proteins from an eight-year-old male donor (FF1) selectively bound by anti-actin antibody: a, untreated control; b, 12-*O*-tetradecanoylphorbol-13-acetate-treated cells

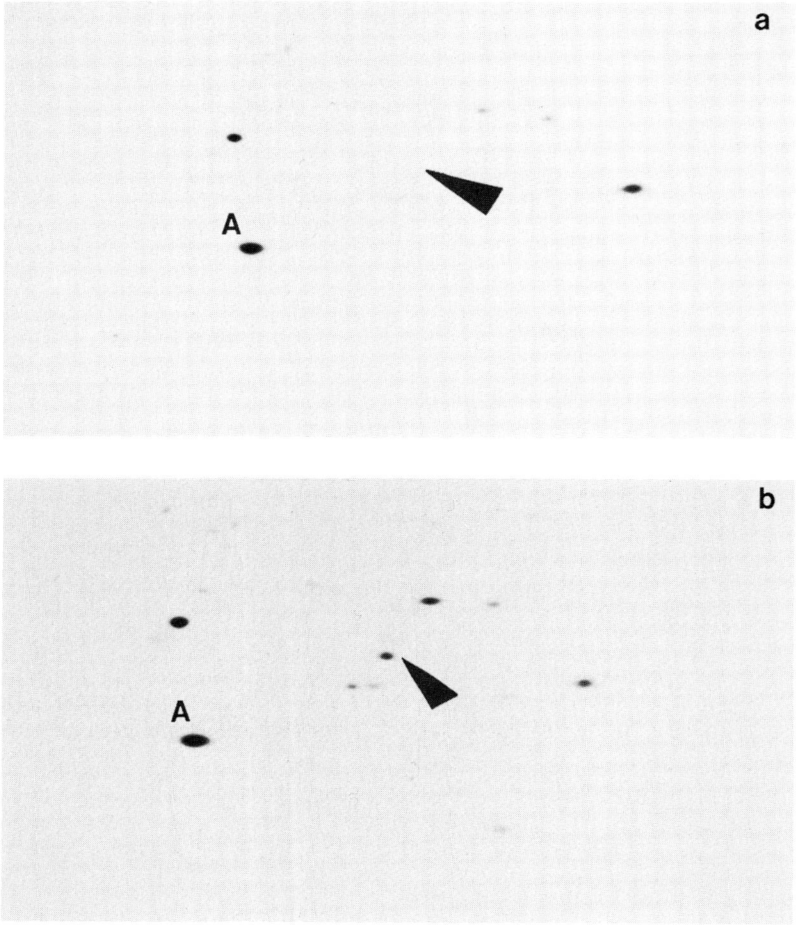


*al.*, 1981), the failure of EGF in our hands to demonstrate the same highly specific effects on protein synthesis, confirms the hypothesis that the stimulation of P44 and P55 synthesis is promoter-specific. Obviously, it is not mediated by either EGF or by an effector mechanism shared by EGF and promoters. However, it is still not clear whether or not this enhanced peptide synthesis is a necessary early step in promotion or whether it represents some form of differentiation effect. The influence of tumour promoters on the process of cell differentiation is well documented (Yamasaki, 1980 and references therein), and Laskin *et al.* (1981) reported the induction by TPA of a marked increase in the synthesis of keratin proteins in mouse epidermis. Such changes have recently been put forward as representing changes in differentiation state (Roop *et al.*, 1983).

Fig. 5. a, response of eight-year-old male donor (FF1) fibroblasts to isoproterenol challenge ($2 \times 10^{-5}$M) in the presence of 200 µg/mL isobutylmethylxanthin; b, dose response of FF1 fibroblast cAMP accumulation to isoprotenerol stimulation in presence of IBMX Incubation after challenge of 10 min; ●, control and O, cells pre-incubated with 12-*O*-tetradecanoylphorbol-13-acetate for 24 h.

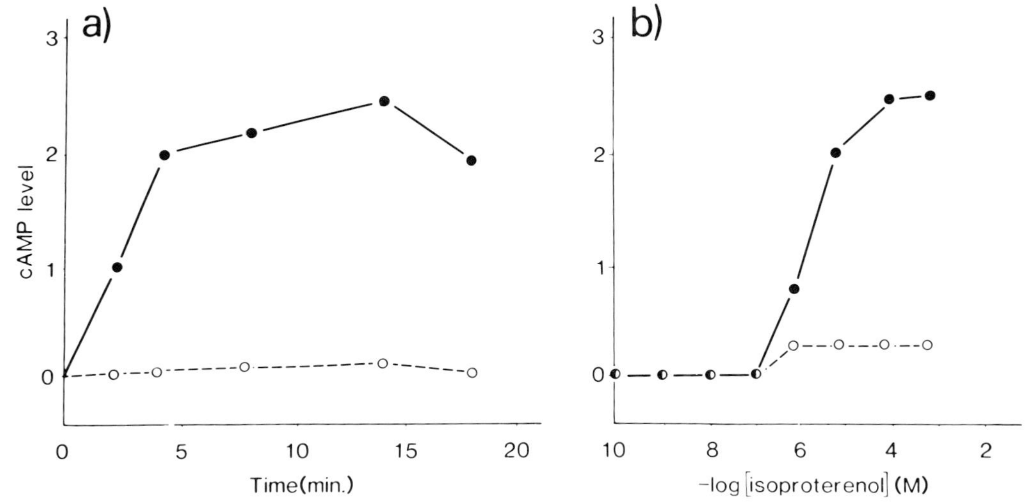


Whether this is a differentiation effect or not, it is becoming increasingly obvious that promoters and transforming growth factors (Reynolds *et al.*, 1981; Roberts *et al.*, 1982) exert their effects at the cell surface, presumably by modulating normal cellular factor control. We know that certain sera and physiological fluids are highly inhibitory to [20–$^{3}$H]-phorbol 12,13-dibutyrate (TPA analogue) receptor binding (Horowitz *et al.*, 1981). In addition, a phorbol ester-binding inhibitory factor, isolated from human placenta (Hamel *et al.*, this volume, p. 157), may have a possible role in regulation of differentiation. Therefore, TPA probably mediates its effect by inhibiting the binding of an endogenous ligand(s) to its own cellular receptor. This modulation of normal cellular control is also confirmed by the effects TPA has on isoproterenol-stimulated cAMP accumulation in human skin fibroblasts (Fig. 5). Parallel studies on the hepatic regulatory enzyme, adenylate cyclase, show that TPA inhibits both glucagon-stimulated and cholera toxin-stimulated cAMP accumulation in isolated rat hepatocytes. Under normal conditions, glucagon exerts its effects on the liver cell by binding to a specific receptor exposed on the cell surface. This receptor-hormone complex interacts *via* a guanyl nucleotide regulatory protein to form a trans bilayer complex with the catalytic unit of adenylate cyclase (Limbird *et al.*, 1980). However, cholera toxin activation of adenylate cyclase is independent of the glucagon receptor; it interacts directly with the guanyl nucleotide regulatory protein involved in coupling. This binding, together with the observation that $^{125}$I-glucagon binding to its receptor is unaffected by TPA, suggests that TPA exerts its effects on this system either at the level of the regulatory protein or directly on the catalytic unit of adenylate cyclase. In any event, this hypothesis implies that TPA exerts its activity at the cytosol surface of the plasma membrane, as neither the catalytic unit nor the regulatory protein is exposed at the external surface of the plasma membrane (Houslay *et al.*, 1980; Houslay & Gordon, 1983). Also, our failure to observe an effect of TPA on adenylate cyclase in purified plasma membranes suggests that cytosol components are involved in mediating the TPA effect.

*In conclusion*

These observations are entirely consistent with recent proposals that TPA mediates its effects *via* a calcium-dependent, phospholipid-dependent protein kinase (Kuo *et al.,* 1980; Castagna *et al.,* 1982; Niedel *et al.,* 1983; Blumberg, this volume p. 139). Under physiological conditions, the activation of this enzyme appears to be linked to receptor-mediated phosphatidyl-inositol breakdown (Castagna *et al.*, 1982), which may, in turn, be provoked by a large number of extracellular messengers.

## REFERENCES

Amtmann, E. & Sauer, G. (1982) Activation of non-expressed bovine papilloma virus genomes by tumour promoters. *Nature, **296**,* 675–676

Bojan, F., Kinsella, A.R. & Fox, M. (1983) Effect of tumour promoter 12-*O*-tetradecanoylphorbol-13-acetate on recovery of methotrexate, *N*-(phosphonacetyl)-L-aspartate- and cadmium-resistant colony-forming mouse and hamster cells. *Cancer Res., **43,*** 5217–5221

Bravo, R., Fey, S.J., Small, J.V., Larsen, P.M. & Celis, J.M. (1981) Co-existence of three major iso-actins in a single sarcoma 180 cell. *Cell, **25**,* 195–202

Brown, K.D., Dicker, P. & Rozengurt, E. (1979) Inhibition of epidermal growth factor binding to surface receptors by tumour promoters. *Biochem. biophys. Res. Commun., **86***, 1037–1043

Castagna, M., Takai, Y., Kaituchi, K., Sano, K., Kikkawa, U. & Nichizuka, Y. (1982) Direct activation of calcium-activated, phospholipid-dependent protein kinase by tumour promoting phorbol esters. *J. biol. Chem., **257***, 7847–7851

Cleveland, D.W., Fischer, S.G., Kirschner, M.W. & Laemmli, U.K. (1977) Peptide mapping by limited proteolysis in SDS and analysis by gel electrophoresis. *J. biol. Chem., **252***, 1102–1106

Colburn, N.Y., Lau, S. & Head, R.A. (1975) Decrease of epidermal histidase activity by tumour promoting phorbol esters. *Cancer Res., **35***, 3154–3159

DiPasquale, A., White, D. & McGuire, P (1978) Epidermal growth factor stimulates putrescine transport and ornithine decarboxylase activity in cultivated human fibroblasts. *Exp. Cell Res., **116***, 317–323

Fisher, P.B., Mufson, R.A., Weinstein, I.B. & Little, J.B. (1981) Epidermal growth factor like tumour promoters enhances viral and radiation-induced cell transformation. *Carcinogenesis, **2***, 183–191

Fujiki, H., Mori, M., Nakaysu, M. Terada, M. & Sugimura, T. (1979) A possible naturally occurring tumour promoter, teleocidin B from Streptomyces. *Biochem. biophys. Res. Commun.*, ***90***, 976–983

Fujiki, H., Mori, M., Nakaysu, M., Terada, M., Sugimura, T. & Moore, R.E. (1981) Indole alkaloids, dihydro-teleocidin B, teleocidin and lyngbyatoxin B, a new class of tumour promoters. *Proc. natl Acad. Sci. USA*, ***78***, 3872–3876

Garte, S.J. & Belman, S. (1980) Tumour promoter uncouples β-adrenergic receptor from adenyl cyclase in mouse epidermis. *Nature*, ***284***, 171–173

zur Hausen, H.Z., O'Neill, F.J. & Freese, U.K. (1978) Persisting onogenic herpes virus induced by the tumour promoter TPA. *Nature*, ***272***, 373–375

Horowitz, A.D., Greenbaum, E. & Weinstein, I.B. (1981) Identification of receptor for phorbol ester tumour promoters in intact mammalian cells and of an inhibitor of receptor binding in biological fluids. *Proc. natl. Acad. Sci. USA*, ***78***, 2315–2319

Houslay, M.D. & Gordon, L.M. (1983) In: Kleinzeuer, A. & Martin, B.R., eds, *Membrane Receptors*, Vol. 1, New York, Academic Press (in press)

Houslay, M.D., Metcalf, J.C., Warren, T.B., Hesketh, T.R. & Smith, G.A. (1976) The glucagon receptor of rat liver plasma membrane can couple to adenylate cyclase without activating it. *Biochem. biophys. Acta*, ***436***, 489–494

Houslay, M.D., Dipple, I. & Elliot, K.R.F. (1980) Guanosine 5′-triphosphate and guanosine 5′-(βγ-imide) triphosphate effect of a collision coupling mechanism between the glucagon receptor and catalytic unit of adenylate cyclase. *Biochem. J.*, ***186***, 649–658

Kuo, J.F., Anderson, R.G.G., Wise, B.C., Mackerlova, L., Salomonsson, I., Brackett, N.L., Katoh, N., Shoji, M. & Wrenn, R.W. (1980) Calcium-dependent protein kinase: widespread occurrence in various tissues and phyla of the animal kingdom and comparison of effects of phospholipid, calmoulin, and trifluoperazine. *Proc. natl Acad. Sci. USA*, ***77***, 7039–7043

Laskey, R.A. & Mills, A.D. (1975) Quantitative film detection of [$^3$H] and [$^{14}$C] in polyacrylamide gels by fluorography. *Eur. J. Biochem.*, ***56***, 335–341

Laskin, J.D., Mufson, R.A., Piccini, L., Engelhardt, D.L. & Weinstein, I.B. (1981) Effects of tumour promoter 12-*O*-tetradecanoyl phorbol-13-acetate on newly synthesised proteins in mouse epidermis. *Cell*, ***25***, 441–449

Leavitt, J. & Kakunaga, T. (1980) Expression of a variant form of actin and additional polypeptide changes following chemical-induced *in vitro* neoplastic transformation of human fibroblasts. *J. biol. Chem.*, ***255***, 1650–1661

Lee, L.S. & Weinstein, I.B. (1978a) Tumour-promoting phorbol esters inhibit binding of epidermal growth factor to cellular receptors. *Science*, ***202***, 313–315

Lee, L.S. & Weinstein, I.B (1978b) Epidermal growth factor, like tumour promoting phorbol esters, induces plasminogen activator activity. *Nature*, ***274***, 696–697

Limbird, L.E., Gill, D.M. & Lefkowitz, R.J. (1980) Agonist-promoted coupling of the β-adrenergic receptor with the guanine nucleotide regulatory protein of the adenylate cyclase system. *Proc. natl Acad. Sci. USA*, ***77***, 775–779

Marks. F. (1976) Epidermal growth control mechanisms; hyperplasia and tumour promotion. *Cancer Res.*, ***36***, 2636–2645

Niedel, J.E., Kuhn, L.J. & Vandenbark, G.R. (1983) Phorbol diester receptor co-purifies with protein kinase C. *Proc. natl Acad. Sci. USA*, ***80***, 36–40

O'Brien, T.G., Simsiman, R.C. & Boutwell, R.K. (1975) Induction of polyamine biosynthetic enzymes in mouse epidermis and their specificity in tumour promotion. *Cancer Res.*, ***35***, 2426–2433

O'Farrell, P.H. (1975) High resolution two-dimensional electrophoresis of proteins. *J. biol. Chem.*, ***250***, 4007–4021

O'Farrell, P.Z, Goodman, H.M. & O'Farrell, P.H. (1977) High resolution two-dimensional gel electrophoresis of basic as well as acidic proteins. *Cell*, ***12***, 1133–1142

Reynolds, F.M., Todaro, G.J., Fryling, C. & Stephenson, J.R. (1981) Human transforming growth factors induce tyrosine phosphorylation of EGF receptors. *Nature*, ***292***, 259–262

Roberts, A.B., Anzano, M.A., Lamb, L.C., Smith, J.M., Frolik, C.A., Marquardt, H., Todaro, G.J. & Sporn, M.B. (1982) Isolation from murine sarcoma cells of novel transforming growth factors potentiated by EGF. *Nature*, ***295***, 417–419

Roop. D.R., Hawley-Nelson, P., Cheng, C.K. & Yuspa, S.H. (1983) Keratin gene expression in mouse epidermis and cultured epidermal cells. *Proc. natl Acad. Sci. USA*, ***80***, 716–720

Rose, S.P., Stahn, R., Passovey, D.V. & Herschman, H. (1976) Epidermal growth factor enhancement of skin tumour induction. *Experientia*, ***32***, 913–919

Shoyab, M., DeLarco, J.E. & Todaro, G.J. (1979) Biologically active phorbol esters specifically alter affinity of epidermal growth factor membrane receptors. *Nature*, ***279***, 387–391

Umezawa, K., Weinstein, I.B., Horowitz, A., Fujiki, H., Matsushima, T. & Sugimura, T. (1981) Teleocidin B and phorbol ester tumour promoters produce similar effects on membranes and membrane receptors. *Nature*, ***290***, 411–413

Varshavsky, A. (1981) Phorbol ester dramatically increases the incidence of methotrexate-resistant mouse cells: possible mechanisms and relevance to tumour promotion. *Cell*, ***25***, 561–572

Weinstein, I.B., Lee, L.S., Fisher, P.B., Mufson, A. & Yamasaki, H. (1979) Action of phorbol esters in cell culture: mimickry of transformation, altered differentiation and effects on cell membranes. *J. Supramol. Struct.*, ***12***, 195–208

Wigler, M. & Weinstein, I.B. (1976) Tumour promoter induces plasminogen activator. *Nature*, ***259***, 232–233

Yamasaki, H. (1980) *Reversible inhibition of cell differentiation by phorbol esters as a possible mechanism of the promotion step of chemical carcinogenesis.* In: Montesano, R., Bartsch, H. & Tomatis, L., eds, *Molecular and Cellular Aspects of Carcinogen Screening Tests (IARC Scientific Publications No. 27)*, Lyon, International Agency for Research on Cancer, pp. 91–111

# CELLULAR RESPONSE TO TUMOUR-PROMOTING AGENTS

# MECHANISMS OF INITIATION AND PROMOTION IN MOUSE EPIDERMIS

S.H. YUSPA

*Laboratory of Cellular Carcinogenesis and Tumor Promotion, National Cancer Institute, Bethesda, MD 20205, USA*

## SUMMARY

Studies performed on mouse skin have indicated that chemical carcinogenesis can be subdivided into two distinct stages — initiation and promotion. Initiation results from exposure to a classical mutagenic carcinogen and is irreversible even after a single exposure. The permanently altered initiated cell and its progeny may never form a tumour or be in any way recognizable in the target tissue. Exposure to tumour promoters permits the expression of the neoplastic change in initiated cells, and tumours develop. In contrast to initiators, promoters must be given repeatedly to be effective; individual exposures are reversible. Studies in mouse skin cell cultures have provided new insights into the changes associated with initiation and promotion. Some carcinogen-treated cells and cells derived from initiated mouse skin are resistant to signals for terminal differentiation and can proliferate under conditions in which normal cells are obliged to cease proliferation and begin their maturation programme. This change is essential for a tumour cell, since it provides it with the ability to grow away from a basement membrane attachment site. In cultured epidermal cells, tumour promoters are capable of stimulating selectively the growth of certain cells, including initiated cells, while inducing simultaneously terminal differentiation in other epidermal cells. The induction of terminal differentiation may be mediated by the phorbol ester receptor. The net effect of these responses to promoters is the clonal expansion of cells stimulated to proliferate. In this way, promoters are capable of increasing the clone size of initiated cells and producing benign tumours. In-vivo studies have indicated that promoters are incapable of accelerating the conversion of benign to malignant tumours. However, exposure of papilloma-bearing mice to genotoxic initiating carcinogens accelerates malignant conversion markedly. Thus, initiation and promotion appear to be relevant to the formation of preneoplastic lesions, but further genetic damage may be required for the carcinogenic event.

## INTRODUCTION

Studies performed in mouse skin have indicated that tumour induction by chemicals can be subdivided into two distinct stages, initiation and promotion. Initiation results from exposure to a classical mutagenic carcinogen and is irreversible even after a single exposure. The permanently altered initiated cell and its progeny may never form a tumour or be in any way recognizable in the target tissue. Exposure to tumour promoters permits the expression of the neoplastic change in initiated cells, and tumours develop. In contrast to initiation, promoters must be given repeatedly to be effective; individual exposures are reversible. Other model systems for chemical carcinogenesis have shown a similar biology, although the initiating and promoting agents involved may be distinct for each tissue. Thus, in experiments with rats, the liver, oesophagus, colon, bladder, mammary gland and trachea, and in mice, the lung and stomach are subject to multistage tumour induction. It is clear from this list that the phenomenon occurs in the epithelium of complex tissues. In most of these tissues, target epithelial cells are organized in a stratifying or maturing arrangement, usually in a terminally differentiating lining epithelium. Such epithelia are often composed of more than one cell type or of cells in differing biological states. It is not clear if tissue complexity is a fundamental requirement for a multistage mechanism or if other, less complex, organ sites have simply not been explored adequately.

Tumours may also be induced in skin by repeated application of initiating agents. Studies comparing tumour induction by initiator-promoter or by repeated initiator application have suggested that the mechanism of cancer induction by each protocol may be different. One-stage protocols generally yield de-novo carcinomas or persistent papillomas, while two-stage protocols yield mostly papillomas which regress (Shubik, 1950; Burns *et al.*, 1976). Carcinomas arise from papillomas late in the two-stage process (Verma & Boutwell, 1980; Hennings *et al.*, 1983). Carcinogenesis involving promoters also differs from repeated initiator application in strain susceptibility and in the types of chemicals which modify each process (Yuspa, 1983). Therefore, mechanistic studies in tumour promotion must be directed at defining pathogenesis based upon the biology of tumour induction by the two-stage protocol, particularly with regard to the formation of benign lesions. It is in this context that our laboratory has approached the elucidation of mechanisms of initiation and tumour promotion in mouse skin.

## MATERIALS AND METHODS

### *Chemicals*

12-*O*-Tetradecanoylphorbol-13-acetate (TPA) was obtained from Chemicals for Carcinogenesis Research, Eden Prairie, MN, USA. Teleocidin B was kindly provided by Dr Hirota Fujiki and Dr Takashi Sugimura of the National Cancer Research Institute, Tokyo, Japan. Benzo[*a*]pyrene (BP), 7,12-dimethylbenz[*a*]anthracene (DMBA) and *N*-methyl-*N'*-nitro-*N*-nitrosoguanidine (MNNG) were obtained from the carcinogen repository of the National Cancer Institute, USA. 4-Nitroquinoline-

*N*-oxide (4-NQO) was from Sigma Chemicals, and urethane was obtained from Coleman, Bell, Matheson. Reagents for the transglutaminase assay were from sources described previously (Yuspa *et al.*, 1980a).

### *Induction of skin tumours*

SENCAR female mice in the resting phase of the hair cycle (6–7 weeks of age) were painted once with 20 μg DMBA in acetone. One week later, TPA (2.5 μg) was applied topically in 200 μL acetone, and this treatment was continued weekly for 10 weeks. At that time, the following treatment was instituted at weekly intervals: acetone, 2.5 μg TPA, 120 μg MNNG topically, 250 μg 4-NQO topically or 20 mg urethane intraperitoneally. Papillomas and carcinomas were recorded weekly and confirmed histologically at sacrifice.

### *Cell culture*

Epidermal cells were prepared from BALB/c newborn mice as described elsewhere (Yuspa *et al.*, 1980b) and plated at $8 \times 10^6$ cells per 100-mm culture dishes or $4 \times 10^6$ cells per 60-mm culture dish. Cultures were grown under reduced calcium conditions in either Medium 199 and 2% Chelex (Chelex, Biorad, Richmond, CA, USA)-treated fetal calf serum (Reheis, Kankakee, IL, USA) (0.07 mM calcium ion) or Eagle's minimal essential medium (MEM) containing non-essential amino acids and 8% Chelex-treated fetal calf serum (0.02 mM calcium ion) (Hennings *et al.*, 1980). This method selects for the basal-cell population (Yuspa *et al.*, 1980b). In order to induce differentiation, the calcium ion concentration was increased to 1.2–1.4 mM by addition of appropriate amounts of 0.3 M calcium chloride. All media contained 1% Antibiotic-Antimycotic Solution (GIBCO, Grand Island, NY, USA).

### *Biochemical assays*

Transglutaminase activity was assayed by measuring the incorporation of $^3$H-putrescine into casein in the presence of frozen-thawed cell lysates. The assay was performed as described previously (Yuspa *et al.*, 1980a). Studies of DNA synthesis measured the incorporation of [methyl-$^3$H]-thymidine into DNA (Hennings *et al.*, 1980).

## RESULTS

### *In-vivo development of squamous-cell carcinomas*

Recent studies in our laboratory demonstrated the importance of recognizing the distinction between tumorigenesis associated with applications of tumour promoters and carcinogenesis associated with other protocols in mouse skin (Hennings *et al.*, 1983). Papillomas were produced on SENCAR mouse skin by a standard initiation-promotion protocol. After 10 weeks of TPA promotion, groups of papilloma-bearing mice were subdivided into five groups of 30 animals each for third-stage treatment. One group received only topical acetone for the remainder of the experiment, while

Table 1. Cancer development at 52 weeks in SENCAR mice

| Stage 3 treatment | Carcinomas (%)[a] | | |
|---|---|---|---|
| | Stage 1 – Stage 2<br>Acetone – Acetone | Stage 1 – Stage 2<br>Acetone – TPA | Stage 1 – Stage 2<br>DMBA – TPA |
| Acetone | – | 5 | 42 |
| TPA (2.5 μg) | – | 4 | 46 |
| MNNG (120 μg) | 14 | 20 | 90 |
| Urethane (20 μg) | 0 | 16 | 70 |
| 4-NQO (250 μg) | 0 | 6 | 66 |

[a] Percentage of mice in each group bearing carcinomas

TPA, 12-*O*-tetradecanoylphorbol-13-acetate; MNNG, *N*-methyl-*N*′-nitro-*N*-nitrosoguanidine; 4-NQO, 4-nitro-quinoline-*N*-oxide

the others received either topical TPA, topical MNNG, topical 4-NQO or systemic urethane once a week. The conversion rate from papilloma to carcinoma was then calculated during a 42-week experimental period (Table 1 and Hennings *et al.*, 1983). In controls without papillomas (uninitiated), the third-stage agents produced no or very few tumours. In papilloma-bearing mice, the conversion rate was low and the values identical to those obtained with either continuous TPA or acetone exposure. Thus, TPA did not enhance conversion from benign to malignant lesions. All three genotoxic carcinogens used in stage 3 markedly enhanced malignant conversion and also accelerated carcinoma development by up to 12 weeks (data not shown). These results indicate that malignant conversion may result from further genetic change in papilloma cells. The ineffectiveness of TPA points to a mechanism of action different from that of mutagenic carcinogens.

*The biological nature of initiation*

The studies described above suggest that the cellular changes associated with initiation of carcinogenesis are most relevant to the preneoplastic state – that is, the papilloma in mouse skin. The monoclonal nature of the papilloma (Iannacone *et al.*, 1978) suggests that it is a clonal expansion of initiated cells. Growth kinetic studies performed on these tumours indicate several differences from normal skin. The labelling index is about ten-fold higher in both benign and malignant skin tumours (Burns *et al.*, 1976). A striking difference from normal is the presence of proliferating cells away from the basement membrane zone in benign tumours, whereas normal cells are obliged to cease proliferation and initiate their programme of terminal differentiation upon leaving the basement membrane. The ability to proliferate under conditions in which normal cells are obliged to differentiate is probably an early event in transformation – perhaps a key change in initiation.

The discovery that extracellular ionic calcium is a key regulator of epidermal growth and differentiation (Hennings *et al.*, 1980) has facilitated experimental approaches to the study of initiation. In medium with reduced calcium concentrations (0.02–0.09 mM), epidermal basal cells are cultivated selectively. These cells have

Fig. 1. Differentiation-resistant colonies induced by carcinogen treatment
Newborn mouse epidermal cells were plated in 0.02 mM calcium medium and treated with *N*-methyl-*N'*-nitro-*N*-nitrosoguanidine (12 mmol/L) (top row) or ethanol (0.1%) (bottom row) for one hour on the third day. After two weeks in 0.02 mM calcium, cultures were switched to 0.1 mM calcium for one week, 0.5 mM calcium for 1 week and 1.2 mM calcium medium for two weeks. Dishes were fixed with 10% formalin and stained with 1% rhodamine.

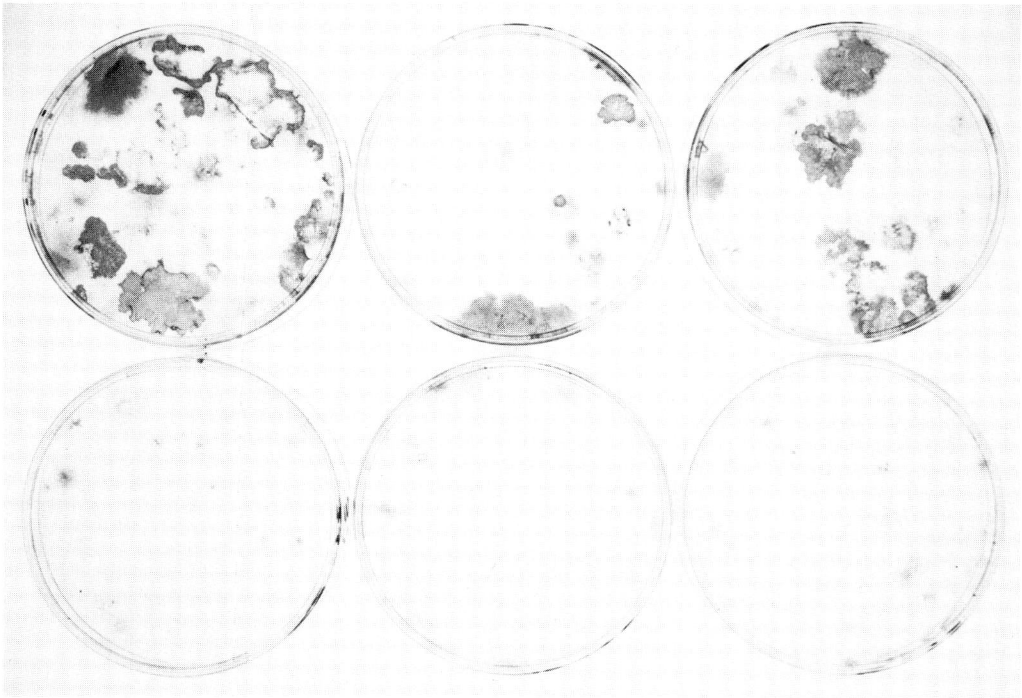

morphological, cell kinetic and marker protein characteristics of basal cells and grow as a monolayer with a high proliferation rate. When the calcium concentration of culture medium is elevated to the levels found in most commercial preparations (1.2–1.4 mM), proliferation ceases and terminal differentiation rapidly ensues, with squamous differentiation and sloughing of cells occurring by 72–96 h. The responses of cultured basal cells to increases in extracellular calcium resemble the changes observed in basal cells *in vivo* as they migrate away from the basement membrane and are committed to differentiate terminally. Therefore, in analogy to in-vivo data, it might be expected that in cell culture carcinogens could alter the basal-cell response to calcium-induced terminal differentiation. In our laboratory we have been studying this model, and some results are presented in Figure 1; others were published previously (Kulesz-Martin *et al.*, 1980).

Basal cells were exposed to carcinogens *in vitro* and subsequently induced to differentiate by calcium. Foci formed which resisted terminal differentiation. Several initiating agents cause the induction of foci, including MNNG, DMBA, BP, 4-NQO, and *N*-acetoxyacetylaminofluorene (N-Ac-AAF). In general, the potency of each agent (DMBA > BP > MNNG > 4-NQO > N-Ac-AAF) *in vitro* paralleled its potency as an initiator in mouse skin. When studied, colony number observed for each agent was proportional to carcinogen dose (Kulesz-Martin *et al.*, 1980). Cells obtained from these colonies have typical keratinocyte morphology, express differentiating functions, synthesize keratin proteins but fail to cease proliferation when signaled to differentiate by calcium ion. Such cells are generally not tumorigenic when tested early after selection in high calcium ion concentrations; but, on prolonged subculture, tumorigenic cell lines evolve. Similar foci can be derived from cell cultures of mouse skin initiated *in vivo* by exposure to DMBA and cultured in 0.02 mM calcium medium for several weeks, followed by selection in 1.2 mM calcium. In these experiments, control skin does not yield colonies (Yuspa & Morgan, 1981). Malignant epidermal cells cultured in the presence of a large excess of normal basal cells in 0.02 mM calcium medium also continue to proliferate and form colonies when switched to 1.2 mM calcium, while normal cells slough from culture as terminally differentiated squamae (Kulesz-Martin *et al.*, 1980). These results suggest that initiation of carcinogenesis results in the ability of initiated cells to resist the signal to cease proliferation in association with terminal differentiation. In normal skin, such a trait alone could not result in a tumour because of the strong regulatory influences of surrounding normal cells (Potten & Allen, 1975).

*The biological nature of promotion*

Analysis of the biochemical changes in mouse skin produced by phorbol esters, and in particular TPA, has been useful in formulating working hypotheses on the mechanism of tumour promotion. A large number of changes occur in response to TPA (Yuspa, 1983). Several occur within a few minutes (in cyclic nucleotides, in prostaglandins); others take hours (changes in RNA and protein synthesis, polyamine synthesis, transglutaminase and histidase activity, histone phosphorylation, phospholipid synthesis) or up to 24 h (DNA synthesis, synthesis of a histidine-rich protein, HRP). The hyperplasia induced by phorbol esters in mouse skin may persist for weeks. Mediation of some responses *via* action at the cell membrane is likely, and a receptor for TPA has been identified in mouse skin (Delclos *et al.*, 1980). The pleiotropic responses of skin to TPA exposure can be divided into major functional groups relating to epidermal proliferation or terminal differentiation. Many of these changes occur with the same temporal sequence. Since terminal differentiation and proliferation are thought to be mutually exclusive in individual epidermal cells, and basal cells appear to be the principal target for TPA action (Lichti *et al.*, 1981), considerable heterogeneity must exist among basal cells in their programme of induced responses. These biochemical and biological observations have guided our studies to elucidate the mechanism of tumour promotion.

Cell culture studies designed to understand the cellular basis for tumour promotion have focused on data derived in-vivo on the heterogeneity of biochemical responses in mouse skin. When the responsiveness of cultured basal cells to TPA was studied, it became clear that a portion of the population was induced to differentiate by the promoter (Fig. 2) (Yuspa *et al.*, 1982). This phenomenon could be detected by

Fig. 2. Schematic presentation of the heterogeneous response pattern induced in cultured mouse basal cells by brief exposures (18 h from zero time in second column) to phorbol ester tumour promoters
Solid circles represent cells induced to differentiate; open circles are cells stimulated to proliferate. The proliferating cells are obviously precursors of the differentiating cells, as seen in the right-hand column. For experimental details see Yuspa *et al.* (1982). TPA, 12-*O*-tetradecanoylphorbol-13-acetate

| **Resting phase** | **Mixed response phase** | **Selective growth phase** | **Recovery phase** |
|---|---|---|---|
| **Untreated** | **TPA (0-24 hours)** | **TPA (24-72 hours)** | **TPA (10 days)** |
| 1. Basal cell characteristics | 1. Increased transglutaminase | 1. Altered basal cell morphology | 1. Basal cell characteristics |
| 2. High proliferation rate | 2. Cornifying cells | 2. Increased proliferation | 2. High proliferation rate |
| 3. Low transglutaminase | 3. Basal cells | 3. Resistant to $Ca^{++}$ induced differentiation | 3. Low transglutaminase |
| 4. Few cornified cells | 4. Low proliferation rate | 4. Resistant to TPA induced differentiation | 4. Few cornified cells |
| 5. Sensitive to $Ca^{++}$ | | 5. Sensitive to TPA stimulated proliferation | 5. Sensitive to $Ca^{++}$ |

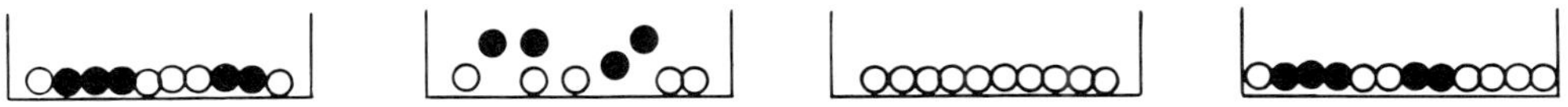

| | | | |
|---|---|---|---|
| Morphologically homogeneous (covert heterogeneity) | Morphologically, pharmacologically heterogeneous | Morphologically, pharmacologically homogeneous | Morphologically homogeneous (covert heterogeneity) |

morphological changes, measurement of the formation of cornified squamae and increase in the activity of the differentiation-associated enzyme epidermal transglutaminase (Yuspa *et al.*, 1980a, 1982). As terminally differentiated cells were sloughed from the culture dish, transglutaminase activity decreased. The basal cells remaining after brief TPA exposure were shown to be transiently resistant to terminal differentiation when cultured in 1.2 mM calcium or when exposed to TPA a second time (Yuspa *et al.*, 1982); however, these cells were stimulated to proliferate by the second exposure to TPA. Thus, two types of responses occur in epidermal basal cells exposed to phorbol esters. In one population, there is the induction of terminal differentiation. In a second population, TPA stimulates proliferation and produces a transient block in response to a differentiation stimulus. The second subpopulation cannot be induced to differentiate by a second TPA exposure if the interval between exposures is short. This response is similar to that of mouse skin *in vivo* after several TPA exposures where proliferative stimulation is the principal effect. Heterogeneity in responsiveness is restored when the culture interval between TPA exposures is prolonged (10 days) (Yuspa *et al.*, 1982). This observation in cell culture is similar to findings *in vivo* when treatment intervals are prolonged.

Recent studies have indicated that other promoting agents which act at the phorbol ester receptor are effective inducers of epidermal transglutaminase and terminal

Fig. 3. Transglutaminase activity after exposure of epidermal cells to 12-*O*-tetradecanoylphorbol-13-acetate (TPA) or teleocidin B
Primary mouse epidermal cells were cultured in 0.07 mM calcium medium for six days and exposed to the indicated concentration of each test agent in 0.1% dimethyl sulfoxide (DMSO) for eight hours. Duplicate dishes were harvested and transglutaminase activity measured in frozen-thawed cell lysates.

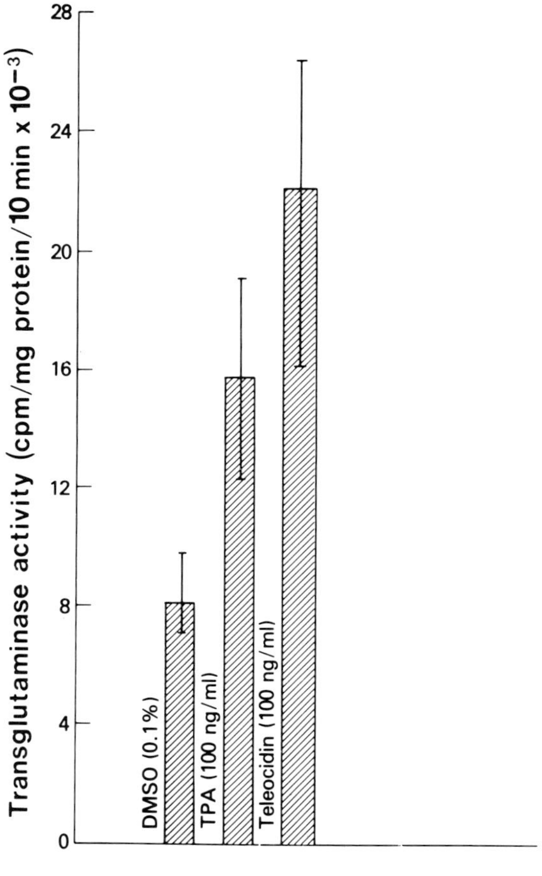


differentiation. Figure 3 shows the response to teleocidin B, a potent tumour promoter for mouse skin which binds with high affinity to the phorbol ester receptor. On a molar basis, teleocidin is a better inducer of transglutaminase activity than TPA. Similar studies have indicated a good correlation for phorbol esters with regard to promoter potency, receptor binding and induction of transglutaminase. However, skin tumour promoters that are not competitive at the phorbol ester receptor do not induce transglutaminase. Figure 4 shows that anthralin is ineffective as an inducer, and similar data were obtained with benzoyl peroxide (data not shown) even at $10^{-5}$ M, a cytotoxic concentration. These results suggest that the phorbol ester receptor is a regulator of epidermal differentiation.

Fig. 4. Transglutaminase activity after exposure of epidermal cells to 12-*O*-tetradecanoylphorbol-13-acetate (TPA) or anthralin
Protocol was the same as that described in the footnote to Figure 3.

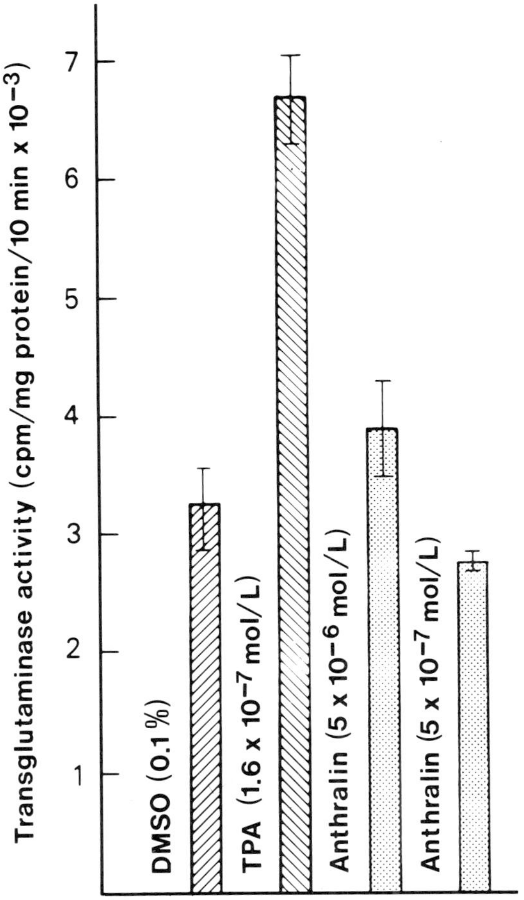


Further support for the inductive nature of phorbol esters for epidermal differentiation comes from studies in which both TPA and calcium ion were combined to induce transglutaminase and terminal differentiation. In this case, there was a rapid acceleration of the differentiation process, including a dramatic increase in transglutaminase activity (Fig. 5) and a rapid decrease as the cells cornified. The results shown in Figure 5 were obtained when TPA and 1.2 mM calcium ion were applied simultaneously; however, similar results were achieved when 1.2 mM calcium were applied first and differentiating cells were challenged up to five hours later with TPA (data not shown). Such cells thus remain responsive to the differentiation signal supplied by TPA. This is markedly different from the response to TPA of differentiating cells in 1.2 mM calcium ion as seen in studies of the induction of ornithine decarboxylase activity (Lichti *et al.*, 1981): in that case, differentiating cells cannot induce ornithine decar-

Fig. 5. Effect of 12-*O*-tetradecanoylphorbol-13-acetate (TPA) on transglutaminase activity in differentiating epidermal cells
Primary epidermal cells were cultured for six days in 0.09 mM calcium medium and maintained in that medium or switched to 1.2 mM calcium plus TPA ($1.6 \times 10^{-7}$ mol/L). Duplicate samples were taken at the indicated intervals. ●, 0.09 mM calcium; △, TPA + 1.2 mM calcium; □, 1.2 mM calcium

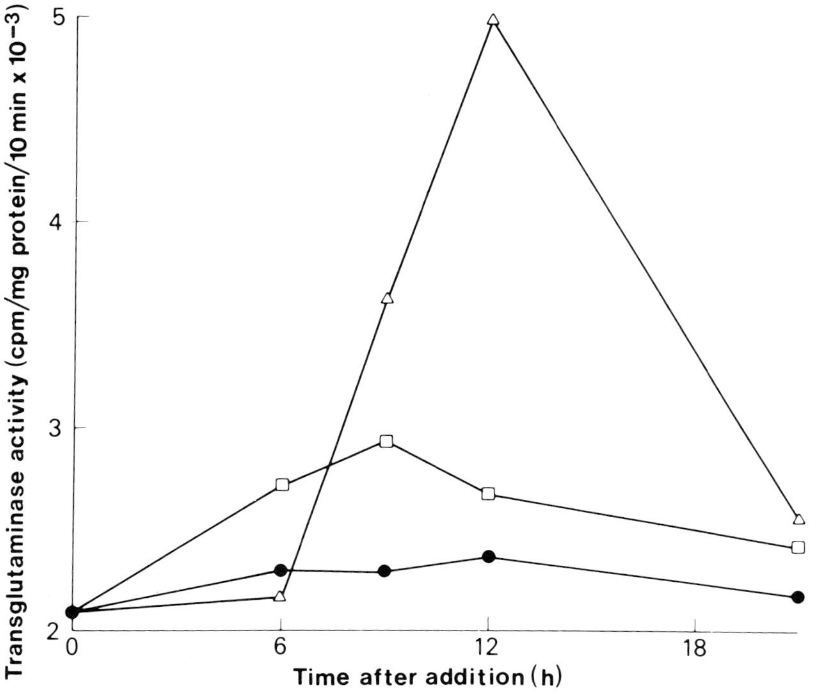


boxylase within a few hours of growth in the higher calcium medium. In other studies, we have found that cells resistant to calcium-induced differentiation in our putative initiation assay are resistant to the differentiation-inducing effects of TPA (Yuspa *et al.*, 1983a), even when cultured in 1.2 mM calcium ion, suggesting a defect in this response pathway.

## DISCUSSION

Multistage carcinogenesis in mouse skin appears to have at least three components, as demonstrated by our studies *in vitro* and *in vivo*. The initial alteration produced by initiators has the characteristics of a genetic change resulting in an uncoupling of the proliferative block associated with induced terminal differentiation. The clonal expansion of this population is accomplished by tumour promoters. In the case of phorbol esters, a receptor-mediated, selective regenerative hyperplasia may be the underlying pharmacological response. The result of these two stages is a premalignant lesion. The conversion of premalignant cells to carcinoma cells is not accomplished by the promoter but may occur spontaneously at a low rate. This low conversion rate can be enhanced significantly by genotoxic carcinogens, suggesting that a further genetic change is required. The high level of proliferation and the large proliferative pool in papillomas may be associated with a finite spontaneous rate of genetic change and malignant conversion in papillomas.

The results obtained from studies in epidermal basal-cell cultures suggest that phorbol esters produce a balanced and programmed heterogeneous response with regard to differentiation and proliferation. The net effect of this type of heterogeneity is to select for and to expand the proliferating population with each exposure to promoter, thus remodelling the target tissue. Clonal selection of carcinogen-altered (differentiation-altered) cells would result if normal basal cells were induced to differentiate while altered (initiated) cells were among those which were stimulated to proliferate. Clonal expansion of initiated cells (with an altered programme of differentiation) resulting from phorbol ester-regulated cell selection would yield benign tumours, which are the major product of two-stage skin carcinogenesis.

The pharmacological basis for the heterogeneity of the epidermal response to phorbol esters could be explained by studies of phorbol ester binding to membrane receptors. In mouse skin, phorbol ester binding to membrane receptors is heterogeneous, with at least two, and possibly three, classes of binding sites (Dunn & Blumberg, 1983). In cultured keratinocytes, subclasses of binding sites can be elicited by inducing terminal differentiation with 1.2 mM calcium ion (Dunn *et al.,* 1983). When cells induced to differentiate by 1.2 mM calcium ion are exposed simultaneously to TPA, there is a marked acceleration of the differentiation response and a recruitment of cells into the differentiating pool (Yuspa *et al.,* 1983b). These findings suggest that the biological and receptor heterogeneity observed in skin is based on a difference in maturation state of epidermal cells. More mature cells respond by accelerated differentiation, while less mature cells are stimulated to proliferate. Studies with a limited number of differentiation-resistant initiated cell lines indicate that these cells are resistant to the differentiative influences of TPA but can be stimulated to proliferate by the promoter (Yuspa *et al.*, 1983a). These results are not influenced by the calcium concentration in the culture medium. The initiated cell lines also appear to have only a single phorbol ester binding component.

The induction of transglutaminase activity and cornification of keratinocyte cell envelopes is part of a programme of changes associated with accelerated epidermal differentiation after exposure to phorbol esters. Other associated changes include rapid migration of cells from the basal layer (Argyris, 1980), accelerated synthesis of higher molecular weight keratins (Steinert & Yuspa, 1978), and increase in synthesis of the histidine-rich protein, fillagrin (Kreig *et al.*, 1974; Balmain, 1978). Phorbol esters also induce differentiation in several cell culture models of tissues other than skin (Diamond *et al.*, 1980) and in human keratinocyte cultures (Hawley-Nelson *et al.*, 1982). Structure-activity studies indicate that receptor binding is critical to these responses, suggesting that the phorbol ester receptor may be a common regulator of differentiation in several cell types. The recent isolation of a soluble phorbol ester binding protein and its probable identification as protein kinase C (Leach *et al.*, 1983; Niedel *et al.*, 1983) could provide a major advance in our understanding of the control of differentiation in epidermis and a variety of other tissues. In this regard, both extracellular calcium ion and TPA induce terminal differentiation in cultured epidermal cells. The finding that protein kinase C requires calcium ion as a cofactor and that TPA also activates this enzyme (Castagna *et al.*, 1982) would indicate a common pathway, through protein kinase C, by which both calcium ion and TPA induce terminal differentiation. This mechanism could be similar to the synergistic action of TPA and calcium ion in activating protein kinase C in the release of serotonin by platelets (Yamanishi *et al.*, 1983).

## ACKNOWLEDGEMENTS

I am indebted to my colleagues Dr Henry Hennings, Dr Ulrike Lichti and Dr Molly Kulesz-Martin for their contributions to these studies and for their discussions in formulating the conclusions. The technical assistance of Theresa Ben and Anne Kilkenny and the secretarial assistance of Margaret Green are also appreciated.

## REFERENCES

Argyris, T.S. (1980) Epidermal growth following a single application of 12-*O*-tetradecanoylphorbol-13-acetate in mice. *Am. J. Pathol.*, ***98***, 639–646

Balmain, A. (1978) *Synthesis of specific proteins in mouse epidermis after treatment with tumor promoter TPA.* In: Slaga, T.J., Sivak, A. & Boutwell, R.K., eds, *Mechanisms of Tumor Promotion and Cocarcinogenesis*, Vol. 2, New York, Raven Press, pp. 153–172

Burns, F.J., Vanderlaan, M., Sivak, A. & Albert, R.A. (1976) Regression kinetics of mouse skin papillomas. *Cancer Res.*, ***36***, 1422–1427

Castagna, M., Takai, Y., Kaibachi, K., Sano, K., Kalekawa, U. & Nishizuka, Y. (1982) Direct activation of calcium activated, phospholipid dependent protein kinase by tumor promoting phorbol esters. *J. biol. Chem.*, ***257***, 7847–7851

Delclos, K.B., Nagle, D.S. & Blumberg, P.M. (1980) Specific binding of phorbol ester tumor promoters to mouse skin. *Cell*, ***19***, 1025–1033

Diamond, L., O'Brien, T.G. & Baird, W.M. (1980) Tumor promoters and the mechanism of tumor promotion. *Adv. Cancer Res.*, ***32***, 1–74

Dunn, J.A. & Blumberg, P.M. (1983) Specific binding of [20–$^{3}$H]-12-deoxyphorbol-13-isobutyrate to phorbol ester receptor subclasses in mouse skin particulate preparations. *Cancer Res.*, ***40***, 4632–4637

Dunn, J.A., Yuspa, S.H. & Blumberg, P.M. (1983) Specific binding of [20–$^{3}$H]-phorbol-12,13-dibutyrate to proliferating and differentiated mouse primary keratinocytes. *Proc. Am. Assoc. Cancer Res.*, ***24***, 111

Hawley-Nelson, P., Stanley, J., Schmidt, J., Gullino, M. & Yuspa, S.H. (1982) The tumor promoter 12-*O*-tetradecanoylphorbol-13-acetate accelerates keratinocyte differentiation and stimulates growth of an unidentified cell type in cultured human epidermis. *Exp. Cell Res.*, ***137***, 155–167

Hennings, H., Michael, D., Cheng, C., Steinert, P., Holbrook, K. & Yuspa, S.H. (1980) Calcium regulation of growth and differentiation of mouse epidermal cells in culture. *Cell*, ***19***, 245–254

Hennings, H., Shores, R., Wenk, M.L., Spangler, E.F., Tarone, R. & Yuspa, S.H. (1983) Malignant conversion of mouse skin tumours is increased by tumour initiators and unaffected by tumour promoters. *Nature*, ***304***, 67–69

Iannaccone, P.M., Gardner, R.L. & Harris, H. (1978) The cellular origin of chemically induced tumors. *J. Cell Sci.*, ***29***, 249–269

Kreig, L., Kuhlman, I. & Marks, F. (1974) Effect of tumor-promoting phorbol esters and acetic acid on mechanisms controlling DNA synthesis and mitosis (chalones) and on the biosynthesis of histidine-rich protein in mouse epidermis. *Cancer Res.*, ***34***, 3135–3146

Kulesz-Martin, M., Koehler, B., Hennings, H. & Yuspa, S.H. (1980) Quantitative assay for carcinogen-altered differentiation in mouse epidermal cells. *Carcinogenesis*, ***1***, 995–1006

Leach, K.L., James, M.L. & Blumberg, P.M. (1983) Characterization of a specific phorbol ester apo-receptor in mouse brain cytosol. *Proc. natl Acad. Sci. USA*, ***80***, 4208–4212

Lichti, U., Patterson, E., Hennings, H. & Yuspa, S.H. (1981) The tumor promoter 12-O-tetradecanoylphorbol-13-acetate induces ornithine decarboxylase in proliferating basal cells but not in differentiating cells from mouse epidermis. *J. Cell Physiol.*, ***107***, 261–270

Niedel, J.E., Kuhn, L.J. & Vandenbark, G.R. (1983) Phorbol diester receptor copurifies with protein kinase C. *Proc. natl Acad. Sci. USA*, ***80***, 36–40

Potten, C.S. & Allen, T.D. (1975) Control of epidermal proliferative units. *Differentiation*, ***3***, 161–165

Shubik, P. (1950) The growth potentialities of induced skin tumors in mice. The effects of different methods of chemical carcinogenesis. *Cancer Res.*, ***10***, 713–717

Steinert, P. & Yuspa, S.H. (1978) Biochemical evidence for keratinization by mouse epidermal cells in culture. *Science*, ***200***, 1491–1493

Verma, A.K. & Boutwell, R.K. (1980) Effects of dose and duration of treatment with the tumor promoting agent, 12-*O*-tetradecanoylphorbol-13-acetate on mouse skin carcinogenesis. *Carcinogenesis*, ***1***, 271–276

Yamanishi, J., Takai, Y., Kaibachi, K., Sano, K., Castagna, M. & Nishizuka, Y. (1983) Synergistic function of phorbol ester and calcium in serotonin release from human platelets. *Biochem. biophys. Res. Commun.*, ***112***, 778–786

Yuspa, S.H. (1983) *Cutaneous carcinogenesis: natural and experimental.* In: Goldsmith, L.A., ed., *Biochemistry and Physiology of the Skin*, Vol. II, New York, Oxford University Press, pp. 1115–1138

Yuspa, S.H. & Morgan, D.L. (1981) Initiation of carcinogenesis in mouse skin is associated with alterations in commitment for terminal differentiation. *Nature*, ***293***, 72–74

Yuspa, S.H., Ben, T.B., Hennings, H. & Lichti, U. (1980a) Phorbol ester tumor promoters induce epidermal transglutaminase activity. *Biochem. biophys. Res. Commun.*, ***97***, 700–708

Yuspa, S.H., Hawley-Nelson, P., Stanley, J.R. & Hennings, H. (1980b) Epidermal cell culture. *Transplant. Proc. 12:* ***Suppl. 1***, 114–122

Yuspa, S.H., Ben, T., Hennings, H. & Lichti, U. (1982) Heterogeneous response in epidermal basal cells exposed to the tumor promoter 12-*O*-tetradecanoylphorbol-13-acetate. *Cancer Res.,* ***42***, 2344–2349

Yuspa, S.H., Kulesz-Martin, M., Ben, T. & Hennings, H. (1983a) Transformation of epidermal cells in culture. *J. invest. Dermatol.,* ***81,*** $144_s$–$149_s$

Yuspa, S.H., Ben, T. & Hennings, H. (1983b) The regulation of epidermal transglutaminase and terminal differentiation by tumor promoters in cultured epidermal cells. *Carcinogenesis,* ***4,*** 1413–1418

# ROLE OF SPECIFIC MEMBRANE AND GENETIC CHANGES IN THE MECHANISM OF TUMOUR PROMOTION. STUDIES WITH PROMOTER-RESISTANT VARIANTS

N.H. COLBURN, L. SRINIVAS, G.A. HEGAMYER, L.D. DION & E.J. WENDEL

*Cell Biology Section, Laboratory of Viral Carcinogenesis, National Cancer Institute-FCRF, Bldg 560, Frederick, MD 21701, USA*

M. COHEN

*Laboratory of Molecular Virology and Carcinogenesis, National Cancer Institute-FCRF, Bldg 560, Frederick, MD 21701, USA*

T.D. GINDHART

*Laboratory of Experimental Pathology, National Cancer Institute-FCRF, Bldg 560, Frederick, MD 21701, USA*

## SUMMARY

Several cell culture model systems in current use for studying tumour promotion mechanism are reviewed briefly. The conclusions that can be drawn from studies with the JB6 mouse epidermal system are summarized. Promoter-induced mitogenic stimulation, epidermal growth factor receptor binding and stimulated hexose transport are apparently not required for promotion of neoplastic transformation in JB6 cells by phorbol esters and other promoters. Phorbol ester receptor binding (or protein kinase C activation) and switched-off collagen synthesis may be required, but definitive proof is not available. Decreased cell surface trisialoganglioside synthesis and one or more genes that determine promotion sensitivity appear to distinguish sensitive from resistant cells and to be required for promotion of neoplastic transformation in JB6 cells.

## INTRODUCTION

Many of the questions posed sometime ago about the mechanism of multistage carcinogenesis remain unanswered. In-vivo studies (Slaga *et al.,* 1980a,b; Furstenberger *et al.,* 1981) have made it possible to characterize substages of tumour promotion or progression with respect to specific inducers or inhibitors, thereby suggesting requirements for certain biochemical events. Several recently developed cell culture systems offer possibilities for discerning rate-limiting events involved in traversing stages of carcinogenesis. As shown in Table 1, several rodent fibroblast and epithelial systems are suitable for the study of tumour promotion. The adenovirus-transformed cells (Fisher *et al.,* 1979, 1982; Babiss *et al.,* 1983), both 10T½ systems (Mondal & Heidelberger, 1976; Mondal *et al.,* 1976; Kennedy *et al.,* 1978; Mordan *et al.,* 1982), the BALB 3T3 cells (Hirakawa *et al.,* 1982), rat tracheal cells (Terzaghi & Nettesheim, 1979; Terzaghi *et al.,* 1982) and JB6 mouse epidermal cells (Colburn *et al.,* 1979–1984) all reach an anchorage-independent and tumorigenic endpoint at the end of the promotion process. All but the JB6 and a subset of the calcium-resistant (Hennings *et al.,* 1980; Yuspa & Morgan, 1981) cells have been obtained after exposure to a known initiator of carcinogenesis. All but the 10T½ RA cells, the calcium-resistant cells and the rat tracheal cells require exposure to specific

Table 1. Cell culture systems available for studying the mechanism of tumour promotion[a]

| System | Initiator(s) | Promoter(s) | References |
|---|---|---|---|
| Adenovirus 5-transformed anchorage-dependent rat embryo fibroblasts | Adenovirus 5 | PDE<br>EGF | Fisher *et al.*, 1979, 1982;<br>Babiss *et al.*, 1983 |
| C3H 10T½ cells | MC<br>UV, X-rays<br>MNNG<br>AFB | PDE | Mondal & Heidelberger, 1976;<br>Mondal *et al.*, 1976<br>Kennedy *et al.*, 1978<br>Boreiko *et al.*, 1982 |
| C3H 10T½ INIT retinyl acetate-dependent cells | MC | Spontaneous: absence of RA | Mordan *et al.*, 1982 |
| BALB 3T3 cells | MC<br>4NQO | PDE<br>Teleocidin | Hirakawa *et al.*, 1982 |
| Calcium-resistant mouse epidermal cell lines | Spontaneous<br>DMBA | ND | Hennings *et al.*, 1980<br>Yuspa & Morgan, 1981 |
| Rat tracheal epithelial cells | MNNG<br>DMBA | ND | Terzaghi & Nettesheim, 1979;<br>Terzaghi *et al.*, 1982 |
| JB6 mouse epidermal cell lines | Spontaneous | PDE<br>Teleocidin<br>EGF<br>TGF<br>Benzoyl peroxide<br>DEHP | Colburn *et al.*, 1979–1984 |

[a] Abbreviations: MC, 3-methylcholanthrene; UV, ultraviolet irradiation; MNNG, *N*-methyl-*N*′-nitro-*N*-nitrosoguanidine; AFB, aflatoxin B; 4NQO, 4-nitroquinoline-*N*-oxide; DMBA, 7,12-dimethylbenz[*a*]anthracene; PDE, phorbol diesters; EGF, epidermal growth factor; RA, retinoic acid; ND, not determined; TGF, transforming growth factors; DEHP, diethylhexylphthalate

promoters to induce neoplastic transformation. The JB6- and the adenovirus-transformed systems offer both sensitive and resistant variants for induction of neoplastic transformation by tumour promoters. The adenovirus-transformed cells, the calcium-resistant epidermal cells, the rat tracheal epithelial cells and the JB6 epidermal cells all retain stable preneoplastic phenotypes over many passages. The adenovirus-transformed cells make it possible to study the regulation of expression of clonal genes for which probes are available. The JB6- and adenovirus-transformed cells have been shown to be sensitive to promotion of transformation, not only by agents that interact with the phorbol ester receptor but also with other classes of agents. In the case of the JB6 cells, these agents include growth factors (Colburn *et al.*, 1980; Colburn & Gindhart, 1981), free radical-generating agents and oxidants (Srinivas & Colburn, 1984b; Gindhart *et al.*, 1984) and liver tumour promoters such as diethylhexylphthalate (DEHP) (Diwan *et al.*, 1983).

Figure 1 illustrates some of the characteristics of the JB6 mouse epidermal system, used in our study of late preneoplastic progression. Sensitive ($P^+$) JB6 clonal lines can be exposed, either in monolayer culture (Colburn *et al.*, 1978) or in soft agar (Colburn *et al.*, 1979), to tumour promoters with resultant induction of anchorage independence and tumorigenicity, which is attained irreversibly. The resistant ($P^-$) variants obtained by cloning the same uncloned JB6 parental cells (Colburn *et al.*, 1980) show an anchorage-independent response that is approximately 0.1 to 1% as high as that of the JB6 $P^+$ lines.

Fig. 1. Clonal variation for promotion of transformation by tumour-promoting phorbol diester

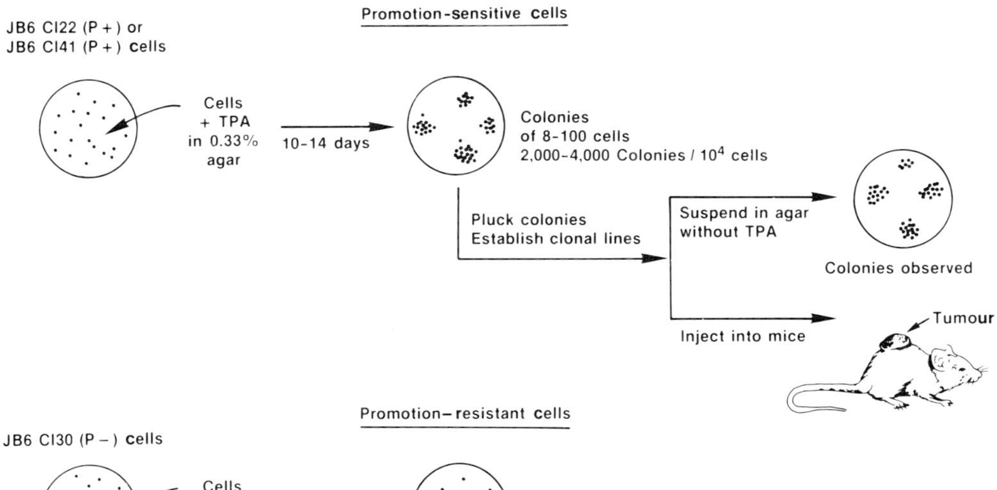

Table 2. Molecular and cellular events implicated in promotion of neoplastic transformation in JB6 mouse epidermal cells[a]

| Event | Evidence | Reference |
|---|---|---|
| *Not required* | | |
| Mitogenic stimulation | $M^-$ $P^+$ variants found | Colburn *et al.*, 1981b |
| | DEHP promotes without mitogenesis | Diwan *et al.*, 1983 & unpublished data |
| EGF receptor binding | $EGF_R^-$ $P^+$ variants found | Colburn *et al.*, 1982a,b |
| Stimulated hexose transport | $\uparrow HX^-$ $P^+$ variants found | Copley *et al.*, 1983 |
| *Possibly required* | | |
| PDE receptor binding | No $PDE_R^-$ variants found | Colburn *et al.*, 1982a, 1983a |
| Switched-off collagen synthesis | No $\downarrow COLL^-$ variants found | Dion *et al.*, 1981, 1982 |
| *Probably required* | | |
| Decreased $G_T$ synthesis | All $P^+$ lines showed $>90\% \downarrow G_T$ All $P^-$ lines did not | Srinivas *et al.*, 1982 |
| | Added $G_T$ specifically blocks promotion | Srinivas *et al.*, 1982; Srinivas & Colburn, 1984b |
| | Selection for $\downarrow G_T^-$ coselected for $P^-$ | Colburn & Srinivas, 1984 |
| One or more $P^+$ genes | Transfection of DNA from $P^+$ but not $P^-$ cells transfers $P^+$ phenotype | Colburn *et al.*, 1983c,d |
| | Transfectable $P^+$ activity is sensitive to DNase and some but not all restriction endonucleases | Table 4 & unpublished data |

[a] Abbreviations: $M^-$, resistant to mitogenic stimulation at plateau density by TPA; $P^+/P^-$, sensitive/resistant to promotion of transformation by phorbol esters and non phorbol tumour promoters; DEHP, diethylhexylphthalate, a liver tumour promoter (Diwan *et al.*, 1983) and promoter of neoplastic transformation in JB6 cells; $EGF^-$, EGF receptorless; $\uparrow HX^-$, resistant to stimulation of hexose transport by phorbol esters; $PDE^-$, phorbol diester receptorless; $\downarrow COLL^-$, resistant to 90% decrease in collagen synthesis by phorbol esters and other tumour promoters; $G_T$, trisialoganglioside; $\downarrow G_T^-$, resistant to $>90\%$ decrease in $G_T$ synthesis by tumour promoters

The work reported in this communication involves the testing of several hypotheses for the events required in promotion of neoplastic transformation in JB6 cells. Two events emerge as likely to be required, namely, a decreased cell-surface trisialoganglioside synthesis and the expression of one or more genes that determine sensitivity to tumour promoters. The evidence is summarized in Table 2.

## RESULTS AND DISCUSSION

### *Responses to tumour promoters that do not discriminate P+ from P− cells and appear not to be required for promotion of transformation*

Mitogenic stimulation occurs in response to a variety of tumour promoters *in vivo* and in cell culture (Colburn *et al.*, 1981b). Since selection for cells resistant to mitogenic stimulation by phorbol esters did not consistently coselect for cells resistant to promotion of neoplastic transformation (Colburn *et al.*, 1981b), we concluded that mitogenic stimulation and promotion in JB6 cells were dissociable. Further support for this conclusion has come from three observations: (1) the selection for 12-*O*-tetradecanoylphorbol-13-acetate (TPA) mitogen-resistant (M-) variants actually produced some anchorage-independent transformants under conditions in which the selected cells were not mitogenically stimulated (Colburn *et al.*, 1981b); (2) nonselective cloning of JB6 cells yielded new M- variants that were promotable (data not shown); and (3) the liver-tumour promoter DEHP promotes anchorage-independence in JB6 cells but does not act as a mitogen (Diwan *et al.*, 1983; and data not shown).

Two other events that also appear to be dissociable from promotion of transformation are epidermal growth factor (EGF) receptor-binding and promoter-stimulated hexose transport (Plagemann & Estensen, 1980). Variants resistant to TPA stimulation of hexose uptake (Copley *et al.*, 1983) and variants that lack EGF receptors (Colburn *et al.*, 1982a) have been found which are sensitive to promotion of transformation. Evidence published elsewhere (Colburn *et al.*, 1983b) suggests that both EGF receptor binding and stimulated hexose uptake may be required for mitogenic stimulation of JB6 cells by TPA.

*Events that do not account for the resistance of P− variants but may nevertheless be required for promotion of transformation*

Virtually all mammalian cells, except erythrocytes, show specific binding of phorbol diesters (PDE) and certain nonphorbol compounds such as teleocidin and lynbyatoxin. The result that has emerged from our laboratory and several others is that attempts to select for PDE receptorless variants by selecting for resistance to induction of various biological responses have consistently failed to yield receptorless variants (Fisher *et al.*, 1981; Butler-Gralla & Herschman, 1981; Colburn *et al.*, 1982a). TPA-resistant (P- and M-) JB6 cells showed both receptor numbers and receptor affinities that were indistinguishable from those of sensitive cells (Colburn *et al.*, 1982a, 1983a). Since biological responses to PDEs do not occur in the absence of phorbol diester receptors, these receptors may be necessary mediators. These data also suggest that the receptor function, presumably protein kinase C activity (see Blumberg *et al.* and Ashendel & Boutwell, this volume), may be required for cell viability.

Another response to phorbol esters that occurs in both P+ and P− cells is a greater than 90% decrease in procollagen synthesis, preceded by a rapid loss of translatable and hybridizable mRNA for collagen (Dion *et al.*, 1981, 1982; Sobel *et al.*, 1983). It is not possible to determine whether this is relevant to promotion, since no JB6 variant has been obtained that is deficient in the collagen switch-off response. Decreased or altered collagen synthesis has been associated with neoplastic transformation (Delclos & Blumberg, 1979; Hata & Peterkofsky, 1977).

*Events that appear to account for the resistance of P− variants and thereby appear to be required for promotion of transformation*

To date, the only biochemical response to TPA that has been found consistently to distinguish P− from P+ JB6 cells is a greater than ten-fold decrease in

Fig. 2. Promotable but not nonpromotable variant cells show decreased trisialoganglioside ($G_T$) Variants selected for their sensitivity or resistance to 12-*O*-tetradecanoylphorbol-13-acetate (TPA) promotion or mitogenesis (Colburn *et al.*, 1981b) were used to study the ganglioside response to TPA. Cells were labelled with [1-$^{14}$C]-glucosamine for the terminal 4 h of the 24-h exposure to TPA at 10 ng/ml (16 nmol/L). Gangliosides were isolated according to the method of Srinivas and Colburn (1981), separated on a silica gel G plate using chloroform: methanol:ammonium hydroxide:water, 60:35:0.5:7.5 (vol/vol) as solvent, visualized by exposure to iodine vapour, and identified by co-chromatography with authentic standards. The iodine-containing bands were scraped from the plate after removing excess iodine by sublimation; gangliosides were extracted with chloroform:methanol:water, 10:10:1 (vol/vol); and radioactivity was determined by liquid scintillation counting. Results are expressed as ganglioside-associated radioactivity in TPA-treated cells as a percentage of untreated control and are given as mean ± range for duplicate dishes.

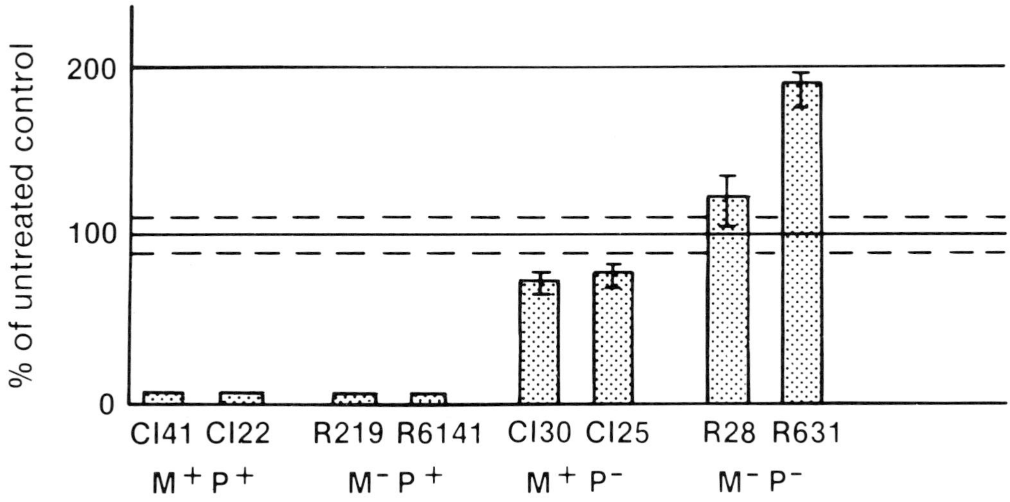


incorporation of $^{14}$C-glucosamine into trisialoganglioside ($G_T$) (Srinivas & Colburn, 1981; Srinivas *et al.*, 1982) (Fig. 2). Decreased $G_T$ synthesis also occurred in response to promoters of other classes, including EGF and benzoyl peroxide (Srinivas & Colburn, 1984a,b; Gindhart *et al.*, 1984). The effects of TPA on ganglioside synthesis were similar in M− and M+ cells. Added $G_T$ specifically blocked promotion of transformation by TPA (Fig. 3); other gangliosides were not inhibitory (Srinivas *et al.*, 1982). A final suggestion that the decrease in $G_T$ synthesis produced by exposure to promoters is relevant to promotion comes from a recent observation that selection of JB6 cells for resistance to the $G_T$ response to TPA coselected for cells resistant to the promotion of transformation response to TPA (Colburn & Srinivas, 1984). That complex gangliosides such as $G_T$ may function to maintain the non-transformed phenotype is suggested by experiments from several laboratories (Brady & Fishman, 1974; Hakomori, 1981).

The expression of one or more genes that determine sensitivity to promotion, designated 'P+ genes', is apparently also required for promotion of neoplastic transformation in JB6 cells. Recent results from our laboratory show that DNA from

Fig. 3. Trisialoganglioside ($G_T$) inhibits promotion of anchorage independence by 12-*O*-tetradecanoylphorbol-13-acetate (TPA) in a concentration-dependent manner
Standard $G_T$ from bovine brain was evaporated under nitrogen to remove the solvent and dissolved in ethanol, which was then evaporated. The ganglioside was dissolved in 1.0 ml of minimal essential medium/8% foetal calf serum and sonicated for three 45-sec periods with cooling. Gangliosides thus packaged into liposomes were added to cells simultaneously with TPA (10 ng/ml) at the time of preparing the soft agar/10% serum suspension. This incorporated $G_T$ was stable for at least 72 h. Colony yield 10 days after induction by TPA was corrected for background (solvent control values). Results are expressed as percent of TPA control colony induction and given as mean ± range for duplicate dishes.

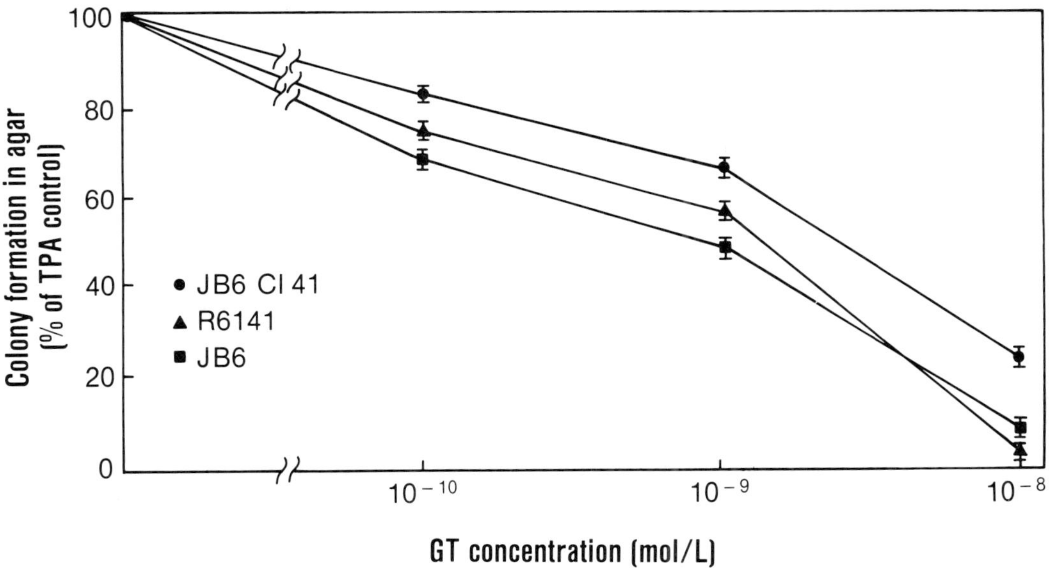


Table 3. Promotability can be transferred by transfection of genomic DNA from $P^+$ into $P^-$ cells[a]

| $P^+$ donor DNA | Recipient cells | Phenotype of recipient cells | No. of expts | Promotion response (TPA[b]-induced agar colonies per $10^5$ cells) |
|---|---|---|---|---|
| JB 6 Cl 41 | JB 6 Cl 30 | $P^-$ | 4 | 440 ± 250 |
| JB 6 Cl 41 | JB 6 Cl 25 | $P^-$ | 3 | 393 ± 102 |
| JB 6 Cl 41 | NIH 3T3 | – | 4 | 10 ± 17 |
| JB 6 Cl 22 | JB 6 Cl 30 | $P^-$ | 4 | 478 ± 164 |
| JB 6 Cl 22 | JB 6 Cl 25 | $P^-$ | 3 | 356 ± 75 |
| JB 6 Cl 22 | NIH 3T3 | – | 4 | 3 ± 6 |

[a] Seven days after transfection of DNA (6 days after subculturing), the transfected JB 6 $P^-$ cells were suspended in 0.33% agar + 12-*O*-tetradecanoyl 13-phorbol acetate (TPA) at $1.6 \times 10^{-8}$M. Results are given as mean number of TPA-induced agar colonies per $10^5$ cells ± standard deviation for the number of independent experiments. $P^+$, promotable to anchorage independence and tumorigenicity by TPA and other tumour promoters, $P^-$, nonpromotable. The NIH 3T3 cells failed to form colonies in agar in the absence or presence of TPA, but their phenotype may differ in several respects from that of JB6 $P^-$ cells (see Colburn *et al.*, 1983c,d).

Table 4. Restriction endonuclease sensitivity of CL 22 $P^{+}$ [a] DNA [b]

| Enzyme | Loss of transfectable $P^{+}$ activity: sensitive (+) or insensitive (−) |
|---|---|
| ECORI | + |
| BAMHI | + |
| HINDIII | + |
| XHOI | + |
| SALI | + |
| PVUII | + |
| BGLI | − |
| BGLII | − |

[a] $P^{+}$, sensitive to promotion of transformation by phorbol esters and nonphorbol tumour promoters
[b] Cl 22 DNA was incubated with the indicated restriction enzymes until hydrolysis was complete, as indicated by sizes of fragments hybridizable with a ribosomal cDNA probe. This was ascertained by choosing the digestion time that resulted in complete cleavage of the Cl 22 DNA ribosomal genes but gave no apparent nuclease activity. Following digestion, the DNA was precipitated with calcium phosphate, transfected into JB6 $P^{-}$ Cl 30 cells and assayed for transfer of $P^{+}$ activity, as described in the footnote to Table 3. +, showed greater than 70% loss of activity in comparison with undigested controls; −, showed less than 10% loss of activity after digestion

P+ cells can transfer promotion sensitivity when transfected into P− cells (Colburn *et al.*, 1983c,d) (Table 3). As shown in Table 4, this activity is sensitive to several restriction endonucleases, including EcoRI and BamHI, but resistant to Bgl I and Bgl II. Lack of inhibitory activity for Bgl I and Bgl II was not due to incomplete digestion. Cloning of the P+ gene(s) using Bgl II restriction fragments is currently underway.

Candidates for the function of the P+ gene(s) include a promoter-inducible neuraminidase that may account for the net decrease in precursor incorporation into $G_T$. It is noteworthy that the 35 000-dalton MEP protein of Gottesman and Sobel (1980) is TPA-inducible and localizes over lysozomes (M. Gottesman, personal communication), suggesting its possible identity as a neuraminidase.

## REFERENCES

Babiss, L.E., Ginsberg, H.S. & Fisher, P.B. (1983) Cold sensitive expression of transformation by host-range mutant of type 5 adenovirus. *Proc. natl Acad. Sci. USA*, ***80***, 1352–1356

Boreiko, C.J., Ragan, D.L., Abernethy, D.J. & Frazelle, J.H. (1982) Initiation of C3H/10T1/2 cell transformation by *N*-methyl-*N′*-nitro-*N*-nitrosoguanidine and aflatoxin $B_1$. *Carcinogenesis*, ***3***, 391–395

Brady, R.O. & Fishman, P.H. (1974) Biosynthesis of glycolipids in virus transformed cells. *Biochim. biophys. Acta*, ***355***, 121–148

Butler-Gralla, E. & Herschman, H.R. (1981) Variants of 3T3 cells lacking mitogenic response to the tumor promoter tetradecanoyl-phorbol-acetate. *J. Cell Physiol.*, ***107***, 59–67

Colburn, N.H. (1979) *The use of tumor promoter responsive epidermal cell lines to study preneoplastic progression. In:* Franks, L.M. & Wigley, C.B., eds, *Neoplastic Transformation in Differentiated Epithelial Cell Systems in vitro,* New York, pp. 113–134

Colburn, N.H. (1980a) Tumor promoter produces anchorage independence in mouse epidermal cells by an induction mechanism. *Carcinogenesis,* ***1***, 951–954

Colburn, N.H. (1980b) *Tumor promotion and preneoplastic progression. In:* Slaga, T.J., ed., *Carcinogenesis. A Comprehensive Survey,* Vol. 5, New York, Raven Press, pp. 33–56

Colburn, N.H. & Gindhart, T. (1981) Specific binding of transforming growth factor correlates with promotion of anchorage independence in EGF receptorless JB6 cells. *Biochem. biophys. Res. Commun.,* ***102***, 799–807

Colburn, N.H. & Srinivas, L. (1984) Selection of JB6 cells for resistance to ganglioside synthesis response to TPA coselects for promotion resistance (submitted for publication)

Colburn, N.H., Vorder Bruegge, W.F., Bates, J. & Yuspa, S.H. (1978) *Epidermal cell transformation* in vitro. In: Slaga, T.J., Sivak, A. & Boutwell, R.K., eds, *Mechanisms of Tumor Promotion and Cocarcinogenesis,* New York, Raven Press, pp. 257–271

Colburn, N.H., Former, B.F., Nelson, K.A. & Yuspa, S.H. (1979) Tumour promoter induces anchorage independence irreversibly. *Nature,* ***281***, 589–591

Colburn, N.H., Kohler, B.A. & Nelson, K.J. (1980) A cell culture assay for tumor-promoter dependent progression toward neoplastic phenotype: Detection of tumor promoters and promotion inhibitors. *Teratog. Carcinog. Mutag.,* ***1***, 87–96

Colburn, N.H., Ozanne, S. Lichti, U., Ben, T., Yuspa, S.H., Wendel, E., Jardini, E. & Abruzzo, G. (1981a) Retinoids inhibit promoter dependent preneoplastic progression in mouse epidermal cell lines. *Ann. N.Y. Acad. Sci.,* ***359***, 251–259

Colburn, N.H., Wendel, E. & Abruzzo, G. (1981b) Dissociation of mitogenesis and late-stage promotion of tumor cell phenotype by phorbol esters: Mitogen resistant variants are sensitive to promotion. *Proc. natl Acad. Sci. USA,* ***78***, 6912–6916

Colburn, N.H., Gindhart, T.D., Hegamyer, G.A., Blumberg, P.M., Delclos, K.B., Magun, B.E. & Lockyer, J. (1982a) Phorbol diester and epidermal growth factor receptors in 12-*O*-tetradecanoylphorbol-13-acetate-resistant and -sensitive mouse epidermal cells. *Cancer Res.,* ***42***, 3093–3097

Colburn, N.H., Wendel, E. & Srinivas, L. (1982b) Response of preneoplastic epidermal cells to tumor promoters and growth factors: use of promoter resistant variants for mechanism studies. *J. Cell Biochem.,* ***18***, 261–270

Colburn, N.H., Gindhart, T.D., Dalal, B. & Hegamyer, G.A. (1983a) In: Langenbach, R., Nesnow, S. & Rice, J., eds, *Organ and Species Specificity in Chemical Carcinogenesis,* New York, Plenum Press, pp. 189–200

Colburn, N.H., Hegamyer, G.A., Wendel, E.J. & Copley, M.P. (1983b) Insertion of EGF receptors restores phorbol ester mitogenic response to mitogen resistant JB6 cells. *Proc. Am. Assoc. Cancer Res.,* ***24***, 108

Colburn, N.H., Talmadge, C.B. & Gindhart, T.D. (1983c) Transfer of sensitivity to tumor promoters by transfection of DNA from sensitive into insensitive mouse JB6 epidermal cells. *Mol. cell. Biol.*, ***3***, 1182–1186

Colburn, N.H., Talmadge, C.B. & Gindhart, T.D. (1983d) Transfer of phorbol ester promotable into nonpromotable cells. *Prog. Nucleic Acid Res. mol. Biol.*, ***29***, 107–110

Copley, M.P., Gindhart, T.D. & Colburn, N.H. (1983) Hexose uptake as an indicator of JB6 mouse epidermal cell resistance to the mitogenic activity of TPA. *J. Cell Physiol.*, ***114***, 173–178

Delclos, K.B. & Blumberg, P.M. (1979) Decrease in collagen production in normal and Rous sarcoma virus transformed chick embryo fibroblasts induced by phorbol myristate-acetate. *Cancer Res.*, ***282***, 589–591

Dion, D.L., DeLuca, L.M. & Colburn, N.H. (1981) Phorbol ester induced anchorage independence and its antagonism by retinoic acid correlates with altered expression of specific glycoproteins. *Carcinogenesis*, ***2***, 951–958

Dion, D.L., Bear, J., Bateman, J., DeLuca, L.M. & Colburn, N.H. (1982) Inhibition by tumor promoting phorbol esters of procollagen synthesis in promotable JB6 mouse epidermal cells. *J. natl Cancer Inst.*, ***69***, 1147–1154

Diwan, B., Ward, J.M., Colburn, N., Spangler, F., Creasia, D., Lynch, P. & Rice, J.M. (1983) Promoting effects of di(2-ethylhexyl)phthalate in mouse liver, skin and JB-6 epithelial cells. *Proc. Am. Assoc. Cancer Res.*, ***24***, 105

Fisher, P.B., Bozzone, J.H. & Weinstein, I.B. (1979) Tumor promoters and epidermal growth factor stimulate anchorage-independent growth of adenovirus-transformed rat embryo cells. *Cell*, ***18***, 695–705

Fisher, P.B., Cogan, U., Horowitz, A.D., Schacter, D. & Weinstein, B. (1981) TPA-resistance in Friend erythroleukemia cells: role of membrane lipid fluidity. *Biochem. biophys. Res. Commun.*, ***100***, 370–376

Fisher, P.B., Babiss, L.E., Weinstein, I.B. & Ginsberg, H.S. (1982) Analysis of type 5 adenovirus transformation with a cloned rat embryo cell line (CREF). *Proc. natl Acad. Sci. USA*, ***79***, 3527–3531

Furstenberger, G.D., Berry, D.L., Sorg, B. & Marks, F. (1981) Skin tumor promotion by phorbol esters is a two-stage process. *Proc. natl Acad. Sci. USA*, ***78***, 7722

Gindhart, T.D., Srinivas, L. & Colburn, N.H. (1984) Benzoyl peroxide promotes transformation in JB6 mouse epidermal cells (submitted for publication)

Gottesman, M.M. & Sobel, M.E. (1980) Tumor promoters and Kirsten sarcoma virus increase synthesis of a secreted glycoprotein by regulating levels of translatable mRNA. *Cell*, ***19***, 449–455

Hakomori, S.I. (1981) Glycosphingolipids in cellular interaction differentiation and oncogenesis. *Ann. Rev. Biochem.*, ***50***, 733–764

Hata, R.I. & Peterkofsky, B. (1977) Specific changes in the collagen phenotype of BALB 3T3 cells as a result of transformation by sarcoma viruses or a chemical carcinogen. *Proc. natl Acad. Sci. USA*, ***74***, 2933–2937

Hennings, H., Michael, D., Cheng, C., Steinert, P., Holbrook, K. & Yuspa, S.H. (1980) Calcium regulation of growth and differentiation of mouse epidermal cells in culture. *Cell*, ***19***, 245–254

Hirakawa, T., Kakunaga, T., Fujiki, H. & Sugimura, T. (1982) A new tumor-promoting agent, dihydroteleocidin B, markedly enhances chemically induced malignant cell transformation. *Science*, ***216***, 527–529

Kennedy, A.R., Mondal, S., Heidelberger, C. & Little, J.B. (1978) Enhancement of X-ray transformation by 12-*O*-tetradecanoyl-phorbol-13-acetate in a cloned line of C3H mouse embryo cells. *Cancer Res.*, ***38***, 439–433

Mondal, S. & Heidelberger, C. (1976) Transformation of C3H/10T$^1/_2$ Cl 8 mouse embryo fibroblasts by ultraviolet radiation and a phorbol ester. *Nature*, ***260***, 710–711

Mondal, S., Brankow, D.W. & Heidelberger, C. (1976) Two-stage chemical oncogenesis in cultures of C3H/10T1/2 cells. *Cancer Res.*, ***36***, 2254–2260

Mordan, L.J., Bergin, L.M., Budnick, J.E.L., Meegan, R.R. & Bertram, J.S. (1982) Isolation of methylcholanthrene-'initiated' C3H/10T$^1/_2$ cells by inhibiting neoplastic progression with retinyl acetate. *Carcinogenesis*, ***3***, 279–285

Plagemann, P.G.W. & Estensen, R.D. (1980) Lack of correlation between effects of tumor promoter TPA on plasminogen activator production, phosphatidyl choline synthesis, and hexose transport in mammalian cell culture systems. *J. Cell Biol.*, ***104***, 105–119

Slaga, T.J., Fisher, S.M., Nelson, K. & Gleason, G.E. (1980a) Studies on the mechanism of skin tumor promotion: Evidence for several stages in promotion. *Proc. natl Acad. Sci. USA*, ***77***, 3659–3663

Slaga, T.J., Klein-Szanto, A.J.P., Fisher, S.M., Weeks, C.E., Nelson, K. & Major, S. (1980b) Studies on mechanisms of action of antitumor-promoting agents: Their specificity in two-stage promotion. *Proc. natl Acad. Sci. USA*, ***77***, 2251–2254

Sobel, M.E., Dion, L.D., Vuust, J. & Colburn, N.H. (1983) Tumor promoting phorbol esters inhibit procollagen synthesis at a pretranslational level in JB6 mouse epidermal cells. *Mol. cell. Biol.*, ***3***, 1527–1532

Srinivas, L. & Colburn, N.H. (1981) Ganglioside changes induced by tumor promoters in promotable JB6 mouse epidermal cells: antagonism by an antipromoter. *J. natl Cancer Inst.*, ***68***, 469–473

Srinivas, L. & Colburn, N. (1984a) Chemically but not Mos transformed epidermal cells show reduced trisialoganglioside synthesis. *Cancer Res.*, ***44***, 1510–1514

Srinivas, L. & Colburn, N.H. (1984b) Preferential oxidation of cell surface sialic acid by periodate leads to promotion of transformation in JB6 cells. *Carcinogenesis*, ***5***, 515–519

Srinivas, L., Gindhart, T.D. & Colburn, N.H. (1982) Tumor promoter resistant cells lack trisialoganglioside response. *Proc. natl Acad. Sci. USA*, ***79***, 4988–4991

Terzaghi, M. & Nettesheim, P. (1979) Dynamics of neoplastic development in carcinogen-exposed tracheal mucosa. *Cancer Res.*, ***39***, 4003–4010

Terzaghi, M., Nettesheim, P. & Riester, L. (1982) Effect of carcinogen dose on the dynamics of neoplastic development in rat tracheal epithelium. *Cancer Res.*, ***42***, 4511–4518

Yuspa, S. & Morgan, D.L. (1981) Mouse skin cells resistant to terminal differentiation associated with carcinogenesis. *Nature*, ***293***, 72–74

# INTERCELLULAR COMMUNICATION, CELL DIFFERENTIATION AND TUMOUR PROMOTION

H. YAMASAKI, T. ENOMOTO & N. MARTEL

*Division of Environmental Carcinogenesis, International Agency for Research on Cancer, Lyon, France*

## INTRODUCTION

Numerous biochemical and biological effects of tumour-promoting phorbol esters, usually 12-*O*-tetradecanoyl phorbol 13-acetate (TPA), have been reported, and yet the mechanism of tumour promotion is not understood (see the proceedings of two previous symposia on tumour promotion: Slaga *et al.*, 1978; Hecker *et al.*, 1982). It is important to recognize that whatever the biochemical mechanism is, the process of tumour promotion should involve cellular events in which a clonal expansion of initiated cells in relation to surrounding normal cells finally takes place. The biological effects of phorbol esters that may elucidate the mechanisms of clonal expansion of initiated cells include modulation of intercellular communication and cell differentiation (for reviews, see Trosko *et al.*, 1982; Yamasaki, 1984).

Gap junction-mediated intercellular communication is considered to play an important role in the control of cell proliferation and differentiation (Loewenstein, 1981). It seems reasonable to assume that interruption of intercellular communication may lead the cell population to an uncontrolled situation, since individual cells can behave independently from each other. Thus, the inhibition of gap junction-meditated intercellular communication by phorbol esters may provide us with a clue to elucidate the mechanisms of action of tumour promoters (Murray & Fitzgerald, 1979; Yotti *et al.*, 1979; Enomoto *et al.*, 1981).

Tumour promoter-mediated modulation of cell differentiation is now well documented on the basis of a variety of model systems of differentiation (Yamasaki, 1984). Prevention of entry of the cell into terminal division by tumour promoters seems to be the simplest way of accumulating initiated cells, provided that their cell proliferation is not inhibited. In view of these considerations, we in our laboratory are studying the mechanisms by which tumour promoters modulate cell differentiation and intercellular communication.

## INHIBITION OF INTERCELLULAR COMMUNICATION BY TUMOUR PROMOTERS

Evidence that tumour promoters can inhibit cell-cell communication was first obtained independently by Yotti *et al.* (1979) and by Murray and Fitzgerald (1979). These investigators found that TPA and related phorbol ester tumour promoters inhibit metabolic cooperation between cells in culture. Although the effects were striking, the metabolic cooperation technique for the study of cell-cell communication has several limitations: (1) since metabolic cooperation represents the transfer between cells of relatively large molecules, the absence of this process is not in itself a demonstration of complete communication incompetence (Loewenstein, 1979); (2) metabolic cooperation is a relatively complex process involving several biochemical reactions; and (3) inhibition of metabolic cooperation may reflect inhibition of previously established and/or de-novo formation of pathways of intercellular communication in cultures, and the procedure used does not distinguish the difference.

### *Inhibition of electrical coupling*

An assay that overcomes the limitations of the metabolic cooperation method involves the passing of pulses of electric current through intracellular microelectrodes from the interior of a cell to an external medium and measurement of the corresponding electrical potential in this cell and in a neighbouring cell (Loewenstein, 1979). A schematic diagram of the method is shown in Figure 1.

Figure 2 illustrates the effect of TPA on electrical coupling between cultured human amniotic membrane cells (FL cells; Fogh & Lund, 1957). Under control conditions, approximately 90% of cell pairs became electrically coupled within 2 h of incubation, and the coupling remained stable for at least another 22 h. When TPA (100 ng/mL) was present at the time of cell plating, almost no electrical cell coupling occurred. This inhibition lasted for at least 24 h, unless TPA was removed from the culture medium. TPA did not change the membrane potential, membrane resistance or growth rate of the cells, suggesting that it can inhibit cell-cell communication without affecting the general properties of the surface membrane. There was a good correlation among various phorbol esters and related compounds tested between their ability to inhibit intercellular transfer of electrical current and their tumour promoting activities (Enomoto *et al.*, 1981).

When TPA was removed from the culture medium, there was a rapid increase in the percentage of electrically coupled cells, indicating that the inhibitory effect of TPA on electrical coupling is reversible (Fig. 2). Figure 2 also illustrates that TPA can disrupt electrical coupling already established between FL cells. It is important to emphasize these effects of TPA on established intercellular communication, since in-vivo tumour promotion experiments are carried out with tissues in which cells are already in communication.

Recently, Blumberg's group demonstrated specific binding of phorbol esters to several cell types (Blumberg *et al.*, 1982). Other investigators have confirmed and extended their findings (Shoyab & Todaro, 1980; Horowitz *et al.*, 1981; Solanki *et al.*,

Fig. 1. Schematic diagram of the bridge circuit used
M, microscope; TR, thermoregulator; E1 and E2, microelectrodes; MZ-4, preamplifier (Nihonkoden); V-comp, voltage compensator; Osc, oscilloscope (Tektronic); S, stimulator; C1 and C2, paired cells; V1 and V2, outputs of changes of membrane potential in paired cells during current flow (from Yamasaki *et al.*, 1983)

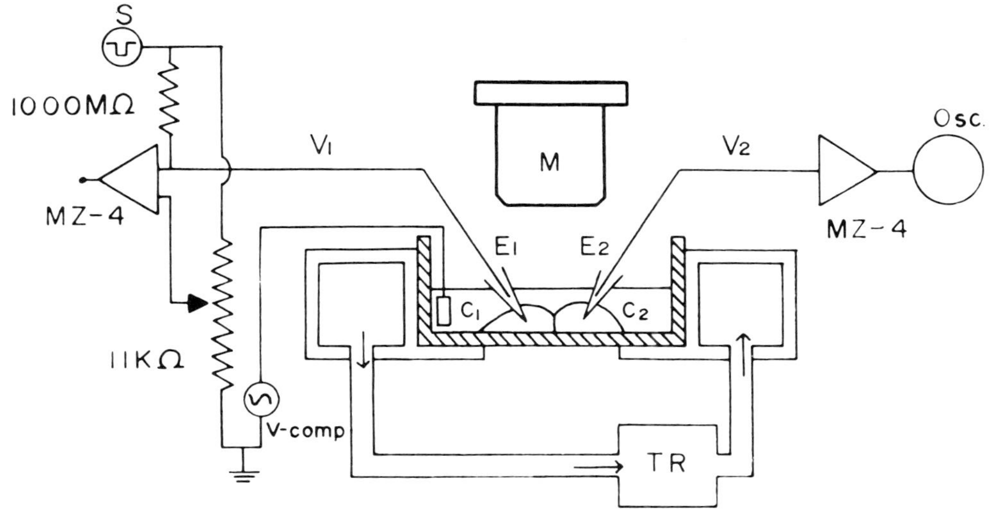


1981). Since the affinity of various phorbol esters and related compounds to the binding sites generally correlated well with their biological activity, it was proposed that these binding sites mediated a pleiotropic effect of phorbol esters (Blumberg *et al.*, 1982). We have demonstrated a class of specific, high-affinity, saturable binding sites for phorbol esters, using $^3$H-phorbol 12,13-dibutyrate (PDBu) in a human amniotic membrane epithelial cell line (FL), in which we also demonstrated reversible inhibition of cell-cell communication by tumour promoters (Yamasaki *et al.*, 1983). The specific binding of $^3$H-PDBu to FL cells was inhibited by TPA, phorbol-12,13-didecanoate, mezerein and ingenol-13,20-dibenzoate but not by phorbol or 4α-phorbol-12,13-didecanoate, and the extent of inhibition of cell coupling and that of $^3$H-PDBu binding by these compounds were in general agreement. Therefore, although quantitative dose-response data on the effect of these chemicals on cell-cell communication are still lacking (due to the laborious nature of its measurement), our results strongly suggest that the inhibition of electrical coupling of FL cells by these tumour promoters is mediated through such specific cellular binding sites.

TPA-mediated inhibition of electrical coupling between FL cells was observed even in the presence of actinomycin D or cycloheximide, indicating that de-novo synthesis of RNA and protein is not required for this effect of TPA (Yamasaki *et al.*, 1983). Taken together with the rapidity of the destruction by TPA of progressing cell coupling, the effect of TPA on intercellular communication appears to be the result of its relatively direct interaction with cell surface membrane. Unwin and Zampighi (1980) proposed a model for gap-junctional structure and its relationship to function, in which an arrangement of six subunits of the gap junction can open or close a central

Fig. 2. Effect of removal and readdition of 100 ng/mL 12-*O*-tetradecanoylphorbol-13-acetate (TPA) on coupling between FL cells
Arrows indicate times of addition or removal of TPA; TPA was removed by carefully washing the cell layers three times with culture medium containing 10% calf serum. ○, control; ●, TPA-treated cells (from Enomoto *et al.*, 1981)

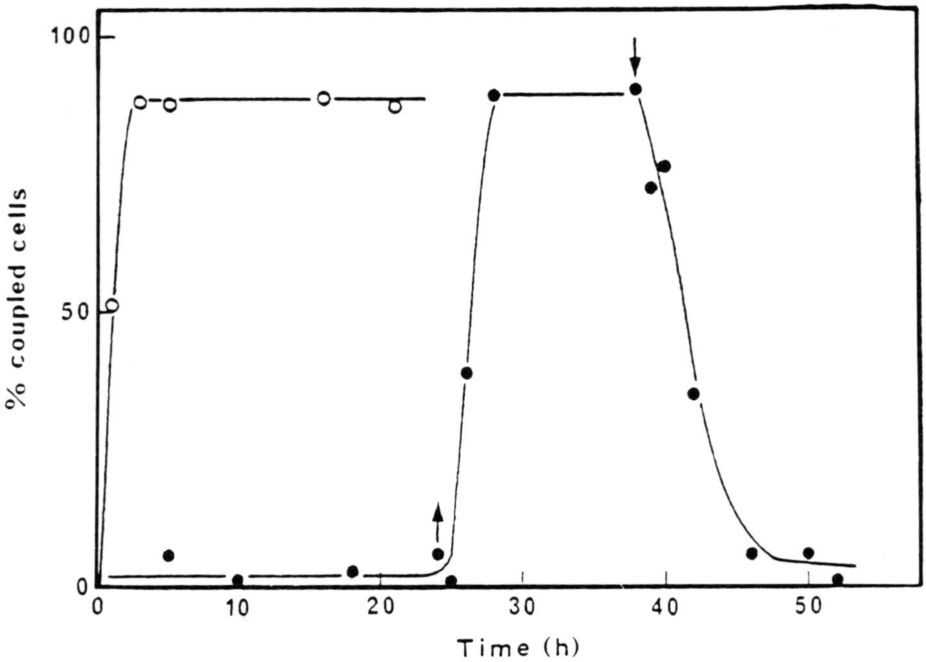


area of the junctional structure, depending on the environmental and physiological status of the cells. According to this model, de-novo synthesis of protein is not necessary to turn on or shut off gap-junctional communication. TPA may close the junctional structure so that no cell-cell communication can occur. This would explain the ready reversibility of the action of TPA and its independence from de-novo protein synthesis.

---

Fig. 3. Pattern of dye transfer in control (0.1% dimethyl sulfoxide) and 12-*O*-tetradecanoylphorbol-13-acetate (TPA)-treated cells
A, Fluorescence photomicrograph of cells cultured in 0.1% dimethyl sulfoxide for 4 h; B, phase-contrast photomicrograph of A; C, cells cultured in 100 ng/mL TPA for 4 h; D, phase-contrast photomicrograph of C.
Cells were injected with dye and photographed 10 min later. Dye was injected *via* capillaries filled with fluorescent Lucifer Yellow CH (molecular weight, 457.3; 10% in 0.33M lithium chloride solution) under a microinjectoscope (Olympus injectoscope) (Yamamoto & Furusawa, 1978). The cells were impaled with capillaries, close to the nucleus, and then dye was injected continuously for 3–5 sec by hand pressure. The capillaries were prepared by an automatic magnetic puller (Narishige, Tokyo). The cells were maintained at room remperature. Transfer of dye into surrounding cells was monitored with a Leitz fluorescence microscope equipped with a blue excitation filter BA 12, a heat-absorbing filter BA 38 and a blue-absorbing barrier filter. × 380

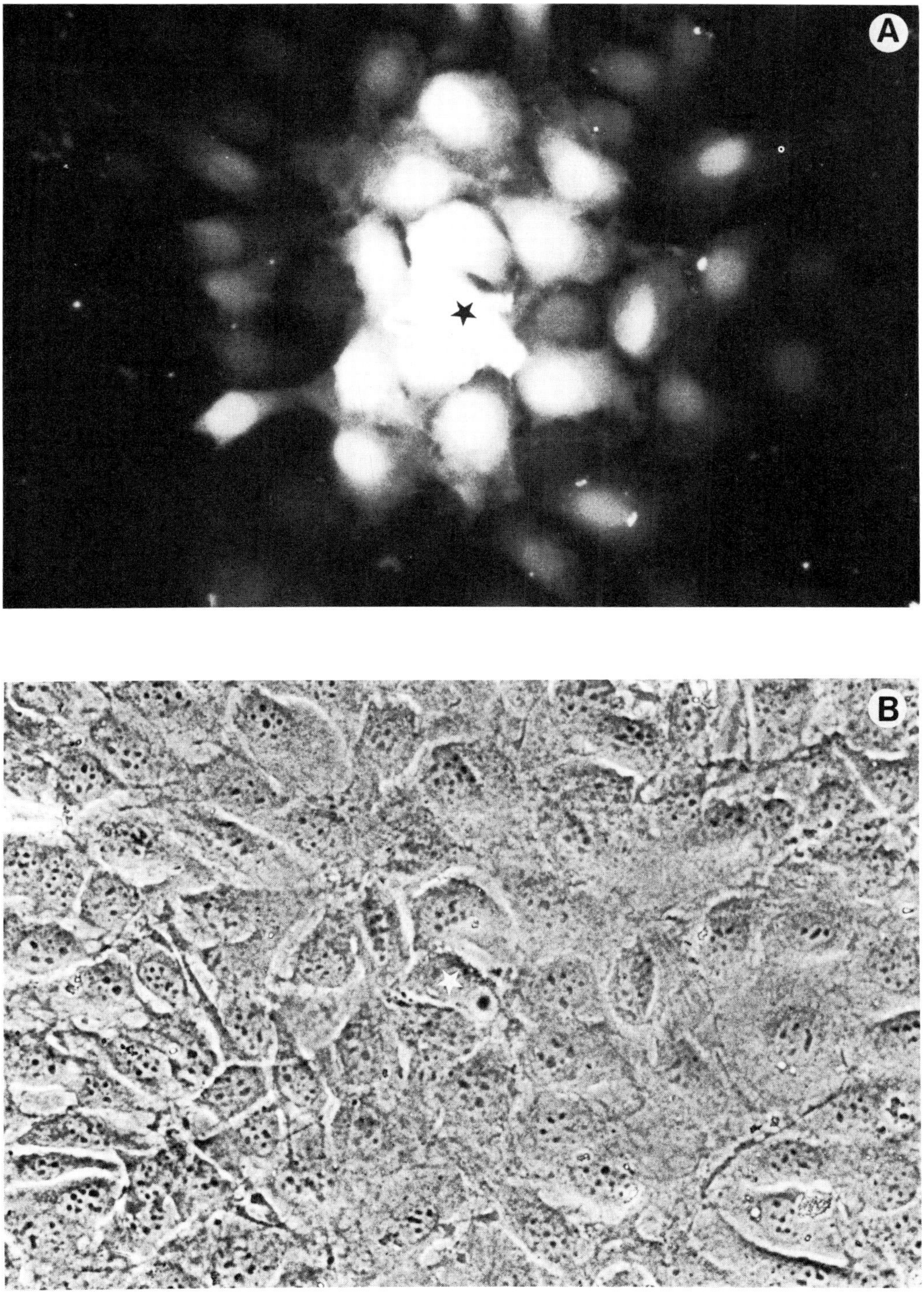
A
B

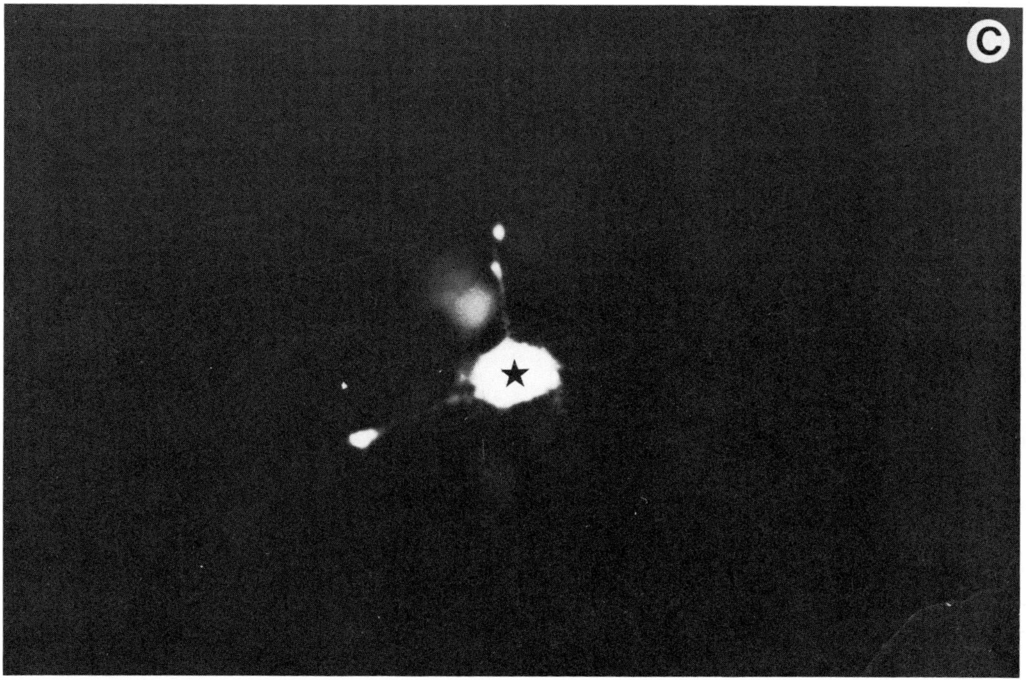
C

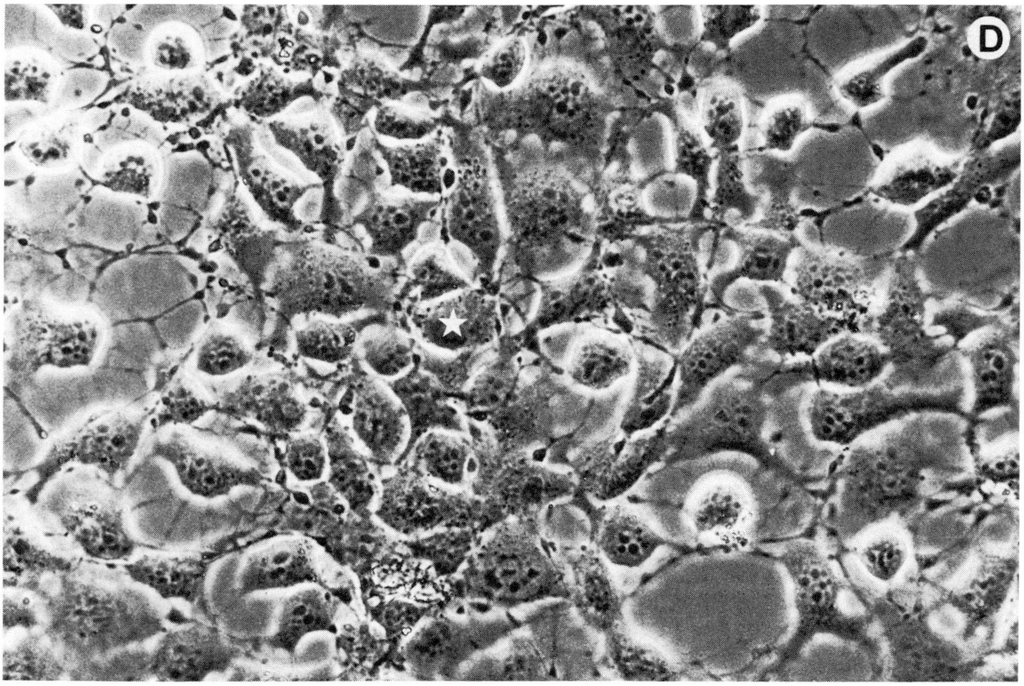
D

More recently, however, Yancey *et al.* (1982) showed by electron microscopy that TPA-treated cells have a decreased number of gap junctions, indicating that TPA inhibits the ability of the cells to form and/or maintain stable gap-junctional contacts. It is not clear from their data whether gap junctions disappear completely or whether they are merely disassembled into individual particles. The results of our work showed that TPA-mediated inhibition of electrical coupling of FL cells is reversible upon the removal of TPA, even in the presence of cycloheximide. If we assume that electrical coupling is also mediated through gap-junctional structures, our results may favour the idea that TPA disassembles the gap-junctional structure into individual particles. Since we have not examined the effect of TPA on gap-junctional structures of FL cells, we cannot draw any conclusion as to the effect of TPA on the structure of FL cell gap junctions.

*Inhibition of dye transfer between cells*

Although the electrophysiological measurements of cell communication described above are ideally suited for detecting the presence or absence of permeable junctions in an isolated system, e.g., paired cells, this laborious method is less suited to a quantitative study of intercellular communication among relatively large cell populations, such as cultured monolayer cells and tissue cells. It is important to study such large cell populations since the carcinogenesis process occurs in complex tissues where intercellular communication is controlled. The problems inherent in the preceding methods can be circumvented when a fluorescent dye is microinjected into a cell and the extent of dye transfer is subsequently determined visually (Loewenstein, 1979). We have investigated the effect of phorbol ester tumour promoters on dye transfer between BALB/c 3T3 A31-1-1 cells using the fluorescent dye Lucifer Yellow CH (Stewart, 1978; Atkinson *et al.*, 1981). Similar studies have been reported in cultured human and mouse cells (Friedman & Steinberg, 1982; Fitzgerald *et al.*, 1983).

When fluorescent Lucifer Yellow CH was microinjected into a BALB/c 3T3 cell in confluent culture, the injected dye was transferred into surrounding cells immediately after injection, and the number of dye-coupled cells that contained a detectable amount of the dye reached a plateau within 5 min after injection (Fig. 3). Thereafter, the extent of dye transfer was constant for at least 15 min (Fig. 4). When, however, the cultures were treated with TPA (100 ng/mL) for 4 h, the number of dye-coupled cells decreased to $2.5 \pm 1.6$ cells by 5 min after injection (Figs 3 & 4), indicating that TPA inhibits dye transfer by more than 90%. The inhibition was constant for at least 20 min after injection (Fig. 4).

Figure 5 shows the effect of the time of TPA treatment on dye transfer. In control cultures (0.1% dimethyl sulfoxide), no significant change in the capacity to transfer dye was observed during the 24-h duration of the experiment. However, when cells were treated with TPA (100 ng/mL), the number of dye-coupled cells decreased to $18.1 \pm 6.0$ and $3.8 \pm 3.0$, respectively, 0.5 h and 1 h later. This inhibition continued for at least 12 h after the addition of TPA, indicating that 1-h treatment of the culture with TPA is sufficient to inhibit maximally dye transfer between BALB/c 3T3 cells. Thereafter, the number of dye-coupled cells was increased slightly: $11.7 \pm 3.6$ and $10.5 \pm 4.0$, respectively, 16 h and 24 h later. This small recovery of dye transfer

Fig. 4. Time course of dye transfer between BALB/c 3T3 cells after dye injection
Cells were cultured with 0.1% dimethyl sulfoxide (○) and 100 ng/mL 12-*O*-tetradecanoylphorbol-13-acetate (●) for 4 h before the dye was microinjected, and the extent of dye transfer was measured as described in the legend to Fig. 3. Each point is the mean (± SD) of 11–26 separate injections.

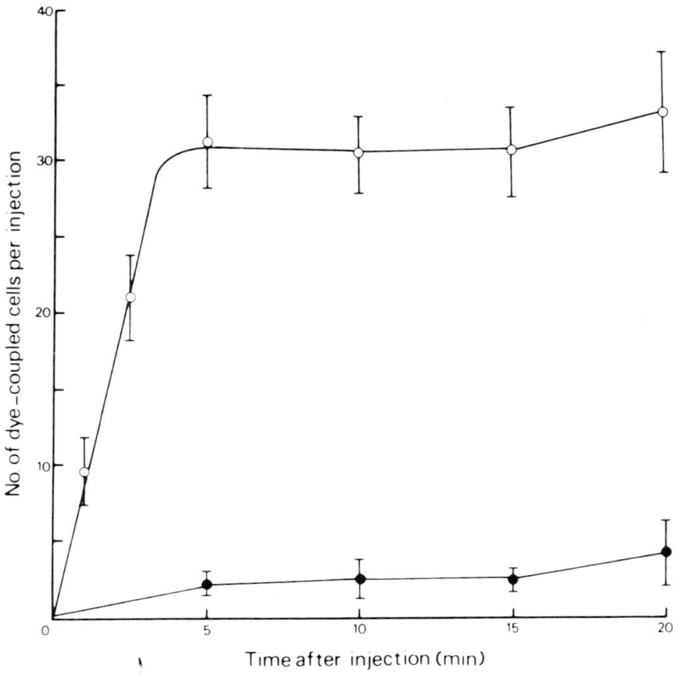


capacity was not apparently due to exhaustion of TPA, because TPA was added at 0, 11 and 20 h in this experiment. Similar recovery from the effect of TPA on intercellular communication has already been reported (Mosser & Bols, 1982; Fitzgerald *et al.*, 1983).

There was a good correlation among the various phorbol esters and related compounds tested between their inhibitory effect on intercellular communication between BALB/c 3T3 cells, their inhibitory effect on specific binding of $^3$H-PDBu to BALB/c 3T3 cells and their tumour-promoting activity on mouse skin (Table 1). These results support our previous conclusion that the inhibition of intercellular communication by phorbol esters is receptor-mediated (Yamasaki *et al.*, 1983).

*Effect of cyclic adenosine-5′-monophosphate (cAMP) on TPA-mediated inhibition of dye transfer*

cAMP has been reported to enhance communicating capacity of some cell lines, including BALB/c 3T3 cells, and it is postulated to be a possible physiological modulator of cell-cell communication (Flagg-Newton *et al.*, 1981; Loewenstein,

Fig. 5. Time course of the effect of 12-*O*-tetradecanoylphorbol-13-acetate (TPA) on dye transfer between BALB/c 3T3 cells
In treated cultures, TPA (100 ng/mL) was added at 0, 12, 24 h; Lucifer Yellow CH solution was microinjected at the times indicated, and the extent of dye transfer was measured 10 min later, as described in the legend to Fig. 3. Each point is the mean (± SD) of 22–35 separate injections. ○, control (0.1% dimethyl sulfoxide); ●, TPA-teated cells

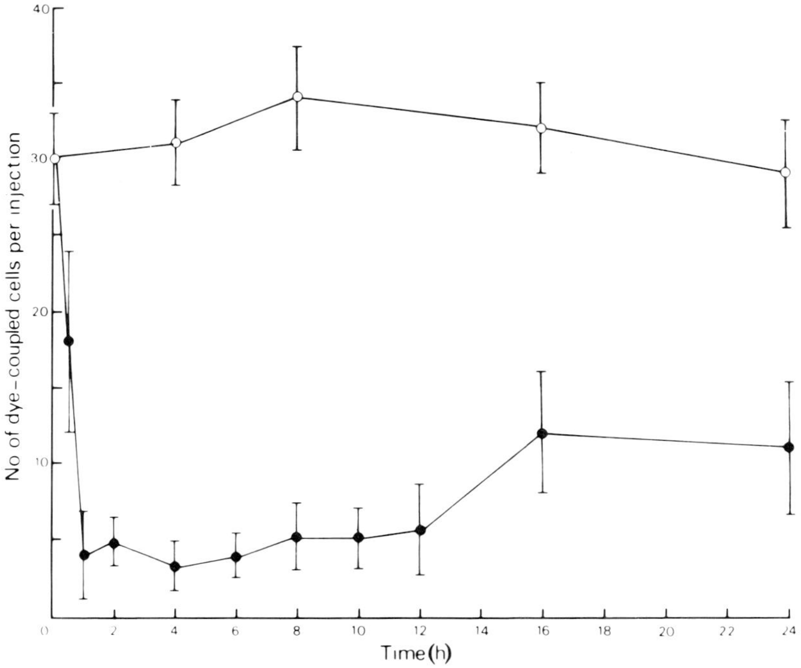


Table 1. Effect of phorbol esters and related compounds on dye transfer and specific binding of $^{3}$H-phorbol-12,13-dibutyrate (PDBu) in BALB/c 3T3 cells

| Compound (100 ng/mL) | No. of dye-coupled cells per injection[a] | Inhibition of $^{3}$H-PDBu binding ($ID_{50}$, ng/mL)[b] |
|---|---|---|
| Control (0.1% dimethylsulfoxide) | 30.5±5.4 | – |
| Phorbol | 30.5±3.4 | >3 000[c] |
| 4α-Phorbol-12,13-didecanoate | 32.3±4.8 | >3 000[c] |
| 4-*O*-Methyl-12-*O*-tetradecanoylphorbol 13-acetate | 30.2±4.5 | >1 000[c] |
| 12-*O*-Tetradecanoylphorbol 13-acetate | 3.2±2.9 | 2.5 |
| Phorbol-12,13-didecanoate | 3.5±1.7 | 11 |
| Phorbol-12,13-dibutyrate | 9.7±4.0 | 20 |
| Mezerein | 8.7±4.0 | 25 |

[a] Cells were cultured for 4 h in medium containing the indicated chemicals; dye transfer was measured 10 min after injection. Data represent the mean (±SD) of 16–32 separate injections
[b] Specific binding of $^{3}$H-PDBu (12 nmol/L) to intact BALB/c 3T3 cells was measured in confluent cultures, and its inhibition by varying concentrations of phorbol derivatives was determined as described previously. $ID_{50}$, the concentration which gives 50% inhibition of specific $^{3}$H-PDBu binding
[c] These compounds did not significantly inhibit $^{3}$H-PDBu binding at the concentration indicated

Fig. 6. Effect of dbcAMP and caffeine on 12-*O*-tetradecanoylphorbol-13-acetate (TPA)-mediated inhibition of dye transfer
Chemicals were added at 0, 12 and 20 h, and dye transfer was assayed as described in the legend to Fig. 3. Data for each point represent the mean (± SD) of 16–34 separate injections. ○, 100 ng/mL TPA + 1.0 mmol/L dbcAMP + 1.0 mmol/L caffeine; □, 1.0 mmol/L dbcAMP + 1.0 mmol/L caffeine; ●, 100 ng/mL TPA

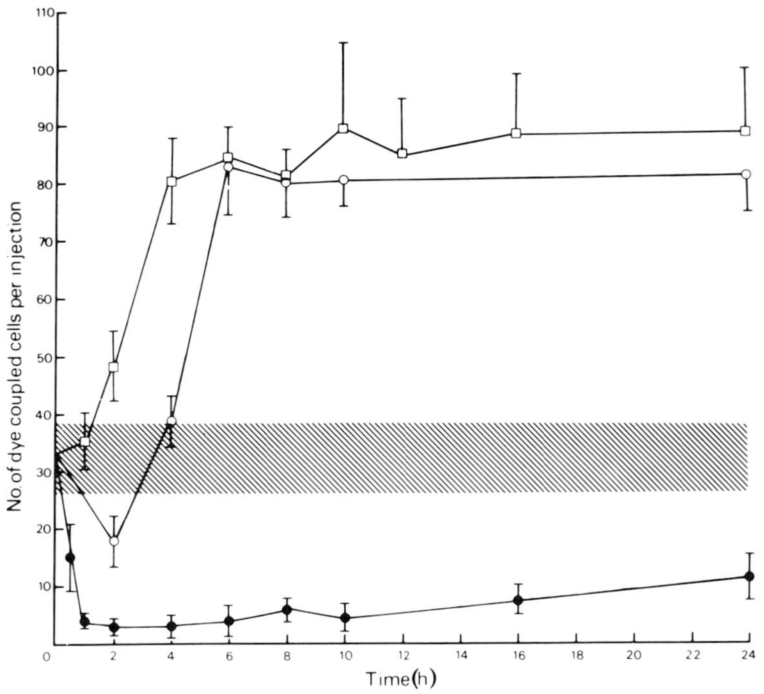


1981). More recently, we have found that cAMP can protect against the inhibitory effect of TPA on electrical communication between human FL cells (unpublished data); moreover, this cyclic nucleotide and diphosphodiesterase inhibitor has been shown to inhibit tumour promotion on mouse skin (Slaga *et al.*, 1982). We therefore investigated the effect of cAMP on TPA-induced inhibition of dye transfer.

As shown in Figure 6, when cells were cultured in medium containing 1.0 mmol/L dbcAMP and 1.0 mmol/L caffeine, the average number of dye-coupled cells increased to 48.3 ± 6.0 and 84.5 ± 5.5, respectively, 2 h and 6 h later, compared to 30.5 ± 5.4 for control cultures. This elevated value remained constant for at least 24 h. These data are similar to those obtained by Flagg-Newton *et al.* (1981), that dbcAMP and caffeine enhance the capacity of dye transfer in cell lines such as BALB/c 3T3 cells. The effect of cAMP on TPA inhibition of dye transfer is also shown in Figure 6. When cells were cultured in TPA-containing medium together with dbcAMP and caffeine, the number of dye-coupled cells decreased to 18.1 ± 5.0, 2 h after treatment, but increased to 39.2 ± 4.7 and 82.8 ± 8.2, respectively, 4 h and 6 h later; the recovered value was maintained for at least 24 h. The average number of dye-coupled cells is almost the same whether they were treated with TPA together with dbcAMP and caffeine or with dbcAMP and caffeine alone, indicating that dbcAMP and caffeine protect against TPA inhibition of intercellular communication between BALB/c 3T3 cells.

## MODULATION OF CELL DIFFERENTIATION BY TUMOUR PROMOTERS

The modulating action of phorbol esters on cellular differentiation is not restricted to a specific cell type or animal species: they modulate the differentiation of cells derived from many species, including mouse, hamster, chick and human (summarized by Yamasaki, 1984). For example, they modulate the differentiation of murine erythroleukaemia cells, murine pre-adipocytes, chick melanoblasts, chick chondroblasts, human promyelocytic leukaemia cells and many other cells in culture. Moreover, they inhibit the development of a nematode, *Caenorhabditis elegans* (Miwa *et al.*, 1982) and the asexual reproduction of hydra (Shiba, 1981).

Reported examples of phorbol ester-modulated cell differentiation systems include both inhibitory and inducing (or stimulating) effects of phorbol esters on cell differentiation. When one attempts to interprete the mechanism of tumour promotion in terms of aberrant differentiation, their dual effects on cell differentiation, inhibition and induction appear confusing. However, when one considers that the induction of cell differentiation leads a cell population to greater maturity and, finally, to cell death, it is reasonable to assume that it is the inhibition of cell differentiation that is responsible for tumour promotion, since accumulation of stem cells is attained (Yamasaki *et al.*, 1982a). It is also possible that tumour promoters induce the terminal differentiation of noninitiated cells and thus provide space for initiated cells to proliferate.

### *Tumour promoter-mediated inhibition of cell differentiation and globin gene expression in Friend erythroleukaemia cells (FELC)*

Rovera *et al.* (1977) found that TPA reversibly inhibits spontaneous differentiation of FELC, and they reported a decreased accumulation of globin molecules and haemoglobin in FELC treated with TPA. From independent studies, we have reported reversible inhibition of both spontaneous and induced differentiation of FELC (Yamasaki *et al.*, 1977). These studies showed that TPA inhibits the accumulation of haemoglobin and of cytoplasmic globin-specific mRNA. Since biochemical and biological events associated with the expression of FELC differentiation are being studied extensively at the cellular and molecular levels, this system is now being widely used to study the mechanism by which TPA and related tumour promoters inhibit cell differentiation. Furthermore, clones of FELC have been isolated that are completely resistant to phorbol ester-mediated inhibition of differentiation and yet retain the capacity to differentiate normally in response to various inducers (Fibach *et al.*, 1978; Yamasaki *et al.*, 1979, 1982a).

Reversibility is one of the most striking features of the tumour promotion process on mouse skin (Boutwell, 1974). Most of the biological and biochemical effects of

Fig. 7. Effect of hexamethylene bisacetamide (HMBA) and 12-*O*-tetradecanoylphorbol-13-acetate (TPA) on accumulation of cytoplasmic globin mRNA and on differentiation of Friend erythroleukaemia cells (FELC)
A, FELC clone TS 19–101 cultured in the presence of 4 mmol/L HMBA; B, FELC clone TS 19–101 grown for 46 weeks (91 serial passages) in the presence of 100 ng/mL TPA and 4 mmol/L HMBA, as described in the legend to Table 2. After the 92nd passage in HMBA and TPA, the cells were washed and inoculated into fresh control medium at a density of $10^5$ cells/mL; and the amount of globin mRNA and the extent of differentiation were scored during the following four days. B+, benzidine-positive

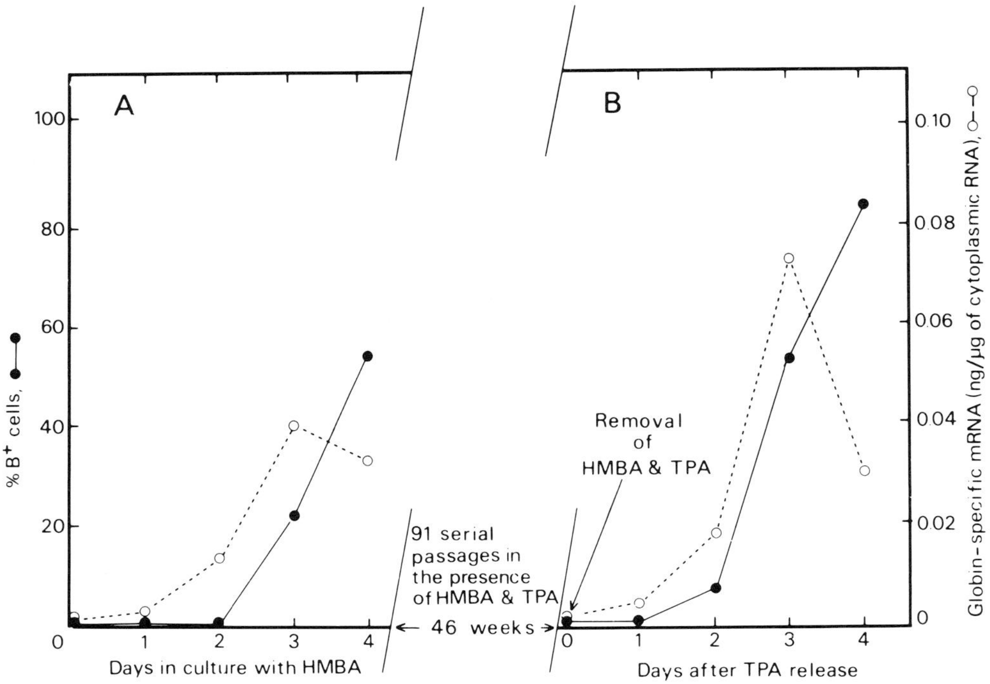


TPA on cell cultures are reversible when TPA is removed from the culture medium (Weinstein *et al.,* 1979), and the reversibility of TPA inhibition of spontaneous and induced differentiation of FELC has been studied extensively (Rovera *et al.,* 1977; Yamasaki *et al.,* 1980, 1982a).

Although FELC lose their ability to divide a few divisions after induction of differentiation (Friend *et al.,* 1971; Fibach *et al.,* 1977), they continue to grow if TPA is present, since their terminal differentiation is inhibited (Yamasaki *et al.,* 1980). We have maintained FELC clone TS-19-101 in the continuous presence of hexamethylene bisacetamide (HMBA) plus TPA for a total of 125 weeks by transferring the cells twice a week to fresh medium containing these compounds. During this period, differentiation, scored by the appearance of benzidine-positive cells, was usually less than 1%, indicating that there was no significant escape of cells from the TPA block during this time. The reversibility of the TPA effect is demonstrated in Table 2: suppression of the expression of erythroid differentiation by TPA for up to 125 weeks

Table 2. Continuous inhibition of hexamethylene bisacetamide (HMBA)-induced differentiation of Friend erythroleukaemia cell (FELC) clone 19–101 by 12-*O*-tetradecanoylphorbol 13-acetate (TPA) and its reversibility

| | Passage in culture medium with HMBA plus TPA | | | | | | | | | | | |
|---|---|---|---|---|---|---|---|---|---|---|---|---|
| Passage no. | 0 | 3 | 8 | 11 | 49 | 73 | 109 | 145 | 161 | 195 | 229 | 239 |
| Total time cultured with HMBA plus TPA (weeks) | 0 | 2.5 | 5 | 6.5 | 25.5 | 37.5 | 55.5 | 73.5 | 81.5 | 98.5 | 115.5 | 125.5 |
| Differentiation (% $B^+$ cells) when resuspended in the presence of: | | | | | | | | | | | | |
| No chemical | <1 | 20 | 29 | 18 | 71 | 65 | 75 | 49 | 40 | 52 | 56 | 62 |
| HMBA | 78 | 97 | 78 | 81 | 10 | 13 | 26 | 10 | 20 | 14 | 14 | 35 |
| TPA | <1 | 7 | 2 | 3 | <1 | <1 | <1 | <1 | <1 | <1 | <1 | <1 |
| HMBA plus TPA | <1 | 10 | 2 | <1 | <1 | <1 | <1 | <1 | <1 | <1 | <1 | <1 |

FELC clone TS 19–101 (a subclone of TS 19–10[19]) were grown and maintained as described in the text. At passage '0', the cells were transferred to a culture medium containing 4 mmol/L HMBA and 100 ng/mL TPA at a cell density of $10^5$ cells/mL. When the cells had grown to confluency ($\sim 1.2$–$2.0 \times 10^6$ cells/mL), they were transferred to medium containing the chemicals at a concentration of $10^5$ cells/mL. Up to the eight passage, the cells grew more slowly than in the absence of HMBA and TPA; but, thereafter, they began to grow at a normal rate, and they were then transferred twice weekly. At passage 39, the cells were frozen in liquid nitrogen. After three months, they were thawed and recovered. The first transfer of cells after this treatment was called the '40th' transfer. At passage 109 the cells were cloned in methyl cellulose, and a subclone (HT-2) was chosen for further transfer. During the procedures of freezing and cloning, the medium always contained 4 mmol/L HMBA and 100 ng/mL TPA. After the numbers of passages indicated, portions of cells were released from the TPA block by washing four times with warm culture medium containing fetal calf serum, with a 30-min incubation at 37°C between the third and fourth washings to obtain complete replacement of TPA. The cells were resuspended in culture medium containing no chemical, HMBA alone, TPA alone, or HMBA plus TPA. Differentiation was scored four days later by the benzidine reaction, as described previously.

(2.5 years) has never led to loss of potential for terminal maturation. HMBA, the usual inducer of differentiation used in these studies, had been observed previously to inhibit terminal maturation after long-term culture of FELC in the presence of TPA (Yamasaki *et al.*, 1980). A similar continuous, yet reversible suppression of induced FELC differentiation by TPA was demonstrated in two other independent experiments, and the suppression was found to be continuous for more than 50 weeks in both cases (Yamasaki *et al.*, 1980, and unpublished results).

Differentiation of FELC can be monitored either by staining them with benzidine or by measuring the accumulation of globin mRNA in cytoplasm prior to the appearance of benzidine-positive (B+) cells (Ostertag *et al.*, 1972; and Fig. 7A). We showed previously that the accumulation of globin mRNA is inhibited only partly when FELC are incubated for three days in the presence of HMBA and TPA (Yamasaki *et al.*, 1977). We now determined the amount of globin mRNA in FELC in which differentiation has been suppressed for 11 months (91 passages) in the presence of an inducer and an inhibitor, TPA (Fig. 7B); only background levels of globin mRNA, i.e., $< 10^{-4}\%$ of the total cytoplasmic RNA, were detected. Globin mRNA accumulated rapidly, however, when TPA was removed by transferring cells to fresh medium (Fig. 7B): three days later, the amount of globin mRNA had increased by 70 fold, to $7.3 \times 10^{-3}\%$.

These results indicate that globin mRNA accumulation in FELC is completely suppressed as long as TPA is present in the culture medium and that, upon removal of TPA from the culture medium, globin mRNA rapidly accumulates and terminal cell differentiation follows. Since cultured FELC exposed to HMBA and TPA for years grow as well as unexposed control cells, we conclude that TPA does not alter the rate of cell division and does not interfere with normal FELC proliferation. These observations suggest that TPA interferes specifically with the expression only of those genes required for terminal differentiation, such as globin gene expression, and not of those necessary for maintenance of cell proliferation.

### *Receptor-occupancy and inhibition of Friend cell differentiation by phorbol esters*

We showed previously, using a technique advanced by Driedger and Blumberg (1980), that specific receptors for phorbol esters are present on FELC (Yamasaki *et al.*, 1982b). There is a good correlation between the inhibitory effect of various phorbol esters on FELC differentiation and their ability to compete for their binding sites, suggesting that tumour-promoting phorbol esters inhibit FELC differentiation through their specific receptors. Down-regulation of the number of receptors can be obtained when FELC cells are exposed to phorbol esters for just a few hours.

In order to determine the long-term effect of TPA on the phorbol ester receptors, the number of receptors on FELC that had been exposed continuously to TPA for 232–235 serial passages was compared with that of unexposed parent cells (Fig. 8). About $2.1 \times 10^5$ binding sites were present on each unexposed cell, whereas only $0.44 \times 10^5$ sites/cell were observed in cells that had been cultured with TPA; thus, approximately 80% of the sites are lost or unavailable for binding on cells exposed continuously to TPA. The affinity constants of the receptors on FELC were similar before and after culture with TPA: 12.2 nmol/L in the control cells and 18.2 nmol/L

Fig. 8. Specific binding of $^{3}$H-phorbol 12, 13-dibutyrate (PDBu) to intact Friend erythroleukaemia cells (FELC) before and after long-term culture in the presence of 12-*O*-tetradecanoylphorbol-13-acetate (TPA)

A, saturation curve with increasing concentrations of $^{3}$H-PDBu; B, Scatchard analysis of specific $^{3}$H-PDBu binding.

About 1–3 × $10^{6}$ cells were incubated in 1 mL of culture medium containing varying amounts of $^{3}$H-PDBu, and specific binding was determined as described previously (Yamasaki *et al.*, 1982b). Each point represents the mean of three independent experiments with duplicate assays. ○, control FELC clone TS 19–101; ●, FELC clone TS 19–101 cultured in the presence of hexamethylene bisacetamide (HMBA) and TPA for 232–235 serial passages, as described in the footnote to Table 2. In order to exclude the possibility that the observed decrease in the number of binding sites was due to the interaction of TPA molecules remaining on the cell surface because of the long-term culture, the cultured cells were washed thoroughly with warm culture medium containing 10% fetal calf serum, as described in the footnote to Table 2, just prior to the binding assay. In order to evaluate the effectiveness of the washing, a parallel culture of FELC was incubated with HMBA and 100 ng/mL $^{3}$H-TPA (Amersham, UK) for up to three weeks, or six passages, washed as above, and the radioactivity in the cells determined: only about 0.05% of the initially bound $^{3}$H-TPA reactivity was recovered.

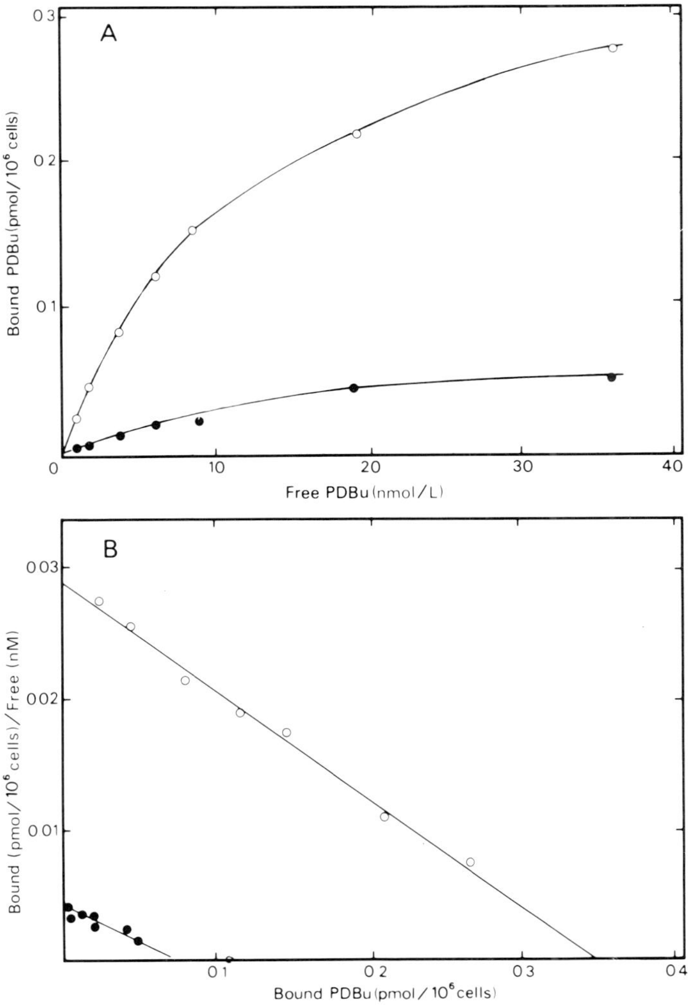

in TPA-exposed FELC (Fig. 8B). We can thus conclude that exposure of FELC to TPA and HMBA for long periods results in extensive homologous down-regulation of phorbol ester receptors.

In order to determine whether down-regulation of phorbol ester receptors alters the response of the cells to TPA, the quantitative effect of TPA on the differentiation of the receptor was studied. TPA was able to inhibit FELC differentiation completely at a dose as low as 10 ng/mL and there was essentially no significant difference in the response to TPA between control FELC and down-regulated FELC (Table 3).

We were interested to see whether such extensive down-regulation of phorbol ester receptors would change the structure-activity relationship of phorbol ester tumour promoters to FELC differentiation. Investigation of the effects of various derivatives of plant diterpenes on FELC differentiation before and after down-regulation of phorbol ester receptors (Table 3) showed that down-regulation does not alter the effect of these tumour promoting compounds on cell differentiation. Therefore, it appears that occupation of only a few receptors of FELC by TPA and other tumour promoters is sufficient to exert an inhibitory effect on the cell differentiation. This finding is in a sharp contrast to the effect of TPA on the stimulation of DNA synthesis in Swiss 3T3 cells (Collins & Rozengurt, 1982): down-regulation of phorbol ester receptors in these cells resulted in a refractoriness to TPA on the stimulation of DNA synthesis. It is important to note that we removed more than 99.95% of TPA molecules by washing prior to the $^{3}$H-PDBu binding assay, whereas only 97% of PDBu was removed in the study with Swiss 3T3 cells (Collins & Rozengurt, 1982). Since those authors used 400 nmol/L PDBu during preincubation, 12 pmol PDBu remained on the cell surface during their $^{3}$H-PDBu assay. Since a maximum of only about 8 pmol PDBu are bound per nontreated $10^6$ Swiss 3T3 cells, it is conceivable that the remaining 12 pmol PDBu disturbed the subsequent binding of $^{3}$H-PDBu and, thus, the response to subsequent addition of PDBu in the uptake of $^{3}$H-thymidine in their system.

Table 3. Quantitative comparative effects of various plant diterpenes on the differentiation of Friend erythroleukaemia cells (FELC) before or after down-regulation of phorbol ester receptors

| Compound | $ID_{50}$ (ng/mL)[a] | |
|---|---|---|
| | FELC cultured in unsupplemented media | FELC cultured with hexamethylene bisacetamide (HMBA) and 12-*O*-tetradecanoylphorbol 13-acetate (TPA) for 129 weeks[b] |
| TPA | 0.92 | 0.50 |
| Phorbol-12,13-didecanoate | 0.49 | 0.40 |
| Phorbol-12,13-butyrate | 4.7 | 7.1 |
| Mezerein | 0.37 | 0.68 |
| 4-*O*-MeTPA | 158 | 110 |
| Phorbol | >1 000 | >1 000 |
| 4α-Phorbol-12,13-didecanoate | >1 000 | >1 000 |

[a] $ID_{50}$, concentration that gives 50% inhibition of HMBA-induced differentiation scored on day 4.
[b] Cells were cultured with 4 mmol/L HMBA and 100 ng/mL TPA, as described in the footnote to Table 2. Prior to the experiments, the cultures were washed thoroughly and resuspended in the presence of 4 mmol/L HMBA and varying amounts of the plant diterpenes indicated

Down-regulation of PDBu binding sites has also been demonstrated in primary mouse epidermal cells (Solanki & Slaga, 1982), GH4Cl rat pituitary cells (Jaken *et al.*, 1981) and human promyelocytic leukaemia cells (Solanki *et al.*, 1981). Although a physiological significance of such down-regulation in the biological effects of phorbol esters is suggested, our present findings indicate that down-regulation does not necessarily alter the response of cells to subsequent treatment with phorbol esters; rather, they suggest that only a few TPA receptors are necessary for TPA inhibition of FELC differentiation.

## POSSIBLE ROLE OF BLOCKED INTERCELLULAR COMMUNICATION AND CELL DIFFERENTIATION IN TUMOUR PROMOTION

Phorbol esters are the first class of compounds with which it has been shown repeatedly that chemicals involved in carcinogenesis inhibit intercellular communication and cell differentiation. The possible role of blocked cell differentiation in tumour promotion has been much discussed previously (Berenblum, 1954; Diamond *et al.*, 1980; Yamasaki, 1984). It has been suggested that intercellular communication plays an important role in the control of cell differentiation (Loewenstein, 1979). Therefore, it is conceivable that tumour promoter-mediated inhibition of intercellular communication is itself the mechanism of modulation of cell differentiation by these chemicals, and, thus, initiated cells can be accumulated (Yamasaki, 1984). The results of in-vivo experiments described by Raick (1973) are consistent with this hypothesis. He examined under the electron microscope morphological changes in mouse skin exposed to TPA and found that TPA appears to induce the appearance of intercellular spaces between epidermal cells. Such changes could be associated with a loss of cell-cell communication. The same author also reported that TPA impairs epidermal cell differentiation; however, when ethyl phenylpropiolate, a hyperplasmiogenic agent without tumour-promoting activity, was used, there was no widening of the intercellular spaces, and no inhibition of cell differentiation was observed (Raick & Burdzy, 1973). These results obtained *in vivo* are consistent with the hypothesis that tumour promotion is related to aberrant cell-cell communication and to aberrant cell differentiation.

Depending on the commitment state of cell differentiation, blocked intercellular communication may either leave the cells in an undifferentiated state or force them into differentiation. The dual effects of TPA – inhibition and stimulation of cell differentiation – can be explained in this way. However, since TPA can influence the differentiation of haematopoietic and leukaemic cells, which exist as single cells, other mechanisms must also be involved.

Since tumour promoters do not usually convert normal cells to tumour cells, normal and initiated cells should differ in their response to tumour promoters. This difference could consist either of preferential recognition of initiated cells by tumour promoters (e.g., altered receptors for tumour promoters) or of a programmation of initiated cells such that interaction with tumour promoters will result in the modulation of specific gene expression. The difference between normal and initiated cells should be determined by the action of initiating carcinogens. It is believed currently that the primary target of initiating carcinogens is DNA, and there is ample evidence to support this idea. If we assume that the mechanism of action of tumour promoters is to modulate differentiation of initiated cells, the action of initiators on the genes involved in cellular commitment of differentiation is probably essential. Recently, Yuspa and Morgan (1981) showed that treatment of mouse dorsal skin with 7,12-dimethylbenz[*a*]anthracene increased the population of epidermal cells that do not differentiate but continue to proliferate under conditions in which normal cells are obliged to differentiate. These results are consistent with the idea that the alteration in commitment to the programme of differentiation is due to initiating carcinogens. They are also consistent with more recent observations that different cellular oncogenes are expressed during different developmental stages (Lane *et al.*, 1982), suggesting that these oncogenes may play an important role in commitment to the programme of cell differentiation.

The idea that the promotion step is due to aberrant differentiation of initiated cells was extended by Matsunaga (1979) to explain the mechanism for the causation of hereditary bilateral retinoblastoma in humans. The initiation step is presumed to be a genetic predisposition, because bilateral retinoblastoma cases usually show autosomal dominant inheritance. His analysis of age-specific incidence data on 244 cases of bilateral retinoblastoma showed a high intraclass correlation of the ages of the patients at the time of diagnosis of the disease in both the right and left eyes. This result argues against the two-mutation theory of the disease proposed by Knudson (1971), in which the occurrence of cancers in both the right and left eyes would not be expected within a short time interval, since somatic cell mutation is a random and rare event. Matsunaga suggests that it is more reasonable to assume that the 'expression of retinoblastoma genes' is largely determined by host factors common to both eyes. He believes that the promotion stage in bilateral retinoblastoma is an error in the process of differentiation.

## ACKNOWLEDGEMENTS

The authors are grateful to Drs Y. Kanno, Y. Shiba, W. Ostertag and A. Fusco for their collaboration during our studies. The continuous encouragement of Drs L. Tomatis, R. Montesano and I.B. Weinstein are deeply appreciated. We thank Miss M. Geesink for typing the manuscript.

## REFERENCES

Atkinson, M.M., Menko, A.S., Johnson, R.G., Sheppard, J.R. & Sheridan, J.D. (1981) Rapid and reversible reduction of junctional permeability in cells infected with a temperature-sensitive mutant of avian sarcoma virus. *J. Cell Biol.*, ***91***, 573–578

Berenblum, I. (1954) A speculative review: the probable nature of promoting action and its significance in the understanding of the mechanisms of carcinogenesis. *Cancer Res.*, ***14***, 471–474

Blumberg, P.M., Declos, K.B., Dunphy, W.G. & Jaken, S. (1982) *Specific binding of phorbol ester tumor promoters to mouse tissue and cultured cells*. In: Hecker, E., Fusenig, N.E., Kunz, W., Marks, F. & Thielmann, H.W., eds, *Carcinogenesis*, Vol. 7, *Cocarcinogenesis and Biological Effects of Tumor Promoters*, New York, Raven Press, pp. 519–535

Boutwell, R.K., (1974) The function and mechanisms of promoters of carcinogenesis. *CRC crit. Rev. Toxicol.*, **2**, 419–443

Collins, M.K.L. & Rozengurt, E. (1982) Binding of phorbol esters to high-affinity sites on murine fibroblastic cells elicits a mitogenic response. *J. cell. Physiol.*, **112**, 42–50

Diamond, L., O'Brien, T.G. & Baird, W.M. (1980) Tumor promoters and the mechanism of tumor promotion. *Adv. Cancer Res.*, **32**, 1–74

Driedger, P.E. & Blumberg, P.M. (1980) Specific binding of phorbol ester tumor promoters. *Proc. natl Acad. Sci. USA*, **77**, 567–571

Enomoto, T., Sasaki, Y., Shiba, Y., Kanno, Y. & Yamasaki, H. (1981) Tumor promoters cause a rapid and reversible inhibition of the formation and maintenance of electrical cell coupling in culture. *Proc. natl Acad. Sci. USA*, **78**, 5628–5632

Fibach, E., Reuben, R., Rifkind, R.A. & Marks, P.A. (1977) Effect of hexamethylene bisacetamide on the commitment to differentiation of murine erythroleukemia cells. *Cancer Res.*, **37**, 440–444

Fibach, E., Yamasaki, H., Weinstein, I.B., Marks, P.A. & Rifkind, R.A. (1978) Heterogeneity of murine erythroleukemia cells with respect to tumor promoter-mediated inhibition of cell differentiation. *Cancer Res.*, **38**, 3685–3688

Fitzgerald, D.J., Knowles, S.E., Ballard, F.J. & Murray, A.W. (1983) Rapid and reversible inhibition of junctional communication by tumor promoter. *Cancer Res.*, **43**, 3614–3618

Flagg-Newton, J.L., Dahl, G. & Loewenstein, W.R. (1981) Cell junction and cyclic AMP: I. Upregulation of junctional membrane permeability and junctional membrane particles by administration of cyclic nucleotide or phosphodiesterase inhibitor. *J. Membrane Biol.*, **63**, 105–121

Fogh, I. & Lund, R. (1957) Continuous cultivation of epithelial cell strain (FL) from human amniotic membrane. *Proc. Soc. exp. Biol. Med.*, **94**, 532–537

Friedman, E.A. & Steinberg, M. (1982) Disrupted communication between late-stage premalignant human colon epithelial cells by 12-*O*-tetradecanoyl phorbol-13-acetate. *Cancer Res.*, **42**, 5096–5105

Friend, C., Scher, W., Holland, J.G. & Sato, T. (1971) Hemoglobulin synthesis in murine virus-induced leukemic cells *in vitro:* Stimulation of erythroid differentiation by dimethylsulfoxide. *Proc. natl Acad. Sci. USA*, **68**, 378–382

Hecker, E., Fusenig, N.E., Kunz, W., Marks, F. & Thielmann, H.W., eds (1982) *Carcinogenesis*, Vol. 7, *Cocarcinogenesis and Biological Effects of Tumor Promoters*, New York, Raven Press

Horowitz, A.D., Greenebaum, E. & Weinstein, I.B. (1981) Identification of receptors for phorbol ester tumor promoters in intact mammalian cells and of an inhibitor of receptor binding in biologic fluids. *Proc. natl Acad. Sci. USA*, **78**, 2315–2319

Jaken, S., Tashjian, A.H., Jr & Blumberg, P.M. (1981) Characterization of phorbol ester receptors and their down modulation in GH4Cl rat pituitary cells. *Cancer Res.*, ***41***, 2175–2181

Knudson, A.G., Jr (1971) Mutation and cancer: Statistical study of retinoblastoma. *Proc. natl Acad. Sci. USA*, ***68***, 820–823

Lane, M.A., Sainten, A. & Cooper, G.M. (1982) Stage-specific transforming genes of human and mouse B- and T-lymphocyte neoplasms. *Cell*, ***28***, 873–880

Loewenstein, W.R. (1979) Junctional intercellular communication and the control of growth. *Biochem. biophys. Acta*, ***560***, 1–65

Loewenstein, W.R. (1981) Junctional intercellular communication: The cell-to-cell membrane channel. *Physiol. Rev.*, ***61***, 829–913

Matsunaga, E. (1979) Hereditary retinoblastoma: Host factors and age at onset. *J. natl Cancer Inst.*, ***63***, 933–939

Miwa, J., Tabuse, Y., Furusawa, M. & Yamasaki, H. (1982) Tumor promoters specifically and reversibly disturb development and behaviour of *Caenorhabditis elegans*. *J. Cancer Res. clin. Oncol.*, ***104***, 81–87

Mosser, D.D. & Bols, N.C. (1982) The effect of phorbol on metabolic cooperation between human fibroblasts. *Carcinogenesis*, ***3***, 1207–1212

Murray, A.W. & Fitzgerald, D.J. (1979) Tumor promoters inhibit metabolic cooperation in coculture of epidermal and 3T3 cells. *Biochem. biophys. Res. Commun.*, ***91***, 395–401

Ostertag, W., Melderis, H., Steinheider, G., Kluge, N. & Dube, S. (1972) Synthesis of mouse hemoglobin and globin mRNA in leukemia in DBA/2 mice. *Nature-New Biol.*, ***239***, 231–234

Raick, A.N. (1973) Ultrastructural, histological and biochemical alterations produced by 12-*O*-tetradecanoyl phorbol-13-acetate on mouse epidermis and their relevance to skin tumor promotion. *Cancer*, ***33***, 269–278

Raick, A.N. & Burdzy, K. (1973) Ultrastructural and biochemical changes induced in mouse epidermis by a hyperplastic agent, ethylphenylpropiolate. *Cancer Res.*, ***33***, 2221–2230

Rovera, G., O'Brien, T.G. & Diamond, L. (1977) Tumor promoters inhibit spontaneous differentiation of Friend erythroleukemia cells in culture. *Proc. natl Acad. Sci. USA*, ***74***, 2894–2898

Shiba, Y. (1981) Modulatory action of 12-*O*-tetradecanoyl phorbol-13-acetate on bud production in hydra. *Wilhelm Roux's Arch.*, ***190***, 305–308

Shoyab, M. & Todaro, G.J. (1980) Specific high affinity cell membrane receptors for biologically active phorbol and ingenol esters. *Nature*, ***288***, 451–455

Slaga, T.J., Sivak, A. & Boutwell, R.K., eds (1978) *Carcinogenesis*, Vol. 2, *Mechanisms of Tumor Promotion and Cocarcinogenesis*, New York, Raven Press

Slaga, T.J., Fischer, S.M., Weeks, C.E., Nelson, K., Mamrack, M. & Klein-Szanto, A.J.P. (1982) *Specificity and mechanisms of promoter inhibitors in multistage promotion in carcinogenesis*. In: Hecker, E., Fusenig, N.E., Kunz, W., Marks, F. & Thielmann, H.W., eds, *Carcinogenesis*, Vol. 7, *Cocarcinogenesis and Biological Effects of Tumor Promoters*, New York, Raven Press, pp. 19–34

Solanki, V. & Slaga, T.J. (1982) The down-regulation of receptors for phorbol ester tumor promoter in primary epidermal cells. *Carcinogenesis*, ***3***, 993–998

Solanki, V., Slaga, T.J., Callaham, M. & Huberman, E. (1981) Down regulation of specific binding of (20-$^3$H)phorbol 12,13-dibutyrate and phorbol ester-induced differentiation of human promyelocytic leukemia cells. *Proc. natl Acad. Sci. USA*, ***78***, 1722–1525

Stewart, W.W. (1978) Functional connections between cells as revealed by dye-coupling with a highly fluorescent naphthalimide tracer. *Cell*, ***14***, 741–759

Trosko, J.E., Yotti, L.P., Warren, S.T., Tsushimoto, G. & Chang, C.C. (1982) *Inhibition of cell-cell communication by tumor promoters*. In: Hecker, E., Fusenig, N.E., Kunz, W., Marks, F. & Thielmann, H.W., eds, *Carcinogenesis*, Vol. 7, *Cocarcinogenesis and Biological Effects of Tumor Promoters*, New York, Raven Press, pp. 565–585

Unwin, P.N.T. & Zampighi, G. (1980) Structure of the junctions between communicating cells. *Nature*, ***283***, 545–549

Weinstein, I.B., Lee, L.S., Fisher, P.B., Mufson, R.A. & Yamasaki, H. (1979) Action of phorbol esters in cell culture: mimicry of transformation, altered differentiation and effects on cell membranes. *J. Supramolec. Struct.*, ***12***, 195–208

Yamamoto, F. & Furusawa, M. (1978) A simple microinjection technique not employing a micromanipulator. *Exp. Cell Res.*, ***117***, 441–445

Yamasaki, H. (1984) *Modulation of cell differentiation by tumor promoters*. In: Slaga, T.J., ed., *Mechanisms of Tumor Promotion*, Vol. 4, *Cellular Responses to Tumor Promoters*, Boca Raton, FL, CRC Press, pp. 1–26

Yamasaki, H., Fibach, E., Nudel, U., Weinstein, I.B., Rifkind, R.A. & Marks, P.A. (1977) Tumor promoters inhibit spontaneous and induced differentiation of murine erythroleukemia cells in culture. *Proc. natl Acad. Sci. USA*, ***74***, 3451–3455

Yamasaki, H., Weinstein, I.B., Fibach, E., Rifkind, R.A. & Marks, P.A. (1979) Tumor promoter-induced adhesion of the DS-19 clone of murine erythroleukemia cells. *Cancer Res.*, ***39***, 1989–1994

Yamasaki, H., Saint-Vincent, L. & Martel, N. (1980) Long-term effect of a tumor promoter, 12-*O*-tetradecanoyl phorbol-13-acetate, on induced differentiation of Friend leukemia cells. *Cancer Res.*, ***40***, 3780–3785

Yamasaki, H., Drevon, C. & Martel, N. (1982a) In vitro *studies on the mechanisms of tumor promoter-mediated inhibition of cell differentiation*. In: Hecker, E., Fusenig, N.E., Kunz, W., Marks, F. & Thielmann, H.W., eds, *Carcinogenesis*, Vol. 7, *Cocarcinogenesis and Biological Effects of Tumor Promoters*, New York, Raven Press, pp. 359–377

Yamasaki, H., Drevon, C. & Martel, N. (1982b) Specific binding of phorbol esters to Friend erythroleukemia cells – General properties, down regulation and relationship to cell differentiation. *Carcinogenesis*, ***3***, 905–910

Yamasaki, H., Enomoto, T., Martel, N., Shiba, Y. & Kanno, Y. (1983) Tumor promoter-mediated reversible inhibition of cell-cell communication (electrical coupling): Relationship with phorbol ester binding and *de novo* macromolecule synthesis. *Exp. Cell Res.*, ***146***, 297–308

Yancey, S.B., Edens, J.E., Trosko, J.E., Chang, C.C. & Revel, J.P. (1982) Decreased incidence of gap junctions between Chinese hamster V-79 cells upon exposure to the tumor promoter 12-*O*-tetradecanoyl phorbol-13-acetate. *Exp. Cell Res.*, ***139***, 329–340

Yotti, L.P., Chang, C.C. & Trosko, J.E. (1979) Elimination of metabolic cooperation in Chinese hamster cells by a tumor promoter. *Science*, **206**, 1089–1091

Yuspa, S.H. & Morgan, D.L. (1981) Mouse skin cells resistant to terminal differentiation associated with initiation of carcinogenesis. *Nature*, **293**, 72–74

# THE USE OF IN-VITRO ASSAYS TO STUDY AND TO DETECT TUMOUR PROMOTERS

J.E. TROSKO, C. JONE & C.C. CHANG
*Department of Pediatrics and Human Development*
*Michigan State University*
*East Lansing, MI 48824, USA*

## INTRODUCTION

One of the major challenges of our era is to be able to predict and to assess the potential health and environmental consequences of the large number of chemicals to which human and other biological organisms are exposed. These chemicals reach human beings *via* the food chain, air, water, occupational setting, drugs and life-style, Part of this exposure has a component of choice, whereas another part does not.

Reliance on human epidemiological evidence of health consequences of past exposure as the only direct means of assessing uniquely human responses to chemicals is clearly not a very practical or reasonable means for this task. The use of animals to test for reproductive, genetic, teratogenic, carcinogenic, mutagenic, and other toxic endpoints presupposes that the data will provide both a qualitative and a quantitative basis for prediction of potential human harm. While this method, in principle, seems to be the only practical alternative for comparison of the effects of chemicals on the whole organism, it is obviously not perfect. The thalidomide case is the most poignant example of the failure of animal tests to predict a human consequence.

There have been attempts to develop many kinds of molecular, biochemical and in-vitro assays to assess the ability of chemicals to affect human health (Hsie *et al.*, 1979; Stich & San, 1981). The primary reason for using this approach is to avoid the relatively high cost of whole animal tests and the time required to assess the chemical. Furthermore, in-vivo assessments rarely give information on the mechanisms of action of these chemicals.

In spite of the inherent limitations of all molecular, biochemical and in-vitro assays to assess potential harm to human health, in our technological societies we have neither the resources nor the time to perform only animal studies. In addition, humane considerations demand that we find alternative ways of testing chemicals. Some of the limitations of any molecular, biochemical or in-vitro assay are as follows: (1) many chemically-induced health disruptions occur in biochemical functions of a higher order which are not found in in-vitro systems (i.e., immunological, neurological, endocrinological-physiological functions not found in organ, tissue or cell culture systems); (2) at present, we have not defined the molecular mechanisms of any disease process in human beings; (3) species, developmental stage, individual tissue, sex factors, individual genetic variability and biological context are factors usually not taken into consideration in these short-term assays; (4) assessment of single chemicals in short-term assays may not mimic the 'real life' exposure *in vivo;* and (5) unless the biological principle of the assay is understood and is related to one aspect of the mechanism of disease causation in humans, in-vitro results have little predictive value in assessing human health risks. For example, although chromosomal changes or sister chromatid exchanges – indicators of *some* mutagens – are found in human cells, there is little one can say about the health consequences of these endpoints.

In spite of these serious and acknowledged limitations, much useful information has been, and will be, obtained from short-term assays.

## INITIATION/PROMOTION MODEL OF CARCINOGENESIS

In order to justify the use of a short-term assay to detect chemicals that affect carcinogenesis, an examination is made here of both the observations related to carcinogenesis and some theories of the mechanisms of carcinogenesis.

It seems trite to note that carcinogenesis is a complex biological process. We do not know if the mechanisms leading to benign tumours also contribute to malignant tumours. Indeed, we do not know if there are universal steps by which cell tumours must pass, or if they are brought about by several different molecular mechanisms or only one mechanism.

However, carcinogenesis does seem to involve an evolution of cellular phenotypes. During the process, a contact-inhibited normal cell stem is converted into a premalignant cell, which has a selective growth advantage over its normal counterpart in a particular environment. During this premalignant stage, additional phenotypic changes occur, giving rise to non-contact-inhibited, invasive and metastatic phenotypes. It is generally assumed that, in spite of the heterogeneity of phenotypes within a tumour (Owens *et al.,* 1982), the cells are of clonal origin (Fialkow, 1974; Nowell, 1976). Characterized as a 'disease of differentiation' (Pierce, 1974) or as 'blocked or partially blocked ontogeny', carcinogenesis is clearly a reflection of abnormal genotypic information and/or expression (Potter, 1978).

The concepts of initiation and promotion were introduced to explain the observations that, in rodent skin, a 'sub-carcinogenic' exposure to a carcinogen, if followed by chronic and regular application of a 'non-carcinogen', gives rise to tumours. Conversion of a single normal cell to a premalignant cell is an operational definition of the initiation process, while the clonal amplification of the initiation process, which ultimately leads to a malignant cell, is the promotion process (Trosko

& Chang, 1980). Additional changes that occur after this event have been described as 'progression' (Pitot *et al.*, 1981).

Clearly, the molecular mechanisms leading to either the initiation or promotion phase are not yet known. Indeed, assuming that most, but not all (Mintz & Illmensee, 1975), cancers can be explained by the initiation and promotion process, it seems that several different mechanisms could lead to a stable alteration of a normal cell genome (i.e., mutations and stable gene modulations) to bring about initiation (Trosko *et al.*, 1983). Most initiators seem, however, to be mutagens (Ames *et al.*, 1973) and/or reagents that can damage DNA (Miller & Miller, 1981). Promotion is, in general, a 'mitogenic' process, whereby proliferation of the initiated cell is, at least, stimulated and, apparently, normal differentiation is prevented (Potter, 1980; Trosko & Chang, 1980; Yuspa & Morgan, 1981). Promoters seem, in general, to be membrane-active components (Weinstein *et al.*, 1980). In fact, there is clear evidence that what might be a tumour promoter in one cell type might not be in another. For example, the tumour-promoting phorbol esters are known to stimulate growth of human epithelial cells but not that of normal human fibroblasts (Lechner & Kaighn, 1980). In addition, normal human melanocytes are stimulated to proliferate in the presence of phorbol esters, but human keratinocytes are killed by phorbol esters (Eisinger & Marko, 1982). The promotion of fibroblast-derived tumours and that of epithelial-derived tumours probably requires quite different agents. If this assessment of tumour promotion is accurate, no single short-term assay can be designed to detect all means of tumour promotion. Some of the requirements or mechanisms of different promoters are: (1) tissue specific receptors (i.e., hormones, growth factors); (2) cell-type specificity; (3) metabolism; (4) accumulation in certain organs; and (5) action as an 'indirect' promoter by cytotoxic action (Trosko *et al.*, 1982).

## INTERCELLULAR COMMUNICATION AND TUMOUR PROMOTION

The literature seems to indicate that once an experimental animal has been initiated, the promotion process can be brought about by agents which are cytotoxic, by physical conditions which bring about regenerative or compensatory hyperplasia (abrasion, wound healing), by hyperplasia-inducing growth factors or hormones, by stimulating hyperplasia and abnormal differentiation by the interference of solid objects in normal growth control or by non-cytotoxic chemicals which can stimulate proliferation in contact-inhibited cells (Trosko *et al.*, 1983). In each case, sustained hyperplasia of the surviving stem cell population, if previously exposed to initiators, can give rise to a 'critical mass' of dysfunctional cells (Trosko & Chang, 1980). Sustained hyperplasia has been implicated as one of the most important biological processes correlated with tumour promotion (Sisskin & Barrett, 1981).

However, this does not mean that short-term assays cannot be used to detect some tumour promoters. A number of observations have been made that, among the many pleiotropic effects of tumour promoters on the molecular, biochemical and cellular levels (Hecker *et al.*, 1982), the phenomenon of inhibited intercellular communication might be one unifying process linking all of the forms of tumour promotion (i.e., regenerative hyperplasia; solid-state stimulated hyperplasia; receptor and non-receptor mediated mitogenesis; etc). In each case, if the ability to retard the growth of an initiated cell is the result of that cell being surrounded by and communicating with its normal neighbours, blockage of that communication by cell removal, cell death or chemical inhibition of intercellular communication will isolate that cell (Potter, 1980; Trosko & Chang, 1980).

Intercellular communication is a concept that describes at least two mechanisms by which cells within and between tissues coordinate their actions in a multicellular organism. The process of intercellular communication has been linked to the regulation of differentiation and proliferation of cells (Loewenstein, 1979; Revel *et al.*, 1980). By inference, interference of the communication between a pluripotent stem cell with differentiated daughter cells or with other target cells would lead to abnormal control of differentiation and proliferation.

Several observations have implicated abnormal intercellular communication with the carcinogenic process: (1) most, if not all, truly malignant cells have abnormal ability to contact-inhibit (Borek, 1966) or to perform gap-junction-mediated communication (Corsaro & Migeon, 1977) [see Trosko *et al.* (1982) for discussions of exceptions]; (2) many non-cytotoxic and non-mutagenic tumour promoters can inhibit intercellular communication (Murray & Fitzgerald, 1979; Yotti *et al.*, 1979; Trosko *et al.*, 1982); (3) non-cytotoxic levels of mutagenic carcinogens do not inhibit intercellular communication (Umeda *et al.*, 1980; Telang *et al.*, 1982); (4) virus-induced cell transformation affects intercellular communication (Steinberg & Defendi, 1981); co-cultivation, fusion or co-injection of transformed cells with normal cells implies that normal cells can suppress the transformed phenotype by cell-cell communication (see Trosko *et al.*, 1983) for review); (5) tumour promoters have been shown to alter proliferation and differentiation patterns in cells (Weinstein *et al.*, 1979); (6) most recently, in human colonic epithelial cells, it has been shown that phorbol esters can, in late-stage benign tumour cells, block gap-junction-mediated intercellular communication (Friedman & Steinberg, 1982).

In view of the observations that sustained hyperplasia is needed for tumour promotion and that inhibited intercellular communication can lead to abnormal proliferation and differentiation, markers that are correlated with these biological phenomena might be used for detecting potential promoters.

Since many types of studies have suggested that several genetic 'hits' occur during the carcinogenic process (Ashley, 1969; Knudson, 1971; Trosko & Chang, 1980), and since mutations occur during DNA replication, promotion of an initiated cell containing a single 'hit' of an allele at a genetic locus would increase the population of these cells. During that increase, more cells will contain this single 'hit'. The chances of incurring a second hit in one cell at the same critical locus is now increased by the promotion process (Trosko & Chang, 1980; Potter, 1982).

In other words, promotion increases the probability of multiple genetic changes by at least two actions, namely, by increasing the number of 'target'-initiated cells and by enhancing mutagenic changes that occur during cell division. Promoters are not mutagenic (Trosko *et al.*, 1983) but they facilitate the changes that are needed to bring about mutagenic events during DNA synthesis by fixing unrepaired DNA lesions caused by mutagens or by enhancing error-prone replication (Weymouth & Loeb, 1978).

## SHORT-TERM ASSAY FOR PROMOTERS

If sustained hyperplasia and inhibited intercellular communication are accepted as obligatory components of tumour promotion, the molecular, biochemical and cellular markers for each of these processes might serve as indicators for the presence of *some* chemicals that are tumour promoters.

In view of previous comments on the various ways in which hyperplasia could be brought about, it must be re-emphasized that it is highly unlikely that any one short-term assay could either detect or distinguish chemicals or conditions which could act as a promoter *via* any of these mechanism (i.e., cell death, specific receptor mediated-mitogenesis, non-receptor-mediated mitogenesis).

Several short-term assays have been proposed for the detection of tumour promoters (Sivak, 1982). Induction of ornithine decarboxylase (ODC) (O'Brien, 1977), induction of anchorage-independence (Colburn *et al.,* 1980), in-vitro enhancement of transformation (Sivak, 1982), activation of Epstein-Barr virus in human lymphoblastoid cells (Ito *et al.,* 1981), alterations of surface-attachment properties of tumour cells (Braun *et al.,* 1981) and inhibition of intercellular communication (Trosko *et al.,* 1983).

Few of these assays can be used to test many non-phorbol ester promoters. The mechanism of action or the mechanistic relationship of the short-term assay to the promotion process *in vivo* for most, if not all, of these assays is not known. For example, the fact that ODC is induced by tumour-promoting phorbol esters gives us few clues as to why the initiated, but not the uninitiated, cell ultimately becomes malignant. (It should be noted that ODC is induced by phorbol ester in both of these kinds of tissue in mouse skin.) Although some have argued that not all promoters induce ODC [i.e., phenobarbital in rat liver is a promoter (Peraino *et al.,* 1980) but not an inducer of ODC (Farwell *et al.,* 1978; Saccone & Pariza, 1978), it should be noted that phenobarbital appears to suppress cell division in normal liver cells (Shinozuka *et al.,* 1982) while it obviously stimulates growth of the initiated cells (Schulte-Hermann *et al.,* 1981). Therefore, while ODC may be an obligatory marker for cell division, *in vivo* it might be practically impossible to distinguish increases in ODC from a few initiated cells in a mass of non-dividing cells.

Various in-vitro assays have been designed to detect chemicals that inhibit intercellular communication. This property of non-cytotoxic levels of chemicals to inhibit intercellular communication *in vivo* has been found to belong to many classes of chemicals known to be promoters of either skin, colon, lung, liver, breast or oesophagus in several species. Several in-vitro techniques have been designed to measure intercellular communication, including: (1) metabolic cooperation between 6-thioguanine-sensitive and -resistant cells (Yotti *et al.,* 1979); (2) autoradiographic detection or detection of radioactive transfer (Murray & Fitzgerald, 1979); (3) co-cultivation of target cells with a communicating population of cells with drug-metabolizing capability (Williams *et al.,* 1981); (4) electrocoupling techniques to measure ionic transfer between cells (Enomoto *et al.,* 1981; Yamasaki *et al.,* 1983); and (5) the use of fluorescent dye transfer (Freidman & Steinberg, 1982).

The use of metabolic cooperation between 6-thioguanine-sensitive and 6-thioguanine-resistant cells has, apart from the aforementioned shortcomings, several advantages over the other techniques. This approach is based on testing chemicals at non-cytotoxic levels. In other words, almost any chemical (mutagen, non-mutagenic cytotoxin, or promoter at cytotoxic levels) could inhibit intercellular communication by inducing cytotoxicity. Most of the other techniques cannot be used to distinguish between the non-cytotoxic and cytotoxic effects.

The metabolic cooperation assay is also quantitative. We feel that it is important to test each chemical in a dose-responsive manner. By doing this, we have made several observations that we consider important to the understanding of mechanisms. The first is that each chemical shown to inhibit intercellular communication at non-cytotoxic doses appears to exhibit a non-effect level. In other words, below a certain concentration, these chemicals are unable to inhibit intercellular communication. The second observation is that above the no-effect level, there is a linear dose-response, until one of several things happens: (1) the chemical becomes cytotoxic, and recovery of 6-thioguanine resistant cells decreases (Tsushimoto *et al.*, 1982a); (2) a plateau of recovery is reached without cytotoxicity (Tsushimoto *et al;* 1982b) and (3) a 'down-regulation' of metabolic cooperation is observed without cytotoxicity (Jone *et al.*, 1982).

Since it has to be assumed that some tumour promoters require metabolism, the in-vitro assay must ultimately include a metabolizing system, similar to that designed by Williams *et al.* (1981). In addition, tissue and species differences probably influence the ability of a chemical to act as a promoter, which implies that, ultimately, human cells from various tissues will have to be used in the assay.

Furthermore, some reports indicate that certain promoters cause effects in epithelial cells which are opposite to those in fibroblast cells. Phorbol ester appear to be fairly cytostatic and cytotoxic to normal human fibroblast cells, whereas the same concentration is not cytotoxic to various human cell types, including epithelial cells (Lechner & Kaighn, 1980; Yotti, 1980; Eisinger & Marko, 1982). Consequently, in-vitro assays utilizing human fibroblasts and epithelial cells might help predict promoters of fibroblast- and epithelial-derived tumours. In addition, the use of cell lines with receptors to growth factors and hormones could be used to study the mechanism by which these molecules act as promoters, possibly by inhibiting intercellular communication (Merk *et al.*, 1980; Meda *et al.*, 1980; Amsterdam *et al.*, 1981; Larsen *et al.*, 1981).

## THE USE OF IN-VITRO INTERCELLULAR COMMUNICATION TO STUDY MECHANISMS OF TUMOUR PROMOTION

To reiterate, no single in-vitro assay can be expected to detect all possible promoters. In addition, no single in-vitro assay can be expected to give all the information necessary to study all the facets of the complex tumour promotion process (Slaga *et al.*, 1980).

In view of the demonstration, in mouse skin at least, of several stages of promotion and according to the concept of promotion as an artificial model to explain what happens after a single initiated premalignant cell is converted to a premalignant cell, we can only surmise that promotion is more than just 'sustained hyperplasia'. In addition, even if inhibition of intercellular communication is a necessary step in isolating the initiated cell from surrounding suppressing normal cells, ultimately, other events must occur during the clonal amplification of initiated cells, which is different from the clonal amplification of normal cells.

We have discussed previously the possibility that 'mitogens' or tumour promoters might have at least three concomitant functions: (1) to send a membrane-triggered signal to the nucleus to activate cell cycle-dependent genes (e.g., the gene for ODC); (2) to make the membrane permeable to the necessary building blocks for macromolecular synthesis (sugars, amino acids, etc); and (3) to isolate the cell from its gap-junction-linked neighbours in order to prevent the transfer of the newly synthesized energy-rich molecules needed for macromolecular synthesis.

The fact that with our in-vitro assay we have demonstrated that tumour promoters cause disappearance of gap-junctions under the same conditions leading to inhibition of metabolic cooperation (Yancey *et al.*, 1982) is consistent with this idea. The fact that the in-vitro assay seems to indicate a no-effect, threshold level before intercellular communication is inhibited might be explained theoretically by the fact that, in a tissue, the initiated cell is probably gap-junctionally linked to cells in three dimensions. It is highly unlikely that the disruption of cell gap-junctions is due to a single molecular 'hit' by a promoter molecule. A certain concentration of the chemical is probably needed to reach a 'critical level' which will set off a physiological reaction to close the gap junctions (Azarnia *et al.*, 1981). These observations are consistent with observations that there appears to be a threshold phenomenon needed for tumour promotion *in vivo* (Boutwell, 1979; Verma & Boutwell, 1980).

The fact that our in-vitro assay seems to indicate a 'down-regulation' of gap-junctional-mediated intercellular communication for promoters that seem to be 'receptor-mediated' (Blumberg, 1981), is consistent with observations of a 'down-regulation' of receptors of 12-*O*-tetradecanoylphorbol-13-acetate (Solanki *et al.*, 1981; Yamasaki *et al*; 1982) and of 'down-regulation' of gap-junction function (Flagg-Newton, 1980).

The fact that gap-junctional intercellular communication is a reversible phenomenon (Enomoto *et al.*, 1981) is also consistent with the general observation that tumour promoters must be applied in a regular, chronic fashion in order to maintain sustained hyperplasia (Boutwell, 1979).

Clearly, many chemicals which are cytotoxic interact with specific cellular receptors or require metabolism prior to action and may act as promoters *in vivo* might not be detected in any specific in-vitro assay to measure intercellular communication. For example, 3,4,5,3′,4′,5′-hexabromobiphenyl does not inhibit intercellular communication in Chinese hamster cells (Tsushimoto *et al.*, 1982a). At non-cytotoxic doses *in vivo*, it is not a liver tumour promoter in rats (Jensen *et al.*, 1983). However, at necrotoxic doses, it can act as a liver promoter, presumably by its indirect action as a stimulator of regenerative hyperplasia (Jensen *et al.*, 1983). Also, diethylstilboesterol does not inhibit intercellular communication in the Chinese hamster lung fibroblast (V79) cell assay (Barrett *et al.*, 1983), due probably to a lack of known diethylstilboestrol receptors in these cells.

## SOME IMPLICATIONS OF INHIBITED INTERCELLULAR COMMUNICATION

If we assume that the results of all the in-vitro studies on tumour promoter-inhibited intercellular communication have some bearing on understanding carcinogenesis, there seem to be two levels of implications. The first level provides a practical means for screening for potential tumour promoters, while the second level leads to an understanding of some mechanistic aspects of the initiation/promotion model of carcinogenesis. The rationale, potential and limitations of the current in-vitro assays for measuring intercellular communication as a means of detecting tumour promoters have been discussed previously.

One additional practical implication seems evident. Multicellular organisms acquired, through evolution, the means to regulate opposing functions of cells (i.e., proliferation and differentiation) in order to be adaptive (i.e., they could develop many adaptive differentiated systems, as well as grow, heal wounds, etc). A wide variety of molecular communication signals (hormones, growth factors, cell-specific 'mitogens', etc), as well as an array of specific receptors for these molecular signals, were developed. However, the signal, once received, seems to be transferred to the responsive centre of the cell by a relatively conserved system (calcium ion, cyclic-AMP, protein kinase, calmodulin-related reactions) in most, if not all, cells.

Environmental chemicals, plant toxins, food components, insect toxins, etc, have evolved to interact with the normal mechanisms of intercellular communication. The organism can respond adaptively to these agents on the basis of the short-term biological consequences (i.e., pain or pain relief, taste aversion or taste stimulation, inflammation or anti-inflammation, growth or differentiation). If, however, the chemical induces prolonged, chronic interference with intercellular communication processes, abnormal regulation of the normal process will occur.

However, the recent demonstration that bladder 'oncogenes' in tumour cells differ from their normal counterparts by a single base change (Reddy *et al.,* 1982; Tabin *et al.,* 1982) now forces us to think seriously of the implications of these results for the biology of the multistage nature of carcinogenesis, both *in vitro* and *in vivo.*

The eloquent results of the molecular studies of 'oncogenes' have led some to claim that it is hard to 'reconcile' these facts with the multistage schema of carcinogenesis (Marx, 1982). Although it would be wrong to assume that all cancers have their origin in a *mutation* in oncogenes, it is only reasonable to assume, together with all the other solid evidence linking mutations with carcinogenesis (Trosko & Chang, 1979), that mutations do play some role. Therefore, the next question has to be, 'What gene, or genes, when mutated (or stably epigenetically altered), contributes to a portion of the carcinogenic process?'

In view of the series of observations linking a lack of intercellular communication with malignancy (Trosko *et al.,* 1983), and the ability of known tumour promoters to inhibit intercellular communication (Murray & Fitzgerald, 1979; Yotti *et al.,* 1979; Trosko *et al.,* 1982), it seems reasonable to implicate the genes that regulate the structure and function of intercellular communication mechanisms (e.g., gap-junction structure and formation in solid tissues) as candidate 'oncogenes'.

If a gene that affects either the regulation or structure of gap-junctions is mutated, clearly dramatic consequences to the regulation of cell proliferation and differentiation can be expected, since, as pointed out before (Trosko *et al.*, 1983), gap-junction-mediated intercellular communication is needed for normal differentiation and proliferation. Cyclic-AMP, calcium ion and pH have been implicated in the regulation of gap-junctions (Loewenstein, 1981; Hooper, 1982). Abnormal cyclic-AMP levels and calcium ion metabolism have been found in many malignant cells (Whitfield *et al.*, 1979). Metabolic-cooperation-deficient cells have also been isolated (MacDonald, 1982; Nakano *et al.*, 1982). To date, no true gap-junction structural mutant has been isolated or characterized; however, one could only assume that the genes for gap-junctions can be mutated. Therefore, in the sense that an 'oncogene' is just a normal gene that has been highly conserved over a long period of evolution because it was needed to perform a sufficiently important function, genes controlling the regulation of gap-junctions surely fit that description.

## ACKNOWLEDGEMENTS

Research was supported by grants from the US Environmental Protection Agency (R808470) and the National Cancer Institute (CA21104).

'Although the information described in this article has been funded wholly or in part by the United States Environmental Protection Agency under assistance agreement R808587010 to James E. Trosko, it has not been subjected to the Agency's required peer and administrative review, and therefore does not necessarily reflect the views of the Agency and no official endorsement should be inferred.'

## REFERENCES

Ames, B.N., Durston, W.E., Yamasaki, E. & Lee, F.D. (1973) Carcinogens are mutagens: A simple test system combining liver homogenates for activation and bacteria for detection. *Proc. natl Acad. Sci. USA*, ***70***, 2281–2285

Amsterdam, A., Knecht, M. & Catt, K. (1981) Hormonal regulation of cytodifferentiation and intercellular communication in cultured granulosa cells. *Proc. natl Acad. Sci. USA*, ***78***, 3000–3004

Ashley, D.J. (1969) The two 'hit' and multiple 'hit' theories of carcinogenesis. *Br. J. Cancer*, ***23***, 313–328

Azarnia, R., Dahl, G. & Loewenstein, W.R. (1981) Cell junction and cyclic AMP: III. Promotion of junctional membrane permeability and junctional membrane particles in a junction-deficient cell type. *J. Membrane Biol.*, ***63***, 133–145

Barrett, J.C., McLachlan, J.A. & Elmore, E. (1983) Inability of diethylstilbestrol to induce 6-thioguanine resistant mutants and to inhibit metabolic cooperation of V79 Chinese hamster cells. *Mutat. Res.*, ***107***, 427–432

Blumberg, P.M. (1981) *In vitro* studies on the mode of action of the phorbol esters, potent tumor promoters: Part 2. *CRC crit. Rev. Toxicol.*, ***9***, 199–234

Borek, C. & Sachs, L. (1966) The difference in contact inhibition of cell replication between normal cells and cells transformed by different carcinogens. *Proc. natl Acad. Sci. USA*, ***56***, 1705–1711

Boutwell, R.K. (1979) The function and mechanism of promoters of carcinogenesis. *CRC crit. Rev. Toxicol.*, ***2***, 419–443

Braun, A.G., Buckner, L.A. & Nichinson, B.B. (1981) Plasma membrane alterations due to promoters and anti-promoters. *Terat. Carcinog. Mutag.*, ***1***, 417–427

Colburn, N.H., Koehler, B.A. & Nelson, K.J. (1980) A cell culture assay for tumor promoter-dependent progression toward neoplastic phenotype: Detection of tumor promoters and promotion inhibitors. *Terat. Carcinog. Mutag.*, ***1***, 87–96

Corsaro, C.M. & Migeon, B.R. (1977) Comparison of contact-mediated communication in normal and transformed human cells in culture. *Proc. natl Acad. Sci. USA*, ***74***, 4476–4480

Eisinger, M. & Marko, O. (1982) Selective proliferation of normal human melanocytes *in vitro* in the presence of phorbol ester and cholera toxin. *Proc. natl Acad. Sci. USA*, ***79***, 2018–2022

Enomoto, T., Sasaki, Y., Shiba, Y., Kanno, Y. & Yamasaki, H. (1981) Tumor promoters cause a rapid and reversible inhibition of the formation and maintenance of electrical coupling in culture. *Proc. natl Acad. Sci. USA*, ***78***, 5628–5632

Farwell, D.C., Nolan, C.E. & Herbst, E.J. (1978) Liver ornithine decarboxylase during phenobarbital promotion of nitrosamine carcinogenesis. *Cancer Lett.*, ***5***, 139–144

Fialkow, P. (1974) The origin and development of human tumors studied with cell markers. *New Engl. J. Med.*, ***29***, 26–35

Flagg-Newton, J.L. (1980) The premeability of the cell to cell membrane channel and its regulation in mammalian cell junctions. *In Vitro*, ***16***, 1043–1048

Friedman, E.A. & Steinberg, M. (1982) Disrupted communication between late-stage premalignant human colon epithelial cells by 12-*O*-tetradecanoyl phorbol-13-acetate. *Cancer Res.*, ***42***, 5096–5105

Hecker, E., Fusenig, N.E., Kunz, W., Marks, F. & Thielmann, H.W., eds (1982) *Carcinogenesis, Vol. 7, Cocarcinogenesis and Biological Effects of Tumor Promoters*, New York, Raven Press

Hooper, M.L. (1982) Metabolic cooperation between mammalian cells in culture. *Biochim. biophys. Acta*, ***651***, 85–103

Hsie, A.W., O'Neill, J.P. & McElheny, V.K., eds (1979) *Mammalian Cell Mutagenesis. The Maturation of Test Systems (Banbury Report 2)*, Cold Spring Harbor, NY, Cold Spring Harbor Laboratory

Ito, Y., Yanase, S., Fujita, J., Harayama, T., Takashima, M. & Imanaka, H. (1981) A short-term *in vitro* assay for promoter substances using human lymphoblastoid cells latently infected with Epstein-Barr virus. *Cancer Lett.*, ***13***, 29–37

Jensen, R.K., Sleight, S.D., Aust, S.D., Goodman, J.I. & Trosko, J.E. (1983) Hepatic tumor promotion by 3,3′,4,4′5,5′-hexabromobiphenyl: The interrelationship between toxicity, induction of microsomal drug metabolizing enzymes and tumor promotion. *Toxicol. appl. Pharmacol.*, ***71***, 163–176

Jone, C.M., Trosko, J.E., Chang, C.C., Fujiki, H. & Sugimura, T. (1982) Inhibition of intercellular communication in Chinese hamster V79 cells by teleocidin. *Gann*, ***73***, 874–878

Knudson, A.G. (1971) Mutation and cancer: Statistical study of retinoblastoma. *Proc. natl Acad. Sci. USA*, ***68***, 820–823

Larsen, W.J., Tung, N.N. & Polking, C. (1981) Response of granulosa cell gap junctions to human chorionic gonadotropin (hCG) at ovulation. *Biol. Reprod.*, ***25***, 1119–1134

Lechner, J.F. & Kaighn, M.E. (1980) EGF growth promoting activity is neutralized by phorbol esters. *Cell Biol. intern. Rep.*, ***4***, 23–28

Loewenstein, W.R. (1979) Junctional intercellular communication and the control of growth. *Biochim. biophys. Acta Cancer Res.*, ***560***, 1–65

Loewenstein, W.R. (1981) Junctional intercellular communication: The cell to cell membrane channel *Physiol. Rev.*, ***61***, 829–913

MacDonald, C. (1982) Genetic complementation in hybrid cells derived from two metabolic cooperation defective mammalian cell lines. *Exp. Cell Res.*, ***138***, 303–310

Marx, J.L. (1982) Cancer cell genes linked to viral oncogenes. *Science*, ***216***, 724

Meda, P., Halban, P., Perrelet, A., Renold, A.S. & Orci, L. (1980) Gap junction development is correlated with insulin content in the pancreatic β cell. *Science*, ***209***, 1026–1028

Merk, F.B., Kwan, P.W.L. & Leav, I. (1980) Gap junctions in the myometrium of hypophysectomized estrogen-treated rats. *Cell Biol. intern. Rep.*, ***4***, 287–294

Miller, E.C. & Miller, J.A. (1981) Search for ultimate chemical carcinogens and their reactions with cellular macromolecules. *Cancer*, ***47***, 2327–2345

Mintz, B. & Illmensee, K. (1975) Normal genetically mosaic mice produced from malignant teratocarcinoma cells. *Proc. natl Acad. Sci. USA*, ***73***, 3585–3589

Murray, A.W. & Fitzgerald, D.J. (1979) Tumor promoters inhibit metabolic cooperation in cocultures of epidermal and 3T3 cells. *Biochem. biophys. Res. Commun.*, ***91***, 395–401

Nakano, S., Bruce, S.A., Ueo, H. & Ts'o, P.O.P. (1982) A qualitative and quantitative assay for cells lacking post-confluence inhibition of cell division: Characterization of this phenotype in carcinogen-treated Syrian hamster embryo cells in culture. *Cancer Res.*, ***42***, 3132–3137

Nowell, P. (1976) The clonal evolution of tumor cell populations. *Science*, ***194***, 23–28

O'Brien, T.G. (1977) The induction of ornithine decarboxylase as an early, possibly obligatory, event in mouse skin carcinogenesis. *Cancer Res.*, ***36***, 2644–2653

Owens, A.H., Coffey, D.S. & Baylin, S.B., eds (1982) *Tumor Cell Heterogeneity Cell Heterogeneity*, New York, Academic Press

Peraino, C., Staffeldt, E.F., Haugen, D.A., Lombard, L.S., Stevens, F.J. & Fry, R.J.M. (1980) Effects of varying the dietary concentration of phenobarbital on its enhancement of 2-acetylaminofluorene-induced hepatic tumorigenesis. *Cancer Res.*, ***40***, 3268–3273

Pierce, G.B. (1974) Neoplasms, differentiation and mutations. *Am. J. Pathol.*, ***77***, 103–118

Pitot, H.C., Goldsworthy, T. & Moran, S. (1981) The natural history of carcinogenesis: Implications of experimental carcinogenesis in the genesis of human cancer. *J. supramol. Struct. cell. Biochem.*, ***17***, 133–146

Potter, V.R. (1978) Phenotypic diversity in experimental hepatomas: The concept of partially blocked ontogeny. *Br. J. Cancer*, ***38***, 1–23

Potter, V.R. (1980) Initiation and promotion in cancer formation: The importance of studies on intercellular communication. *Yale J. Biol. Med.*, ***53***, 367–384

Potter, V.R. (1982) A new protocol and its rationale for the study of initiation and promotion of carcinogenesis in rat liver. *Carcinogenesis*, ***3***, 1375–1379

Reddy, E.P., Reynolds, R.K., Santos, E. & Barbacid, M. (1982) A point mutation is responsible for the acquisition of transforming properties by the $T_{24}$ human bladder carcinoma oncogene. *Nature*, ***300***, 149–152

Revel, J.-P., Yancey, S.B., Meyer, D.J. & Nicholson, B. (1980) Cell junctions and intercellular communications. *In vitro*, ***16***, 1010–1017

Saccone, G.T.P. & Pariza, M.W. (1978) Effects of dietary butylated hydroxytoluene and phenobarbital on the activities of ornithine decarboxylase and thymidine kinase in rat liver and lung. *Cancer Lett.*, ***5***, 145–152

Schulte-Hermann, R., Ohde, G., Schuppler, J. & Timmermann-Trosiener, I. (1981) Enhanced proliferation of putative preneoplastic cells in rat liver following treatment with the tumor promoters phenobarbital, hexachlorocyclohexane, steroid compounds and nafenopin. *Cancer Res.*, ***41***, 2556–2562

Shinozuka, H., Lombardi, B. & Abanobi, S.E. (1982) A comparative study of the efficacy of four barbiturates as promoters of the development of α-glutamyltranspeptidase-positive foci in the liver of carcinogen-treated rats. *Carcinogenesis*, ***3***, 1017–1020

Sisskin, E.E. & Barrett, J.C. (1981) Hyperplasia of Syrian hamster epidermis induced by single but not multiple treatments with 12-*O*-tetradecanoyl phorbol-13-acetate. *Cancer Res.*, ***41***, 346–350

Sivak, A. (1982) An evaluation of assay procedures for detection of tumor promoters. *Mutat. Res.*, ***98***, 377–387

Slaga, T.J., Fischer, S.M., Nelson, K. & Gleason, G.L. (1980) Studies on the mechanism of skin tumor promotion: Evidence for several stages in promotion. *Proc. natl Acad. Sci. USA*, ***77***, 3659–3663

Solanki, V., Slaga, T.J., Callaham, M. & Huberman, E. (1981) Down regulation of specific binding of (20-$^{3}$H)phorbol 12,13-dibutyrate and phorbol ester-induced differentiation of human promyelocytic leukemia cells. *Proc. natl Acad. Sci. USA*, ***78***, 1722–1725

Steinberg, M. & Defendi, V. (1981) Patterns of cell communication and differentiation in SV40 transformed human keratinocytes. *J. cell. Physiol.*, ***109***, 153–159

Stich, H.F. & San, R.H.C. (1981) *Short-term Tests for Chemical Carcinogens*, New York, Springer-Verlag

Tabin, C.J., Bradley, S.M., Bargman, C.I., Weinberg, R.A., Papageorge, A.G., Scolnick, E.M., Dhor, R., Lowy, D.R. & Chang, E.H. (1982) Mechanism of activation of a human oncogene. *Nature*, ***300***, 143–149

Telang, S., Tong, C. & Williams, G.M. (1982) Epigenetic membrane effects of a possible tumor promoting type on cultured liver cells by the non-genotoxic organochlorine pesticides chlordane and heptachlor. *Carcinogenesis*, **3**, 1175–1178

Trosko, J.E. & Chang, C.C. (1979) *Chemical carcinogenesis as a consequence of alterations in the structure and function of DNA*. In: Grover, P., ed., *Chemical Carcinogens and DNA*, Vol. II, Boca Raton, FL, CRC Press, pp. 181–260

Trosko, J.E. & Chang, C.C. (1980) An integrative hypothesis linking cancer, diabetes, and atherosclerosis: The role of mutations and epigenetic changes. *Med. Hypotheses*, **6**, 455–468

Trosko, J.E., Jone, C., Aylsworth, C. & Tsushimoto, G. (1982) Elimination of metabolic cooperation is associated with the tumor promoters, oleic acid and anthralin. *Carcinogenesis*, **3**, 1101–1103

Trosko, J.E., Chang, C.C. & Medcalf, A. (1983a) Mechanisms of tumor promotion: Potential role of intercellular communication. *Cancer Invest.*, **1**, 511–526

Trosko, J.E., Jone, C. & Chang, C.C. (1983b) The role of tumor promoters on phenotypic alterations affecting intercellular communication and tumorigenesis. *Ann. N. Y. Acad. Sci.*, **407**, 316–327

Tsushimoto, G., Trosko, J.E., Chang, C.C. & Aust, S.D. (1982a) Inhibition of metabolic cooperation in Chinese hamster V79 cells in culture by various polybrominated biphenyl (PBB) congeners. *Carcinogenesis*, **3**, 181–185

Tsushimoto, G., Trosko, J.E., Chang, C.C. & Matsumura, F. (1982b) Inhibition of intercellular communication by chlordecone (Kepone) and Mirex in Chinese hamster V79 cells *in vitro*. *Toxicol. appl. Pharmacol.*, **64**, 550–556

Umeda, M., Noda, K. & Ono, T. (1980) Inhibition of metabolic cooperation in Chinese hamster cells by various chemicals including tumor promoters. *Gann*, **71**, 614–620

Verma, A.K. & Boutwell, R.K. (1980) Effects of dose and duration of treatment with the tumor-promoting agent, 12-*O*-tetradecanoylphorbol-13-acetate on mouse skin carcinogenesis. *Carcinogenesis*, **1**, 271–276

Weinstein, I.B., Lee, L.S., Fisher, P.B., Mufson, A. & Yamasaki, H. (1979) Action of phorbol esters in cell culture: Mimicry of transformation altered differentiation and effects on cell membranes. *J. supramol. Struct.*, **2**, 194–208

Weinstein, I.B., Mufson, R.A., Lee, L.S., Fisher, P.B., Laskin, J., Horowitz, A.D. & Ivanovic, V. (1980) *Membrane and other biochemical effects of the phorbol esters and their relevance to tumor promotion*. In: Pullman, D., Ts'o, P.O.P. & Gelboin, H., eds, *Carcinogenesis: Fundamental Mechanisms and Environmental Effects*, Amsterdam, Reidel, pp. 543–563

Weymouth, L.A. & Loeb, L.A. (1978) Mutagenesis during *in vitro* DNA synthesis. *Proc. natl Acad. Sci. USA*, **75**, 1924–1928

Whitfield, J.F., Boynton, A.L., MacManus, J.P., Sikorska, M. & Tsang, B.K. (1979) The regulation of cell proliferation by calcium and cyclic AMP. *Mol. cell. Biochem.*, **27**, 155–179

Williams, G.M., Telang, S. & Tong, C. (1981) Inhibition of intercellular communication between liver cells by the liver tumor promoter 1,1,1-trichloro 2,2-bis(*p*-chlorophenyl)ethane. *Cancer Lett.*, **11**, 339–344

Yamasaki, H., Drevon, C. & Martel, N. (1982) Specific binding of phorbol esters to Friend erythroleukemia cells — general properties, down regulation and relationship to cell differentiation. *Carcinogenesis,* ***3,*** 905–910

Yamasaki, H., Enomoto, T., Martel, N., Shiba, Y. & Kanno, Y. (1983) Tumor promoter-mediated reversible inhibition of cell-cell communication (electrical coupling): relationship with phorbol ester binding and *de novo* marcromolecule synthesis. *Exp. Cell Res.,* ***146,*** 297–308

Yancey, S.B., Edens, J.E., Trosko, J.E., Chang, C.C. & Revel, J.-P. (1982) Decreased incidence of gap junctions between Chinese hamster V79 cells upon exposure to the tumor promoter 12-*O*-tetradecanolyphorbol-13-acetate. *Exp. Cell Res.,* ***139,*** 329–340

Yotti, L.P. (1980) *The Elimination of Metabolic Cooperation in Chinese Hamster Cells by Tumor Promoters,* Ph.D. Thesis, Michigan State University

Yotti, L.P., Chang, C.C. & Trosko, J.E. (1979) Elimination of metabolic cooperation in Chinese hamster cells by a tumor promoter. *Science,* ***206,*** 1089–1091

Yuspa, S.H. & Morgan, D.L. (1981) Mouse skin cells resistant to terminal differentiation associated with initiation of carcinogenesis. *Nature,* ***293,*** 72–74

# INTERACTION OF PHORBOL DERIVATIVES WITH REPLICATING CELLS

V. KINZEL, J. RICHARDS, K. GOERTTLER & H. LOEHRKE

*Institute of Experimental Pathology, German Cancer Research Center Heidelberg, Federal Republic of Germany*

G. FÜRSTENBERGER & F. MARKS

*Institute of Biochemistry, German Cancer Research Center Heidelberg, Federal Republic of Germany*

## SUMMARY

The significance of the interaction of phorbol derivatives with replicating cells has been studied in HeLa cells and in tumour promotion experiments. Dose-response relationships for the radiomimetic activity of phorbol derivatives in HeLa cells (Kinzel *et al.*, 1980) were obtained by analysis of the degree of transient blockage in G2 phase of the cell cycle. HeLa cells are shown to be one order of magnitude more sensitive to 12-*O*-tetradecanoylphorbol-13-acetate (TPA) than to equally mitogenic and irritant but much less promoting derivatives. The susceptibility of HeLa cells reflects the promoting capacity of these compounds. Studies on effects of modifiers on TPA-induced G2 blockage indicate that the influence of TPA, even in a single cell cycle phase, may be the result of a 'multiple site' attack. The significance of the interaction of TPA with replicating mouse epidermal cells in tumour promotion has been demonstrated in animal experiments after initiation with 7-12-dimethylbenz[*a*]anthracene by using a two-stage protocol which effects promotion with a single dose of TPA followed by repeated treatment with 12-*O*-retinoylphorbol-13-acetate (Fürstenberger *et al.*, 1981). A single dose of the inhibitor of DNA synthesis, hydroxyurea, given to groups of mice at different times before and after treatment with TPA interferes with tumour formation; almost complete inhibition is observed after 18 h. The interaction of TPA with DNA-synthesizing cells seems to be of crucial importance to the first stage of tumour promotion.

## INTRODUCTION

The mechanisms at the cellular and the molecular levels by which the tumour promoter 12-*O*-tetradecanoylphorbol-13-acetate (TPA) converts initiated but phenotypically normal cells into visible tumours is not yet understood. The discovery of phorbol derivatives such as 12-*O*-tetradeca-2-*cis*, 4-*trans*-6,8-tetraenoyl-phorbol-13-acetate ($Ti_8$) (Fürstenberger & Hecker, 1977) and 12-*O*-retinoylphorbol-13-acetate (RPA) (Fürstenberger *et al.*, 1981), which are as effectively mitogenic and irritant as TPA but lack almost completely promoting capacity, illustrates the fact that hyperplasia and inflammation are not sufficient conditions to bring about tumour promotion. Despite their differential promoting capacity, TPA, $Ti_8$ and RPA cause almost identical biochemical responses in mouse skin (Fürstenberger *et al.*, 1979, 1981; Marks *et al.*, 1979, 1982).

We have proposed that the particular, additional activity of TPA, as compared to those of other compounds, may lie in a specific interaction with replicating cells; we have shown that, in HeLa cells (which have no target for mitogenic activity), TPA causes transient alterations in the cell cycle similar to those observed after X-irradiation (Kinzel *et al.*, 1980, 1981a,b, 1982a). Data published by a number of groups indicate that mouse epidermal cells that are engaged in the replication cycle at the time of application of TPA react in a fashion similar to that of HeLa cells *in vitro* (Raick, 1973; Astrup & Iversen, 1981). Therefore we investigated the biological significance of the interaction of phorbol derivatives with replicating cells. The problem was approached by cell culture studies, as well as by promotion experiments in animals.

By adopting methods from radiobiology, we were able to establish dose-response relationships for the radiomimetic activity of TPA in the HeLa cell system (Kinzel *et al.*, 1982b). In this study, we have used the culture system to compare the efficiency of the compounds $Ti_8$, RPA and 4-*O*-methyl-12-*O*-tetradecanoyl-phorbol-13-acetate (4-O-Me-TPA) with that of TPA. In addition, the application of response modifiers was expected to provide some information on the mechanisms involved in the radiomimetic activity of TPA.

In order to evaluate the significance of cell culture data in tumour promotion, we carried out animal experiments designed to elucidate the interaction of TPA with DNA-synthesizing epidermal cells. The two-stage protocol for tumour promotion (Fürstenberger *et al.*, 1981) which effects the first stage, also called conversion (Boutwell, 1964), allowed us to approach this problem. The protocol is based on a single application of TPA followed by repeated treatments with RPA. The data indicate that the cell cycle alterations caused by TPA reflect a critical event in the first stage of tumour promotion.

## MATERIALS AND METHODS

The phorbol esters TPA and 4-*O*-Me-TPA were generous gifts from Professor Dr E. Hecker (German Cancer Research Center). $Ti_8$ and RPA were prepared as reported previously (Fürstenberger & Hecker, 1977; Sorg *et al.*, 1982). The phorbol derivatives were dissolved in analytical grade acetone (Merck, Darmstadt) and kept at −70 °C in dark bottles until use. Solutions were protected from direct light during handling.

7,12-Dimethylbenz[*a*]anthracene (DMBA) (Sigma, Munich), soya bean trypsin inhibitor (Serva, Heidelberg) and amethopterin (Lederle, Munich) were obtained from the quoted sources. Several batches of freshly synthesized hydroxyurea (HU) were kindly provided by Dr M. Wiessler (German Cancer Research Center); [methyl-$^3$H]-thymidine (specific activity 40–60 Ci/mmol) was purchased from NEN (Dreieich).

Cloned HeLa cells were cultivated routinely as monolayers in Eagle's minimal essential medium containing Earle's salts supplemented with 10% calf serum (not heat inactivated). Cells were kept in plastic bottles gassed with 95% air and 5% carbon dioxide in a humidified incubator at 37 °C. The cells, which were checked routinely, were free of *Mycoplasma*. Sixteen hours before the addition of compounds for experiments, the cells were transferred to plastic petri dishes in fresh medium. Partial synchronization with amethopterin and release by thymidine was carried out as described earlier (Kinzel *et al.*, 1981b).

Different concentrations of phorbol derivatives in acetone (final concentration, 0.2%) were added directly to the cultures, which were kept carefully in slow motion in order to allow an even distribution of the compounds.

Movement of cells out of G2 phase was analysed by counting mitotic figures. The method and the validity of the analysis for quantifying the influence in G2 have been described in detail elsewhere (Kinzel *et al.*, 1982b, 1984). For determination of cells in S phase by $^3$H-thymidine incorporation and autoradiography, cultures were treated, processed, and analysed as described earlier (Kinzel *et al.*, 1981a).

NMRI mice (female, eight weeks old, from Süddeutsche Versuchstierfarm) were initiated by intragastric application, through a stomach tube, of 50 μg/g body weight DMBA dissolved in sesame oil. One week later, one topical application of 20 nmol TPA in 100 μL of acetone was made to the shaved back of the animals. After one more week, mice were treated twice weekly with 10 nmol RPA dissolved in 100 μL acetone for 20 weeks. Groups of 20 animals received a single application of HU (0.5 mg/g body weight dissolved in physiological sodium chloride solution) intraperitoneally at various times before and after application of TPA, as indicated below. One control group did not receive HU (TPA/RPA control), another control group received neither HU nor TPA (RPA control). Papilloma formation was recorded weekly. RPA treatment was continued for 20 weeks and then stopped. Starting at week 21, the animals received twice weekly 10 nmol TPA, in order to elicit the remaining potential of initiated cells to form papillomas.

## RESULTS AND DISCUSSION

### *Comparison of biological activity of phorbol derivatives in HeLa cells and that in mice*

Among the different cell cycle alterations caused by TPA in HeLa cells (Kinzel *et al.*, 1980, 1981a,b), the pronounced response of cells in G2 phase proved to represent

Table 1. Comparison of the biological activities of phorbol derivatives[a] in HeLa cultures and with that in mouse skin

| Phorbol derivative | HeLa cells not affected in G2 (%) by the following concentrations (M) | | | | Equieffective dose[b] for | | | |
|---|---|---|---|---|---|---|---|---|
| | | | | | HeLa cells in G2 | Mouse skin | | |
| | $10^{-6}$ | $10^{-7}$ | $10^{-8}$ | $10^{-9}$ | ($M \times 10^{-8}$) | Promoting | Mitogenic | Irritant |
| TPA | ND | 15 | 26 | 62 | 1 | 1 | 10 | 0.016 |
| $Ti_8$ | ND | 29 | 38 | 71 | 10 | 10 | 9 | 0.03 |
| RPA | ND | 26 | 46 | 78 | >10 | >10 | 6 | 0.04 |
| 4-*O*-Me-TPA | 51 | 87 | 92 | 97 | >500 | >400 | 400 | 2.3 |

[a] TPA, 12-*O*-tetradecanoylphorbol-13-acetate; $Ti_8$, 12-*O*-tetradeca-2-*cis*,4-*trans*-6,8-tetraenoylphorbol-13-acetate; RPA, 12-*O*-retinoylphorbol-13-acetate; 4-*O*-me-TPA, 4-*O*-methyl-TPA
[b] Equieffective dose for HeLa cells: for calculation, see Kinzel *et al.* (1982b)
equieffective dose: promotion: nmol/animal/application
mitogenicity: for calculation, see Fürstenberger *et al.* (1983); nmol/animal
irritation: $ID_{50}^{24}$ nmol/ear measured by ear reddening
ND, not determined

an accurate quantitative basis for the establishment of dose-response relations (Kinzel *et al.*, 1982b, 1984). The method consists of the analysis of mitotic cells at various times after treatment and the determination of the percentage of unaffected cells. This parameter is virtually free of background effects and has been shown to depend on the dose of X-rays (Dewey & Highfield, 1976), as well as on the dose of TPA (Kinzel *et al.*, 1982b). The values for this parameter in HeLa cells treated with TPA, $Ti_8$, RPA and 4-*O*-Me-TPA are shown in Table 1. A detailed analysis of a number of experiments (Kinzel *et al.*, 1984) shows that TPA is one order of magnitude more active than $Ti_8$ and RPA. In view of the radiomimetic activities of these compounds, the involvement of free radicals must be taken into consideration. In this connection, the ten-fold difference in the activity of TPA *versus* that of $Ti_8$ and RPA may be explained by the conjugated double bonds in the retinoyl and the tetradecatetraenoyl moiety in the latter compounds, which may have a 'quenching' effect on free radicals.

In addition, for comparison of the biological activity of these compounds in HeLa cells with that exerted in mouse skin, equipotent doses have been plotted (Table 1) according to irritant, mitogenic and promoting capacity. The cell culture data correspond to the promoting activity of these compounds. These data substantiate the suitability of HeLa cells as a model for studying trigger mechanisms of TPA-effected promotion, even though this cell represents a transformed cell line.

*Further analysis of the cell cycle responses induced by TPA*

In order to localize the TPA-sensitive transition point in G2, a fine-line analysis for $10^{-8}$ mol/L and $10^{-7}$ mol/L TPA was carried out during the first two hours of treatment. The data indicate that the cells are inhibited approximately 30 min before they enter visible mitosis. This 30-min period was observed whether TPA was present continuously or for a period as short as one min (Fig. 1). Unlike irradiated cells, TPA-treated cells recover from this blockage, even in the continued presence of the active

Fig. 1. Influence of length of treatment with $10^{-8}$ mol/L 12-*O*-tetradecanoylphorbol-13-acetate (TPA) on mitotic activity of HeLa cells
HeLa monolayer cells were treated with TPA either for 1 min (○), 5 min (■), 30 min (◆), 60 min (△), 120 min (□) or continuously (●). After the periods indicated, TPA-containing media were carefully removed and replaced by conditioned media from untreated sister plates. Mitotic activity was related to that of a control group which received acetone.

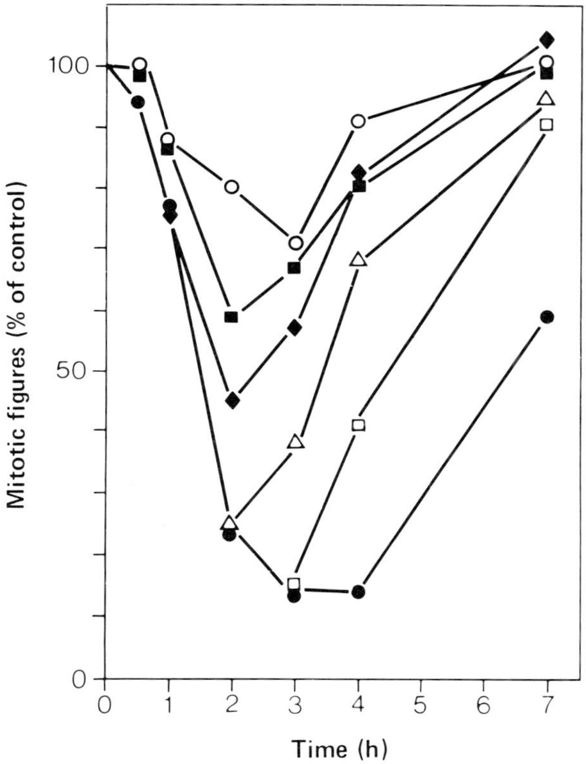


principle. This fact indicates that TPA acts for only a limited period of time, probably by triggering cellular activities. After their termination, cells begin to recover from G2 blockage. It should be noted that TPA-induced G1 blockage and delayed traverse through S phase last much longer (Kinzel *et al.*, 1981a). Pulse treatment of HeLa cells with TPA has been carried out in order to evaluate the influence of the length of treatment on recovery from G2 blockage. With $10^{-7}$ mol/L TPA, no difference in the mitotic curves was seen, whether the cells were treated for 10 sec or continuously (data not shown). This result indicates that the majority of the cells responding to TPA were in the same sensitive part of the cell cycle; the response was not a sequential one caused by continuous movement of cells into the sensitive phase. With $10^{-8}$ mol/L TPA, recovery does depend on the length of treatment. At shorter pulse length (one and five min), the system may not have been fully equilibrated with TPA, thus reflecting results obtained with smaller concentrations of TPA. After one and two hours, however, equilibration of the system with TPA should have taken place.

Fig. 2. Influence of soya bean trypsin inhibitor (STI) on 12-*O*-tetradecanoylphorbol-13-acetate (TPA)-induced alterations of mitotic activity in HeLa cells
HeLa monolayer cells were treated with $10^{-8}$ mol/L TPA for 30 min. The medium was replaced by fresh medium containing 0.25 mg/mL STI (▲), 1 mg/mL STI (■) or no additions (●). Mitotic activity was related to that of a group which received acetone.

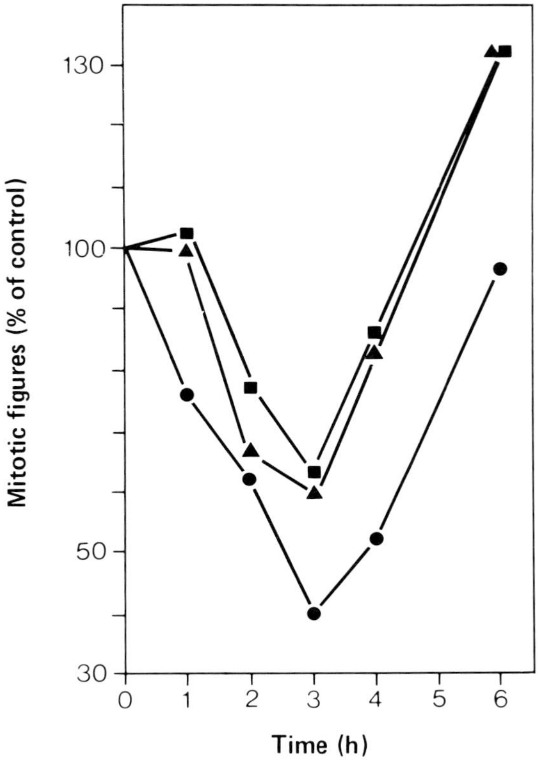


Nevertheless, under these circumstances, the cells recovered earlier. With continuous treatment, a different quality in TPA activity, which delays recovery from G2 blockage, may become effective. The possibility that the G2 delay, as well as the other cell cycle alterations, are triggered *via* more than one pathway is supported by studies with modifiers (see below).

In order to gain insight into the mechanisms by which TPA induces cellular responses, we began to study the influence of tumour promotion modifiers. An analysis of the action of retinoic acid has already been published (Kinzel *et al.*, 1982c). The action of the protease inhibitor, soya bean trypsin inhibitor (STI), is reported in this paper. The effect of STI on TPA-induced G2-delay (Fig. 2) is three-fold: (1) the onset of the TPA action is delayed by approximately 30 min, in such a way that the decrease of mitotic activity becomes visible after 60 min, at the earliest; (2) the recovery starts earlier; (3) the percentage of unaffected cells increases. Since STI sometimes has a stimulatory effect on mitotic activity, we still hesitate to take the

Fig. 3. Influence of soya bean trypsin inhibitor (STI) on 12-*O*-tetradecanoylphorbol-13-acetate (TPA)-induced alterations in labelling index with radioactive thymidine
HeLa monolayer cells were treated at zero time with $10^{-8}$ mol/L TPA (●), at −1 h with 0.5 mg/mL STI (□) or with STI plus TPA (■). $^3$H-Thymidine (1.25 μCi/mL) was added 30 min prior to the indicated times. The labelling indices were analysed from 3 dishes per group (± SD) and related to those of a control group which received acetone.

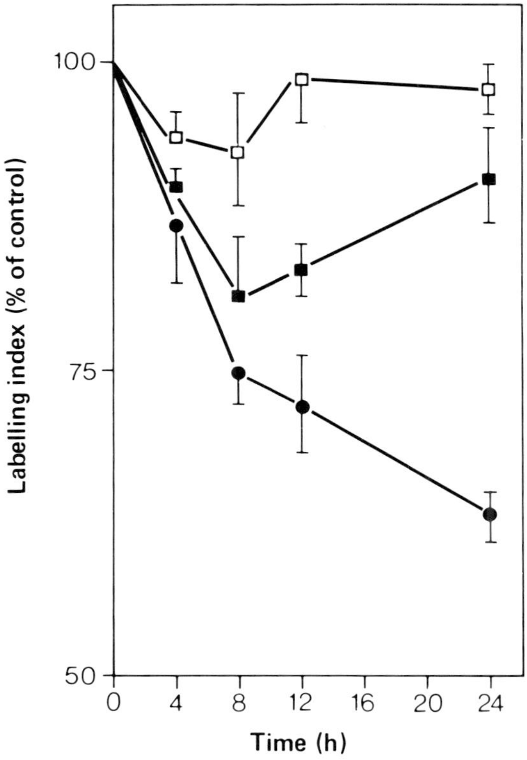


results as an indication of the involvement of proteolytic activity at the cell surface during early events triggered by TPA.

The influence of STI on TPA-induced G1 blockage in asynchronous HeLa cultures, as indicated by the decrease in the labelling index with radioactive thymidine, is shown in Figure 3. Up until eight hours after addition of STI plus TPA, the labelling index in this group followed that of the groups treated with TPA. Beyond eight hours, the labelling index in the TPA-group continued to decrease, whereas the index in the STI plus TPA group started to approach control values, indicating a recovery from G1 blockage. The delayed movement of cells through S phase in the presence of TPA (Kinzel *et al.*, 1980, 1981a,b) was not altered by STI, as indicated by thymidine incorporation rates.

In experiments with partially synchronized cells (Fig. 4), mitotic activity arose earlier in the groups that received acetone or acetone plus STI (Fig. 4A) than in those

Fig. 4. Influence of soya bean trypsin inhibitor (STI) on the effectiveness of 12-*O*-tetradecanoylphorbol-13-acetate (TPA) in partially synchronized HeLa cells
Amethopterin block was released at zero time by addition of thymidine. One hour prior to release, STI (0.5 mg/mL) and at the release, TPA ($10^{-8}$ mol/L) were added; acetone (○), STI (□), TPA (●), STI + TPA (■). A, Mitotic activity per 1500 cells; B, cell counts (mean of 2 dishes)

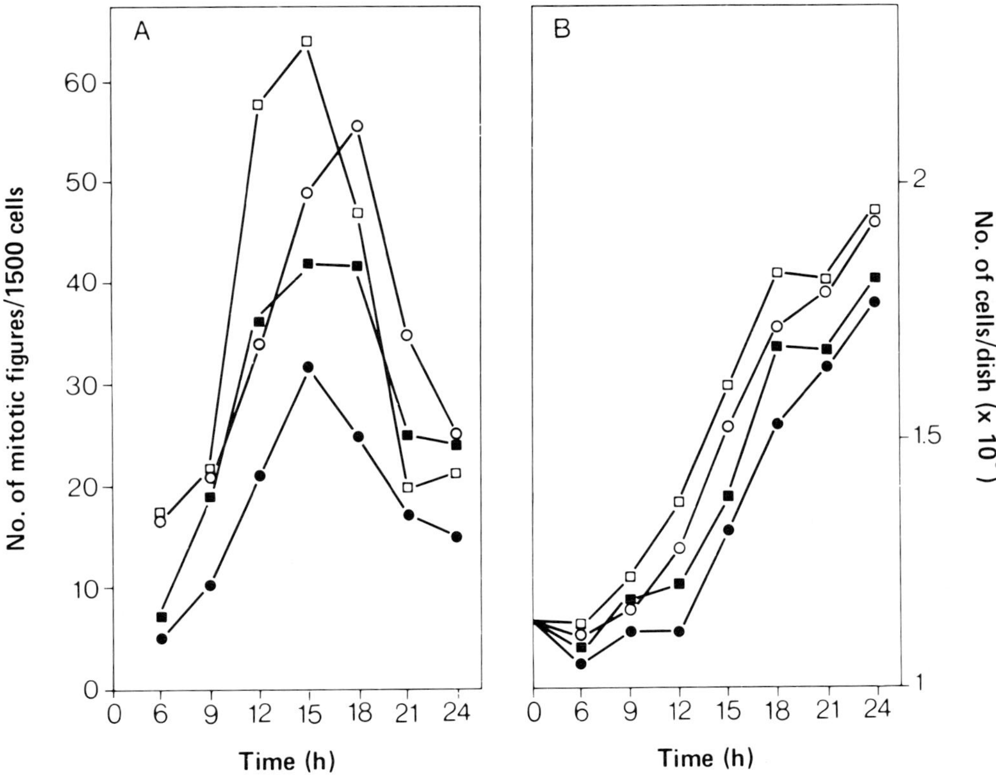


in the TPA group. STI appeared to decrease the efficacy of TPA. The increase in cell number in the various groups (Fig. 4B) supports the results shown in Figure 4A. In view of the above-mentioned data and the stimulatory activity of STI itself, seen also in Figure 4B, this compound does not seem to act by reversing the delayed traverse through S phase, but rather by weakening the effect of TPA in G2 cells.

The fact that STI interferes with certain, but not all, influences of TPA on the cell cycle of HeLa cells indicates that different cell cycle alterations are triggered *via* different mechanisms. So far, it has been impossible to eliminate completely by a single modifier the effect of TPA on the cell cycle. This finding is demonstrated by tests with a number of compounds known to counteract promotion, as well as with known radioprotective agents (Kinzel *et al.*, unpublished data). This fact may support the view that even in a single cell cycle phase, the influence of TPA is the result of a 'multiple site' attack by the promoter on the cellular level.

*Tumour promotion experiments*

What is the significance of the cell cycle alterations in replicating HeLa and in mouse epidermal cells (Raick, 1973; Astrup & Iversen, 1981) after application of TPA for tumour promotion? Animal experiments were used to approach this question. Interaction of TPA with DNA-synthesizing cells was given particular attention, for two reasons: (1) the TPA-induced delay in the passage of cells through S phase (Kinzel *et al.*, 1980, 1981a,b) resembles closely that observed after irradiation, i.e., after application of a tumorigenic principle; Kaufmann and Schwarz (1981) have shown that TPA, like irradiation, inhibits replicon initiation but not replicon elongation; (2) it is known that carcinogens transform cells more effectively during G1/S and early S phase than in the resting phase (Bertram & Heidelberger, 1974; Marquardt, 1974). If the interaction of TPA with replicating cells during S phase is significant, the degree of tumour formation should be altered by a modifier of DNA synthesis. HU was chosen for this purpose, because it inhibits rapidly DNA synthesis in mouse epidermis (Süss & Maurer, 1968) and it is also rapidly metabolized and/or excreted. The two-stage protocol of Fürstenberger *et al.* (1981) was used for promotion; this protocol separates the first stage (induced by a single dose of TPA) from the second stage (caused by repeated applications of RPA), which is characterized by mitogenesis and irritation. HU was given once at various times relative to TPA (for details, see Materials and Methods). The results are shown in Table 2. Clear-cut inhibition of tumour formation was observed when HU was given one hour before TPA. However, the effectiveness of TPA was almost completely abolished when HU was given 18 h later. These values are close to those obtained in the RPA control. In spite of the treatment, the initiated mouse epidermal cells did not lose their potential of conversion by a subsequent treatment with TPA in the absence of HU. In these groups, the kinetics of tumour formation were similar to those of the TPA/RPA control; this result indicated that HU did not inhibit tumorigenesis by damaging initiated cells.

The degree of inhibition of tumorigenesis by HU given at various times relative to TPA correlates with the percentage of epidermal cells in S phase after a single treatment of mouse skin with TPA. In both cases, the maximum is observed at more than 18 h. The promoter, TPA, seems to generate its own target population of cells that are most sensitive to critical attack, resulting in the conversion of initiated cells.

Table 2. Inhibition of tumour formation during the first stage of promotion by hydroxyurea (HU)

| Tumour formation (20th week) | TPA/RPA control | RPA control | Time of application of HU relative to TPA (h) | | | |
|---|---|---|---|---|---|---|
| | | | −1 | +12 | +18 | +48 |
| Tumour incidence (tumour bearers/survivors, %) | 95 | 22 | 79 | 60 | 33 | 94 |
| Tumour yield (papillomas/survivors) | 7.2 | 1.1 | 4.5 | 1.8 | 1.6 | 4.3 |

TPA, 12-*O*-tetradecanoylphorbol-13-acetate; RPA, 12-*O*-retinoylphorbol-13-acetate

The above data seem to indicate that the memory for TPA in initiated cells of NMRI mice (Fürstenberger *et al.*, 1983) probably becomes established during DNA synthesis. A mechanism for tumour promotion, according to the two-stage concept, is proposed through its action on DNA synthesis. The first administration of TPA changes initiated but phenotypically normal cells into the tumour phenotype; this event requires the mitogenic and irritant activity of RPA to become visible.

## CONCLUSIONS

In replicating cells, a single dose of TPA causes cell cycle alterations similar to those observed after irradiation. These alterations seem to be triggered by TPA *via* more than one metabolic route, as indicated by studies with modifiers. A single dose of TPA is sufficient to effect the first stage of tumour promotion (conversion) by establishing a 'memory' in initiated cells. A single dose of the inhibitor of DNA synthesis, HU, inhibits TPA-induced conversion. This inhibition by HU does not prevent a subsequent conversion by TPA in the absence of HU, thus indicating that HU does not act by damaging initiated cells. The degree of inhibition of tumour formation by HU is correlated with the percentage of epidermal cells in S phase during and after application of TPA, thereby indicating that TPA, by its mitogenic activity, generates a particularly large target fraction of cells in S phase. Disturbance of the interaction of TPA with cells in S phase by HU cannot be overcome by the mitogenesis and irritation elicited subsequently by RPA. Cell-cycle alterations – particularly those in S phase – induced by TPA may thus reflect important events during the conversion phase of tumour promotion.

## ACKNOWLEDGEMENTS

This work was supported by the Deutsche Forschungsgemeinschaft. The technical assistance of G. Bender and B. Hesse is appreciated.

## REFERENCES

Astrup, E.G. & Iversen, O.H. (1981) Cell population kinetics in hairless mouse epidermis following a single topical application of 12-*O*-tetradecanoyl-phorbol-13-acetate I. *Carcinogenesis*, ***2***, 999–1006

Bertram, J.S. & Heidelberger, C. (1974) Cell cycle dependency of oncogenic transformation induced by *N*-methyl-*N'*-nitro-*N*-nitrosoguanidine in culture. *Cancer Res.*, ***34***, 526–537

Boutwell, R.K. (1964) Some biological aspects of skin carcinogenesis. *Prog. exp. Tumor Res.*, ***4***, 207–250

Dewey, W.C. & Highfield, D.P. (1976) $G_2$ block in Chinese hamster cells induced by X-irradiation, hyperthermia, cycloheximide, or actinomycin-D. *Radiat. Res.*, ***65***, 511–528

Fürstenberger, G. & Hecker, E. (1977) New highly irritant euphorbia factors of *Euphorbia tirucalli* L. *Experientia*, ***33***, 986–988

Fürstenberger, G., deBravo, M., Bertsch, S. & Marks, F. (1979) The effect of indomethacin on cell proliferation induced by chemical and mechanical means in mouse epidermis. *Res. Commun. Chem. Pathol. Pharmacol.*, ***24***, 533–541

Fürstenberger, G., Berry, D.L., Sorg, B. & Marks, F. (1981) Skin tumor promotion by phorbol esters is a two-stage process. *Proc. natl Acad. Sci. USA*, ***78***, 7722–7726

Fürstenberger, G., Sorg, B. & Marks, F. (1983) Tumor promotion by phorbol esters in skin: evidence for a memory effect. *Science*, ***220***, 89–91

Kaufmann, W.K. & Schwartz, J.L. (1981) Inhibition of replicon initiation by 12-*O*-tetradecanoylphorbol-13-acetate. *Biochem. biophys. Res. Commun.*, ***103***, 82–89

Kinzel, V., Richards, J. & Stöhr, M. (1980) Tumor promoter TPA mimics irradiation effects on the cell cycle of HeLa cells *Science*, ***210***, 429–431

Kinzel, V., Richards, J. & Stöhr, M. (1981a) Early effects of the tumor-promoting phorbol ester 12-*O*-tetradecanoylphorbol-13-acetate on the cell cycle traverse of asynchronous HeLa cells. *Cancer Res.*, ***41***, 300–305

Kinzel, V., Richards, J. & Stöhr, M. (1981b) Responses of synchronized HeLa cells to the tumor-promoting phorbol ester 12-*O*-tetradecanoylphorbol-13-acetate as evaluated by flow cytometry. *Cancer Res.*, ***41***, 306–309

Kinzel, V., Stöhr, M. & Richards, J. (1982a) *Early changes in the cell cycle traverse of HeLa cells induced by tumor promoter TPA resemble irradiation effects.* In: Hecker, E., Fusenig, N.E., Kunz, W., Marks, F. & Thielmann, H.W., eds, *Carcinogenesis, Vol. 7, Cocarcinogenesis and Biological Effects of Tumor Promoters,* New York, Raven Press, pp. 435–438

Kinzel, V., Düzgün, F. & Richards, J. (1982b) Measurement of the response of HeLa cells towards the radiomimetic activity of 12-*O*-tetradecanoylphorbol-13-acetate. *Cancer Lett.*, ***17***, 45–50

Kinzel, V., Krombholz-Nolinski, I., Stöhr, M. & Richards, J. (1982c) Effects of retinoic acid and tumor promoter 12-*O*-tetradecanoylphorbol-13-acetate (TPA) on the cell cycle of HeLa cells. *Int. J. Cancer*, ***29***, 93–99

Kinzel, V., Richards, J., Marks, F. & Fürstenberger, G. (1984) Radiomimetic activity of phorbol esters exerted in HeLa cells in comparison with the tumor promoting capacity of these compounds. *Cancer Res.*, ***44***, 139–143

Marks, F., Bertsch, S. & Fürstenberger, G. (1979) Ornithine decarboxylase activity, cell proliferation, and tumor promotion in mouse epidermis *in vivo*. *Cancer Res.*, ***39***, 4183–4188

Marks, F., Berry, D.L., Bertsch, S., Fürstenberger, G. & Richter, H. (1982) *On the relation between epidermal hyperproliferation and skin tumor promotion.* In: Hecker, E., Fusenig, N.E., Kunz, W., Marks, F. & Thielmann, H.W., eds, *Carcinogenesis,* Vol. 7, *Cocarcinogenesis and Biological Effects of Tumor Promoters,* New York, Raven Press, pp. 331–346

Marquardt, H. (1974) Cell cycle dependence of chemically induced malignant transformation *in vitro*. *Cancer Res.,* ***34,*** 1612–1615

Raick, A.N. (1973) Ultrastructural, histological, and biochemical alterations produced by 12-*O*-tetradecanoylphorbol-13-acetate on mouse epidermis and their relevance to skin tumor promotion. *Cancer Res.,* ***33,*** 269–286

Sorg, B., Fürstenberger, G., Berry, D.L., Hecker, E. & Marks, F. (1982) Preparation of retinoic acid esters of phorbol derivatives. *J. Lipid Res.,* ***23,*** 443–447

Süss, R. & Maurer, H.R. (1968) Reduced binding of carcinogenic hydrocarbons to DNA of mouse skin during inhibition of DNA synthesis. *Nature,* ***217,*** 752–753

# EFFECT OF 12-*O*-TETRADECANOYLPHORBOL-13-ACETATE ON SELECTION OF DRUG-RESISTANT PHENOTYPES IN RODENT CELLS

F. BOJAN[1], A.R. KINSELLA & M. FOX

*Paterson Laboratories,*
*Christie Hospital and Holt Radium Institute,*
*Manchester M20 9BX, UK*

## SUMMARY

The effect of the tumour promoter 12-*O*-tetradecanoylphorbol-13-acetate (TPA) on the selection of drug-resistant phenotypes in hamster and mouse cells has been studied. TPA increased considerably the incidence of methotrexate (MTX)-, *N*-(phosphonacetyl)-L-aspartate- and cadmium-resistant 3T6 and 3T3 mouse cell clones, but it had little effect on V79 and CHO hamster cells. The MTX-resistant V79 hamster cell clones, selected with or without TPA, lost their resistance within 15 cell cycles, however, 50% of the 3T6 mouse cell clones selected and maintained in the presence of TPA preserved their resistance for more than 15 cell cycles. A number of the MTX-resistant 3T6 clones overproduced dihydrofolate reductase enzyme; however, their frequency was lower among the clones selected in the presence of TPA.

## INTRODUCTION

In-vitro resistance of rodent cells to the specific dihydrofolate reductase (DHFR) inhibitor, methotrexate (MTX), has been shown to be due to an increase in the number of DHFR gene copies per cell, resulting in an overproduction of the DHFR enzyme (Schimke *et al.*, 1977; Alt *et al.*, 1978; Milbrandt *et al.*, 1981). Recently, it has been found that the tumour promoter 12-*O*-tetradecanoylphorbol-13-acetate (TPA) can increase the incidence of MTX-resistant mouse cells (Varshavsky, 1981a). Varshavsky (1981a,b) has proposed that TPA acts as a 'locus-unspecific firone' which

[1] Permanent address: Department of Hygiene, University Medical School, H-4012 Debrecen, Hungary

can increase—through extra rounds of DNA replication—the frequency of amplification of not only the DHFR gene but also that of any gene, including the transforming gene(s). Thus, an increase in the dosage of the transforming gene(s) may lead to phenotypic changes—among them, malignant transformation. In order to test this hypothesis of tumour promotion, three questions have been investigated in the present study.

(1) If TPA can increase randomly the frequency of gene amplification, it should increase the incidence of not only MTX- but also *N*-(phosphonacetyl)-L-aspartate (PALA)- and cadmium-resistant cells, because, *in vitro,* PALA- and cadmium-resistance have also been found to be due to gene amplification (Wahl *et al.,* 1979; Beach & Palmiter, 1981). Moreover, in recovery of drug-resistant cells, a species-specific difference could be expected in the presence of TPA in view of its species-specific promoting effect (Shubik *et al.,* 1960; Goerttler *et al.,* 1980).

(2) Malignant transformation is known to be an irreversible process. Therefore, gene amplification, provided it is involved in transformation, should be a stable phenomenon. Thus, TPA should increase the stability of MTX resistance, at least in a proportion of colonies.

(3) If the stable MTX resistance is due to DHFR gene amplification, the MTX-resistant cells should overproduce the DHFR enzyme.

## MATERIALS AND METHODS

### *Cells*

V79 and CHO Chinese hamster and 3T6 and 3T3 mouse cells were cultured in Dulbecco's modification of Eagle's minimal essential medium (DMEM, Flow Laboratories Ltd, Irvine, UK) supplemented with penicillin (100 U/mL), streptomycin (50 μg/mL) and 10% fetal bovine serum for hamster cells or 10% calf serum for mouse cells. The cells were grown in a humidified incubator at 37 °C with 5% carbon dioxide in air, gas phase.

### *Chemicals*

TPA (Sigma Chemical Co., St Louis, MO, USA) was dissolved in dimethylsulfoxide (DMSO). Stock MTX (Lederle, Gosport, UK), PALA (NSC 224131), thymidine and hypoxanthine (Sigma) solutions were made up in phosphate-buffered saline (PBS), pH 7.2. Cadmium sulfate (Hopkin & Williams Ltd, Chadwell Heath, UK) was dissolved in distilled water. Fluorescein isothiocyanate-conjugated MTX (F-MTX) was kindly provided by A. McGown (Paterson Laboratories, Manchester, UK). [3′,5′,7-$^3$H]MTX with specific activity of 8.8 GBq/mmol was purchased from Amersham International (Amersham, UK).

### *Colony formation assay*

All experiments were commenced before the cells reached confluency. The dishes (9-cm diameter) were seeded with $5 \times 10^5$ cells in DMEM supplemented with 1%

serum, and the cells were allowed to attach for four hours. After attachment, this medium was replaced by a medium containing 10% serum and different concentrations of MTX, PALA or cadmium. The plates were incubated for 10–20 days. The colonies were stained with 0.5% crystal violet after fixation with 10% formaldehyde. Two sets of experiments were performed, with five plates per point. In Figures 1–3, the incidence of drug-resistant cells is defined as the ratio of the number of colonies to the number of cells initially seeded.

*Isolation of colonies*

V79 and 3T6 cell colonies, selected after exposure to 200 nmol/L and 150 nmol/L MTX, respectively, were isolated using silicone-greased plastic isolation rings. After isolation, the putative MTX-resistant hamster and mouse cell colonies were allowed to grow in MTX-free medium for one and two weeks, respectively, before retesting for phenotypic stability, as follows: The clones were subcultured at 1–5 × $10^4$ cells per 6-cm dish and exposed to a second challenge with the same doses of MTX; hamster cells were observed for two weeks and mouse cells for three weeks subsequently. Surviving and evenly growing clones were considered to have stable resistance to MTX.

*Determination of DHFR level*

In order to quantitate the DHFR level in MTX-resistant 3T6 mouse cell clones, the DHFR was saturated with F-MTX and the degree of fluorescence emission from individual cells was analysed according to the method of Kaufman *et al.* (1978). Cells were grown in MTX-free medium for at least six days. Then the exponentially growing cells were fed with 2 mL DMEM containing 3 × $10^{-5}$ mol/L F-MTX, thymidine and hypoxanthine and incubated for 22 hours. The cells were then rinsed and incubated in 5 mL DMEM for two hours to allow for the efflux of unbound F-MTX. The cells were gently trypsinized, resuspended in DMEM and centrifuged at 800 r.p.m. for 5 min. The pellet was suspended in cold PBS, the cell number was adjusted to 1 × $10^6$ cells/mL, and the samples were kept at 4 °C until they were analysed for fluorescence. A fluorescence-activated cell sorter (Becton-Dickinson FACS IV; laser power, 220 mW; photo multiplier tube, 700 V) in analyser mode was used to analyse the cells for scattergated fluorescence. In each determination, at least 30 000 cells were run at a flow rate of approximately 500 cells/sec. The DHFR level was expressed as both the channel number of peak of fluorescence histogram and the mean fluorescence channel number (MFCh), determined from computerized integration of the fluorescence histograms.

*Determination of MTX uptake*

MTX uptake was measured using $^3$H-MTX, according to the method of Herman *et al.* (1981). Exponentially growing 3T6 mouse cells (1–2 × $10^6$ cells per 25-cm$^2$ flask) were exposed to 1 × $10^{-6}$ mol/L $^3$H-MTX for varying times. After treatment, cells were washed twice with PBS and lysed in 2 mL of 1% Triton X-100 and 1 mL of 1N potassium hydroxide; then, 1 mL of lysate was solubilized in 10 mL toluene

Fig. 1. Effect of 12-*O*-tetradecanoylphorbol-13-acetate (TPA) on incidence of methotrexate-resistant colony formation in mouse and hamster cells
○, without TPA; ●, with 0.1 μg/mL TPA

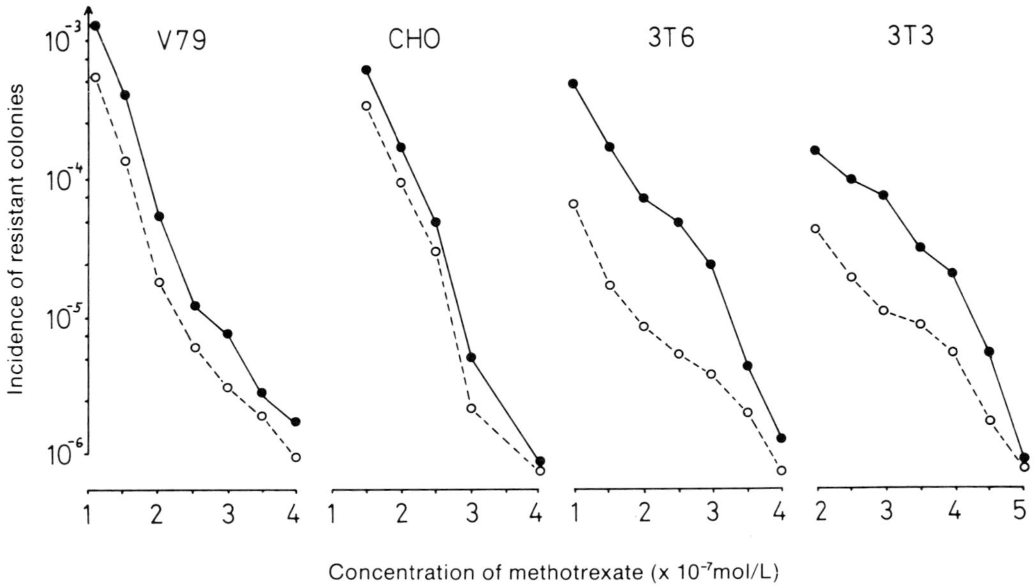


Fig. 2. Effect of 12-*O*-tetradecanoylphorbol-13-acetate (TPA) on incidence of *N*-(phosphonacetyl)-L-aspartate-resistant colony formation in mouse and hamster cells
○, without TPA; ●, with 0.1 μg/mL TPA

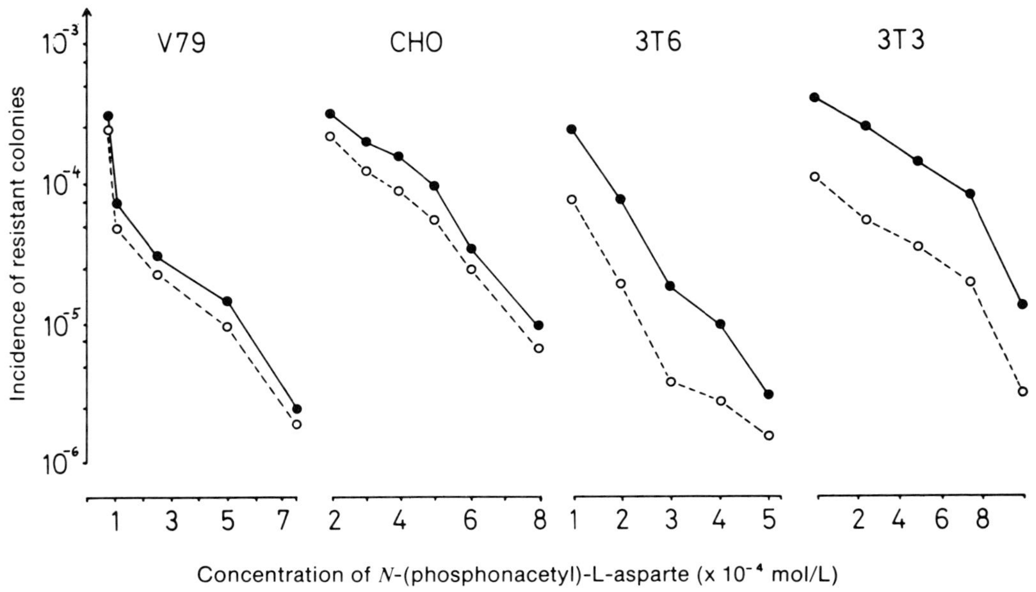

Fig. 3. Effect of 12-*O*-tetradecanoylphorbol-13-acetate (TPA) on incidence of cadmium-resistant colony formation in mouse and hamster cells
○, without TPA; ●, with 0.1 μg/mL TPA

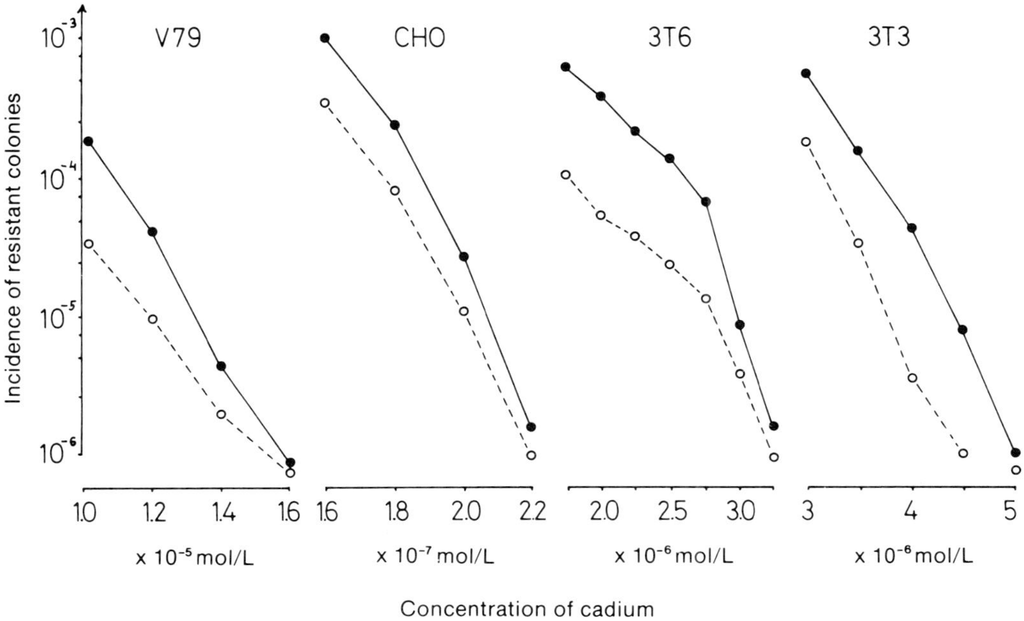


Fig. 4. Level of dihydrofolate reductase in 3T6 mouse cell clones resistant to 150 nmol/L methotrexate and selected without (○) or in the presence of 0.1 μg/mL 12-*O*-tetradecanoylphorbol-13-acetate (●)
+, control 3T6 cell populations; means ± SD; MFCh, mean fluorescence channel number

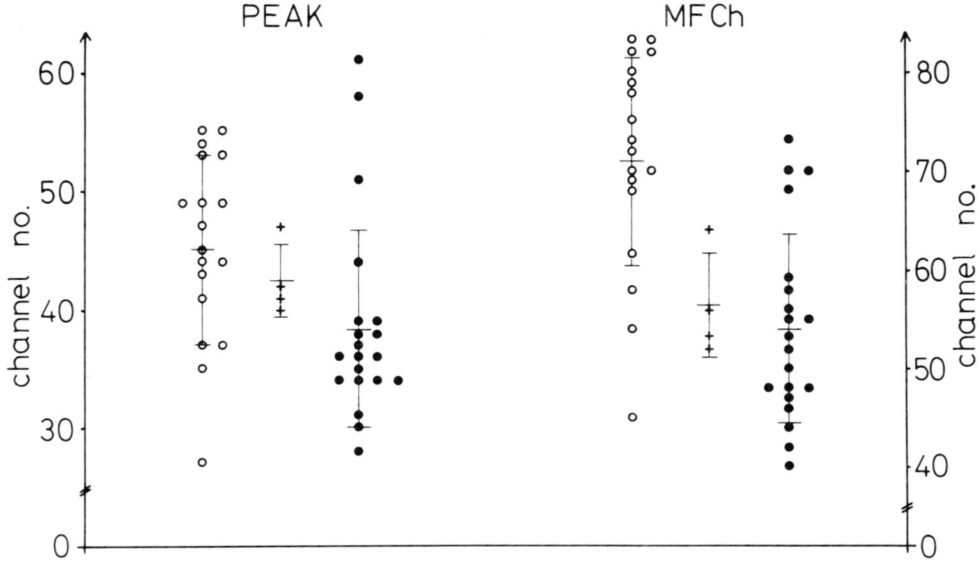

phosphor. Samples were counted in a Packard-Tricarb liquid scintillation counter (18% efficiency for tritium).

## RESULTS AND DISCUSSION

In the first series of experiments, the effect of TPA on the incidence of MTX-, PALA- and cadmium-resistant colony formation was studied in V79 and CHO hamster and 3T6 and 3T3 mouse cells. We found that TPA increased the incidence of MTX-resistant hamster cells by not more than three-fold (Fig. 1). However, the overall recovery of MTX-resistant mouse cells was three- to ten-fold higher in the presence of TPA (Fig. 1). Varshavsky (1981a) observed that TPA could increase the incidence of MTX-resistant 3T6 cells by up to 100-fold. In our experiment the effect of TPA was not so dramatic.

TPA did not increase the frequency of PALA-resistant hamster cells to any significant extent, but it enhanced the incidence of PALA-resistant mouse cells by three- to four-fold (Fig. 2). The overall effect of TPA on the incidence of cadmium-resistant cells was also species-dependent (Fig. 3): TPA increased the number of cadmium-resistant cells to a greater extent in mouse than in hamster cells, although it also had a notable effect on V79 cells at the lowest concentration of cadmium.

The observation that TPA treatment had a considerably greater overall effect on the recovery of drug-resistant mouse cells than hamster cells is in good agreement with in-vivo reports: TPA is a potent tumour promoter in mouse skin, but it is ineffective as a promoter in hamster skin (Shubik *et al.*, 1960; Goerttler *et al.*, 1980). Consistent with this finding, Shoyab *et al.* (1982) failed to detect any notable activity of phorbol-12,13-diester 12-ester hydrolase in mouse skin. This enzyme, however, shows high activity in hamster skin, and it is thought to convert the biologically active phorbol-12,13-diesters, among them TPA, to the inactive phorbol-13-monoester. According to the in-vivo results, one can suppose that *in vitro* hamster cells retain their ability to inactivate TPA whereas mouse cells are not able to produce this enzyme to detoxify the TPA.

These initial observations of the influence of TPA on the recovery of MTX-, PALA- and cadmium-resistant mouse cells could therefore be consistent with a role for TPA in gene amplification.

In the second series of experiments, the stability of the MTX resistance of isolated V79 and 3T6 clones was studied. The results, summarized in Table 1, show that the MTX-resistance of hamster cells was not stable, irrespective of the presence of TPA during the selection. All 115 V79 clones lost their resistance within approximately 15 cell cycles. However, 27.6% of mouse clones selected without TPA and 50.4% of the clones selected in the presence of TPA survived the second MTX exposure and grew evenly after a period of approximately 15 cell cycles in MTX-free medium. These results show that TPA can facilitate not only the development but also the stabilization of the new drug-resistant phenotype.

If the stable MTX resistance of the 3T6 mouse cell clones is due to gene amplification, then the quantity of DHFR gene product should be elevated in those cells. The DHFR level was quantitated by FACS analysis in 38 3T6 clones with stable resistance

Fig. 5. Effect of 12-*O*-tetradecanoylphorbol-13-acetate (TPA) on methotrexate (MTX) uptake by 3T6 mouse cells

●, untreated control; ○, dimethyl sulfoxide-treated control; □, 0.1 μg/mL TPA during MTX uptake; ■, 1.0 μg/mL TPA during MTX uptake; +, 0.1 μg/mL TPA pretreatment for 48 h and during MTX uptake

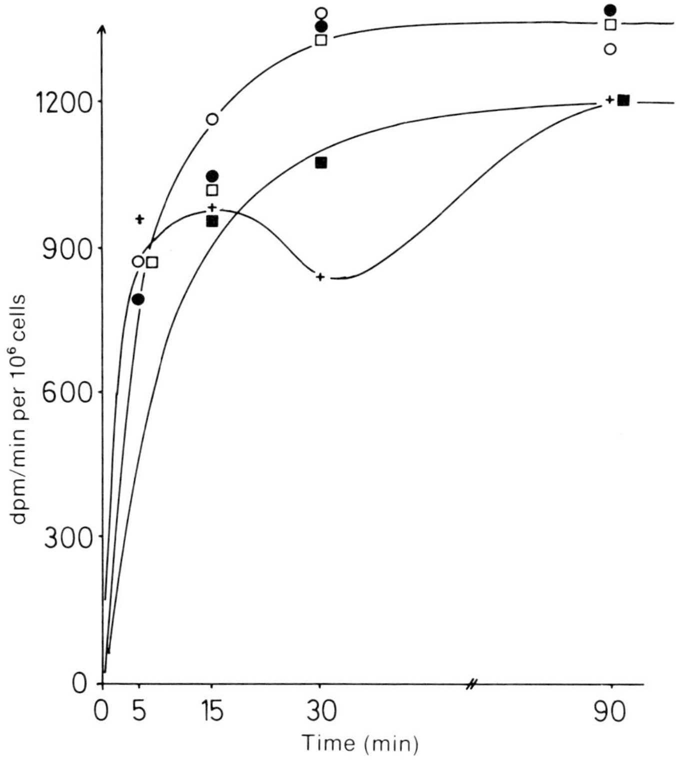


Table 1. Stability of methotrexate (MTX)-resistance of V79 hamster and 3T6 mouse cell clones[a]

| Cell line | Conditions of selection | No. of isolated clones | No. of clones surviving second MTX exposure |
|---|---|---|---|
| V79 | MTX | 57 | 0 |
| | MTX + TPA | 58 | 0 |
| 3T6 | MTX | 83 | 23 |
| | MTX + TPA | 107 | 54 |

[a]Isolated V79 colonies resistant to 200 nmol/L MTX and 3T6 colonies resistant to 150 nmol/L MTX were allowed to grow in MTX-free medium for 7 and 14 days, respectively. The clones were then exposed again to the same MTX concentrations as used for the selection. 0.1 μg/mL 12-*O*-tetradecanoylphorbol-13-acetate (TPA) was used.

to 150 nmol/L MTX (Fig. 4), 18 of which were selected without TPA and 20 in its presence. In comparison with the control 3T6 cell populations, a number of MTX-resistant clones were found with elevated DHFR level, expressed as either the peak channel number of fluorescence histograms or the mean fluorescence channel numbers. However, among the clones selected in the presence of TPA, the frequency of clones with an increased DHFR level was lower than it was among the clones selected without TPA; and TPA seemed to have increased the incidence of clones emitting a lower intensity of fluorescence. These results suggest that the overproduction of the DHFR enzyme is not the only means of developing MTX resistance in 3T6 mouse cells, in contrast to the observation of Varshavsky (1981a). These findings do not appear to be consistent with a role for TPA in gene amplification.

Finally, we investigated the uptake of tritiated MTX by normal 3T6 cells, in order to explain the development of MTX resistance in clones without elevated DHFR levels. Application of 1.0 μg/mL TPA together with MTX, or 0.1 μg/mL TPA for 48 hours before and during MTX-exposure, decreased MTX uptake (Fig. 5). This decrease in MTX uptake in the presence of TPA could result in an intracellular level of MTX lower than that in the absence of TPA. Due to this lower intracellular level, it may be supposed that more cells can survive the first and second exposure to the same extracellular concentration of MTX. The in-vitro uptake of MTX at concentrations as low as $1 \times 10^{-6}$ mol/L seems to be a carrier-mediated and energy-dependent process (Warren *et al.,* 1978). We think that TPA might damage this active transport of MTX.

In conclusion, we have tested the gene amplification hypothesis of tumour promotion. The potent tumour promoter TPA increased considerably the incidence of MTX-, PALA- and cadmium-resistant mouse cells and the stability of the MTX resistance of mouse cells, but analysis of MTX-resistant mouse cells suggests that this is not due to amplification of the target gene product, as demonstrated by the low recovery of MTX-resistant clones with an elevated DHFR level.

## ACKNOWLEDGEMENTS

The authors wish to thank Dr Alan McGown for the F-MTX and Mrs Sally Haran and Mr Mike Hughes for their excellent technical assistance. This work was supported by grants from the Cancer Research Campaign and the Wellcome Trust, UK.

## REFERENCES

Alt, F.W., Kellems, R.E., Bertino, J.R. & Schimke, R.T. (1978) Selective multiplication of dihydrofolate reductase genes in methotrexate-resistant variants of cultured murine cells. *J. biol. Chem.*, ***253***, 1357–1370

Beach, L.R. & Palmiter, R.D. (1981) Amplification of the metallothionein-I gene in cadmium-resistant mouse cells. *Proc. natl Acad. Sci. USA*, ***78***, 2110–2114

Goerttler, K., Loehrke, H., Schweizer, J. & Hesse, B. (1980) Two-stage tumorigenesis of dermal melanocytes in the back skin of the Syrian golden hamster using systemic initiation with 7,12-dimethylbenz(*a*)anthracene and topical promotion with 12-*O*-tetradecanoylphorbol-13-acetate. *Cancer Res.*, ***40***, 155–161

Herman, T.S., Cress, A.E., Sweets, C. & Gerner, E.W. (1981) Reversal of resistance to methotrexate by hyperthermia in Chinese hamster ovary cells. *Cancer Res.*, ***41***, 3840–3843

Kaufman, R.J., Bertino, J.R. & Schimke, R.T. (1978) Quantitation of dihydrofolate reductase in individual parental and methotrexate-resistant murine cells. *J. biol. Chem.*, ***253***, 5852–5860

Milbrandt, J.D., Heintz, N.H., White, W.C., Rothman, S.M. & Hamlin, J.L. (1981) Methotrexate-resistant Chinese hamster ovary cells have amplified a 135-kilobase-pair region that includes the dihydrofolate reductase gene. *Proc. natl Acad. Sci. USA*, ***78***, 6043–6047

Schimke, R.T., Alt, F.W., Kellems, R.E., Kaufman, R.J. & Bertino, J.R. (1977) Amplification of dihydrofolate reductase genes in methotrexate-resistant cultured mouse cells. *Cold Spring Harbor Symp. quant. Biol.*, ***42***, 649–657

Shoyab, M., Warren, T.C. & Todaro, G.J. (1982) Phorbol-12,13-diester 12-ester hydrolase may prevent tumour promotion by phorbol diesters in skin. *Nature*, ***295***, 152–154

Shubik, P., Pietra, G. & Della Porta, G. (1960) Studies of skin carcinogenesis in the Syrian golden hamster. *Cancer Res.*, ***20***, 100–105

Varshavsky, A. (1981a) Phorbol ester dramatically increases incidence of methotrexate-resistant mouse cells: Possible mechanisms and relevance to tumour promotion. *Cell*, ***25***, 561–572

Varshavsky, A. (1981b) On the possibility of metabolic control of replicon 'misfiring': Relationship to emergence of malignant phenotypes in mammalian cell lineages. *Proc. natl Acad. Sci. USA*, ***78***, 3673–3677

Wahl, G.M., Padgett, R.A. & Stark, G.R. (1979) Gene amplification causes overproduction of the first three enzymes of UMP synthesis in *N*-(phosphonacetyl)-L-aspartate-resistant hamster cells. *J. biol. Chem.*, ***254***, 8679–8689

Warren, R.D., Nichols, A.P. & Bender, R.A. (1978) Membrane transport of methotrexate in human lymphoblastoid cells. *Cancer Res.*, ***38***, 668–671

# INTERACTION OF TUMOUR PROMOTERS WITH HOST GENES, VIRUSES AND THE IMMUNE SYSTEM

# INITIAL CELLULAR TARGETS AND EVENTUAL GENOMIC CHANGES IN MULTISTAGE CARCINOGENESIS

I. B. WEINSTEIN, S. GATTONI-CELLI, P. KIRSCHMEIER, M. LAMBERT, W. HSIAO, J. BACKER & A. JEFFREY

*Division of Environmental Sciences and Cancer Center, Institute of Cancer Research, Columbia University, New York, NY 10032, USA*

## INTRODUCTION

Studies in experimental animals and in humans indicate that most tumours evolve through a multistage process that can occupy a considerable fraction of the lifespan of the species. In some instances, the process can be divided into at least three stages, initiation, promotion and progression, although even these stages are often divisible into substages (Foulds, 1969, 1975; Slaga *et al.*, 1980; Hecker *et al.*, 1982). These basic phenomena are also frequently apparent during transformation of cells in culture, whether the process is induced by chemical carcinogens or by certain oncogenic viruses (Barrett & Ts'o, 1978; Fisher *et al.*, 1979; Morris, 1981; Weinstein, 1981; Weinstein *et al.*, 1982). Multistage carcinogenesis and tumour progression are often thought of in terms of a series of successive mutations and selections, eventually resulting in the clonal outgrowth of a fully malignant tumour. This may, however, be an over-simplification. As discussed in detail elsewhere (Weinstein, 1981, 1983), we think that a more suitable model is the multistage process that occurs during normal embryologic development, in which new stem-cell populations emerge and develop into specialized cells and tissues. There is considerable evidence that the successive stages in carcinogenesis may involve qualitatively different events, that they can be enhanced or inhibited by quite different types of environmental and host factors, and that at least the early stages are often reversible (Weinstein, 1981; Hecker *et al.*, 1982; Weinstein *et al.*, 1982).

## EARLY EVENTS IN THE ACTION OF INITIATING CARCINOGENS

It is now known that several types of chemicals that initiate the carcinogenic process yield highly reactive species or metabolites that bind covalently to cellular

DNA (Miller, 1978; Weinstein, 1981). Although there is considerable evidence that damage to DNA can play a critical role in carcinogenesis, the subsequent biochemical events that lead to the conversion of a normal cell to a cancer cell are not known with certainty. There has been a tendency to think that chemical carcinogenesis involves simple, random point mutation resulting from errors in replicating carcinogen-damaged DNA. Several features of the carcinogenic process, particularly the high efficiency of carcinogen-induced cell transformation, the latent period and the multistep aspects suggests that, although random point mutations may play a role, other types of genomic changes are also important. Other mechanisms by which carcinogen-induced DNA damage could induce genomic changes include induction of gene rearrangements or gene amplification. Consistent with these possibilities is the increasing evidence that gene amplification and gene rearrangements occur in several normal systems undergoing development and differentiation. Complex biochemical mechanisms must regulate the latter genomic changes. It is possible, therefore, that carcinogen-DNA interactions might disrupt these mechanisms and thus produce stable aberrations in the control of gene expression (Weinstein, 1981; Weinstein *et al.*, 1982). Consistent with this possibility is increasing evidence that fully established tumours may carry several types of amplified genes, including amplified oncogenes (Cooper, 1982; Duesberg, 1983; Weinstein, 1983).

We have recently used a model system that demonstrates rather dramatically the ability of certain carcinogens to induce a much more complex change in DNA replication than random point mutation (Lambert *et al.*, 1983). The system is one in which DNA damage induces asynchronous replication of an integrated viral genome. In these studies, we employed a cell line, ts-A H3, the DNA of which contains 1.3 viral equivalents of polyoma DNA derived from a virus that carries a temperature-sensitive large T-antigen. We exposed these cells to 0.25 μg/mL benzo[*a*]pyrene (BP) for 24, 48 or 72 h at either 33 °C or 39 °C. The extrachromosomal DNA was then extracted by the method of Hirt, subjected to electrophoresis in 1% agarose, transferred onto nitrocellulose paper, and then hybridized with a $^{32}$P-labelled probe of polyoma DNA prepared by nick-translation. Figure 1 (lanes 1, 3, 5) indicates that, as expected, simply shifting the temperature from 39 °C to 33 °C (in the absence of BP treatment) resulted in increasing production of free polyoma DNA during the subsequent 72 h. The addition of BP at the time of the temperature shift (Fig. 1, lanes 2, 4, 6) led to a marked enhancement in production of free polyoma DNA; however, when cells were simply maintained at 39 °C, either in the absence or presence of BP, and the DNA present in the Hirt extract analysed at 24, 48 or 72 h, no free polyoma DNA was detected (Fig. 1, lanes 7–10). Thus, both the spontaneous production of free polyoma DNA and the production induced by BP are dependent on the function of the T-antigen of polyoma virus, since in these cells the T-antigen functions at 33 °C but not at 39 °C.

Further studies using the highly reactive carcinogenic metabolite of BP, BP dihydrodiol 9,10 epoxide (BPDE), on a rat cell line transformed by wild-type polyoma virus demonstrated that the enhancement of polyoma DNA synthesis persists for at least five days after a single exposure to BPDE, despite the rapid decay of this compound. In addition, enhanced synthesis of polyoma DNA could be induced by fusion of normal rat fibroblasts previously exposed to BPDE with

Fig. 1. Blotting patterns obtained with extrachromosomal DNA from ts-a H3 cells and a polyoma DNA probe
Extrachromosomal DNA was extracted by the Hirt procedure, separated by gel electrophoresis, blotted and hybridized to a $^{32}$P-labelled polyoma DNA probe, described previously (Hennings *et al.*, 1983). In lanes 1, 3 and 5, the cells were shifted from 39 °C to 33 °C and the DNA was extracted at 24, 48 or 72 h after the temperature shift, respectively. In lanes 2, 4 and 6, the procedure was the same except that benzo[*a*]pyrene (BP) (0.25 µg/mL) was added to the cultures at the time of the temperature shift. In lane 7, cells were grown continuously at 39 °C. In lanes 8, 9 and 10, cells were grown at 39 °C in the presence of BP (0.25 µg/mL) for 24, 48 or 72 h, respectively. In lanes 2, 4 and 6, the procedure was the same except that BP (0.25 µg/mL) was added to the cultures at the time of the temperature shift. In lane 7, cells were grown continuously at 39 °C. In lanes 8, 9 and 10 cells were grown at 39 °C in the presence of BP (0.25 µg/mL) for 24, 48 or 72 h, respectively. All lanes were loaded with equivalent amounts of Hirt-extract DNA. The arrows on the left side of the figure indicate the positions of supercoiled (Form I, lower arrows) and relaxed (Form II, upper arrows) molecules of the two major species of free polyoma DNA produced by ts-a H3 cells (Hennings *et al.*, 1983). The arrow on the right indicates the position of the small amount of chromosomal DNA that contaminates the Hirt extract. For additional details see Lambert *et al.* (1983).

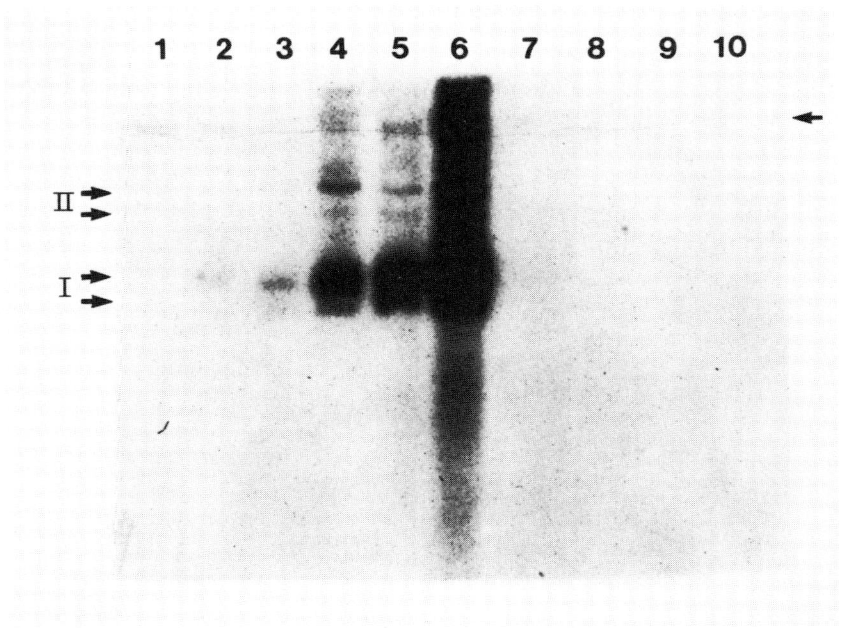


polyoma-transformed rat fibroblasts not exposed to BPDE. It appears, therefore, that the carcinogen enhancement of polyoma DNA replication is not due to direct damage to the integrated polyoma virus DNA, but may instead involve the induction of a cellular factor(s) that can function in 'trans' to enhance asynchronous replication of polyoma DNA (Lambert *et al.*, 1983).

Our results are consistent with other evidence that a variety of DNA-damaging agents can enhance the asynchronous replication of integrated polyoma or SV40 virus

DNA sequences in mammalian cells (Lavi & Etkin, 1981; Lambert *et al.,* 1983). Presumably they do so by enhancing in-situ replication (Botchan *et al.,* 1978) and/or the excision and extrachromosomal replication of these DNA sequences. It is not clear, however, to what extent carcinogens might induce the asynchronous replication of cellular genes, since we found that BP enhancement of polyoma virus DNA production is strictly dependent on the function of the polyoma virus T-antigen (Lambert *et al.,* 1983). Furthermore, we found that, under conditions in which BP induced the production of extrachromosomal copies of polyoma DNA, it did not induce the production of DNAs homologous to the endogenous genomes of two rat retroviral sequences, the 30S and rat leukaemia virus (Lambert *et al.,* 1983). Nevertheless, the ability of carcinogens to induce, *via* an indirect mechanism, the extrachromosomal production of certain viral DNAs is of interest since it demonstrates the complexity of events that may occur when cells are exposed to environmental carcinogens.

## MECHANISM OF ACTION OF TUMOUR PROMOTERS

Tumour promoters can be defined as compounds that have very weak or no carcinogenic activity when tested alone but that markedly enhance tumour yield when applied repeatedly following a low or suboptimal dose of a carcinogen (initiator) (Weinstein, 1981; Hecker *et al.,* 1982). Most of our information on the mechanism of action of this class of agents derives from studies on the potent skin tumour promoter 12-*O*-tetradecanoyl phorbol-13-acetate (TPA), and related phorbol esters. At the biochemical level, it appears that the major difference between initiators and the phorbol ester tumour promoters is that, whereas initiators (or their metabolites) bind covalently to cellular DNA, the primary site of action of the phorbol ester tumour promoters appears to be cell membranes. The phorbol ester tumour promoters can exert highly pleiotropic effects on the growth, function and differentiation of a variety of cell types. We have found it convenient to classify these effects into three categories: (1) mimicry and enhancement of transformation, (2) modulation of differentiation, and (3) membrane effects (for review, see Weinstein, 1981; Hecker *et al.,* 1982; Weinstein *et al.,* 1982).

Utilizing $^{3}$H-phorbol dibutyrate (PDBu), several laboratories have obtained direct evidence for specific, high-affinity, saturable 'phorboid receptors' in membrane preparations and intact cells from various avian, rodent and human tissues (Delclos *et al.,* 1980; Horowitz *et al.,* 1981; Hecker *et al.,* 1982). We have determined the binding constants and receptor numbers in several types of tissue culture cells (Table 1) (Horowitz & Weinstein, 1982; Greenebaum *et al.*, 1983). In general, one or two classes of $^{3}$H-PDBu receptors are found in each cell type. In most cases, a high affinity site, with a dissociation constant ($K_D$) in the range of 3 to 17 nM is present at 0.1–4 $\times$ $10^5$ sites per cell. When a second, lower affinity site is observed the $K_D$ is 300 nM or greater, and the number of sites is greater than 1 $\times$ $10^6$ per cell. Some variation in receptor number occurs within a cell line, depending on the growth state of the cells at the time of assay. When only one binding site is detected, the affinity for PDBu appears to be lower ($K_D$ of 12–41 nM), but the number of sites is, in general, higher.

Table 1. Characterization of phorboid receptors in various cell types

| Code | Cell type[a] | Phorboid receptors | | | |
|---|---|---|---|---|---|
| | | $K_{D1}$ | | $K_{D2}$ | |
| | | (nM) | Number/cell | (nM) | Number/cell |
| CREF N | Rat embryo fibroblast | 8 | $1.6 \times 10^5$ | 710 | $2.8 \times 10^6$ |
| CREF A | Rat embryo fibroblast | 7 | $3.8 \times 10^5$ | 1 700 | $4 \times 10^6$ |
| CREF A2 | Variant of CREF A | 18 | $1 \times 10^6$ | – | – |
| E-11 | Adenovirus-transformed rat embryo fibroblast | 11 | $1.5 \times 10^5$ | 1 100 | $1.4 \times 10^6$ |
| K-22 | Rat liver epithelial cell | 26 | $2.5 \times 10^5$ | 1 450 | $9.4 \times 10^6$ |
| TS 19-10 | TPA-sensitive Friend erythroleukaemia cells | 8 | $3 \times 10^4$ | 800 | $3 \times 10^6$ |
| TR 19-4 | TPA-resistant Friend erythroleukaemia cells | 8 | $3 \times 10^4$ | 800 | $3 \times 10^6$ |
| B-35 | ENU-transformed rat neuronal cell | 25 | $4.1 \times 10^5$ | – | – |
| B-103 | ENU-transformed rat neuronal cell | 36 | $4.5 \times 10^5$ | – | – |
| B-49 | ENU-transformed rat cell with neuronal and glial characteristics | 9 | $1.6 \times 10^5$ | 330 | $5.4 \times 10^6$ |
| B-15 | ENU-transformed rat glial cell | 40 | $1.5 \times 10^6$ | – | – |
| B-92 | ENU-transformed rat glial cell | 37 | $1.4 \times 10^6$ | – | – |
| SC-9 | RSV-transformed rat cerebellar cells | 15 | $1.8 \times 10^5$ | 700 | $4.4 \times 10^6$ |
| WC-5 | RSV-transformed rat cerebellar astrocyte | 3 | $2 \times 10^4$ | 380 | $1.3 \times 10^6$ |
| Ker | Normal human keratinocytes | 37 | $1.3 \times 10^6$ | 4 880 | $7 \times 10^7$ |
| 5K-MEL21 | Human metastatic melanoma | 6 | $5.6 \times 10^5$ | 900 | $8 \times 10^6$ |

We thank Dr G. Giotta of the Salk Institute for cell lines B-35 through WC-5. Lines B-35 through B-92 were isolated by Dr D. Schubert of the Salk Institute.

[a] TPA, 12-*O*-tetradecanoylphorbol 13-acetate; ENU, *N*-ethyl-*N*-nitrosourea; RSV, Rous sarcoma virus

[b] $K_D$, constant of dissociation. For specific references and details, see Fisher *et al.* (1979); Horowitz *et al.* (1981, 1982); Greenebaum *et al.* (1983); Horowitz *et al.* (1983).

It is of interest that, in two rat brain tumour cell lines displaying glial-like properties, as many as $2 \times 10^6$ high-affinity sites per cell are present. This observation is in accord with the results of Nagle *et al.* (1981), showing that brain tissue contains a very large number of phorboid receptors. We have also demonstrated the presence of PDBu receptors in normal human keratinocytes and in normal and transformed human melanocytes (Greenebaum *et al.*, 1983).

In general, the abilities of a series of phorbol esters to compete with $^3$H-PDBu for binding to cell surface receptors correlates with their known potencies in cell culture and with their activities as tumour promoters on mouse skin (Delclos *et al.*, 1980; Horowitz *et al.*, 1981; Hecker *et al.*, 1982; Horowitz & Weinstein, 1982). These results provide evidence that the phorboid receptors mediate the biological action of the phorbol esters. We have also found that the antileukaemic plant diterpenes gnidilatin and gnilatimacrin are potent inhibitors of $^3$H-PDBu binding (Horowitz & Weinstein, 1982). As discussed below, it appears that the phorboid receptors also mediate the

TPA-like effects of two new classes of tumour promoters, teleocidin (and structurally related indole alkaloids) and aplysiatoxin.

Until recently, the phorbol esters were the only class of skin tumour promoters that showed marked structure-function specificity and that were active at nanomolar concentrations. T. Sugimura, H. Fujiki, R.E. Moore and their colleagues have found, however, that the indole alkaloids teleocidin (isolated from *Streptomyces*) and dihydroteleocidin and a polyacetate compound aplysiatoxin (isolated from a marine algae) are potent tumour promoters on mouse skin (Sugimura, 1982). Teleocidin and aplysiatoxin also induce many of the same effects as TPA in cell culture, including effects on growth, differentiation and membrane structure and function (for reviews see Fisher *et al.,* 1982; Hecker *et al.,* 1982; Sugimura, 1982; Horowitz *et al.,* 1983). The chemical structures of teleocidin and aplysiatoxin are quite different from those of the phorbol esters; however, the fact that these compounds share similar biological effects suggested to us that they might act by binding to the phorboid receptors. Indeed, in collaborative studies (Umezawa *et al.,* 1981; Horowitz *et al.,* 1983) we have found that both teleocidin and aplysiatoxin are potent inhibitors of the binding of $^{3}$H-PDBu to membrane receptors. These two compounds are also equipotent with TPA in inhibiting binding to $^{125}$I-epidermal growth factor receptor and in stimulating the release of $^{3}$H-arachidonic acid and $^{3}$H-choline from prelabelled cellular phospholipids.

These results prompted us to study the stereochemistry of these compounds to see if they display structural similarities (Horowitz *et al.,* 1983). All three types of compound are amphiphilic, since they have both hydrophobic and hydrophilic domains. In the case of the phorbol esters, there is evidence that all of the biologically active compounds have a highly hydrophobic residue on the 12 position, although the precise chemical structure of this residue is not critical (Hecker *et al.,* 1982; Horowitz *et al.,* 1983). Presumably, this region of the molecule is required for a relatively non-specific hydrophobic interaction with a region on the phorboid receptor or with the adjacent lipid microenvironment. The saturated six-membered ring of teleocidin and the side chain attached to the polyacetate ring of aplysiatoxin might play analogous roles. Extensive structure-activity studies of the phorbol esters on mouse skin and in cell culture indicate that the region of the molecule containing the 3-keto, 4-OH and 6-$CH_2OH$ residues displays marked structural and steric specificity (Hecker *et al.,* 1982; Horowitz *et al.,* 1983). Our model-building studies indicate that the nine-membered lactam region of teleocidin and the macrocyclic polyacetate ring system of aplysiatoxin can assume conformations that are remarkably similar to the corresponding region present in the biologically active phorbol esters. We postulate, therefore, that the respective regions of the phorbol esters, teleocidin and aplysiatoxin, form highly specific chemical bonding and/or steric interactions with the phorboid receptors. These relationships for a phorbol ester and teleocidin are displayed in Figure 2. Additional compounds are being examined to obtain further data relevant to this hypothesis. Information of this type could make it possible to design rationally compounds that would act either as agonists or as blockers of the phorboid receptor system.

Certain findings lead us to suggest that there may be heterogeneity (or subclasses) of the receptors for phorbol esters and related tumour promoters. Scatchard analyses

Fig. 2. Perspective drawings of 12-*O*-tetradecanoylphorbol-13-acetate (TPA) (top) and dihydroteleocidin B (bottom)
The dotted lines connect heteroatoms the spatial positions of which correspond with one another and which represent residues that could form hydrogen bonds with a putative receptor. The hydrophobic $R_1$ residue on TPA (myristate) and the hydrophobic ring system on the right side of dihydroteleocidin B might interact with a separate hydrophobic domain of the receptor or with its lipid microenvironment. For further details, see text and Horowitz *et al.* (1983). The stereochemistry of dihydroteleocidin is not known and has been drawn arbitrarily to maximize the similarity to TPA.

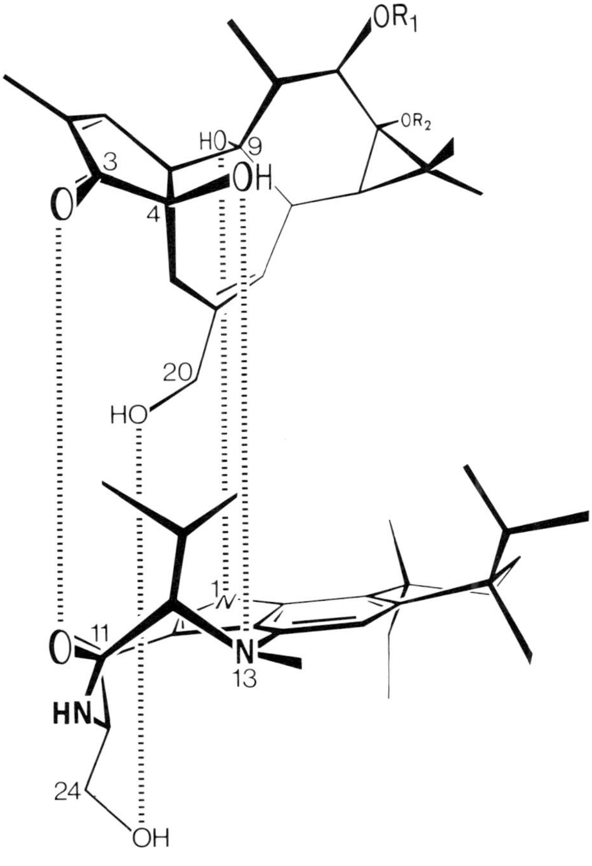


of ³H-PDBu receptor binding to intact cells are consistent with the hypothesis that there are at least two classes of binding sites (Horowitz *et al.*, 1981; Horowitz & Weinstein, 1982; Weinstein *et al.*, 1982, see also Table 1). Although the compound mezerein is equipotent with TPA with respect to certain biological effects, it competes less well than TPA in inhibiting ³H-PDBu-receptor binding and is also much weaker than TPA as a complete tumour promoter on mouse skin (Delclos *et al.*, 1980; Slaga *et al.*, 1980; Horowitz *et al.*, 1981). Therefore, some cell types may have a subset of receptors that discriminate between TPA and mezerein. Differential effects of aplysiatoxin and debromoaplysiatoxin are also consistent with the idea of receptor heterogeneity (Horowitz *et al.*, 1983). A recent study with C3H 10T½ cells indicates that the dose-response curves for TPA, PDBu and teleocidin inhibition of the binding of $^{3}$H-PDBu to high-affinity receptors are quite different from those obtained when the same compounds were tested for their ability to alter membrane lipid fluidity, as measured with fluorescence polarization probes (Tran *et al.*, 1983). It is possible that some of the biological effects of these tumour promoters are due to direct interaction with lipid domains in cell membranes. Indeed, specific binding of these compounds to synthetic phospholipid membranes has been demonstrated (Deleers *et al.*, 1982; Tran *et al.*, 1983). Studies are required to determine the biological significance of these findings. Receptor heterogeneity could contribute to the tissue specificity of these compounds as tumour promoters and could also explain other specific biological effects.

A major limitation in our knowledge of the action of phorbol ester tumour promoters is the mechanism by which they induce their highly pleiotropic effects following receptor binding. Elsewhere, we have reviewed the known effects of these compounds on ion flux (sodium, rubidium, calcium), nutrient uptake, phospholipid metabolism and induction of specific enzymes (Weinstein, 1981; Weinstein *et al.*, 1982). In view of the pleiotropic effects of protein kinases and the evidence that the products of certain oncogenes are protein kinases, an attractive mechanism for mediating the cellular effects of tumour promoters would be through specific protein kinases (Weinstein, 1981; Weinstein *et al.*, 1982). The recent finding of Castagna *et al.* (1982) that low concentrations of TPA stimulate the in-vitro activity of protein kinase C, a phospholipid-dependent protein kinase, is of considerable interest. Further evidence that a phospholipid-protein kinase C may be the actual receptor, and the effector, for TPA and related tumour promoters has been obtained recently from several laboratories (for review see Weinstein, 1983).

Although nuclear events are usually emphasized in the action of chemical carcinogens, there is evidence that carcinogens can also cause extensive damage to mitochondrial DNA (Weinstein, 1981; Backer & Weinstein, 1982). In addition, we have obtained evidence that the potent tumour promoter TPA impairs mitochondrial respiration in intact fibroblasts (Backer *et al.*, 1982) and also accelerates the hydrolysis of ATP by isolated rat liver mitochondria (Backer & Weinstein, 1983). It is possible, therefore, that disturbances in mitochondrial energy metabolism, and/or related disturbances in intracellular ion homeostasis, may play an important role at specific stages of the carcinogenic process.

Since, with repeated applications, BP and certain other polycyclic aromatic hydrocarbon (PAH) carcinogens can act as complete carcinogens on mouse skin, it seemed possible that these compounds might induce certain effects on membranes that are similar to those induced by the phorbol ester tumour promoters (Ivanovic & Weinstein, 1982). We have indeed found that the exposure of C3H 10T½ cells to BP and certain other PAHs led to a loss of epidermal growth factor-receptor binding (Ivanovic & Weinstein, 1982). There is evidence that these compounds can also mimic other effects of TPA, including increases in membrane phospholipid turnover (for review, see Ivanovic & Weinstein, 1982). We have obtained indirect evidence that these responses are mediated *via* the *Ah* receptor system (Ivanovic & Weinstein, 1982). Our results have recently been confirmed and extended (Karenlampi *et al.*, 1983; Hudson *et al.*, 1983). Our findings may also be relevant to recent studies indicating that 2,3,7,8-tetrachlorodibenzo-*para*-dioxin (TCDD), which binds to the *Ah* receptor, acts as a potent mouse skin tumour promoter in an appropriate strain of mice (Poland *et al.*, 1982).

Although our group has stressed the membrane and 'epigenetic' effects of tumour promoters, other investigators have provided evidence that the phorbol ester tumour promoters can also produce chromosomal aberrations and DNA damage, perhaps *via* activated forms of oxygen (Kinsella & Radman, 1978; Nagasawa & Little, 1979; Birnboim, 1982; Dzarlieva & Fusenig, 1982; Emerit & Cerutti, 1982; Troll *et al.*, 1982). It is necessary, however, to determine whether or not these effects are prominent only in certain cell types (i.e., macrophages, leucocytes and lymphocytes), whether or not they occur at non-toxic concentrations, and whether they can be causally associated with tumour promotion in the intact animal. We would also stress that since the process of tumour promotion on mouse skin is often reversible (Hecker *et al.*, 1982), it seems unlikely that the critical events occurring during tumour promotion involve DNA damage and chromosomal aberrations. It is possible, of course, that with prolonged exposure to TPA the latter effects might occur and contribute to the process of tumour progression. A related question is whether tumour promoters act entirely *via* inductive or hormone-like effects, thus mediating clonal expansion of previously mutated cells, or whether they can themselves produce stable and heritable changes in cell phenotype. Although most of the pleiotropic effects produced by tumour promoters in cell culture are dependent upon the continuous presence of the promoter (Weinstein, 1981; Hecker *et al.*, 1982), there are a few examples in which the action of tumour promoters is associated with irreversible effects. These include: (1) the enhancement of anchorage-independent growth of either adenovirus-transformed rat fibroblasts (Fisher *et al.*, 1979) or of certain murine epidermal cell lines (Colburn *et al.*, 1979); and (2) enhancement of the outgrowth of cell variants displaying amplified genes for dihydrofolate reductase (Varshavsky, 1981). The mechanism by which tumour promoters produce these irreversible effects is not known. These phenomena may be relevant to our understanding of how tumours can eventually evolve to a stage where they become autonomous of tumour promoters, growth factors and/or specific hormones. It is of interest that recent studies show that DNA-damaging agents are more effective than tumour promoters in enhancing the progression of papillomas to carcinomas on mouse skin (Hennings *et al.*, 1983). This suggests that the evolution of a fully malignant tumour during multistage carcinogenesis may involve more than one cycle of damage to DNA, rather than a simple linear sequence of DNA damage induced by the initiator and subsequent non-genomic effects induced by the promoter. This is, however, a highly speculative area, since even less is known about the mechanism of tumour progression than about the earlier stages of initiation and promotion. It will be important to focus on this question in future studies, because, at a clinical level, the major challenges presented by tumours relate to invasion and metastasis, aspects of the tumour phenotype that probably result from the process of tumour progression.

## CELLULAR GENES INVOLVED IN CHEMICAL CARCINOGENESIS

In contrast to oncogenic viruses, chemical carcinogens, radiation and tumour promoters cannot introduce new genetic information into cells. During the transformation process, they must, therefore, call upon genes already present in the target cells to bring about and to maintain the transformed state. Until recently, there did not appear to be a direct method available for the identification of these cellular genes. However, recent findings with retroviruses may provide direct approaches to this problem.

Studies of the RNA acute leukaemia and sarcoma viruses have led to the idea that these viruses arose by recombination of replication-proficient retroviruses with specific oncogenes (also called 'protooncogenes') endogenous to normal vertebrate species (for reviews, see Bishop, 1982; Weiss *et al.*, 1982). The proviral DNAs of retroviruses are flanked by long terminal repeat sequences (LTR) which contain strong promoter signals for enhancing transcription (Blair *et al.*, 1981; Hayward *et al.*, 1981; Bishop, 1982; Weiss *et al.*, 1982). It is possible that cellular homologues of the viral oncogenes or of the LTR sequences are involved in the transformation of cells by non-viral agents. Perhaps the DNA damage induced by chemical carcinogens or radiation triggers alterations in the state of integration and/or causes a switch-on in the constitutive expression of these DNA sequences, in the absence of a virus vector (Weinstein, 1981; Gattoni-Celli *et al.*, 1982; Kirschmeier *et al.*, 1982; Weinstein *et al.*, 1982). In studies described below, we have explored this hypothesis.

### *Studies on the cellular oncogene c-mos*

We utilized a cloned DNA fragment representing a portion of the oncogene (v-mos) of Moloney murine sarcoma virus as a probe to determine whether or not transformation of rodent cells by chemical carcinogens or radiation is associated with alterations in the state of integration or transcription of the normal cellular sequence (c-mos) that is homologous to the v-mos gene (Gattoni-Celli *et al.*, 1982). Our results with a series of transformed murine embryo fibroblast lines were, however, entirely negative (Gattoni-Celli *et al.*, 1982). More recently (Gattoni-Celli *et al.*, 1983), we have extended our studies on the c-mos oncogene to a murine myeloma cell line designated P3-X63-Ag-653 (abbreviated P3), which was derived from the MOPC 21 myeloma (Kearney *et al.*, 1979). The latter tumour is of interest since it was originally induced by the intraperitoneal injection of a rather simple chemical agent, mineral oil (Potter *et al.*, 1975). DNA samples obtained from P3 cells and various other cell types were cleaved with specific restriction endonucleases, electrophoresed through a 1% agarose gel, blot hybridized by the Southern procedure with a probe specific for c-mos, and radioautographs of the filters were made (Gattoni-Celli *et al.*, 1983). Figure 3 indicates that with DNA from the murine fibroblast cell line NIH 3T3, cleavage with the restriction enzymes EcoRI, Hind III, Sac I or Xba I gave single bands homologous to the c-mos probe, the sizes of which were 14.5, 8.7, 6.6 and 2.8 kb, respectively. Identical results were obtained with DNA samples from the BALB/c 3T3 fibroblast cell line, two carcinogen-induced transformants of this cell line and several normal murine tissues (data not shown). In P3 DNA, however, there

Fig. 3. Southern blot patterns of the c-mos sequences in the genome of NIH 3T3 (c) and murine myeloma cells (P3)
Chromosomal DNAs were digested with the restriction endonucleases (New England Biolabs) shown in the figure, using the conditions suggested by the manufacturer. The DNAs (10 μg/lane) were electrophoresed through a 1% agarose gel, transferred onto nitrocellulose filter paper and hybridized with a $^{32}$P-labelled probe prepared from an Ava I-Hind III c-mos specific fragment contained in the plasmid pMS1, kindly provided by Dr George Vande Woude. After hybridization, the blots were subjected to autoradiography. The molecular weights of the normal and rearranged c-mos alleles are shown by the arrows. For additional details, see Gattoni-Celli *et al.* (1983).

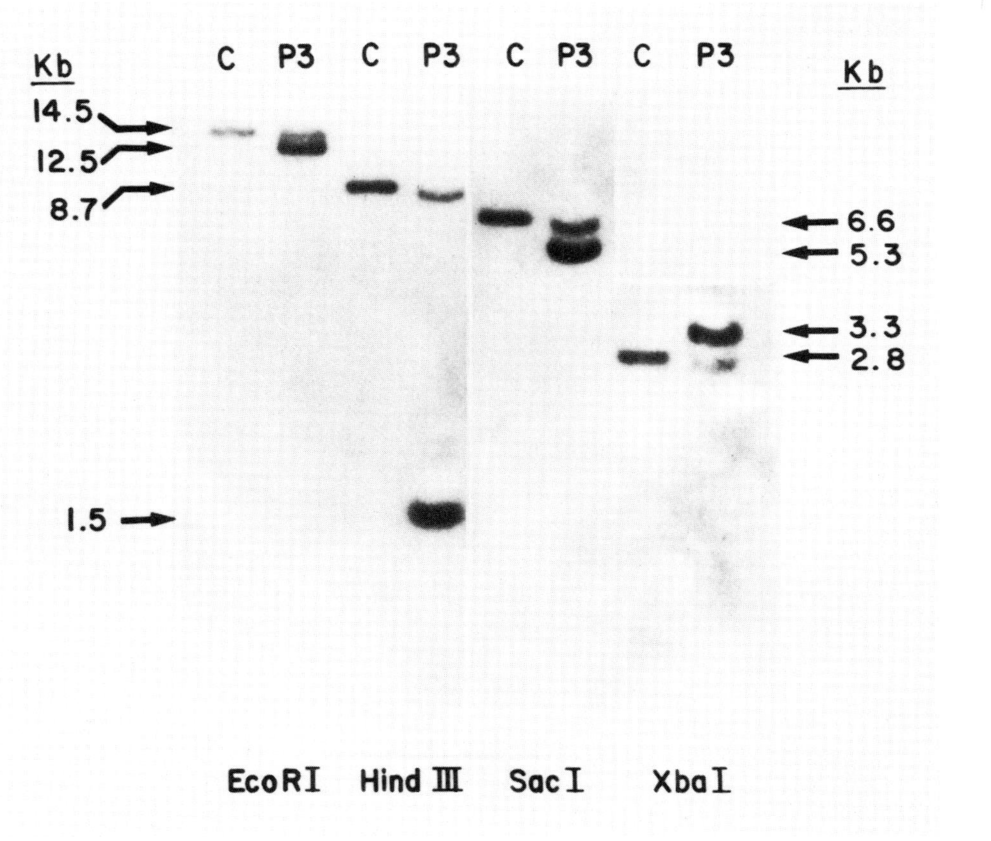


appears to be rearrangement of at least one of the c-mos alleles, since two rather than one c-mos homologous bands were obtained with all four of the restriction enzymes. Thus, EcoRI digestion yielded 14.5 and 12.5 kb bands, Hind III gave 8.7 and 1.5 kb bands, Sac I gave 6.6 and 5.5 kb bands and Xba gave 3.3 and 2.8 kb bands (Fig. 3).

Since the P3 line is used routinely to produce hybridomas that synthesize monoclonal antibodies, it was of interest to determine whether the rearranged c-mos sequence was maintained in the hybridomas. We examined three hybridoma cell lines (kindly provided by Drs L. Cleveland and B. Erlanger) and found that all three contained the altered c-mos allele (Gattoni-Celli *et al.,* 1983). As with the parental P3 cells (Fig. 3), the additional band seen on Southern blots was more intense than the normal band, suggesting that the rearranged c-mos locus is amplified in the P3 and in the hybridoma cell lines. Our finding that the altered c-mos allele persists in the hybridoma cell lines, even after prolonged serial passage, suggests that this altered oncogene may play a role in the continuous growth and/or constitutive immunoglobulin production characteristic of these hybridomas. We are currently examining this possibility.

In normal adult murine tissues and in several previously examined carcinogen-transformed mouse embryo fibroblast cell lines, the c-mos locus is hypermethylated and transcriptionally silent (Gattoni-Celli *et al.,* 1982). However, utilizing the isoschizomer pair of restriction enzymes, Hpa II and Msp I, we have obtained evidence that the c-mos locus is hypomethylated in P3 and in the hybridoma cell lines (Gattoni-Celli *et al.,* 1983, and unpublished data). Furthermore, analysis of the poly $A^+$ RNA fraction of P3 and the hybridoma cells by the Northern technique indicates that the c-mos locus is transcribed in these cells (Gattoni-Celli *et al.,* 1983).

Rechavi *et al.* (1982) have found that in a separate mouse myeloma, designated XRPC 24, which was originally induced by pristane (2,6,10,14-tetramethylpentadecane), the c-mos gene is also rearranged and transcriptionally active. Furthermore, they have cloned the rearranged c-mos gene present in the XRPC24 myeloma and found that it transformed mouse fibroblasts (Rechavi *et al.,* 1982). Their sequence studies indicate that it differs from the normal c-mos by the presence at the 5' end of a 159-base-pair insertion, which is derived from murine intracisternal A particle DNA, although the insert is oriented in a direction opposite to that of c-mos (Rechavi *et al.,* 1982; Kuff *et al.,* 1983a). A comparison of their restriction map with our results suggests that the rearranged c-mos allele found in P3 cells was derived by a similar mechanism (Gattoni-Celli *et al.,* 1983). Yet, it is clear that the two myelomas were derived independently, using two different chemicals (M. Potter, personal communication). Kuff *et al.* (1983b) have also detected the insertion of an A particle LTR sequence within a 'K' light chain intron of a murine hybridoma. Since the genome of *Mus musculus* contains about 1 000 copies of these A particle sequences (Kuff *et al.,* 1981), it is possible that they may play a rather frequent role in producing gene rearrangements.

### *Studies related to LTR sequences*

We have also pursued an alternative approach to identifying retrovirus-related sequences that might be involved in radiation and chemical carcinogenesis. Several types of evidence indicate that the LTR regions of the proviral DNA copies of these viruses play a crucial role in enhancing transcription, and that the specific sequences involved (so called 'enhancer sequences') are present in the U3 portion of the LTR sequence (Blair *et al.,* 1981; Weiss *et al.,* 1982). The LTR sequence also has structural features similar to transposable elements of bacteria, suggesting that LTR sequences might be involved in gene transposition (Blair *et al.,* 1981; Weiss *et al.,* 1982). They could act, therefore, as mobile promoters capable of enhancing the transcription of sequences adjacent to sites into which they might become integrated. Consistent with

Fig. 4. Northern blot analysis showing hybridization of the long terminal repeat (LTR) to the poly $A^+$ RNA from normal, transformed and drug-induced murine cells.
The gels contained poly $A^+$ RNAs from the following cell lines: lane a, C3H 10T½ JL#2 (ultraviolet-transformed); lane b, C3H 10T½ CB#2 (benzo[*a*]pyrene-transformed); lane c, C3H 10T½ JL#1 (X-ray-transformed); lane d, C3H 10T½ CB#1 (X-ray-transformed); lane 3, C3H 10T½ JL#3 (methylcholanthrene-transformed); and lane f, normal C3H 10T½. Poly $A^+$ RNA was isolated from these cells, denatured with 50% formamide-6% formaldehyde at 65 °C and separated on a 0.8% agarose gel containing 6% formaldehyde and 20 mmol/L morpholinopropane sulfonic acid at pH 7.0. The RNA was then transferred to nitrocellulose sheets (BA 85, Schleicher and Schuell) and hybridized to a $^{32}$P-labelled LTR probe. (For additional details, see Kirschmeier *et al.*, 1982.)

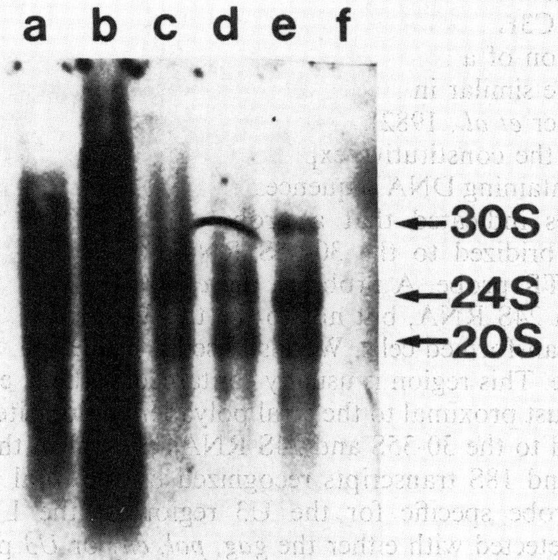


this possibility are recent studies indicating that the insertion of the LTR sequence of an avian leucosis virus at specific sites into the host cell DNA activates transcription of a flanking host oncogene sequence designated c-myc, and that this is responsible for the induction of avian lymphomas (Hayward *et al.*, 1981; Payne *et al.*, 1982). Normal murine cells contain a large number of copies of DNA sequences homologous to the LTR sequence of murine retrovirus proviral DNA (Weiss *et al.*, 1982; and our unpublished data). This suggests that, if damage to cellular DNA caused the rearrangement and/or activation of these endogenous LTR sequences, this event could lead to the constitutive expression of host genes the products of which might contribute to the multistage process of malignant cell transformation (Kirschmeier *et al.*, 1982).

To test this hypothesis, we examined whether there are differences between normal C3H 10T½ cells transformed by radiation or chemical carcinogens in terms of the expression of RNA species containing sequences homologous to a probe prepared to the LTR sequence of Moloney murine sarcoma virus (Kirschmeier *et al.*, 1982). The poly $A^+$ RNA fraction was purified from these cells, separated by gel electrophoresis and then hybridized by the Northern blotting technique to a $^{32}P$-labelled DNA probe specific for LTR sequences (Fig. 4). The poly $A^+$ RNA from normal C3H 10T½ cells showed negligible hybridization to the LTR probe (Fig. 4, lane f); however, the poly $A^+$ RNA from five different transformed C3H 10T½ cell lines (Fig. 4, lanes a–e) showed appreciable hybridization to this probe. At least five distinct poly $A^+$ RNA species, ranging from about 38S to 18S, were detected in the transformed lines. Three additional carcinogen-transformed C3H 10T½ cell lines gave similar results. The exposure of normal C3H 10T½ cells to either bromodeoxyuridine or 5-azacytidine induced the expression of a series of poly $A^+$ RNAs that were homologous to the LTR probe and were similar in size to those found in the transformed C3H 10T½ cell lines (Kirschmeier *et al.*, 1982). Thus, it appears that the unusual aspect in the transformed cells is the constitutive expression of these transcripts rather than the presence of LTR-containing DNA sequences that are unique to the transformed cells.

Additional studies indicated that a probe for the *gag-pol* region of murine retroviruses also hybridized to the 30-35S RNAs, but not to the 24-18S RNAs detected with the LTR probe. A probe to the *env* region hybridized to the 30-35S RNAs and also to a 24S RNA, but not to the the 20-18S RNAs detected with the LTR probe in the transformed cells. We also used a probe specific to the U3 region of the LTR sequence. This region is usually contained at the 3′ end of virally-related messages since it is just proximal to the viral polyadenylation site. We found that the U3 probe hybridized to the 30-35S and 24S RNAs present in the transformed cells. However, the 20S and 18S transcripts recognized by the total LTR probe did not hybridize to the probe specific for the U3 region of the LTR. No significant hybridization was detected with either the *gag, pol, env* or *U3* probes with the poly $A^+$ RNA from normal C3H 10T½ cells (Kirschmeier *et al.*, 1982). We suspect that the 20S and 18S transcripts reflect the expression of non-virally related host sequences that utilize virally-related LTR sequences as promoters. We are currently analysing the possible role of these mRNAs in initiation or maintenance of the transformed state in rodent systems.

Studies in progress utilizing Southern blot analyses indicate that normal C3H 10T½ cells contain over 30 copies of sequences homologous to our LTR probe. We have been unable, however, to detect any evidence for rearrangement or amplification of these sequences in the carcinogen- or radiation-transformed cells. Thus, the mechanism for the constitutive expression of the RNAs described above in the transformed cells is not apparent at the present time. We suspect that this may reflect a gross disturbance in mechanisms controlling the transcription of specific enhancer sequences (see 'Discussion'), but this requires further study.

As part of our interest in LTR sequences, we have recently developed a transfection and expression vector, in which specific genes can be conveniently inserted between a 5′ and 3′ LTR sequence present in the vector (Perkins *et al.*, 1983). This construct can then be transfected into rodent cells, and the inserted gene will then be expressed in the recipient cells, utilizing the transcription signals present in the LTR sequences of the vector. The vector also permits the encapsidation of RNA sequences into virus-like particles which then mediate gene transfer with extremely high efficiency. This should greatly facilitate the further analysis of genes involved in chemical carcinogenesis.

## DISCUSSION

Given the complexity of the multistep carcinogenic process, it would not be surprising if the evolution and maintenance of fully malignant cancer cells involved changes in multiple types of cellular genes. In the present paper, we have described rearrangement and transcriptional activation of the oncogene c-mos in a cell line derived from a murine myeloma. There are numerous previous reports of alterations in several other cellular oncogenes (particularly in the ras family of oncogenes) in various types of rodent and human tumours (for reviews, see Bishop, 1982; Cooper, 1982; Reddy *et al.*, 1982; Tabin *et al.*, 1982; Duesberg, 1983; Gattoni-Celli *et al.*, 1983; Klein, 1983). Most of these studies were performed with fully malignant tumour cells, and, therefore, it is not known at which stage in the carcinogenic process these changes occurred.

In considering the possible involvement of cellular oncogenes in chemical carcinogenesis, it is important to stress that they differ in several respects from their viral homologues. For example, the cellular oncogenes usually contain introns; they are not necessarily flanked by LTR sequences; and they may contain coding sequences that differ appreciably from the corresponding viral oncogenes (Weiss *et al.*, 1982; Duesberg, 1983). Therefore, we believe that it is likely that cellular oncogenes will be expressed at lower levels and under a greater degree of host control in carcinogen-induced tumours than the corresponding oncogenes introduced into cells by the acute transforming viruses. For this reason, cell transformation induced by a chemical carcinogen might often depend on changes in the function of multiple cellular oncogenes, as well as other types of host genes, rather than a single dominant gene. The oncogenes present in the acute transforming viruses have had time to evolve, and may have undergone selection, to produce a dominant phenotype. If oncogenes present in normal cellular DNA do play a role in chemical carcinogenesis, we think that it is unlikely that they do so by undergoing the full evolution in structure that occurred in the origin of viral oncogenes.

Consistent with this formulation is the increasing evidence that a given tumour may display alterations in more than one cellular oncogene (Diamond *et al.*, 1983; Duesberg, 1983). Thus, in addition to the rearrangement and expression of the c-mos sequence seen in certain murine myelomas (Rechavi *et al.*, 1982; Gattoni-Celli *et al.*, 1983), these same cells display chromosomal translocations involving the oncogene c-myc (Klein, 1983). Furthermore, the types of changes seen in cellular oncogenes in various tumours include: simple point mutations, sequence deletions, sequence insertions, gene amplification and gross translocations (Bishop, 1982; Cooper, 1982; Reddy *et al.*, 1982; Tabin *et al.*, 1982; Duesberg, 1983; Gattoni-Celli *et al.*, 1983;

Klein, 1983). At the present time, it is difficult to relate these qualitatively different changes to the action of specific initiating agents, tumour promoters or other agents that might be involved in the multistage carcinogenic process.

Furthermore, it is already clear that the repertoire of genomic changes that occurs during malignant cell transformation is not confined to the known oncogenes. Diamond *et al.* (1983) have found that certain lymphomas display alterations in a family of genes that appear to code for polypeptide growth factors. Specific cellular DNA sequences involved in mammary tumorigenesis also appear to be unrelated to the known oncogenes (Lane *et al.,* 1981; Nusse & Varmus, 1982). Moreover, the constitutive expression of a series of poly $A^+$ RNAs that contain LTR-like sequences that we have observed in murine cells transformed by carcinogens or radiation (Kirschmeier *et al.,* 1982) suggests that carcinogenesis can also involve a more widespread disturbance in mechanisms controlling gene transcription. There is increasing evidence that mammalian cells contain several classes of DNA sequences that control gene transcription, i.e., 'enhancer' sequences, and that disturbances in the function of one or more of these types of sequences could, in a broader sense, account for the aberrations in gene regulation and cellular differentiation seen in cancer.

Alterations in the state of methylation of specific DNA sequences may also play an important role in chemical carcinogenesis. The following findings are consistent with this: (1) The DNAs of certain tumours show evidence of hypomethylation (Lu *et al.,* 1983); (2) carcinogens can interfere with DNA methylation, at least in in-vitro model systems (Jones & Taylor, 1980); and (3) the drug 5-azacytidine, which interferes with DNA methylation, enhances cell transformation (Jones & Taylor, 1980; Hsiao, W., Gattoni-Celli, S. & Weinstein, I.B., unpublished data). These changes could perturb gene expression, since there is considerable evidence that in mammalian cells transcriptionally-active genes are often hypomethylated (Razin & Riggs, 1980).

Unfortunately, our current understanding of the biochemical effects of initiating carcinogens and of tumour promoters is limited to describing the initial encounters between these agents and target cells. Entirely new approaches will be required to understand the possible relationship of these early effects to the multifaceted types of genomic changes described above which are seen in fully evolved cancer cells.

## ACKNOWLEDGEMENTS

This research was supported by DHS, NCI Grants CA 021111 and CA 26056, a grant from the National Foundation for Cancer Research, and funds from the Dupont Company and the Alma Toorock Memorial for Cancer Research. The authors wish to acknowledge the valuable collaboration with Drs T. Sugimura and H. Fujiki of the National Cancer Center Research Institute, Tokyo; I. Umezawa of the Cancer Institute, Tokyo; and R.E. Moore, University of Hawaii in the studies on teleocidin and aplysiatoxin. We are grateful to L. Cleveland and B. Erlanger for providing cell lines and to G. Vande Woude for providing c-mos probes. We thank P. Kelly for assistance in preparing this manuscript.

## REFERENCES

Backer, J.M. & Weinstein, I.B. (1982) Interaction of benzo[a]pyrene and its dihydrodiol epoxide with nuclear and mitochondrial DNA in C3H 10T½ cell cultures. *Cancer Res.*, ***42***, 2764–2769

Backer, J. & Weinstein, I.B. (1983) A phorbol ester tumor promoter accelerates hydrolysis of ATP by isolated rat liver mitochondria. *Proc. Am. Assoc. Cancer Res.*, ***24***, 109

Backer, J.M., Boersig, M.R. & Weinstein, I.B. (1982) Inhibition of respiration by a phorbol ester tumor promoter in murine cultured cells. *Biochem. biophys. Res. Commun.*, ***105***, 855–866

Barrett, J.C. & Ts'o, P.O.P. (1978) Evidence for the progressive nature of neoplastic transformation *in vitro*. *Proc. natl Acad. Sci. USA*, ***75***, 3761–3765

Birnboim, H.C. (1982) Factors which affect DNA strand breakage in human leukocytes exposed to a tumor promoter, phorbol myristate acetate. *Can. J. Physiol. Pharmacol.*, ***60***, 1359–1366

Bishop, J.M. (1982) Oncogenes. *Sci. Am.*, ***246***, 81–91

Blair, D.G., Oskarsson, M., Wood, T.G., McClements, W.L., Fischinger, P.J. & Vande Woude, G.F. (1981) Activation of the transforming potential of a normal cell sequence: A molecular model for oncogenesis. *Science*, ***212***, 941–943

Botchan, M., Topp, W. & Sambrook, J. (1978) Studies on SV40 excision from cellular chromosomes. *Cold Spring Harbor Symp. Quant. Biol.*, ***43***, 709–719

Castagna, M., Takai, U., Kaibuchi, K., Sano, K., Kikkawa, U. & Nishizuka, Y. (1982) Direct activation of calcium-activated, phospholipid-dependent protein kinase by tumor promoting phorbol esters. *J. biol. Chem.*, ***257***, 7847–7851

Colburn, N.H., Former, B.F., Nelson, K.A. & Yuspa, S.H. (1979) Tumor promoter induces anchorage independence irreversibly. *Nature*, ***281***, 589–591

Cooper, G.M. (1982) Cellular transforming genes. *Science*, ***218***, 801–806

Delclos, K.B., Nagle, D.S. & Blumberg, P.M. (1980) Specific binding of phorbol ester tumor promoters to mouse skin. *Cell*, ***19***, 1025–1032

Deleers, M., Ruysschaert, J.M. & Malaisse, W.J. (1982) Interaction between phorbol esters and phospholipid in a monolayer model membrane. *Chem.-biol. Interactions*, ***42***, 271–278

Diamond, A., Cooper, G.M., Ritz, J. & Lane, M.A. (1983) Identification and molecular cloning of the human Blym transforming gene activated in Burkitt's lymphomas. *Nature*, ***305***, 112–116

Duesberg, P.H. (1983) Retroviral transforming genes in normal cells? *Nature*, ***304***, 219–225

Dzarlieva, R.T. & Fusenig, N.E. (1982) Tumor promoter 12-*O*-tetradecanoyl-phorbol-13-acetate enhances sister chromatid exchanges and numerical and structural chromosome aberrations in primary mouse epidermal cell cultures. *Cancer Lett.*, ***16***, 7–17

Emerit, I. & Cerutti, P.A. (1982) Tumor promoter phorbol 12-myristate 13-acetate induces a clastogenic factor in human lymphocytes. *Proc. natl Acad. Sci. USA*, ***79***, 7509–7513

Fisher, P.B., Bozzone, J.H. & Weinstein, I.B. (1979) Tumor promoters and epidermal growth factor stimulate anchorage-independent growth of adenovirus transformed rat embryo cells. *Cell, **18,*** 695–705

Fisher, P.B., Mufson, R.A., Miranda, A.F., Fujiki, H., Sugimura, T. & Weinstein, I.B. (1982) Phorbol ester tumor promoters and teleocidin have similar effects on cell transformation, differentiation and phospholipid metabolism. *Cancer Res., **42,*** 2829–2835

Foulds, L. (1969, 1975) *Neoplastic Development,* Vols 1 and 2, New York, Academic Press

Gattoni-Celli, S., Kirschmeier, P., Weinstein, I.B., Escobedo, J. & Dina, D. (1982) Cellular Moloney murine sarcoma ('c-mos') sequences are hypermethylated and transcriptionally silent in normal and transformed rodent cells. *Mol. cell. Biol., **2,*** 42–51

Gattoni-Celli, S., Hsiao, W.-L. & Weinstein, I.B. (1983) Rearranged c-mos locus in a MOPC-21 murine myelome cell line and its persistence in hybridomas. *Nature, **306,*** 795–796

Greenebaum, E.M., Nicolaides, M., Eisinger, M., Vogel, R.H. & Weinstein, I.B. (1983) Binding of phorbol dibutyrate and epidermal growth factor to cultured human epidermal cells. *J. natl Cancer Inst., **70,*** 435–441

Hayward, W.S., Neel, B.G. & Astrin, S.M. (1981) Activation of a cellular *onc* gene by promoter insertion in ALV-induced lymphoid leukosis. *Nature, **290,*** 475–480

Hecker, E., Fusenig, N.E., Kunz, W., Marks, F. & Thielmann, H.W., eds (1982) *Carcinogenesis: A Comprehensive Survey,* Vol. 7, New York, Raven Press

Hennings, H., Shores, R., Wenk, M.L., Spangler, E.F., Tarone, R. & Yuspa, S. (1983) Malignant conversion of mouse skin tumours is increased by tumour initiators and unaffected by tumour promoters. *Nature, **304,*** 67–69

Horowitz, A. & Weinstein, I.B. (1982) *Receptor binding and cellular effects of tumor promoters.* In: Powles, T.J., Bockman, R., Honn, K. & Ramwell, P., eds, *Prostaglandins and Cancer: First International Conference,* New York, Alan R. Liss, Inc., pp. 217–238

Horowitz, A., Greenebaum, E. & Weinstein, I.B. (1981) Identification of receptors for phorbol ester tumor promoters in intact mammalian cells and of an inhibitor of receptor binding in biologic fluids. *Proc. natl Acad. Sci. USA, **78,*** 2315–2319

Horowitz, A., Fujiki, H., Weinstein, I.B., Jeffrey, A., Okin, E., Moore, R.E. & Sugimura, T. (1983) Comparative effects of aplysiatoxin, debromoaplysiatoxin and teleocidin on receptor binding and phospholipid metabolism. *Cancer Res., **43,*** 1529–1535

Hudson, L.G., Toscano, W.A. & Greenlee, W.F. (1983) Regulation of epidermal growth factor binding in human malignant keratinocytes by 2,3,7,8-tetrachlorodibenzo-*p*-dioxin. *Fed. Proc., **42,*** 1351

Ivanovic, V. & Weinstein, I.B. (1982) Benzo[a]pyrene and other inducers of cytochrome, $P_1$-450 inhibit binding of epidermal growth factor to cell surface receptors. *Carcinogenesis, **3,*** 505–510

Jones, P.A. & Taylor, S.M. (1980) Cellular differentiation, cytidine analogs and DNA methylation. *Cell, **20,*** 85–93

Karenlampi, S.O., Eisen, H.J., Hankinson, O. & Nebert, D. (1983) Effects of cytochrome P1-450 inducers on the cell surface receptors for epidermal growth factor, phorbol 12,13-dibutyrate or insulin of cultured murine hepatoma cells. *J. biol. Chem.*, ***258***, 10378–10383

Kearney, J.F., Radbruch, A., Liesegang, B. & Rajewsky, K. (1979) A new mouse myeloma cell line that has lost immunoglobulin expression but permits the construction of antibody-secreting hybrid cell lines. *J. Immunol.*, ***123***, 1548–1550

Kinsella, A.R. & Radman, M. (1978) Tumor promoter induces sister chromatid exchanges: relevance to mechanisms of carcinogenesis. *Proc. natl Acad. Sci. USA*, ***75***, 6149–6153

Kirschmeier, P., Gattoni-Celli, S., Dina, D. & Weinstein, I.B. (1982) Carcinogen and radiation transformed C3H 10T½ cells contain RNAs homologous to the LTR sequence of a murine leukemia virus. *Proc. natl Acad. Sci. USA*, ***79***, 273–277

Klein, G. (1983) Specific chromosomal translocations and the genesis of B-cell-derived tumors in mice and men. *Cell*, ***32***, 311–315

Kuff, E.L., Smith, L.A. & Lueders, K.K. (1981) Intracisternal A-particle genes in Mus musculus: A conserved family of retrovirus-like elements. *Mol. cell. Biol.*, ***1***, 216–227

Kuff, E.L., Feenstra, A., Lueders, K., Rechavi, G., Givol, D., & Canaani, E. (1983a) Homology between an endogenous viral LTR and sequences inserted in an activated cellular oncogene. *Nature*, ***302***, 547–548

Kuff, E.L., Feenstra, A., Lueders, K., Smith, L., Hawley, R., Hozumi, N. & Shulman, M. (1983b) Intracisternal A-particle genes as movable elements in the mouse genome. *Proc. natl Acad. Sci. USA*, ***80***, 1992–1996

Lambert, M.E., Gattoni-Celli, S., Kirschmeier, P. & Weinstein, I.B. (1983) Benzo(a)pyrene induction of extrachromosomal viral DNA syhthesis in rat cells transformed by polyoma virus. *Carcinogenesis*, ***4***, 587–594

Lane, M.A., Sainten, A. & Cooper, G.M. (1981) Activation of related transforming genes in mouse and human mammary carcinomas. *Proc. natl Acad. Sci. USA*, ***78***, 5185–5189

Lavi, S. & Etkin, S. (1981) Carcinogen-mediated induction of SV40 DNA synthesis in SV40 transformed hamster embryo cells. *Carcinogenesis*, ***2***, 417–423

Lu, L.J.W., Randerath, E. & Randerath, K. (1983) DNA hypomethylation in Morris hepatomas. *Cancer Lett.*, ***19***, 231–239

Miller, E. (1978) Some current perspectives on chemical carcinogenesis in humans and experimental animals: Presidential address. *Cancer Res.*, ***38***, 1479–1496

Morris, A.G. (1981) Neoplastic transformation of mouse fibroblasts by murine sarcoma virus: A multi-step process. *J. gen. Virol.*, ***53***, 39–45

Nagasawa, H. & Little, J.B. (1979) Effect of tumor promoters, protease inhibitors, and repair processes on x-ray-induced sister chromatid exchanges in mouse cells. *Proc. natl Acad. Sci. USA*, ***76***, 1943–1947

Nagle, D.S., Jaken, S., Castagna, M. & Blumberg, P.M. (1981) Variation with embryonic development and regional localization of specific [$^3$H]phorbol 12,13-dibutyrate binding to brain. *Cancer Res.*, ***41***, 89–93

Nusse, R. & Varmus, H. (1982) Many tumors induced by the mouse mammary tumor virus contain a provirus integrated in the same region of the host genome. *Cell*, ***31***, 99–109

Payne, G.S., Bishop, J.M. & Varmus, H.E. (1982) Multiple arrangements of viral DNA and an activated host oncogene in bursal lymphomas. *Nature*, ***295***, 209–214

Perkins, A., Kirschmeier, P., Gattoni-Celli, S. & Weinstein, I.B. (1983) Development of a new transfection vector containing LTR sequences. *Mol. cell. Biol.*, ***3***, 1123–1132

Poland, A., Palen, D. & Glover, E. (1982) Tumor promotion of TCDD in skin of HRS/J hairless mice. *Nature*, ***300***, 271–273

Potter, M., Pumphrey, J.G. & Bailey, D.W. (1975) Genetics of susceptibility to plasmacytoma induction. Balb/CAuN(c), C57B1/GN(B6), C57BL/Ka(BK), (CXB6),$F_1$, (CXBK)$F_1$, and CXB recombinant-inbred strains. *J. natl Cancer Inst.*, ***54***, 1413–1417

Razin, A. & Riggs, A.D. (1980) DNA methylation and gene function. Science, **210,** 604–610

Rechavi, G., Givol, D. & Canaani, E. (1982) Activation of a cellular oncogene by DNA rearrangement: possible involvement of an IS-like element. *Nature*, ***300***, 607–611

Reddy, E.P., Reynolds, R.K., Santos, E. & Barbacid, M. (1982) A point mutation is responsible for the acquisition of transforming properties by the T24 human bladder carcinoma oncogene. *Nature*, ***300***, 149–152

Slaga, T.J., Fisher, S.M., Nelson, K. & Gleason, G.L. (1980) Studies on the mechanism of skin tumor promotion: Evidence for several stages in promotion. *Proc. natl Acad. Sci. USA*, *77*, 3659–3663

Sugimura, T. (1982) Potent tumor promoters other than phorbol esters and their significance. *Gann*, ***73***, 499–507

Tabin, C.J., Bradley, S.M., Bargmann, C.I. & Weinberg, R.A. (1982) Mechanism of activation of a human oncogene. *Nature*, ***300***, 143–149

Tran, P.L., Castagna, M., Sala, M., Vassent, G., Horowitz, A.D., Schachter, D. & Weinstein, I.B. (1983) Differential effects of tumor promoters on phorbol ester receptor binding and membrane fluorescence anisotropy in C3H 10T½ cells. *Eur. J. Biochem.*, ***130***, 155–160

Tran, P.L., Ter-Minassian, L., Madelmont, G. & Castagna, M. (1983) *Biochim. biophys. Acta*, *727*, *31–xx*

Troll, W., Witz, G., Goldstein, B., Stone, D. & Sugimura, T. (1982) *The role of free oxygen radicals in tumor promotion and carcinogenesis.* In: Hecker, E., Fusenig, N.E., Kunz, W., Marks, F. & Thielmann, H.W. eds, *Carcinogenesis*, Vol. 7, *Cocarcinogens and Biological Effects of Tumor Promoters*, New York, Raven Press, pp. 593–597

Umezawa, K., Weinstein, I.B., Horowitz, A., Fujiki, H., Matsushima, T. & Sugimura, T. (1981) Similarity of teleocidin B and phorbol ester tumor promoters in effects on membrane receptors. *Nature*, ***290***, 411–413

Varshavsky, A. (1981) Phorbol ester dramatically increases incidence of methotrexate-resistant mouse cells: Possible mechanisms and relevance to tumor promotion. *Cell*, ***25***, 561–572

Weinstein, I.B. (1981) Current concepts and controversies in chemical carcinogenesis. *J. Supramol. Struct. cell. Biochem.*, ***17***, 99–120

Weinstein, I.B. (1983) Protein kinase, phospholipid and control of growth. *Nature*, ***302***, 750

Weinstein, I.B., Horowitz, A.D., Fisher, P.B., Ivanovic, V., Gattoni-Celli, S. & Kirschmeier, P. (1982) *Mechanisms of multistage carcinogenesis and their relevance to tumor cell heterogeneity*. In: Owens, A.H., Jr, Coffey, D.S. & Baylin, S.B., eds, *Tumor Cell Heterogeneity: Origins and Implications*, New York, Academic Press, pp. 201–238

Weiss, R., Teich, N., Varmus, H. & Coffin, J., eds (1982) *Molecular Biology of Tumor Viruses*, 2nd ed., *RNA Tumor Viruses*, Cold Spring Harbor, NY, Cold Spring Harbor Laboratory

# ENHANCEMENT OF PRIMATE RETROVIRUS SYNTHESIS BY TUMOUR PROMOTERS

V. WUNDERLICH, G. SYDOW & L. BAUMBACH

*Central Institute for Cancer Research,*
*Academy of Sciences of the GDR,*
*Berlin, German Democratic Republic*

## SUMMARY

The tumour promoters 12-*O*-tetradecanoylphorbol-13-acetate (TPA) and teleocidin were found to be effective in stimulating the synthesis of primate retroviruses in chronically infected human cells. Production of baboon endogenous virus, simian sarcoma virus of woolly monkeys, Mason-Pfizer virus of rhesus monkeys and of a type D isolate from a human cell line was evaluated by assaying particle-associated reverse transcriptase activities in culture fluids of cells grown in the presence or absence of tumour promoters. Both TPA and teleocidin caused a significant but transient increase in virus production, as well as cytomorphological changes in the following infected cell types: human embryonic kidney, Tu 197 human ovarian carcinoma cells, NC 37 human lymphoblastoid line. However, infected A 204 human rhabdomyosarcoma cells were not modified by these promoters. The stimulation of virus production reached its maximum after two to four days, at which time virus production was three to forty times higher than that in controls. The optimal concentration of tumour promoters was 5–10 ng/mL. 12-*O*-Retinoylphorbol-13-acetate produced a similar but somewhat weaker effect. Control experiments demonstrated that enhancement was specific to those viruses that chronically infected each cell type.

## INTRODUCTION

The induction of cancer in man is thought to be the final result of complex interactions between initiators and factors that favour tumour development. Viruses associated with human lymphomas and leukaemias, such as Epstein-Barr virus and the recently discovered human T-cell leukaemia virus, may be considered etiological agents of the respective diseases. However, even these viruses require certain cofactors to produce cancer in a multi-step process. Tumour promoters, are among such cofactors. Studies by zur Hausen *et al.* (1978) first demonstrated that persistent genomes of oncogenic herpesviruses can be induced by 12-*O*-tetradecanoylphorbol-13-acetate (TPA) and related compounds. The importance of tumour promoters in viral carcinogenesis has been shown convincingly in studies with papillomaviruses (Amtmann *et al.,* 1983).

The modifying effect of tumour promoters on virus expression is not as well established with retroviruses as with DNA tumour viruses. Only a few papers report a tumour promoter-mediated stimulation of murine retroviruses of type B (Arya, 1980) and type C morphology (Hellman & Hellman, 1981; Lipp *et al.,* 1982; Hoshino *et al.,* 1983). In order to approach the situation in man, we have asked whether tumour promoters influence the expression of primate retroviruses in persistently infected human cells (Wunderlich *et al.,* 1981, 1982).

## MATERIALS AND METHODS

### *Viruses*

Human cell cultures were infected with one of the following viruses: the endogenous baboon virus (BaEV), the sarcoma virus of woolly monkeys (SSV), both of type C morphology, the Mason-Pfizer monkey virus (MPMV), a type D retrovirus, and another type D retrovirus termed PMFV, which was originally isolated in this institute from a continuous human cell line. The PMFV was shown to be closely related to but different from the MPMV (Wunderlich *et al.,* 1983). SSV, BaEV and MPMV were originally obtained from Dr J. Gruber, Office of Program Resources and Logistics, National Cancer Institute, USA.

### *Cells*

Viruses were adapted to grow in either human embryonic kidney (HEK), Tu 197 human ovarian carcinoma, NC 37 human lymphoblastoid, or A 204 human rhabdomyosarcoma cells. Treatment of infected cells with one of the tumour promoters was started three days after retrypsinization.

### *Chemicals*

Stock solutions of TPA, 12-retinoylphorbol-13-acetate (RPA) and teleocidin were diluted with cell culture medium just before use.

### *Assays*

Virus production was assayed by measuring particle-associated reverse transcriptase in 24-h supernatants, as described elsewhere (Wunderlich *et al.,* 1981, 1982). Results were expressed as relative virus production, defined as the ratio of reverse transcriptase activities in the culture fluids of cells grown with tumour

Fig. 1. Effect of tumour promoters on relative virus production during cultivation of virus-infected Tu 197 cells for several days
Medium with or without 12-*O*-tetradecanoylphorbol-13-acetate (TPA) or teleocidin was changed daily, and extracellular reverse transcriptase activities and number of cells were determined. BaEV, baboon endogenous virus; MPMV, Mason-Pfizer monkey virus; PMFV, virus of permanent human cell line

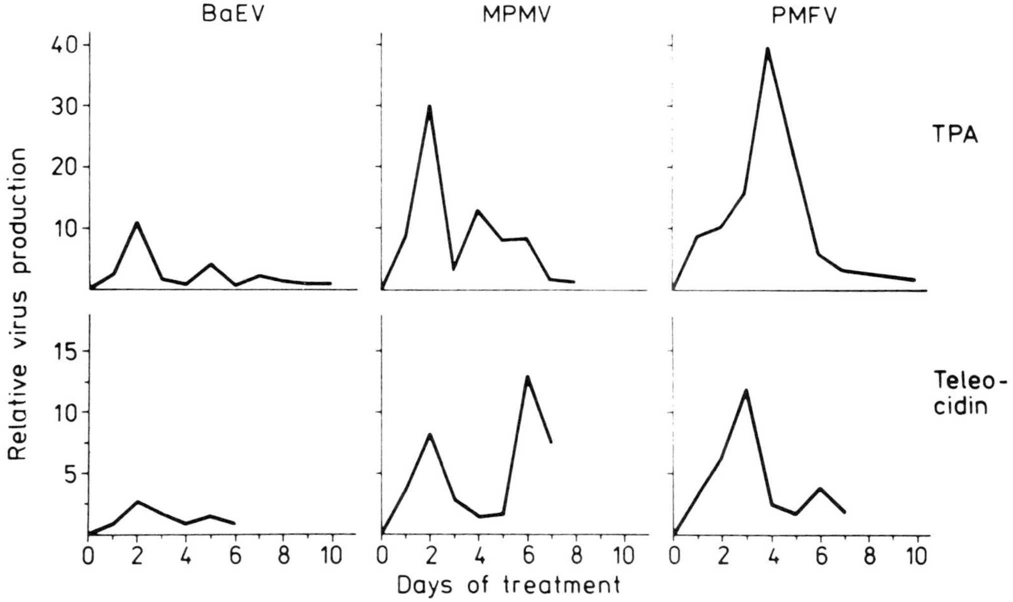


promoter to activities of cells grown without the respective tumour promoter. In every case, the reverse transcriptase activity was adjusted according to the number of cells in culture.

## RESULTS AND DISCUSSION

When confluent cells were treated with one of the tumour promoters, typical morphological alterations appeared within a few hours. Alterations included a tendency to shrinkage and rounding-up of the cells and an increased prominence of cell membrane contours. After removal of tumour promoters, these changes were completely reversed. Human embryonic kidney, Tu 197 and NC 37 cells, but not A 204 cells, responded to treatment with altered morphology.

Addition of varying concentrations of TPA to the growth medium of virus-producing cells led to a marked increase in relative virus production, as measured by the reverse transcriptase activity of extracellular viral particles. This effect was dose-dependent, with an optimal stimulatory concentration of 5 ng/mL.

Further experiments showed that there was only a transient stimulation of retrovirus synthesis. When virus-producing cells were cultivated in the presence of

TPA for eight to ten days, with daily changes of medium and determination of extracellular virus production, maximal stimulation occurred at between two to four days (Fig. 1). Thereafter, the cells gradually lost the ability to increase viral synthesis in response to freshly added TPA. Viral production returned to the basal level regardless of the initial value of that level. However, after a TPA-free interval of about ten days, including one retrypsinization, viruses could again be stimulated in a similar manner.

During a cultivation period of eight to ten days, the presence of TPA did not affect the growth behaviour of the cells.

Similar TPA-induced enhancements of virus production have been observed with all primate retroviruses tested so far (Fig. 1; results with SSV not shown). Stimulation was possible in chronically infected human embryonic kidney, Tu 197 and NC 37 cells. However, at the same TPA concentrations, no significant increase of virus synthesis occurred in infected A 204 cells.

We performed experiments to demonstrate that the increase of reverse transcriptase activity was specific for enhancement of each virus which chronically infects the cells. For example, the assay was specifically inhibited when disrupted particles from MPMV-infected cells were preincubated with a monospecific antiserum against the reverse transcriptase of MPMV. The increase in amounts of virus after treatment was confirmed independently by electron microscopic analysis (courtesy of Dr M. Rudolph). Other controls showed that no virus could be induced by TPA in cells that were not chronically infected with one of the viruses.

Results similar to those obtained with TPA were observed with the newly developed semisynthetic RPA (Fürstenberger *et al.*, 1981). The stimulation of viruses was less pronounced than with TPA and it was again transient.

We tested another tumour promoter, the indole alkaloid teleocidin, which has an entirely different chemical structure from that of TPA (Fujiki *et al.*, 1981). The results obtained with this agent were virtually identical to those obtained with TPA. Again, most of the infected cells responded to teleocidin with a significant (around ten-fold) but transient stimulation of synthesis of each of the four primate retroviruses (Fig. 1). Striking morphological alterations of the cells also appeared within a few hours of addition of teleocidin (Fig. 2). The optimal dose of teleocidin was 10 ng/mL. Parallel cultures treated with identical concentrations of either teleocidin or TPA showed a similar response of increased virus synthesis. As with TPA, A 204 cells failed to respond to teleocidin.

Thus, we have demonstrated that stimulation of retroviral synthesis by tumour promotors depends on the particular cell line. The basal level of virus production and the number of cell passages do not influence the response. Enhanced virus synthesis can be induced in both primary and continuous human cell cultures, as well as in cells of a more fibroblastic or epithelioid appearance. The mechanism for stimulation of virus synthesis is not known.

A more detailed analysis of uninfected and infected Tu 197 cells provided an interesting result. Episomal SV40-related sequences were detected in the cells, both by spot hybridization and Southern blot experiments. In uninfected Tu 197 cells, these sequences are not expressed as SV40 T-antigen. However, after chronic infection of the cells with a retrovirus (PMFV), approximately 5% of the cells were positive for

Fig. 2. Morphological effect of teleocidin on Tu 197 cells infected with PMFV (virus of permanent human cell line) (x 144)
Teleocidin (5 ng/mL) was added to cell cultures 5 days after seeding. Left, control; right, teleocidin, 24 h after addition

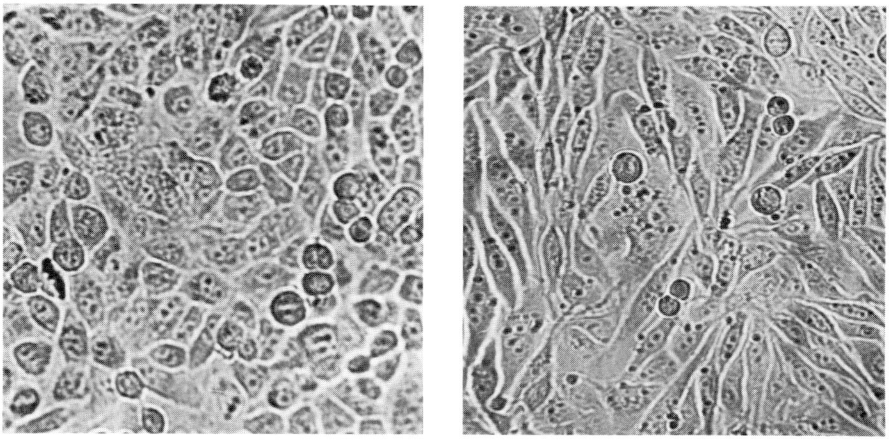

T-antigen in immunofluorescence assays (H. Prokoph *et al.*, unpublished data). Addition of TPA to uninfected Tu 197 cells caused a very large amplification of SV40-like genomes, but only a small, if any, increase in the expression of T-antigen was observed. In contrast, addition of TPA to retrovirus-infected Tu 197 cells produced a large increase in the expression of T-antigen, as well as in the viral genomes; approximately 95% of the cells scored as positive for T-antigen (S. Scherneck & W. Zimmermann, unpublished data). This system may represent a very good model of interaction of retroviruses and usually non-expressed papovaviruses in human cells, which seems to be significantly influenced by tumour promoters.

Our results demonstrate the activation of primate retroviruses by tumour promoters. They complement similar findings with murine retroviruses and a number of DNA tumour viruses. These studies are presumably relevant to elucidation of the multifactorial causation of naturally occurring tumours, in that they indicate a possible synergism of tumour viruses and tumour promoters. The fact that the stimulation reported here occurred in human cells persistently infected with retroviruses isolated originally from nonhuman primates and from a human cell line is potentially significant in the study of human exposure to environmental tumour-promoting agents.

## ACKNOWLEDGEMENTS

The authors are grateful to Professor E. Hecker, Dr H. Fujiki, Dr G. Fürstenberger and Dr F. Marks for generously providing TPA, teleocidin and RPA. They also thank Mrs K. Rücker and H. Sydow for skilful assistance.

## REFERENCES


Amtmann, E., Wayss, K. & Volm, M. (1983) Tumor induction in the rodent *Mastomys natalensis* by activation of latent papillomavirus genomes with a tumor promoter. *J. Cancer Res. clin. Oncol.*, ***105***, A 43

Arya, S.K. (1980) Phorbol ester-mediated stimulation of the synthesis of mouse mammary tumour virus. *Nature*, ***284***, 71–72

Fujiki, H., Mori, M., Nakayasu, M., Terada, M., Sugimura, T. & Moore, R.E. (1981) Indole alkaloids: dihydroteleocidin B, teleocidin, and lungbyatoxin A as members of a new class of tumor promoters. *Proc. natl Acad. Sci. USA*, ***78***, 3872–3876

Fürstenberger, G., Berry, D.L., Sorg, B. & Marks, F. (1981) Skin tumor promotion by phorbol esters is a two-stage process. *Proc. natl Acad. Sci. USA*, ***78***, 7722–7726

zur Hausen, H., O'Neill, F.J., Freese, U.K. & Hecker, E. (1978) Persisting oncogenic herpesvirus induced by the tumour promoter TPA. *Nature*, ***272***, 373–375

Hellman, K.B. & Hellman, A. (1981) Induction of type C retrovirus by the tumor promoter TPA. *Int. J. Cancer*, ***27***, 95–99

Hoshino, H., Miwa, M. & Fujiki, H. (1983) A new tumor promoter, dihydroteleocidin B, enhances cell growth and the production of murine leukemia virus by fibroblasts. *Int. J. Cancer*, ***31***, 509–513

Lipp, M., Scherer, B., Lips, G., Brandner, G. & Hunsmann, G. (1982) Diverse effects: augmentation, inhibition, and non-efficacy of 12-*O*-tetradecanoylphorbol-13-acetate (TPA) on retrovirus genome expression *in vivo* and *in vitro*. *Carcinogenesis*, ***3***, 261–265

Wunderlich, V., Baumbach, L. & Sydow, G. (1981) Phorbolester-induced expression of primate retroviruses (in German). *Arch. Geschwulstforsch.*, ***51***, 615–622

Wunderlich, V., Baumbach, L. & Sydow, G. (1982) Tumor promoter-stimulated synthesis of Mason-Pfizer monkey virus. *J. Cancer Res. clin. Oncol.*, ***102***, 271–275

Wunderlich, V., Uckert, W. & Sydow, G. (1983) Biochemical studies of primate retroviruses. *Arch. Geschwulstforsch.*, ***53***, 267–278

# INTERACTION OF TUMOUR-PROMOTING AGENTS WITH IMMUNOFUNCTIONAL CELLS *IN VITRO* AND *IN VIVO*

C.S. BAXTER, R.A. SCHOOF & A.T. LAWRENCE

*Department of Environmental Health,*
*University of Cincinnati College of Medicine,*
*Cincinnati, OH 45267, USA*

## INTRODUCTION

The existence of immunological antitumour defence mechanisms *in vivo* has current support from several directions. These elements of support include excess cancer incidence in patients immunosuppressed for tissue transplantation (Daynes *et al.*, 1979) and in those affected with acquired immunodeficiency syndrome (AIDS) (Grange & Jones, 1978), as well as facilitation of cancer expression in mice by suppressor T-lymphocyte populations (Fisher & Kripke, 1982). A current hypothesis with regard to mechanisms of carcinogenesis is that immunological involvement arises in the later stages of this apparently multistage process. Multistage cancer models in experimental animals may therefore be especially appropriate for assessing the role of antitumour immunity in carcinogenesis and the stages at which it is most active.

In the last few years, there has been an explosion of interest in the interactions of tumour-promoting agents with cellular components of the immune response in the late stages of chemical carcinogenesis. The majority of studies have been performed *in vitro* (Baxter, 1983). Although, to date, there is no direct evidence that the immune system plays a role in tumour promotion, the following findings are indicative of such a role in multistage carcinogenesis in mouse skin:

(1) Tumour-promoting agents applied topically induce inflammation, immunofunctional cell infiltration and systemic effects on the immune system (Janoff *et al.*, 1970; Klassen *et al.*, 1970; Van Duuren *et al.*, 1973; Schoof *et al.*, 1983).

(2) Promoting agents inhibit killing of tumour cells by cytotoxic immunofunctional cells *in vitro* (Fish *et al.*, 1981a; Keller *et al.*, 1982) and resistance to tumour cell growth *in vivo* (Keller *et al.*, 1982; Dean *et al.*, 1982).

Specific immunofunctional cell responses may provide valuable model systems for studying the interaction of promoters with responsive cells of other kinds. Changes in cell division rate and differentiation have been shown to be common responses to active phorbol diesters of both epidermal and immunofunctional cells (Raick, 1974; Mastro & Mueller, 1974; Fibach *et al.*, 1980; Fish *et al.*, 1981b). In addition, specific immunofunctional cell responses and tumour promotion appear to be regulated by the same biochemical mechanisms. Immunofunctional cell responses to tumour-promoting agents have been examined extensively *in vitro*. In order to assess more directly the role of these responses to carcinogenesis, we began preliminary studies to determine the effect of topically-applied tumour-promoting agents on the immune system *in vivo*.

## RESULTS

### *Response of splenic lymphocytes to phorbol diesters* in vitro

Prior to these experiments, we reported that, whereas active phorbol diester promoting agents such as 12-*O*-tetradecanoylphorbol-13-acetate (TPA) had little mitogenic activity toward splenic T-lymphocytes from BALB/c mice, they strongly potentiated the effects of mitogenic lectins such as phytohaemagglutinin (Fish *et al.*, 1981b). Subsequently, we also found this to be true of *Staphylococcal* enterotoxin A (SEA), a mitogen for T-lymphocytes both *in vitro* and *in vivo* (Fig. 1). As with other mitogens, the degree of potentiation showed a dose-effect relationship with TPA concentration, and it was greatest at lower mitogen concentrations (Fish *et al.*, 1981b). The observed comitogenic effect of phorbol diesters was, furthermore, inhibited by certain agents also found to inhibit tumour promotion, such as retinoic acid and difluoromethylornithine (Slaga *et al.*, 1980; Takigawa *et al.*, 1982) (Fig. 2), although these agents did not affect mitogenesis caused by the lectins themselves.

### *Response of splenocytes to topically-administered phorbol diesters*

In order to determine whether effects similar to those described above would occur following topical application of phorbol diesters to mouse skin, TPA was applied to the shaved back skin at doses in the range used in standard two-stage tumorigenesis protocols. In contrast to its effects *in vitro,* TPA at doses above 1 μg was itself mitogenic for splenocytes, as demonstrated by increased cell numbers and $^3$H-thymidine uptake in suspensions of cells harvested 48 h after promoter application (Fig. 3). Effects similar to those observed with TPA were seen with the phorbol diesters phorbol-12,13-didecanoate and -dibenzoate, reflecting the relative promoting activities *in vivo* of TPA and its analogues (data not shown). Topical application also increased cell division in peripheral lymph nodes and thymus (data not shown).

The mitogenic activity of TPA for splenocytes was considerably greater after a second application than after a single one (Fig. 4). Furthermore, the maximum mitogenic response generally occurred 48 h after each TPA treatment, and it decreased thereafter. Further treatment with TPA twice-weekly for eight weeks resulted in a persistently elevated level of mitogenesis that was above the level in acetone-treated or in untreated controls (Fig. 5). However, at the same time point, inflammation induced by the diester had essentially resolved. The finding that TPA-induced inflammation was maximal at a time (two weeks) when the mitogenic effects

Fig. 1. Comitogenic effect of 12-*O*-tetradecanoylphorbol-13-acetate (TPA) with *Staphylococcal* enterotoxin A (SEA) *in vitro*
●, acetone control; x, 1 ng/mL TPA; △, 10 ng/mL TPA; □, 100 ng/mL TPA
Acetone or TPA and SEA were added to quadruplicate cultures of 5 × $10^5$ spleen cells to yield the concentrations indicated. Cultures were incubated for 48 h with 0.5 μCi $^3$H-thymidine ($^3$H-TdR) added for the last 4 h

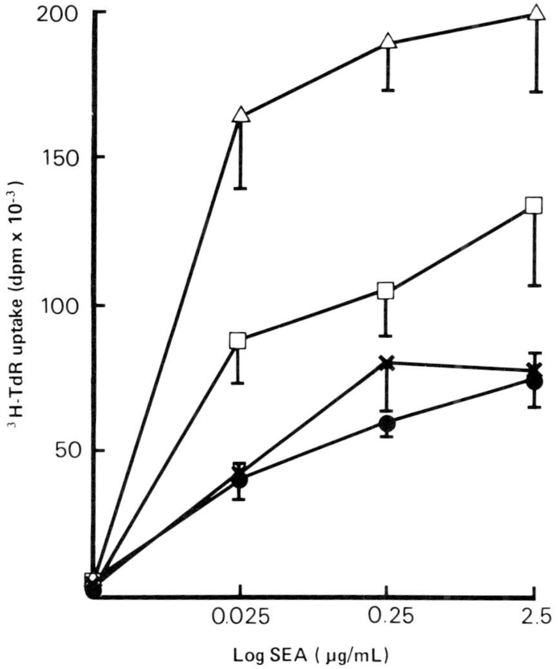


of TPA were submaximal (Fig. 5) further indicated that the two responses are not directly related. Although the findings described above were made in BALB/c mice, similar ones were made in mice of the CD-1 and SENCAR strains (data not shown).

In order to ascertain whether TPA exhibited comitogenic activity with lymphocyte mitogens, as observed *in vitro*, mice were injected retro-orbitally, 48 h before sacrifice, with SEA, a T-cell mitogen *in vivo* as well as *in vitro* (D.L. Archer, personal communication). The activities of TPA and SEA *in vivo*, on the one hand, were essentially additive (Table 1). The activities of TPA and retinoic acid, on the other hand, appeared less than additive at the concentrations used (Table 2); retinoic acid alone had some mitogenic activity following topical administration, an interesting finding in that retinoic acid has recently been reported to have promoting activity in CD-1 mice (Hennings *et al.*, 1982).

The finding that the activities of TPA and SEA are additive suggested that the two agents act on distinct cell populations. In order to verify this hypothesis, cells from the spleens of mice treated topically with TPA were treated with antithymocyte serum and complement in order to lyse T-cells prior to incubation with $^3$H-thymidine in an

Fig. 2. Inhibition by difluoromethylornithine (DFMO) and retinoic acid of comitogenesis induced by 12-*O*-tetradecanoylphorbol-13-acetate (TPA)
○, 0.06% phytohaemagglutinin (PHA) + DFMO; □, PHA + retinoic acid; filled symbols: as above with TPA (1 μg/mL)
Mitogenesis values for cultures containing PHA, TPA and the highest inhibitor concentrations were not significantly different from corresponding controls containing PHA and inhibitor only.

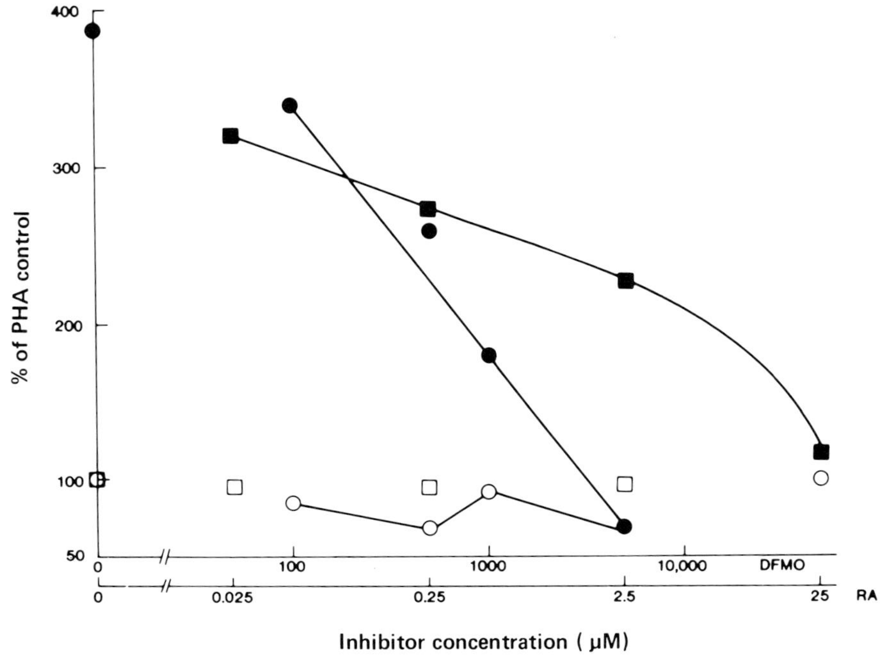


Table 1. Additive effects in mouse spleen of 12-*O*-tetradecanoylphorbol-13-acetate (TPA) and *Staphylococcal* enterotoxin A (SEA) *in vivo*

| Treatment | $^3$H-Thymidine uptake[a] | Percent change | p value[b] |
|---|---|---|---|
| Acetone | 6 318 ± 431 | | |
| SEA, 20 μg | 22 471 ± 553 | +257 | 0.0001[c] |
| TPA, 6 μg | 15 376 ± 1 089 | +143 | 0.0001[c] |
| SEA + TPA | 28 332 ± 1 843 | +348 | 0.0041[d] |

[a] dpm/0.5 × 10$^6$ cells (±SEM)
[b] From two-way analysis of variance
[c] Probability of no treatment effect
[d] Probability of no interaction between treatments
Mice were sacrificed two days after the end of a two-week course of TPA treatment or two days after retro-orbital injection of SEA.

Fig. 3. Dose-dependence of stimulation of splenic mitogenesis by 12-*O*-tetradecanoylphorbol-13-acetate (TPA)
$^3$H-TdR, Tritiated thymidine
Twice weekly for two weeks, TPA in 100 μL acetone or acetone alone was applied to dorsal skin of BALB/c mice. Mice were sacrificed two days after the last treatment, and spleens from three mice were pooled. Using analysis of variance with orthogonal contrasts, the best fit was obtained with a cubic contrast.

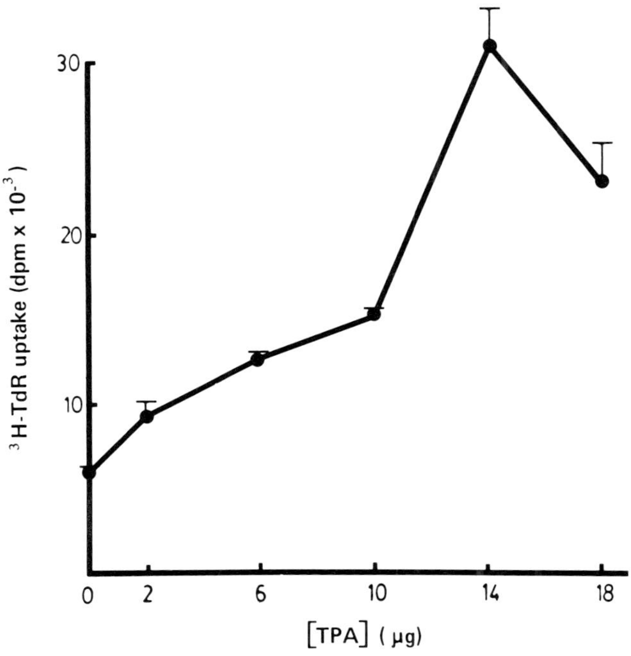


Table 2. Spleen cell mitogenesis: Interaction of retinoic acid (RA) and 12-*O*-tetradecanoylphorbol-13-acetate (TPA)

| Treatment | $^3$H-Thymidine uptake[a] | Percent stimulation | p value[b] |
|---|---|---|---|
| Acetone | 3 182 ± 298 | | |
| RA, 10 μg | 6 971 ± 358 | 119 | 0.0001[c] |
| TPA, 6 μg | 11 191 ± 1 181 | 252 | 0.0001[c] |
| RA + TPA | 12 337 ± 782 | 288 | 0.0007[d] |

[a] dpm/0.5 × $10^6$ cells (±SEM)
[b] From two-way analysis of variance
[c] Probability of no treatment effect
[d] Probability of no interaction between treatments
Mice were sacrificed two days after the end of a two-week course of treatment. RA and TPA were applied concurrently, each in 200 μL acetone.

Fig. 4. Stimulation of spleen cell mitogenesis after first and second treatments with 12-*O*-tetradecanoylphorbol-13-acetate; $^{3}$H-TdR, tritiated thymidine
●, acetone; x, 6 µg TPA
TPA in 100 µL acetone or acetone alone was applied to dorsal skin of BALB/c mice. Mice were sacrificed daily. Spleens from three mice were pooled. Significant differences were found on all days except day 1 ($p < 0.05$, unpaired t tests).

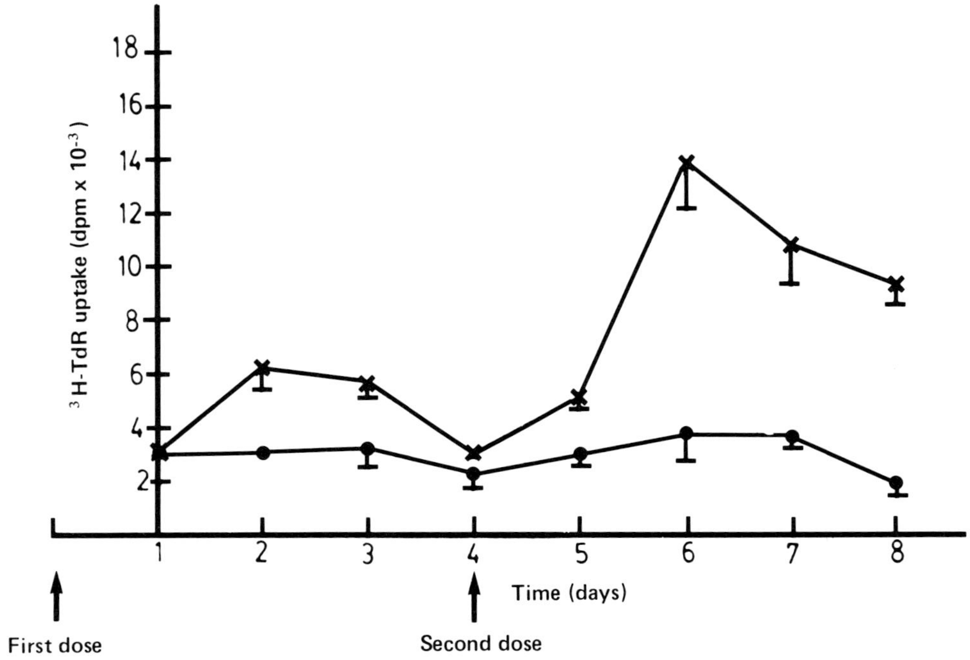


Table 3. Splenic T-cell lysis[a] in mice treated with 12-*O*-tetradecanoylphorbol-13-acetate (TPA)

| Treatment | Complement control | 1:100 ATS |
|---|---|---|
| Acetone | 3 924 ± 202 | 2 177 ± 107 |
| 14 µg TPA | 12 915 ± 1 056 | 12 854 ± 887 |
| 20 µg SEA | 48 667 ± 1 440 | 20 681 ± 1 835 |

[a] $^{3}$H-Thymidine uptake, dpm/0.5 × $10^{6}$ cellls (±SEM); ATS, antithymocyte serum; SEA, *Staphylococcal* enterotoxin A
Splenic T-lymphocytes were lysed by incubation with complement and ATS. Mice were sacrificed two days after the end of a two-week course of TPA treatment or two days after retro-orbital injection of SEA.

assay for DNA synthesis. As expected for SEA, a specific T-cell mitogen, this treatment resulted in a strong decrease in $^{3}$H-thymidine uptake (Table 3). The response of cells from TPA-treated animals was unaffected, suggesting that the T-

Fig. 5. Effects of 12-*O*-tetradecanoylphorbol-13-acetate (TPA) on splenic mitogenesis after extended treatment
$^{3}$H-TdR, tritiated thymidine; ●, acetone; ■, 6 μg TPA
Mice (six to eight weeks old) were treated twice weekly with TPA in acetone or acetone alone, and sacrificed two days after the second treatment on the week indicated. Significant effects were found at all time points ($p < 0.05$, unpaired t tests).

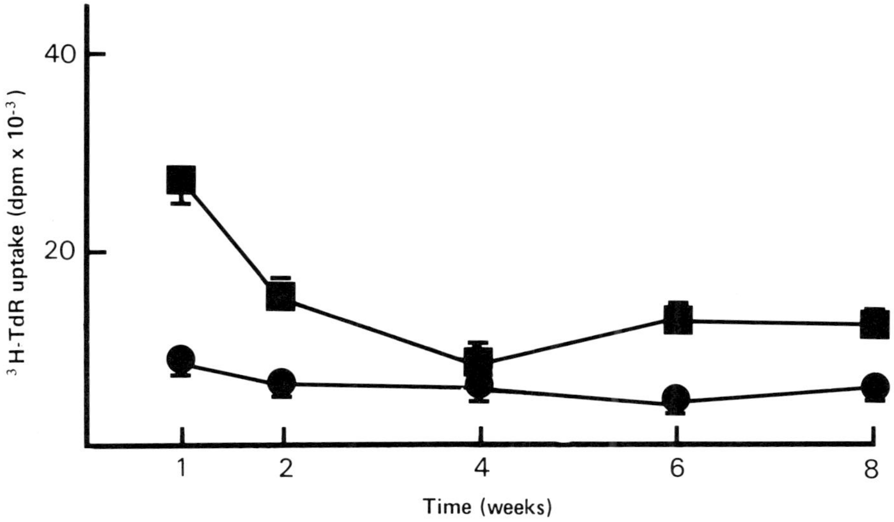


lymphocyte was not the target for TPA following topical application. Although the evidence available to date is not conclusive, it has been proposed that it is this cell population that responds to TPA in leucocyte cultures, where it is mitogenic *per se* (Abb *et al.*, 1979; Andreotti, 1982). In order to identify further the responsive cell following TPA exposure *in vivo*, synthesis of γ interferon, an activity specific to T-cells, was examined. As anticipated, SEA induced interferon synthesis strongly, but TPA was again without effect (Table 4).

These findings suggested that the target cell for the effects of topically-administered TPA was not of T-lymphocyte origin. This proposal was also borne out by the finding that thymectomized mice were responsive to topical phorbol diesters (data not shown). In order to identify further the nature of the responding cell, spleen cells were submitted to gel filtration over Sephadex G10, a procedure that is known to remove adherent cells, including macrophages (Ly & Mishell, 1974). As seen in Table 5, this procedure resulted in a sharp decrease in the ability of cells from TPA-, but not SEA-treated mice to incorporate $^{3}$H-thymidine. This finding indicated that the responding cell population was of macrophage or neutrophil origin, and it verified the lack of involvement of SEA-responsive T-lymphocytes.

*Spleen haematopoietic response to TPA*

Macrophages and granulocytes are generally non-dividing cells; hence, the observed stimulation of DNA synthesis in spleen cells was not readily attributable to

Fig. 6. A, preparation of mouse lung conditioned medium (MLCM) (Stuart & Hamilton, 1980); B, assay for granulocyte/macrophage precursor cells
For the assay, $2 \times 10^5$ spleen cells were plated in 1 mL soft agar with 10% fetal calf serum (FBS) and 1–1.5% MLCM; after eight days the colonies formed ($\geq$ 50 cells) were stained and counted.

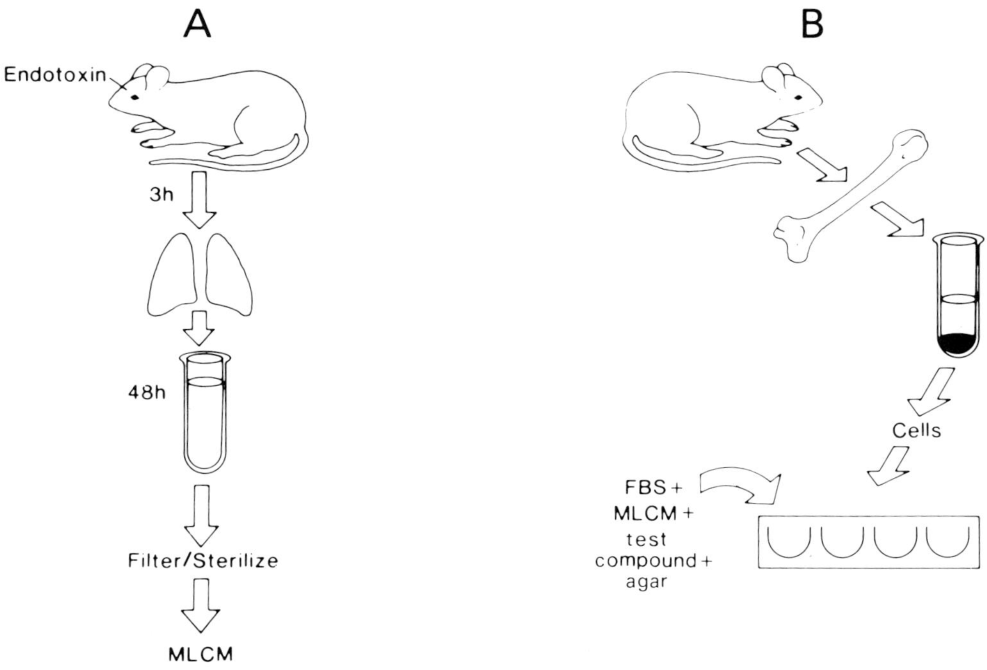


Table 4. Effects of 12-*O*-tetradecanoylphorbol-13-acetate (TPA) and a T-cell mitogen on γ-interferon production

| Treatment | Interferon activity (units/ml)[a] |
|---|---|
| Acetone | 11 |
| *Staphylococcal* enterotoxin A (SEA) (20 μg) | 125 ± 50 |
| TPA (14 μg), 4 × twice weekly | 11 |
| SEA + TPA | 107 ± 56 |

[a] 1 unit/ml = concentration that decreases the number of plaque-forming units of vesicular stomatitis virus by 50%
Cultures of $1.5 \times 10^7$ spleen cells were established from mice 6 h after the last TPA treatment, and 2 h after retro-orbital injection of SEA. Interferon concentration was measured after 24 h of culture.

induction of cell division in these cell populations. In order to determine whether the observed response to TPA involved granulocyte/macrophage precursor cells (CFU-GM), spleen cells were incubated in semisolid medium containing a colony-stimulating factor (CSF). This factor was derived from a medium conditioned by lung

Fig. 7. Effect of 12-*O*-tetradecanoylphorbol-13-acetate (TPA) on proliferation and maturation of granulocyte/macrophage precursor cells *in vitro*
MLCM, mouse lung conditioned medium
Increasing molar concentrations of TPA were added directly to plates set up as shown in Fig. 6. Each point represents three replicate cultures. Colonies were counted after eight days.

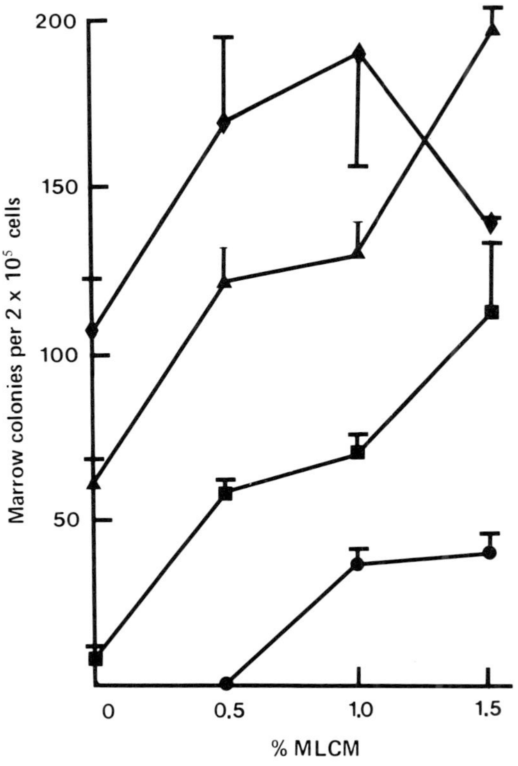


Table 5. Ability of spleen cells from mice treated with 12-*O*-tetradecanoylphorbol-13-acetate (TPA) or *Staphylococcal* enterotoxin A (SEA) to incorporate $^3$H-thymidine[a] after removal of adherent cells with Sephadex G10 column

| Treatment | Controls | Cells recovered from column |
|---|---|---|
| Acetone | 6 359 ± 646 | 5 571 ± 972 |
| 14 μg TPA | 22 541 ± 1 508 | 8 389 ± 854 |
| 20 μg SEA | 60 093 ± 5 547 | 57 258 ± 1 882 |

[a] $^3$H-thymidine uptake, dpm/0.5 × 10$^6$ cells (± SEM)
Adherent spleen cells were removed by passage through a Sephadex G-10 column. Mice were sacrificed two days after the end of a two-week course of TPA treatment or two days after retro-orbital injection of SEA.

Fig. 8. Effect of topically-applied 12-*O*-tetracecanoylphorbol-13-acetate (TPA) on behaviour of granulocyte/macrophage precursor cells
□, acetone; ■, TPA; MLCM, mouse lung conditioned medium
SENCAR mice were painted 1, 2 or 4 times with TPA (3 μg) or acetone. Forty-eight h after the last treatment, spleens were excised and cells plated in soft agar as shown in Fig. 6. Each experimental group contained two animals.

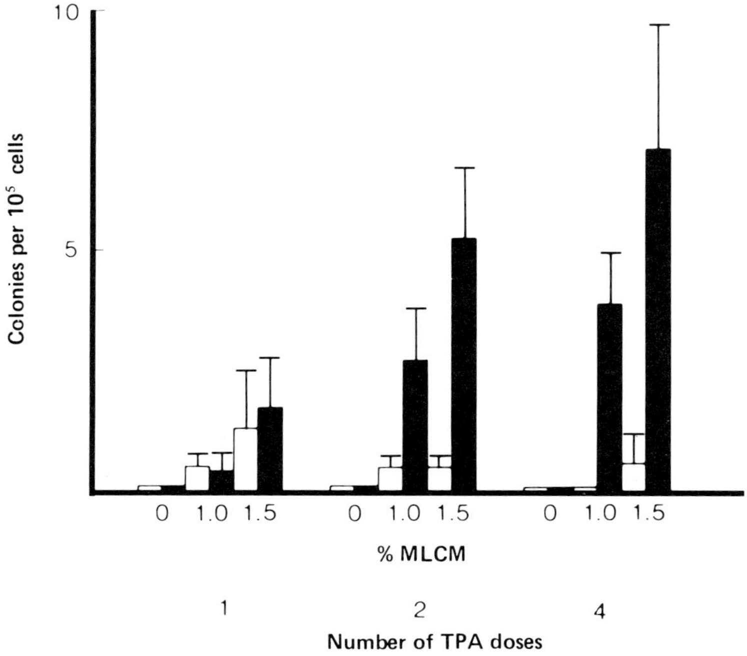


tissue from mice treated with endotoxin (Fig. 6). CSF is a peptide growth factor which induces differentiation of CFU-GM to granulocyte, macrophage and mixed colonies under these conditions. In agreement with the findings of others (Slaga *et al.*, 1981; Troll *et al.*, 1982), TPA added to splenocyte cultures *in vitro* mimicked CSF, and it was also synergistic with the peptide factor (Fig. 7). When incubated with CSF in semisolid medium, spleen cells from mice treated topically with TPA generated many more colonies than those from acetone-treated or completely untreated animals (Fig. 8). This finding was thus consistent with the proposal that TPA increases the number of CFU-GM in spleens of treated animals, probably by stimulation of proliferation of appropriate precursor stem cells.

## CONCLUSION

Inflammation and resulting immunofunctional cell infiltration have been obvious responses to topically-applied carcinogens and tumour-promoting agents since development of the earliest experimental models of carcinogenesis. Although not all inflammatory stimuli are complete carcinogens or tumour-promoting agents, all tumour-promoting agents for the skin are highly inflammatory in conventional mouse strains. Certain non-promoting inflammatory agents are, nevertheless, able to complete the tumorigenic process following brief treatment with other agents capable of completing the earliest stages.

Despite the existence of this knowledge, there have been few efforts to identify and clarify the role of the immune system in multistage mouse skin cancer models (Schinitsky *et al.*, 1973; Schoof *et al.*, 1983). In this respect, no attempt has been made to identify effects of promoting agents or their non-promoting analogues on immunological functions of cells in peripheral or primary lymphoid tissues, or in the skin itself. In this study, we reported that topical application of tumour-promoting agents does result in systemic effects on lymphoid tissues, inducing cell proliferation in the spleen, thymus and peripheral lymph nodes. Although TPA induced inflammation concurrently, a direct correlation between this response and splenic mitogenesis was not indicated, since the two effects were not maximal concurrently, and mitogenesis persisted when inflammation had resolved. More work is clearly needed to define the role of inflammation in systemic effects of TPA and in tumour promotion.

In comparison with its effects on splenocytes *in vitro,* the activity of TPA towards these cells following topical application was different in several respects. Although TPA was unable to induce mitogenesis in splenocyte suspensions *in vitro,* it was active following topical application, but it appeared to affect an adherent cell type—presumably of the macrophage or neutrophil lineage. TPA effects were thus additive with those of a T-cell mitogen also administered *in vivo,* and not synergistic, as observed *in vitro.* Where TPA has been reported to have mitogenic activity *in vitro,* moreover, such as in human peripheral leucocytes (Abb *et al.*, 1979; Andreotti, 1982), the responding cell has been identified tentatively to be of the helper T-cell lineage. The failure of this cell type to respond to topical TPA application was indicated by equivalent activity of TPA in normal and thymectomized mice, as well as the reduction of mitogenic capacity in spleen cultures treated with agents specifically lytic for T-cells. The above findings, together with the observation that all-*trans*-retinoic acid is inhibitory towards TPA-induced comitogenesis *in vitro* but not towards mitogenesis *in vivo,* suggest that in-vitro responses of immunofunctional cells to promoting agents do not necessarily reflect those occurring *in vivo.* Therefore, estimation of the role of the immune response in multistage models of carcinogenesis based on information from the interaction of promoting agents with immunofunctional cells *in vitro* must be made with caution.

Stimulation by TPA of granulocyte/macrophage colony formation in the presence of CSF suggests that topical application of this agent increases the size of the CFU-GM progenitor population in the spleen. Concurrent increase in cell division and cellularity in the spleen and lymph nodes would indicate, therefore, that the splenic haematopoietic response generates increased numbers of neutrophils and macrophages for subsequent transport to the lymph nodes and eventually to the skin. Although immune infiltration of the skin has long been recognized, the invading cell types have not been clearly characterized. The above proposal must await the results of further study for verification. Should macrophages and neutrophils be the major infiltrating cell types, an interesting model for promoter action could be envisaged; active oxygen species, already known to be released by the above cells on exposure to phorbol esters, could enhance carcinogenesis in neighbouring epidermal cells *via* genetic modification or possibly epigenetic modulation. Evidence for a role of oxygen reduction products and peroxidized compounds in tumour promotion has, indeed, been mounting in the recent past (Slaga *et al.,* 1981; Troll *et al.,* 1982).

## ACKNOWLEDGEMENTS

The work described herein was supported by grants CA24022 and ES07073 from the US Department of Health and Human Services. We wish to thank Dr D. Archer, US Food and Drug Administration, for invaluable discussions.

## REFERENCES

Abb, J., Bayliss, G.J. & Deinhardt, F. (1979) Lymphocyte activation by the tumor-promoting agent 12-*O*-tetradecanoylphorbol-13-acetate (TPA). *J. Immunol., **122,*** 1639–1642

Andreotti, P.E. (1982) Phorbol ester tumor promoter modulation of allo-antigen-specific T lymphocyte responses. *J. Immunol., **129,*** 91–96

Baxter, C.S. (1983) Interaction of phorbol diesters and other tumor-promoting agents with immunofunctional cells *in vitro. CRC Crit. Rev. Toxicol.* (in press)

Daynes, R.A., Harris, C.C., Connor, R.J. & Fichwald, E.J. (1979) Skin cancer development in mice exposed chronically to immunosuppressive agents. *J. natl Cancer Inst., **62,*** 1075–1081

Dean, J.H., Luster, M.I., Boorman, G.A. & Lauer, L.D. (1982) Procedures available to examine the immunotoxicity of chemicals and drugs. *Pharmacol. Rev., **34,*** 137–142

Fibach, E., Marks, P.A. & Rifkind, R.A. (1980) Tumor promoters enhance myeloid and erythroid colony formation by normal mouse hematopoietic cells. *Proc. natl Acad. Sci. USA, **77,*** 4152–4155

Fish, L.A., Baxter, C.S. & Bash, J.A. (1981a) Inhibition of macrophage-induced tumor cell cytostasis and cytolysis by tumor-promoting phorbol diesters. *Toxicology, **19,*** 127–138

Fish, L.A., Baxter, C.S. & Bash, J.A. (1981b) Murine lymphocyte comitogenesis by phorbol esters, and its inhibition by retinoic acid and inhibitors of polyamine biosynthesis. *Toxicol. appl. Pharmacol., **58,*** 39–47

Fisher, M.S. & Kripke, M.L. (1982) Suppressor T-lymphocytes control the development of primary skin cancers in ultraviolet-irradiated mice. *Science, **216,*** 1133–1134

Grange, R.W. & Jones, E.W. (1978) Kaposi's sarcoma and immunosuppressive therapy: an appraisal. *Clin. exp. Dermatol., **3,*** 135–146

Hennings, H., Wenk, M.L. & Donahoe, R. (1982) Retinoic acid promotion of papilloma formation in mouse skin. *Cancer Lett.*, ***16***, 1–5

Janoff, A., Klassen, A. & Troll, W. (1970) Local vascular changes induced by the cocarcinogen, phorbol myristate acetate. *Cancer Res.*, ***30***, 2568–2571

Keller, R., Keist, R., Adolf, W., Opferkuch, H.J., Schmidt, R. & Hecker, E. (1982) Tumor-promoting diterpene esters prevent macrophage activation and suppress macrophage tumoricidal capacity. *Exp. Cell Biol.*, ***50***, 121–134

Klassen, A., Janoff, A. & Troll, W. (1970) Possible role of a neutral protease in tumor promotion by phorbol ester. *Proc. Am. Assoc. Cancer Res.*, ***11***, 44

Ly, I.A. & Mishell, R.I. (1974) Separation of mouse spleen cells by passage through columns of Sephadex G-10. *J. Immunol. Methods*, ***5***, 239

Mastro, A.M. & Mueller, G.C. (1974) Synergistic action of phorbol esters in mitogen-activated lymphocytes. *Exp. Cell Res.*, ***88***, 40–46

Raick, A.N. (1974) Cell differentiation and tumor-promoting activity in skin carcinogenesis. *Cancer Res.*, ***34***, 2915–2925

Schinitsky, M.R., Thyman, L.R., Blazkovec, A.A. & Burkholder, P.M. (1973) Vaccination and skin tumor promotion with croton oil in mice. *Cancer Res.*, ***33***, 659–663

Schoof, R.A., Lawrence, A.T. & Baxter, C.S. (1983) Effects on murine immune functions of topically-administered phorbol diesters. *Proc. Am. Assoc. Cancer Res.*, ***24***, 105

Slaga, T.J., Klein-Szanto, A.J.P., Fischer, S.M., Weeks, C.E., Nelson, K. & Major, S. (1980) Studies on mechanism of action of anti-tumor-promoting agents: Their specificity in two-stage promotion. *Proc. natl Acad. Sci. USA*, ***77***, 2251–2254

Slaga, T.J., Klein-Szanto, A.J.P., Triplett, L.L., Yotti, L.P. & Trosko, J.E. (1981) Skin tumor-promoting activity of benzoyl peroxide, a widely used free radical-generating agent. *Science*, ***213***, 1023–1025

Stuart, R.K. & Hamilton, I.A. (1980) Tumor-promoting phorbol esters stimulate hematopoietic colony formation *in vitro*. *Science*, ***208***, 402–404

Takigawa, M., Verma, A.K., Simsiman, R.C. & Boutwell, R.K. (1982) Polyamine biosynthesis and skin tumor promotion: inhibition of 12-*O*-tetradecanoylphorbol-13-acetate-promoted mouse skin tumor formation by the irreversible inhibitor of ornithine decarboxylase α-difluoromethylornithine. *Biochem. biophys. Res. Commun.*, ***105***, 929–973

Troll, W., Witz, G., Goldstein, B., Stone, D. & Sugimura, T. (1982) *The role of free oxygen radicals in tumor promotion and carcinogenesis*. In: Hecker, E., Fusenig, N.E., Kunz, W., Marks, F. & Thielmann, H.W., eds, *Carcinogenesis, A Comprehensive Survey*, Vol. 7, New York, Raven Press, pp. 593–597

Van Duuren, B.L., Sivak, A., Segal, A., Seidman, J. & Katz, C. (1973) Dose-response studies with a pure tumor-promoting agent, phorbol myristate acetate. *Cancer Res.*, ***33***, 2166–2170

# STIMULATION OF MACROPHAGE ACTIVITY BY 12-*O*-TETRADECANOYLPHORBOL-13-ACETATE

D. GEMSA, U. STAAR, W. GRIMM, G. HAUSMANN, C.F. KÖRNER & K. RESCH

*Department of Molecular Pharmacology, Medical School of Hanover, Hanover, Federal Republic of Germany*

P.H. KRAMMER

*Institute of Immunology and Genetics, German Cancer Research Center, Heidelberg, Federal Republic of Germany*

## SUMMARY

Treatment of resident murine peritoneal macrophages with 12-*O*-tetradecanoyl phorbol-13-acetate (TPA) rapidly converted the cells to tumour cytostatic and cytolytic effector cells, as determined by growth inhibition or lysis of T-lymphoma cells (Eb, EL4) *in vitro*. The effective TPA concentrations were $10^{-8}$ to $10^{-7}$M. Macrophages became cytotoxic as early as one to two hours after exposure to TPA, and tumour cytotoxicity persisted up to 48 hours. TPA did not interfere with the action of the lymphokine macrophage activating factor (MAF) but acted in synergy with it. Generation of antitumour-active macrophages by TPA was accompanied by other metabolic and functional changes, such as an enhancement of the hexose monophosphate shunt, glucosamine incorporation, RNA and protein synthesis, release of prostaglandin $E_2$, thromboxane and prostacyclin, as well as pinocytosis. These data show that TPA may be a valuable model substance to complement studies of MAF; furthermore, use of TPA may help to clarify the role of activated macrophages during tumour promotion and tumour defense.

## INTRODUCTION

Activated macrophages express enhanced microbicidal and tumoricidal activity, which is accompanied by a variety of metabolic changes (Cohn, 1978; Karnovsky & Lazdins, 1978; North, 1978). Thus, macrophages are activated by lymphokines (macrophage activating factor; MAF) secreted by T-lymphocytes following antigen or mitogen stimulation. Although the biological effects of MAF are well-characterized, it is still ill-defined biochemically. Furthermore, the nature of macrophage activation by MAF is unknown. The study of macrophage activation mechanisms with chemically well-defined compounds and comparison of the effects of these compounds on macrophage activation with the effects of MAF is, therefore, worthwhile.

The tumour promoter 12-*O*-tetradecanoyl 13-phorbol acetate (TPA) is an especially suitable tool for the analysis of macrophage biochemistry and function, because of the following effects: enhancement of oxygen consumption, glucose metabolism and hydrogen peroxide formation (Nathan & Root, 1977; Hoidal *et al.*, 1978; Johnston *et al.*, 1978; Nathan *et al.*, 1979); induction of prostaglandin and plasminogen activator release (Vassalli *et al.*, 1977; Brune *et al.*, 1978); stimulation of pinocytosis and phagocytosis (Laskin *et al.*, 1980; Phaire-Washington *et al.*, 1980); and enhancement of tumour-cell killing by leukaemic cells and natural killer cells (Kolb *et al.*, 1981; Weinberg, 1981; Ramos *et al.*, 1983). In this report, we present evidence that TPA can activate resident peritoneal macrophages to high tumour cytotoxicity.

## MATERIALS AND METHODS

### *Animals*

C57Bl/6 and DBA/2 mice were obtained from Zentrale Versuchstieranstalt, Hanover, Federal Republic of Germany, and used for experiments at eight to ten weeks of age.

### *Harvest and cultivation of macrophages*

Resident peritoneal macrophages were harvested from mice after an intraperitoneal injection of 3 ml of physiological saline containing heparin (5 units/ml). Fifty to sixty percent of the cells were macrophages, as determined by carbon particle phagocytosis or by staining for non-specific esterase (Gemsa *et al.*, 1973; Seitz *et al.*, 1982). After washing, peritoneal cells were suspended in either Dulbecco's modified Eagle's medium (DMEM) containing 10% heat-inactivated fetal calf serum, RPMI 1640 containing 5% heat-inactivated fetal calf serum or RPMI 1640 containing 0.05% lactalbumin hydrolysate. All media were supplemented with 50 units/ml penicillin, 50 μg/ml streptomycin and 50 mM HEPES buffer, and cell cultures were maintained at 37 °C in an atmosphere of 5% carbon dioxide/95% air. In all experiments, macrophages were enriched (>95%) by adherence to culture plates. Non-adherent cells were removed by three washes with medium.

### *Determination of hexose monophosphate shunt (HMPS) activity*

The conversion of [1-$^{14}$C]-glucose to $^{14}$C-carbon dioxide by C57Bl/6 macrophages was done by a method described previously (Gemsa *et al.*, 1973). Briefly, after 18 h preincubation, purified macrophages (3 × $10^6$) were incubated in 2 ml glucose- and serum-free DMEM in glass tubes. After start of incubation, 2 μCi [1-$^{14}$C]-glucose (NEN, Dreieich, Federal Republic of Germany; specific activity, 56.8 mCi/mmol) was added for 60 min at different time periods. Glass tubes were closed tightly with sleeve-type rubber stoppers equipped with a centre well. Further procedures to measure $^{14}$C-carbon dioxide production were described in detail elsewhere (Gemsa *et al.*, 1973).

*Incorporation of $^{14}$C-glucosamine in macrophages*

C57Bl/6 macrophages (2 × $10^6$/ml DMEM) were incubated in glass scintillation vials for 18 h prior to the experiment. After TPA treatment for 3 h, the adherent macrophage layer was washed four times, and fresh DMEM was added containing 5 μCi $^{14}$C-glucosamine (Amersham-Buchler, Braunschweig, Federal Republic of Germany; specific activity, 19 Ci/mmol). After an additional incubation for 10 h, macrophages were washed and then lysed in 1 ml Soluene (Packard Instruments, Downers Grove, IL, USA). Incorporated radioactivity was determined in a liquid scintillation counter.

*Determination of RNA and protein synthesis*

Macrophages from DBA/2 mice (0.5 × $10^6$/0.5 ml RPMI 1640) were plated in 16-mm wells of 24 Multiwell culture plates (Falcon 3047, Oxnard, CA, USA). A sterilized 15-mm coverslip was placed at the bottom of each well. After incubation with or without TPA for 12 h, the medium was exchanged with fresh RPMI 1640, and the macrophage monolayers were pulsed for 4 h with either 4 μCi $^3$H-uridine (Amersham-Buchler, Braunschweig, Federal Republic of Germany; specific activity, 28.3 Ci/mmol) or 4 μCi $^3$H-leucine (Amersham-Buchler, Braunschweig, Federal Republic of Germany; specific activity, 68 Ci/mmol). Coverslips were then removed, washed five times in warm (25–30 °C) 0.9% saline, air-dried, lysed in 0.5 ml of cold 0.2% aqueous sodium dodecyl sulfate, and 0.05 ml fetal calf serum was added as carrier protein. RNA was precipitated by incubation with an equal volume of 20% aqueous trichloroacetic acid in an ice-bath for 20 min. Protein was similarly precipitated, except for an incubation at room temperature for 3 h. Precipitates were washed three times with 5 ml cold 5% aqueous trichloroacetic acid and then counted in a liquid scintillation counter. Results are expressed as cpm of radioactive label incorporated into precipitable material.

*Determination of prostanoids by radioimmunoassay*

Macrophages from DBA/2 mice (0.5 × $10^6$/0.5 ml RPMI 1640 with 0.05% lactalbumin hydrolysate) were cultured with or without TPA ($10^{-8}$M) in 24 Multiwell culture plates. At the end of the incubation, the culture supernatant was removed, rendered cell-free by centrifugation and the concentration of prostaglandin $E_2$ ($PGE_2$), thromboxane $B_2$ ($TXB_2$) and 6-keto prostaglandin $F_{1\alpha}$ (6-keto $PGF_{1\alpha}$) was determined by radioimmunoassay, as outlined previously (Gemsa *et al.*, 1978; Seitz *et al.*, 1982).

*Assay of pinocytic activity*

The pinocytic activity of C57Bl/6 macrophages was determined by measuring the uptake of horseradish peroxidase (HRPO) according to the method described by Steinman and Cohn (1972). Briefly, purified macrophages ($1 \times 10^6$) were incubated in glass tubes in 1 ml DMEM containing 1 mg HRPO (Boehringer, Mannheim, Federal Republic of Germany). After addition of TPA, macrophages were incubated for 60 min at 37 °C in a rotating water-bath. At the end of incubation, the cells were washed five times in 5 ml 0.9% saline, and the cell pellet was lysed by addition of 2 ml 0.05% Triton X-100 and subsequent sonication. The activity of HRPO pinocytosed by macrophages was determined in a Gilford spectrophotometer, using the assay system outlined by Steinman and Cohn (1972).

*Tumour growth inhibition assay (GIA)*

The tumour cytostatic activity of macrophages was tested in tumour growth inhibition assays (GIA). Two types of assay were used, as reported previously (Kirchner *et al.*, 1975; Gemsa *et al.*, 1981).

(1) Purified C57Bl/6 macrophages, $3 \times 10^6$ per 60-mm Petri dish, were incubated with various concentrations of TPA and for different time periods, as indicated below. After removal of the TPA-containing medium, the plates were washed several times with warm DMEM, and $1 \times 10^6$ T-lymphoma cells (EL4) in 5 ml fresh DMEM were added (macrophage:tumour ratio, 3:1). The degree of tumour growth was assayed after 24 h by a 4-h pulse with 10 μCi $^3$H-thymidine (Amersham-Buchler, Braunschweig, Federal Republic of Germany; specific activity, 400 mCi/mmol). The nonadherent EL4 tumour cells were then removed, washed several times on membrane filters with distilled water and the radioactivity determined by liquid scintillation spectroscopy. Incorporation of $^3$H-thymidine into tumour DNA in the presence of unstimulated macrophages was arbitrarily set as 100% (control); thus, growth inhibition of tumour cells is expressed as a reduction of $^3$H-thymidine incorporation when compared to the 100% value of the control. Since macrophages did not display DNA synthesis *in vitro,* all $^3$H-thymidine incorporation could be accounted for by EL4 cells. Growth inhibition of EL4 cells by macrophages was also determined by enumerating the tumour cells at the end of incubation, using a Coulter counter (Coulter Electronics, Harpenden, UK).

(2) Purified DBA/2 macrophages ($4 \times 10^4$) were incubated with Eb lymphoma cells ($2 \times 10^4$) in a total volume of 0.2 ml RPMI 1640 (macrophage:tumour ratio, 2:1) in flat-bottomed microtitre plates at 37 °C, with or without TPA. The assay was terminated at 48 h after a 4-h pulse with $^3$H-thymidine. The tumour cells were harvested by an automatic cell harvester, and incorporation of $^3$H-thymidine into tumour DNA was measured by liquid scintillation spectroscopy. Growth inhibition of Eb lymphoma cells is expressed as reduction of $^3$H-thymidine incorporation when compared to $^3$H-thymidine incorporation of tumour cells co-cultured with unstimulated, resident macrophages which lack cytostatic activity.

*Tumour cytolysis assay*

DBA/2 macrophages ($0.2 \times 10^6$/0.2 ml) were incubated in round-bottomed microtitre plates for 24 h with or without TPA. Prior to addition of tumour cells, the preincubation medium was carefully removed and replaced by fresh RPMI 1640 containing $4 \times 10^4$ $^3$H-thymidine-labelled Eb tumour cells (macrophage: tumour ratio, 5:1). After incubation for 24 or 48 h, the plates were centrifuged for 3 min at $300 \times g$, and 0.1 ml incubation medium was removed so that the amount of $^3$H-thymidine release could be determined by liquid scintillation spectroscopy. Percent specific lysis was calculated by the formula:

$$\% \text{ specific lysis} = \frac{\text{experimental cpm} - \text{control cpm}}{\text{maximum cpm} - \text{control cpm}} \times 100,$$

where experimental cpm is counts released in wells containing macrophages and tumour cells; control cpm is release of $^3$H-thymidine from target cells cultured without macrophages; and maximum cpm is the maximal radioactivity released from labelled tumour cells incubated for 60 min in water or 1% Triton X-100.

*Macrophage activating factor (MAF)*

The characteristics of MAF secretion by T-cell clone 96 were published recently (Gemsa *et al.*, 1983; Krammer *et al.*, 1983). Growth of this T-cell clone is dependent on interleukin-2. T-cell clone 96 has been passaged in tissue culture for more than two years. MAF secretion was induced by pulsing the cells with concanavalin A for 3 h, washing, and culturing for 24 h in medium free of both interleukin-2 and concanavalin A.

*Reagents*

TPA was kindly provided by Dr E. Hecker, German Cancer Research Center, Heidelberg, Federal Republic of Germany. It was dissolved in dimethyl sulfoxide, and stock solutions were maintained in the dark at −70 °C. The final concentration of dimethylsulfoxide in the incubation medium did not exceed 0.001% (v/v) and did not affect cell viability. $PGE_2$, $TXB_2$ and 6-keto-$PGF_{1\alpha}$ required for the radioimmunoassay were generously donated by Dr J. Pike, Upjohn Co., Kalamazoo, MI, USA.

## RESULTS

Incubation of macrophages with TPA rapidly induced morphological changes, characterized by cell spreading and formation of intracellular granules (Brune *et al.*, 1978; Hoidal *et al.*, 1978). In addition, glucose metabolism, as determined by the activity of the HMPS, was stimulated during the first hour of exposure to TPA (Fig. 1), and persisted for more than 3 h. TPA showed an effect on HMPS activity at concentrations as low as $10^{-9}$ mol/L, and peak stimulation was found at concentrations of $10^{-8}$ and $10^{-7}$ mol/L.

Fig. 1. Stimulation of the hexose monophosphate shunt (HMPS) by 12-*O*-tetradecanoylphorbol-13-acetate (TPA)
Macrophages (3 × $10^6$/2 ml) were incubated with TPA at indicated concentrations. Conversion of [1-$^{14}$C]-glucose to $^{14}$C-carbon dioxide ($^{14}CO_2$) was determined between 0 and 1 h (○), 1 and 2 h (△), or 2 and 3 h (□) after exposure to TPA. $^{14}CO_2$ formation of untreated macrophages was arbitrarily set as 100% (control). Values are the means ± SD of four separate incubations. Reproduced, with permission, from Grimm *et al.* (1980).

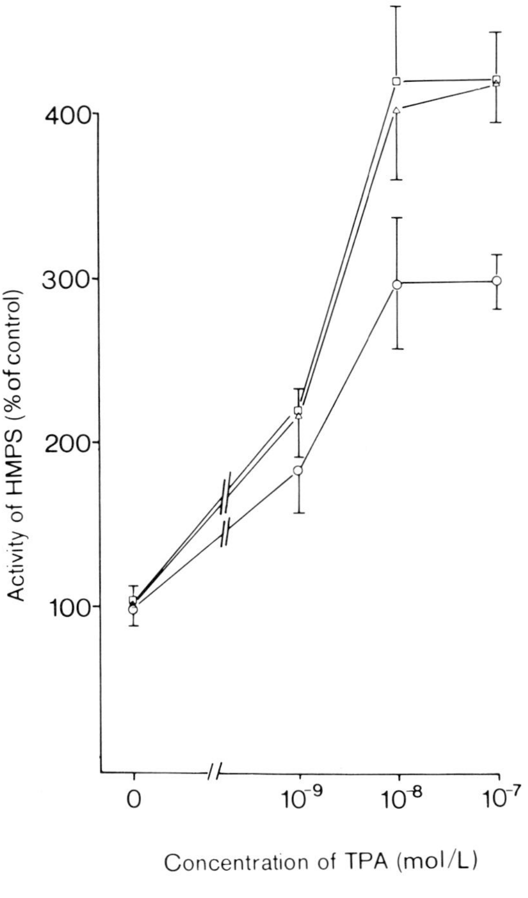


Activation of macrophages had previously been associated with enhanced incorporation of glucosamine into cell membranes (Hammond & Dvorak, 1972). Therefore, we queried whether glycoprotein synthesis was also enhanced after TPA treatment. TPA stimulated $^{14}$C-glucosamine incorporation at concentrations between $10^{-9}$ to $10^{-7}$ mol/L (Fig. 2); this effect is similar to those observed after treatment of macrophages with the lymphokine MAF (Gemsa *et al.*, 1983). In addition, TPA enhanced RNA and protein synthesis after one day of incubation, and the effect persisted for more than two days (Fig. 3).

Tumour- and inflammation-inducing phorbol esters can stimulate arachidonic acid metabolism (Brune *et al.*, 1978). Treatment of macrophages with TPA rapidly

Fig. 2. Stimulation of glucosamine incorporation into macrophages by 12-*O*-tetradecanoylphorbol-13-acetate (TPA)
After treatment of macrophages (2 × $10^6$/ml) with TPA at the concentrations indicated, the adherent cells were washed and incubations were continued for 10 h in 1 ml Dulbecco's modified Eagle's medium containing 5 μCi $^{14}$C-glucosamine. Incorporation of $^{14}$C-glucosamine into untreated macrophages (1.42 × $10^4$ cpm) was set arbitrarily as 100% (control). Values are the means ± SD of four separate incubations. Reproduced, with permission, from Grimm *et al.* (1980).

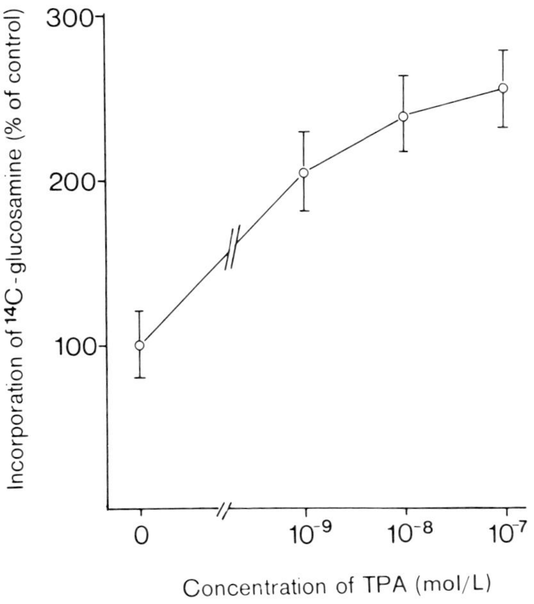


induced synthesis of the cyclooxygenase products $TXB_2$, $PGE_2$ and 6-keto-$PGF_{1\alpha}$ (metabolite of prostacyclin) (Fig. 4). TPA also induced rapid formation of intracellular granules, characteristic of stimulation of pinocytic activity. In fact, increased uptake of HRPO was found with a TPA concentration of $10^{-8}$ mol/L (Fig. 5).

We also determined whether TPA could activate tumour cytostasis of macrophages. When resident macrophages were incubated with tumour cells, no inhibition of tumour growth occurred (Fig. 6A). However, pretreatment of macrophages for 3 h with TPA before addition of tumour cells resulted in a marked inhibition of EL4 proliferation. Effective TPA concentrations were found to be between $10^{-8}$ to $10^{-7}$ mol/L, whereas concentrations of around $10^{-9}$ mol/L were inefficient. The TPA derivative, 4-*O*-methyl TPA, which lacks tumour-promoting and inflammation-inducing properties, did not generate tumour cytostatic macrophages. In order to exclude the possibility that TPA treatment of macrophages caused an artefact by suppressing $^3$H-thymidine incorporation into EL4 tumour cells, the number of tumour cells in the GIA was counted after 24 h of incubation (Fig. 6B).

Fig. 3. Enhancement of RNA and protein synthesis by 12-*O*-tetradecanoylphorbol-13-acetate (TPA) Macrophages ($0.5 \times 10^6$/0.5 ml) were incubated with TPA at the concentrations indicated. After 12 h of incubation, RNA (A) and protein synthesis (B) were determined by measuring incorporation of $^3$H-uridine and $^3$H-leucine. Values are the means ± SD of four separate incubations.

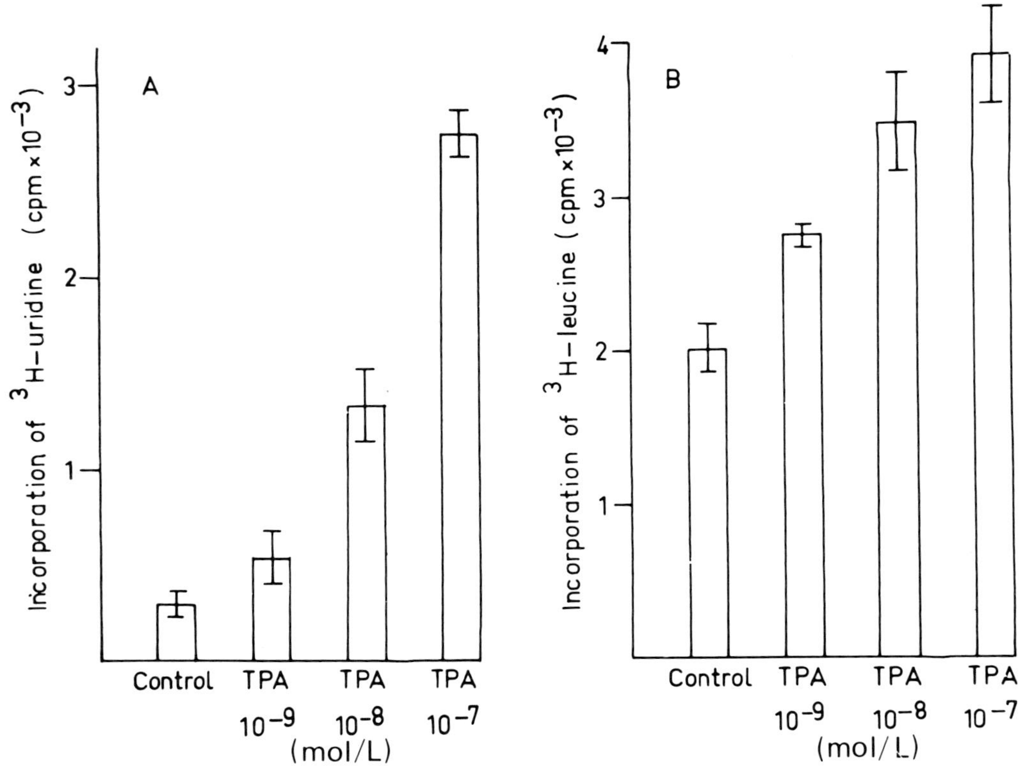


A similar inhibition of growth was found, demonstrating that incorporation of $^3$H-thymidine into tumour DNA is a reliable test for assessing tumour proliferation. Furthermore, 24-h culture supernatants of TPA-treated and untreated macrophages inhibited tumour growth by no more than 20%, indicating that release of ‘cold’ thymidine or arginase was not involved in tumour cytostasis.

TPA converted resident macrophages to tumour cytostatic effector cells in a short period of time, i.e., within one hour (Fig. 7). The cytostatic activity persisted for up to 48 h, although the level declined continuously (Fig. 8).

These findings indicate that TPA can efficiently activate macrophages. It was, therefore, considered especially worthwhile to compare TPA activity with that of MAF. Both were efficient in generating tumour cytostatic macrophages, and,

Fig. 4. Induction of prostanoid synthesis by 12-*O*-tetradecanoylphorbol-13-acetate (TPA) Macrophages ($0.5 \times 10^6$/0.5 ml) were cultured for indicated time intervals with TPA ($10^{-8}$ mol/L) and release of prostaglandin $E_2$ (●), thromboxane $B_2$ (▽) and 6-ketoprostaglandin $F_{1\alpha}$ (○) was determined by radioimmunoassay. Prostanoid release from unstimulated control cells was approximately 10% of the release found after TPA stimulation. Values are the means ± SD of four separate incubations.

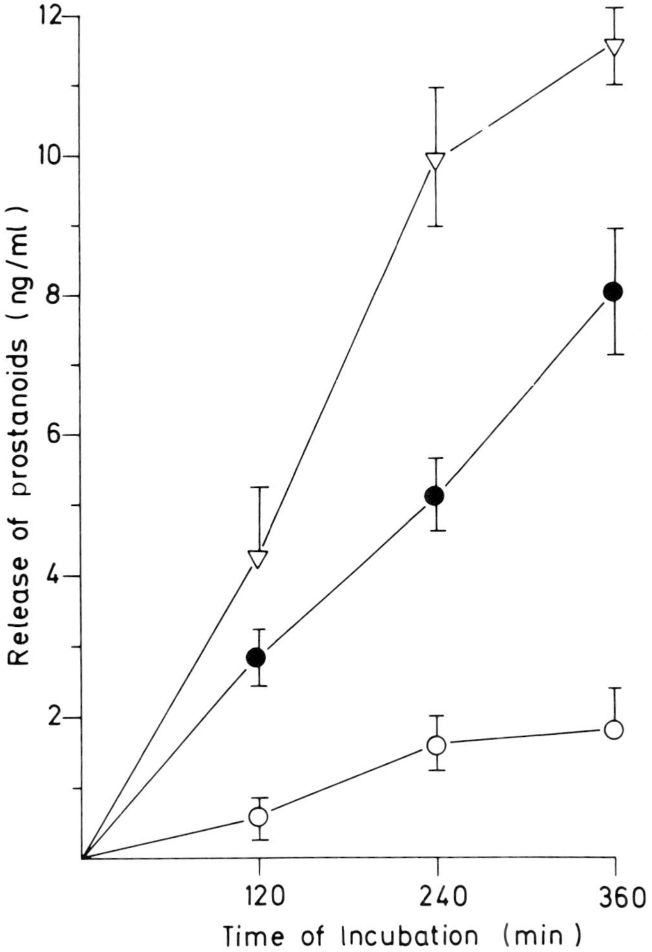


furthermore, an additive effect was observed when TPA and MAF were used together (Fig. 9).

TPA was capable not only of inducing tumour cytostatic macrophages but also of generating tumour cytolytic macrophages (Fig. 10). Again, an additive effect was observed when macrophages were incubated with both TPA and MAF.

Fig. 5. Effect of 12-*O*-tetradecanoylphorbol-13-acetate (TPA) on pinocytosis of horseradish peroxidase (HRPO)
Macrophages ($1 \times 10^6$) were incubated for 60 min with TPA at the concentrations indicated in 1 ml medium containing 1 mg HRPO. Uptake of HRPO by untreated macrophages (116 ± 6 ng) was set arbitrarily as 100% (control). Values are the means ± SD of four separate incubations. Reproduced, with permission, from Grimm *et al.* (1980).

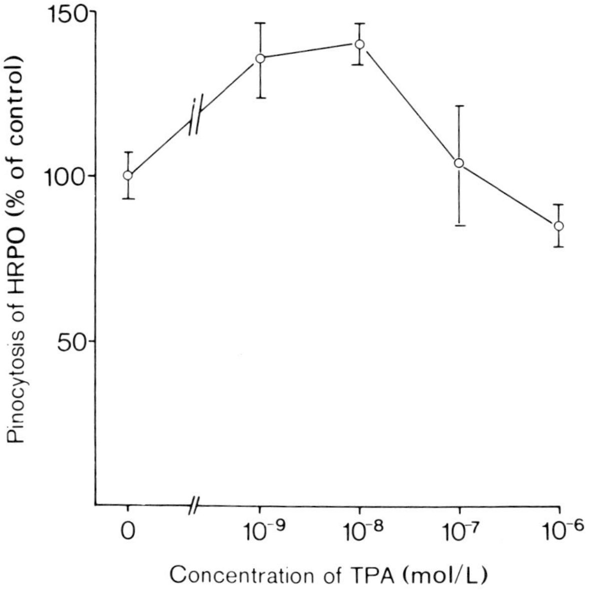


## DISCUSSION

Our data indicate that the well-known tumour promoter, TPA, is capable of activating resident macrophages. These observations can be compared with the finding of a stimulatory capacity of TPA in other systems: mitogenicity in lymphocytes (Whitfield *et al.*, 1973; Touraine *et al.*, 1977; Abb *et al.*, 1979), enhanced oxygen consumption, glucose metabolism and hydrogen peroxide formation in phagocytes (Nathan & Root, 1977; Hoidal *et al.*, 1978; Johnston *et al.*, 1978; Nathan *et al.*, 1979), induction of plasminogen activator and prostaglandin release in macrophages (Vassalli *et al.*, 1977; Brune *et al.*, 1978), stimulation of pinocytosis and phagocytosis (Laskin *et al.*, 1980; Phaire-Washington *et al.*, 1980), and elevation of natural killer cell activity (Kolb *et al.*, 1981; Ramos *et al.*, 1983). Further information on the generally enhancing effects of TPA has been summarized recently in an extensive review (Mastro, 1982).

One basic mechanism of action of TPA appears to be a pronounced membrane perturbation, leading to rapid spreading, granule formation and prostaglandin synthesis in macrophages, and to stimulation of phospholipid metabolism in lymphocytes (Wertz & Mueller, 1978). Therefore, TPA would be a suitable model

Fig. 6. Induction of tumour cytostatic macrophages by 12-*O*-tetradecanoylphorbol-13-acetate (TPA) Macrophages ($3 \times 10^6$/5 ml) were treated for 3 h with either TPA at indicated concentrations, or with 4-*O*-methyl TPA ($10^{-7}$ mol/L), or with the solvent (0.001% dimethyl sulfoxide) alone (control). After four washings, the macrophage cultures were incubated with $1 \times 10^6$ EL4 tumour cells for 24 h in tumour growth inhibition assay. At the end of the incubation, proliferation of EL4 cells was assessed either by a 4-h pulse with $^3$H-thymidine (A) or by enumeration of tumour cells grown from an initial inoculum of $1 \times 10^6$ (B). Incorporation of $^3$H-thymidine into tumour DNA in the presence of control macrophages ($1.8 \times 10^4$ cpm) was set arbitrarily as 100%. Values are the means ± SD of four separate incubations. Reproduced, with permission, from Grimm *et al.* (1980).

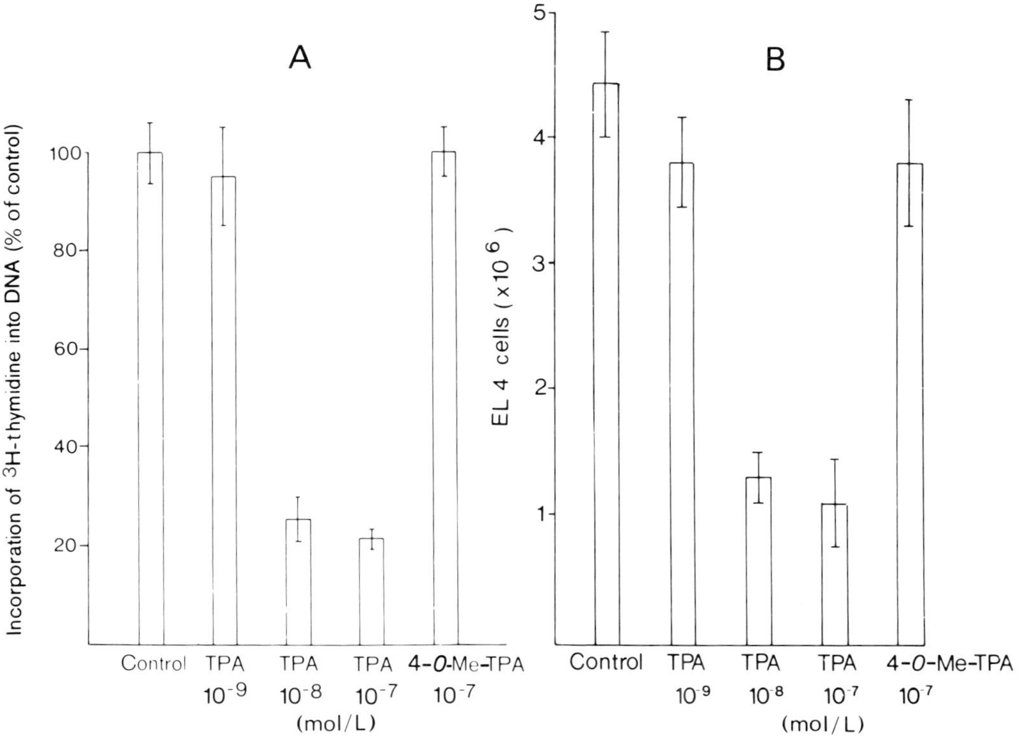


compound for (1) studying macrophage stimulation/activation at a biochemical level, (2) comparing its activity to that of MAF, and (3) analysing macrophage-tumour cell interactions.

Our findings demonstrate that TPA is a potent enhancer of resident macrophage metabolism. Stimulation of the HMPS was an early event in activation and persisted for at least three hours. Incorporation of $^{14}$C-glucosamine was markedly elevated by TPA, as by MAF (Hammond *et al.*, 1975; Gemsa *et al.*, 1983). We also found enhanced RNA and protein synthesis, as well as increased prostanoid release. This finding agrees with results obtained recently with some MAFs which are a

Fig. 7. Time course of induction of tumour cytostatic macrophages by 12-*O*-tetradecanoylphorbol-13-acetate (TPA)
Macrophages ($3 \times 10^6$/5 ml) were treated for the time intervals indicated with $10^{-8}$mol/L TPA. After four washings, the cultures were incubated with $1 \times 10^6$ EL4 tumour cells for 24 h in a tumour growth inhibition assay. Incorporation of $^3$H-thymidine into tumour DNA in the absence of control macrophages ($2.25 \times 10^4$ cpm) was set arbitrarily at 100%. Values are the means ± SD of four separate incubations. Reproduced, with permission, from Grimm *et al.* (1980).

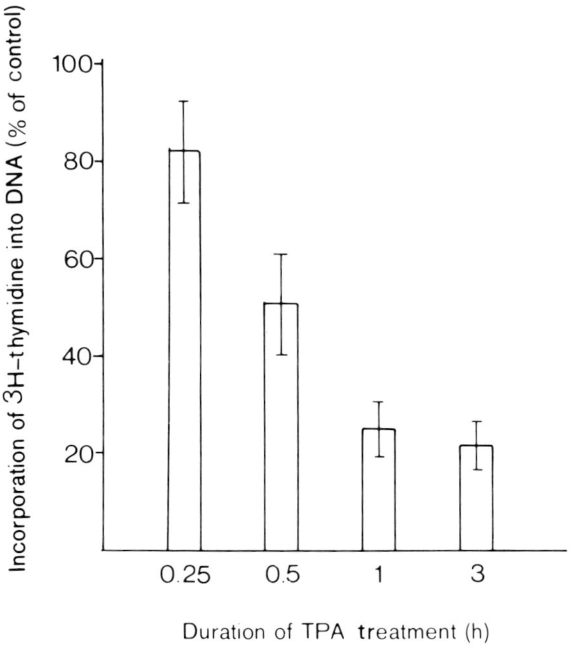


heterogeneous group of lymphokines (Gemsa *et al.*, 1983): glucose metabolism and pinocytic activity were stimulated during the first hour of exposure to TPA. Stimulation of pinocytosis appears to mirror the rapid formation of vacuoles observed microscopically.

It is important to know whether metabolic stimulation of macrophages by TPA is followed by enhanced tumour cytotoxicity, the hallmark of macrophage activation. Our studies showed that treatment of resident macrophages with TPA induced marked tumour cytostasis. It could be argued that cytostasis assays, such as the GIA, are prone to artefacts, since release of 'cold' thymidine or arginase by macrophages may interfere with the assay or may deplete the incubation medium of essential arginine. However, in the experiments reported here, the tumour cytostatic activity of TPA-treated macrophages could also be demonstrated by a decrease in the number of tumour cells. Furthermore, supplementation of the medium with arginine did not abolish tumour cytostasis.

Fig. 8. Persistence of tumour cytostatic activity of macrophages after a single 12-*O*-tetradecanoylphorbol-13-acetate (TPA) treatment
Macrophages ($3 \times 10^6$/5 ml) were treated for 3 h with $10^{-8}$ mol/L TPA or solvent alone (control). After four washings, macrophage cultures were incubated with $1 \times 10^6$ EL4 cells in a tumour growth inhibition assay at the indicated time intervals after TPA treatment. Incorporation of $^3$H-thymidine into tumour DNA in the presence of control macrophages ($1.72 \times 10^4$ cpm) was set arbitrarily at 100%. Values are the means $\pm$ SD of four separate incubations. Reproduced, with permission from Grimm *et al.* (1980).

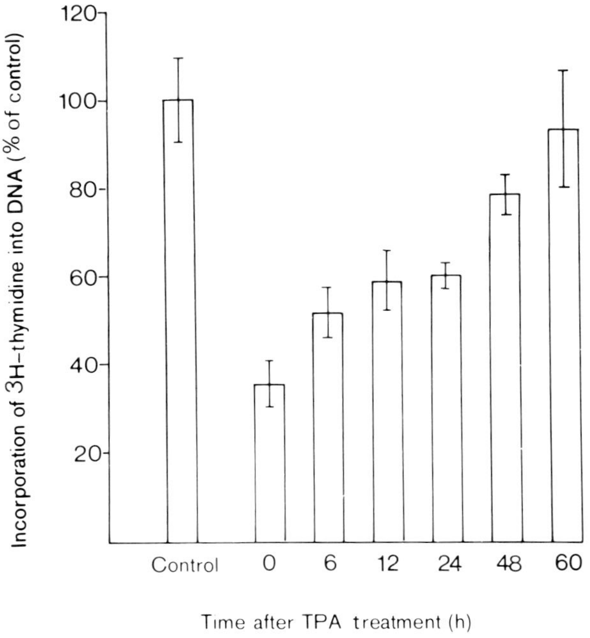


TPA also induced tumour cytolytic macrophages at concentrations somewhat higher than those needed for induction of tumour cytostasis. TPA is highly lipophilic and difficult to remove from the cell surface by washing; however, a direct cytostatic or cytolytic effect on tumour cells could be excluded, since growth of Eb and of EL4 was unaffected by concentrations of $10^{-9}$ to $10^{-7}$mol/L. Although it is unlikely, this finding does not preclude the hypothesis that TPA, enriched on the macrophage surface and present in a toxic form, may have caused tumour cell damage or growth inhibition.

The mechanism of tumour cytotoxicity by TPA-treated macrophages is unclear. TPA may trigger the release of hydrogen peroxide from macrophages (Nathan *et al.*, 1979); however, previous reports demonstrated that hydrogen peroxide was released only from macrophages preactivated *in vivo*. In our experiments, resident, unstimulated macrophages were used; moreover, the tumour cells would have had to

Fig. 9. Comparison of induction of tumour cytostatic macrophages by 12-*O*-tetradecanoylphorbol-13-acetate (TPA) and by macrophage activating factor (MAF)
Macrophages ($4 \times 10^4$) were incubated with Eb lymphoma cells ($2 \times 10^4$) in 0.2 ml medium with or without the addition of TPA ($10^{-8}$ mol/L) and MAF (1%). After 48 h, proliferation of Eb lymphoma cells was determined in the tumour growth inhibition assay by $^3$H-thymidine incorporation into tumour DNA. Values are the means ± SD of four separate incubations.

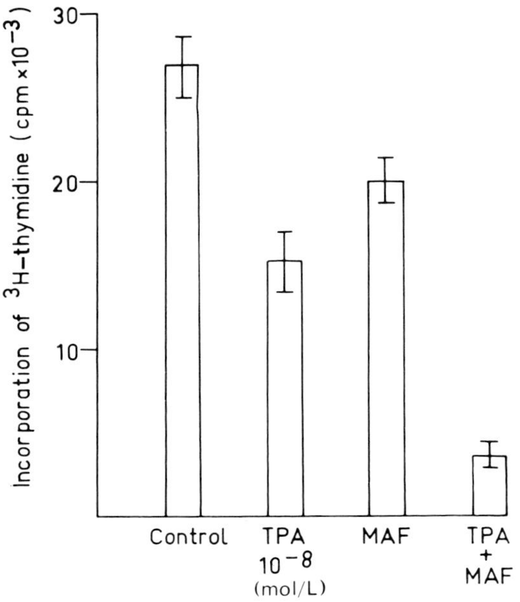


be particularly hydrogen peroxide-sensitive in order to be lysed within four hours of incubation, and tumour lysis was not detectable before 16 h of exposure to TPA-treated macrophages.

Our observations and those of others (Schultz *et al.,* 1980; Laskin *et al.,* 1981; Weinberg, 1981) indicate that TPA is capable of generating tumour cytotoxic macrophages, although other workers have reported opposite results (Keller, 1979; Fish *et al.,* 1981; Keller *et al.,* 1982). At present, it is difficult to reconcile these findings, unless the contradictions can be explained by differences in animal systems, in modes of prestimulation of macrophages, in target cell sensitivities or in the doses of TPA used to treat macrophages. Schultz *et al.* (1980) stated that an activated macrophage may be a 'two-edged sword', i.e., the mode and strength of activation may determine whether stimulation or inhibition of tumour cell growth occurs.

Our findings do not support the data published by Keller *et al.* (1982) demonstrating that TPA interferes directly with the activation and effector phase of tumour cytotoxic macrophages. In our hands, TPA activation of macrophages was further enhanced by MAF from a T-cell clone (Gemsa *et al.,* 1983), suggesting an additive or synergistic action of the two compounds. Thus, the hypothesis that

Fig. 10. Comparison of induction of tumour cytolytic macrophages by 12-*O*-tetradecanoylphorbol-13-acetate (TPA) and by macrophage activating factor (MAF)
Macrophages ($0.2 \times 10^6$/0.2 ml) were preincubated for 24 h with TPA ($10^{-7}$ mol/L) and MAF (5%). After four washings, macrophage cultures were incubated with $4 \times 10^4$ $^3$H-thymidine labelled Eb tumour cells, and, after 48 h, specific $^3$H-thymidine release was determined. Values are the means ± SD of four separate incubations.

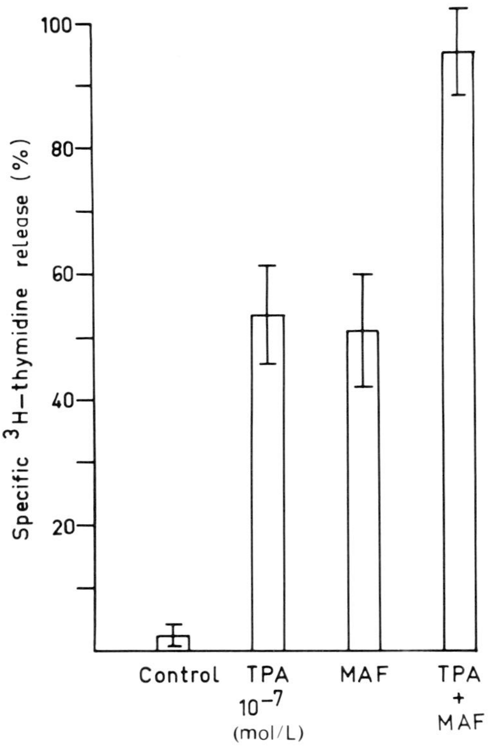


tumour promoters act by interfering with natural anti-tumour effector systems (e.g., MAF-activated macrophages) may have to be re-evaluated.

A number of questions remain open with regard to TPA-induced macrophage activation: (1) TPA may activate macrophages to tumour cytotoxicity by altering membrane fluidity, thus facilitating cell-to-cell contact between macrophage effector cells and tumour target cells. (2) TPA may activate certain enzyme systems or metabolic pathways required for macrophage tumour cytotoxicity, by-passing stimulation of receptors for physiological (e.g., MAF) macrophage activation. (3) TPA may have a high affinity for MAF receptors and may thereby mimic the action of MAF in the same way that opiates bind to endorphin receptors. (4) TPA may bind to and stimulate part of a receptor common to many different receptors, which would explain the multitude of TPA effects observed in various cell systems (Mastro, 1983). (5) TPA may have a structural resemblance to the active receptor-binding moiety of MAF and may thereby mimic the action of MAF.

Recently, specific receptors for phorbol esters have been described on leucocytes (Sando *et al.,* 1981) and on other cells (Shoyab & Todaro, 1980; Horowitz *et al.,* 1981). Furthermore, protein kinase C has been identified as the possible phorbol ester receptor (Castagna *et al.,* 1982; Niedel *et al.,* 1983). Macrophages may be particularly suitable test cells for the study of the biochemical events following TPA receptor binding, since, upon activation with TPA and/or MAF, they respond with a large spectrum of activities. TPA may also be used as an additional or alternative agent to complement studies of lymphokines as typical macrophage-activating compounds. In addition, the investigation of the effects of TPA on macrophages may offer insights into the role of macrophages and their products during tumour promotion. Such studies may help to resolve the apparent paradox that TPA can act both as a tumour promoter and as a stimulator of natural anti-tumour defense mechanisms.

## REFERENCES

Abb, J., Bayliss, G.J. & Deinhardt, F. (1979) Lymphocyte activation by the tumor-promoting agent 12-*O*-tetradecanoylphorbol-13-acetate (TPA). *J. Immunol.,* ***122,*** 1639–1642

Brune, K., Kalin, H., Schmidt, R. & Hecker, E. (1978) Inflammatory, tumor initiating and promoting activities of polycyclic aromatic hydrocarbons and diterpene esters in mouse skin as compared with their prostaglandin releasing potency *in vitro. Cancer Lett.,* ***4,*** 333–342

Castagna, M., Takai, Y., Kaibuchi, K., Sano, K., Kikkawa, U. & Nishizuka, Y. (1982) Direct activation of calcium-activated, phospholipid-dependent protein kinase by tumor-promoting phorbol esters. *J. biol. Chem.,* ***257,*** 7847–7851

Cohn, Z.A. (1978) The activation of mononuclear phagocytes: fact, fancy, and future. *J. Immunol.,* ***121,*** 813–816

Fish, L.A., Baxter, C.S. & Bash, J.A. (1981) Inhibition of macrophage-induced tumor cell cytostasis and cytolysis by tumor-promoting phorbol diesters. *Toxicology,* ***19,*** 127–138

Gemsa, D., Woo, C.H., Fudenberg, H.H. & Schmid, R. (1973) Erythrocyte catabolism by macrophages in vitro. The effect of hydrocortisone on erythrophagocytosis and on the induction of heme oxygenase. *J. clin. Invest.,* ***52,*** 812–822

Gemsa, D., Seitz, M., Kramer, W., Till, G. & Resch, K. (1978) The effects of phagocytosis, dextran sulfate, and cell damage on $PGE_1$ sensitivity and $PGE_1$ production of macrophages. *J. Immunol.,* ***120,*** 1187–1194

Gemsa, D., Kramer, W., Napierski, I., Bärlin, E., Till, G. & Resch, K. (1981) Potentiation of macrophage tumor cytostasis by tumor-induced ascites. *J. Immunol.,* ***126,*** 2143–2150

Gemsa, D., Debatin, K.-M., Kramer, W., Kubelka, C., Deichmann, W., Kees, U. & Krammer, P.H. (1983) Macrophage-activating factors from different T cell clones induce distinct macrophage functions. *J. Immunol.,* ***131,*** 833–844

Grimm, W., Bärlin, E., Leser, H.-G., Kramer, W. & Gemsa, D. (1980) Induction of tumor cytostatic macrophages by 12-*O*-tetradecanoyl phorbol-13-acetate (TPA). *Clin. Immunol. Immunopathol.*, ***17***, 617–628

Hammond, M.E. & Dvorak, H.F. (1972) Antigen-induced stimulation of glucosamine incorporation by guinea pig peritoneal macrophages in delayed hypersensitivity. *J. exp. Med.*, ***136***, 1518–1532

Hammond, M.E., Selvaggio, S.S. & Dvorak, H.F. (1975) Antigen-enhanced glucosamine incorporation by peritoneal macrophages in cell-mediated hypersensitivity. I. Studies on biology and mechanism. *J. Immunol.*, ***115***, 914–921

Hoidal, J.R., Repine. J.E., Beall, G.D., Rasp, F.L. & White, J.G. (1978) The effect of phorbol myristate acetate on the metabolism and ultrastructure of human alveolar macrophages. *Am. J. Pathol.*, ***91***, 469–482

Horowitz, A.D., Greenebaum, E. & Weinstein, I.B. (1981) Identification of receptors for phorbol ester tumor promoters in intact mammalian cells and of an inhibitor of receptor binding in biologic fluids. *Proc. natl Acad. Sci. USA*, ***78***, 2315–2319

Johnston, R.B., Godzik, C.A. & Cohn, Z.A. (1978) Increased superoxide anion production by immunologically activated and chemically elicited macrophages. *J. exp. Med.*, ***148***, 115–127

Karnovski, M.L. & Lazdins, J.K. (1978) Biochemical criteria for activated macrophages. *J. Immunol.*, ***121***, 809–813

Keller, R. (1979) Suppression of natural antitumour defense mechanisms by phorbol esters. *Nature*, ***282***, 729–731

Keller, R., Keist, R., Adolf, W., Opferkuch, H.J., Schmidt, R. & Hecker, E. (1982) Tumor-promoting diterpene esters prevent macrophage activation and suppress macrophage tumoricidal capacity. *Exp. Cell Biol.*, ***50***, 121–134

Kirchner, H., Muchmore, A.V., Chused, T.M., Holden, H.T. & Heberman, R.B. (1975) Inhibition of proliferation of lymphoma cells and T lymphocytes by suppressor cells from spleens of tumor-bearing mice. *J. Immunol.*, ***114***, 206–210

Kolb, J.-P. B., Senik, A. & Castagna, M. (1981) In vitro stimulation of mouse NK cell activity by phorbol esters: A pathway different from interferon-induced activation. *Cell Immunol.*, ***65***, 258–271

Krammer, P.H., Kaltmann, B., Echtenacher, B., Gemsa, D., Hamann, U., Hültner, L., Kees, U., Kubelka, C. & Marcucci, F. (1983) Immune interferon, macrophage activating factors, and colony stimulating factors secreted by T cell clones in limiting dilution microcultures, long term cultures, and by T cell hybridomas. *Immunol. Rev.*, ***76***, 5–28

Laskin, D.L., Laskin, J.D., Weinstein, I.B. & Carchman, R.A. (1980) Modulation of phagocytosis by tumor promoters and epidermal growth factor in normal and transformed macrophages. *Cancer Res.*, ***40***, 1028–1035

Laskin, D.L., Laskin, J.D., Kessler, F.K., Weinstein, I.B. & Carchman, R.A. (1981) Enhancement of macrophage-induced cytotoxicity by phorbol ester tumor promoters. *Cancer Res.*, ***41***, 4523–4528

Mastro, A.M. (1982) Phorbol esters: Tumor promotion, cell regulation, and the immune response. *Lymphokines*, ***6***, 263–313

Nathan, C.F. & Root, R.K. (1977) Hydrogen peroxide release from mouse peritoneal macrophages. Dependence on sequential activation and triggering. *J. exp. Med.*, ***146***, 1648–1662

Nathan, C.F., Brukner, L.H., Silverstein, S.C. & Cohn, Z.A. (1979) Extracellular cytolysis by activated macrophages and granulocytes. *J. exp. Med.*, ***149***, 84–99

Niedel, J.E., Kuhn, L.J. & Vandenbark, G.R. (1983) Phorbol diester receptor copurifies with protein kinase C. *Proc. natl Acad. Sci. USA*, ***80***, 36–40

North, R.J. (1978) The concept of the activated macrophage. *J. Immunol.*, ***121***, 806–809

Phaire-Washington, L., Wang, E. & Silverstein, S.C. (1980) Phorbol myristate acetate stimulates pinocytosis and membrane spreading in mouse peritoneal macrophages. *J. Cell Biol.*, ***86***, 634–640

Ramos, O.F., Masucci, M.G., Bejarano, M.T. & Klein, E. (1983) The tumor promoter phorbol-12,13-dibutyrate $P(Bu)_2$ stimulates cytotoxic activity of human blood lymphocytes. *Immunobiology*, ***165***, 403–414

Sando, J.J., Hilfiker, M.L., Salomon, D.S. & Farrar, J.J. (1981) Specific receptors for phorbol esters in lymphoid cell populations: Role in enhanced production of T-cell growth factor. *Proc. natl Acad. Sci. USA*, ***78***, 1189–1193

Schultz, R.M., Chirigos, M.A. & Olkowski, Z.L. (1980) Stimulation and inhibition of neoplastic cell growth by tumor promoter-treated macrophages. *Cell. Immunol.*, ***54***, 98–106

Seitz, M., Deimann, W., Gram, N., Hunstein, W. & Gemsa, D. (1982) Characterization of blood mononuclear cells of rheumatoid arthritis patients. I. Depressed lymphocyte proliferation and enhanced prostanoid release from monocytes. *Clin. Immunol. Immunopathol.*, ***25***, 405–416

Shoyab, M. & Todaro, G.J. (1980) Specific high affinity cell membrane receptors for biologically active phorbol and ingenol esters. *Nature*, ***288***, 451–455

Steinman, R.M. & Cohn, Z.A. (1972) Interaction of soluble horseradish peroxidase with mouse peritoneal macrophages *in vitro*. *J. Cell Biol.*, ***55***, 186–204

Touraine, J.-L., Hadden, J.W., Touraine, F., Hadden, E.M., Estensen, R. & Good, R.A. (1977) Phorbol myristate acetate: A mitogen selective for a T-lymphocyte subpopulation. *J. exp. Med.*, ***145***, 460–465

Vassalli, J.-D., Hamilton, J. & Reich, E. (1977) Macrophage plasminogen activator: Induction by concanavalin A and phorbol myristate acetate. *Cell*, ***11***, 695–705

Weinberg, J.B. (1981) Tumor cell killing by phorbol ester-differentiated human leukemia cells. *Science*, ***213***, 655–657

Wertz, P.W. & Mueller, G.C. (1978) Rapid stimulation of phospholipid metabolism in bovine lymphocytes by tumor-promoting phorbol esters. *Cancer Res.*, ***38***, 2900–2904

Whitfield, J.F., MacManus, J.P. & Gillan, D.J. (1973) Calcium-dependent stimulation by a phorbol ester (PMA) of thymic lymphoblast DNA synthesis and proliferation. *J. Cell Physiol.*, ***82***, 151–156

# MODELS OF MULTI-STAGE CARCINOGENESIS IN EPIDEMIOLOGY

# EPIDEMIOLOGICAL DATA AND MULTISTAGE CARCINOGENESIS

N.E. DAY

*Unit of Biostatistics, International Agency for Research on Cancer, 150 cours Albert Thomas, 69372 Lyon Cedex 08, France*

## SUMMARY

The purpose of this review has been to demonstrate that a wide range of epidemiological phenomena can be described in terms of simple multistage models of carcinogenesis. The relationship of cancer risk with the different time variables considered corresponds closely with the behaviour predicted by theories of multistage process. Furthermore, the different behaviour associated with different agents enables one to attempt some classification as to how an agent is acting. There is considerable conformity between the tentative classification one might propose for the few agents for which epidemiological data are adequate, and the activity seen experimentally for these agents.

The purpose of using multistage models in epidemiology is not simply descriptive. A distant goal would be the use of experimental information on mechanisms of action for the prediction of human risk. Information currently available is clearly insufficient, but the consistency seen between the epidemiological and experimental results suggests that some progress may be possible.

## INTRODUCTION

Multistage theories of carcinogenesis have two major roots, one experimental, one epidemiological. For many years, the early experimental work on tumour promotion in the mouse skin was looked upon as an oddity of no general significance, and the models of multistage carcinogenesis proposed in an epidemiological setting to explain the generally similar shape of age-incidence curves were not regarded as fruitful in a broader setting. In more recent years, however, it has become clear both that, in many organ systems, the multistage nature of the carcinogenic process can be demonstrated experimentally and that, in epidemiology, multistage models are capable of drawing into a single coherent framework a much wider array of observation than population age-incidence curves. The epidemiological formulation of multistage models may appear unduly mathematical, but the abstraction is necessary to provide the link between qualitative description of events at the cellular level and quantitative description of cancer risk in human populations.

The experimental demonstration of the multistage nature of tumour induction has followed a direct approach. Event A followed by event B induces tumours while A or B alone does not, where A and B can probably be further subdivided into sequential series of events. Each event can be described relatively well, and the name attached to it, 'initiation' or 'promotion', for example, can be well defined. By contrast, in epidemiology causative events rarely occur in such well identifiable sequence, equivalent, for example, to that of an initiation-promotion experiment. The reasoning that leads one to think that the cancer induction process is multistage is indirect. Thus, although one may conclude that a certain agent plays a role late in the induction of a certain tumour, the epidemiological evidence alone would usually be insufficient to justify use of the term 'promotion' in the strict experimental sense. This is especially true now that a late-stage effect for initiating agents has been demonstrated (Scherer & Emmelot, this volume). The lack of a clear one-to-one relationship between experimentally-demonstrated stages and epidemiologically-inferred stages suggests that, in epidemiology, the use of the terms 'initiation' and 'promotion' is best avoided, and the less specific terms 'early-' and 'late-stage' action are to be preferred.

In this paper, we consider first the area in which multistage models have made their greatest impact in epidemiology – the role of time and age in determining cancer risk. We then look at a particular cancer, that of the female breast, to indicate how further elaboration of these concepts can provide a coherent description of a wide range of risk factors.

## THE ROLE OF TIME AND AGE IN DETERMINING CANCER RISK

### *General considerations*

We start by reviewing some of the relevant epidemiological data. For many tumours, the most striking differences in risk between different sections of the population are related to age. For the more common cancers, there are differences of several hundred fold between the incidence in the young and in the old (Waterhouse *et al.,* 1982). For many cancers, especially those of epithelial origin which are not hormone-dependent, there is a striking similarity in the form of the relationship between age and incidence (Fig. 1) (Cook *et al.,* 1969). There are, however, some major exceptions; but these exceptions, when examined more closely, are often cancers that comport rapid temporal changes in risk. Lung cancer is an example. When age-incidence curves for lung cancer are considered cross-sectionally, so that the incidence at different ages refers to different groups of individuals who were probably at different underlying risk, a different picture from that shown in Figure 1 is seen. When incidence at different ages is considered in the same groups of

Fig. 1. Age-specific incidence of stomach cancer in three populations
From Waterhouse *et al.* (1976). Number of cases shown by each point. ▲, Japan (Miyagi); X, UK (Birmingham); ●, US (Connecticut)

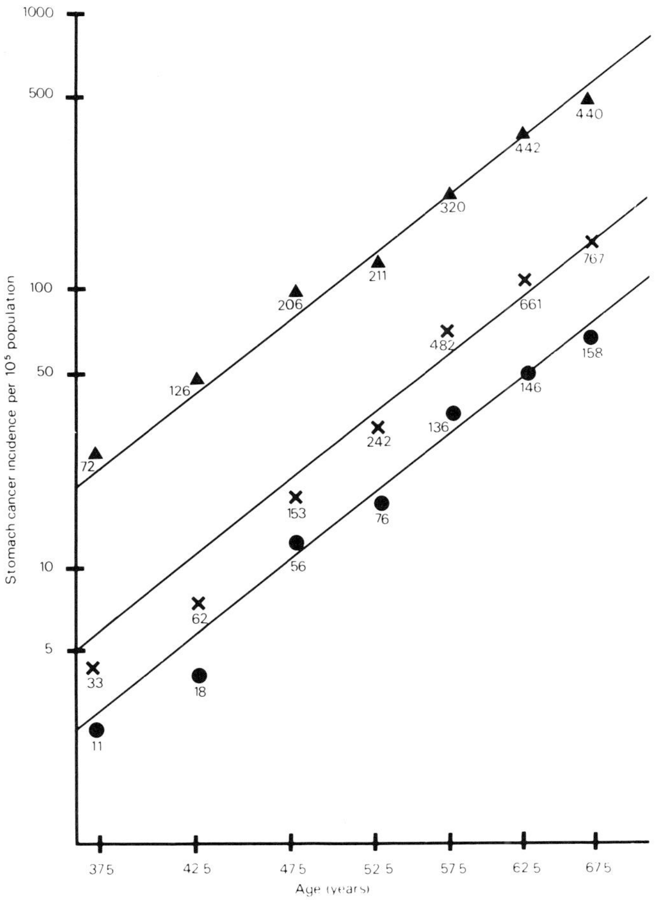


individuals, i.e., on a cohort basis, an altered pattern emerges. Rates increase in a manner parallel to that seen for other cancers, as a power of age (Doll, 1971) (usually between the fourth and fifth). Extension of this approach has demonstrated a similar finding for other cancers, of the larynx, for example, or malignant melanoma (Boyle *et al.,* 1983). The degree of consistency is such that the interest now lies in cancers for which the change of risk with age is clearly of a different pattern. Breast cancer is considered in detail in a later section. Childhood tumours, which might be thought to represent a different type of process, have been considered in multistage terms (Moolgavkar & Venzon, 1979), but with different dynamics for the cell population at risk. An intriguing similarity of age curves is seen for those of cancer of the uterine

Fig. 2. Age-specific incidence of nasopharyngeal carcinoma among Singapore Chinese males (○) and of carcinoma of the cervix uteri among Danish females (●)

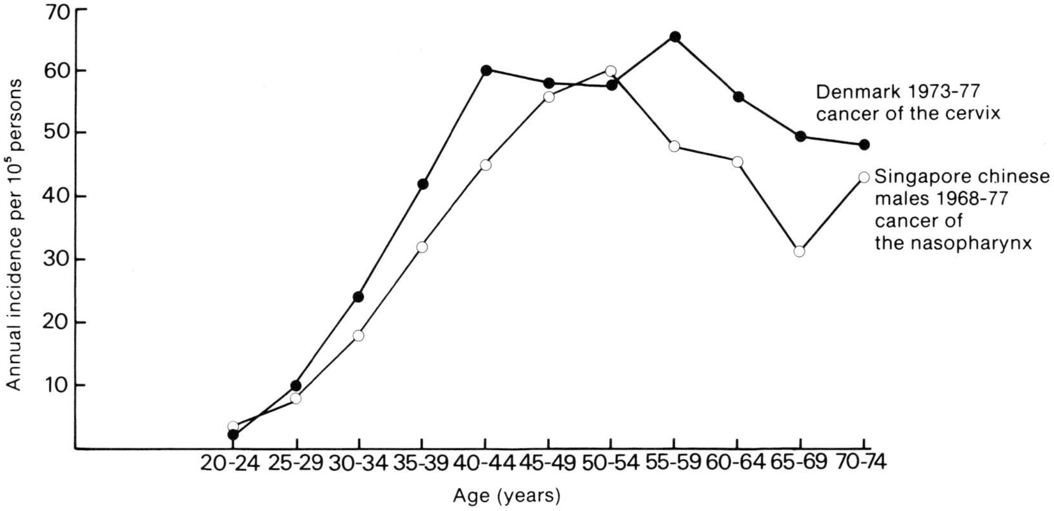


Fig. 3. Age-specific mortality rates from lung cancer for smokers and non-smokers From Doll (1971). ●, cigarette smokers by duration of smoking; ○, cigarette smokers by age; x, non-smokers by age

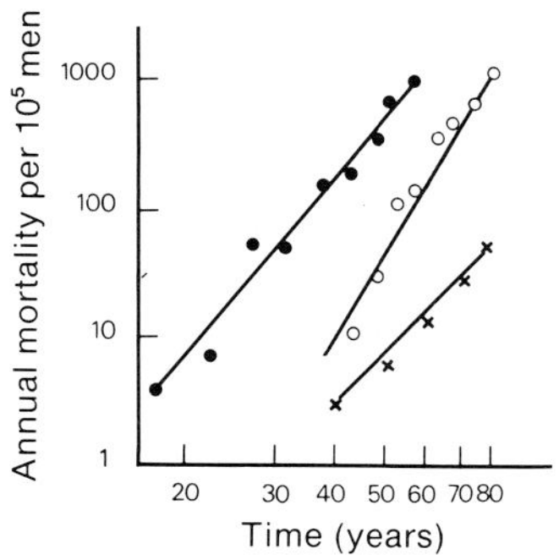


cervix and of cancer of the nasopharynx among the Chinese (Fig. 2) (Shanmugaratnam *et al.*, 1983). The great majority of tumours at these two sites are carcinomas; both have been related to viruses.

Provocative as this consistency of behaviour may be, it can be related to the carcinogenic process only in general terms, since the causative agents have not been specified, nor how exposure to these agents may have varied over time. It is assumed for most tumours that, at least within birth cohorts, exposure is fairly constant over time.

For specific exposures, known to cause particular tumours, and for which the excess risk has been followed over time, a picture emerges, that, although more complex, is of considerably more interest. Different epidemiological behaviour is seen for different agents, and these differences can be seen as the natural consequences of multistage carcinogenesis, which we now explore.

*Exposures of limited duration*

Between single-shot and continuous lifetime exposures, one can clearly consider a wide range of types of intermittent or limited exposure. We consider continuous exposure of limited duration and concentrate on what appear to be two features of particular importance – the age at which exposure starts and the time period after exposure stops. For both situations, it is of critical importance to consider at what stage in the carcinogenic process the exposure acts.

For continuous exposure throughout life, excess incidence of many tumours is related to some power of age:

$$I(t) \ \alpha \ (\text{age})^{k-1}$$

in the traditional Armitage-Doll formulation (Armitage & Doll, 1961) of a k-stage process (see Fig. 1). More recent models that allow for differential growth rates for 'initiated' cells, and age dependence of the number of cells at risk, are perhaps more biologically appealing, but they require more specific parameters the values of which are at present unobservable. In many respects, both models give similar results. We use, as a descriptive tool, the Armitage-Doll model.

If a cancer is rare in the absence of the exposure of interest, then, for exposures starting, say, in early adult life and then remaining continuous, the analogous expression becomes:

$$\text{incidence} \ \alpha \ (\text{duration of exposure})^{k-1}.$$

Such behaviour is seen for lung cancer among cigarette smokers (Doll, 1971) and for mesothelioma among asbestos-exposed workers (Peto *et al.,* 1982) and corresponds closely to the age-related risk for skin tumours among mice following skin painting with benzo[*a*]pyrene (Peto *et al.,* 1975).

(i) *Age at start of exposure*

If, however, there is a spontaneous incidence of the disease unrelated to the exposure in question, then the relationship of the excess risk to time since the exposure started will depend on how the exposure acts in relation to the agents underlying the spontaneous risk. If the exposure makes its greatest contribution early in the carcinogenic process, one type of behaviour will be seen; if at a late stage, then a different behaviour will be observed. In particular, if the exposure acts predominantly at the first stage, then for continuous exposure starting at some time $t_0$, one expects the associated excess incidence to be a function, as before, of duration of exposure:

$$\text{excess incidence } \alpha \text{ (duration of exposure)}^{k-1}.$$

When the exposure acts at a late stage (in terms of the Armitage-Doll model at the penultimate stage), then excess risk following the start, at time $t_0$, of continuous exposure rises as a function of

$$(\text{age})^{k-1} - (t_0)^{k-1}.$$

Examination of these two expressions indicates a clear difference. Excess risk associated with early-stage agents will rise more rapidly than the general increase in risk with age, whereas for late-stage agents the excess risk rises in parallel with the general increase in incidence [i.e., the term $(t_0)^{k-1}$ has little weight once age, say, is more than twice $t_0$]. The difference in epidemiological behaviour of the effect of age at first exposure can be expressed by saying that, for a given duration of exposure, with early-stage agents the *absolute* excess risk is independent of the age at which exposure starts, whereas with late-stage agents it is the *relative* excess risk (relative to the risk among the non-exposed) that is roughly independent of age.

A more rapid rise in incidence among the exposed is exactly what is seen for lung cancer (see Fig. 3) (Doll, 1971) among cigarette smokers, when compared with lung cancer among non-smokers. The incidence rises as the fourth to fifth power of duration of smoking, similar to the age curve among non-smokers. In addition, the absolute excess risk of lung cancer for cigarette smokers changes little with the age at which smoking was started, given the duration of smoking (Table 1). Both these aspects of the relationship between smoking and lung cancer suggest that cigarette smoke is responsible for most of the early-stage events leading to lung cancer among smokers.

Table 1. Effect of age at starting to smoke on mortality from lung cancer (from Appendix Table D of Kahn, 1966)

| Age at starting to smoke (years) | Annual mortality rates per $10^5$ population Age (years) | |
|---|---|---|
| | 55–64 | 65–74 |
| <15 | 251 | 478 |
| 15–19 | 168 | 350 |
| 20–24 | 99 | 241 |
| 25+ | 53 | 162 |

Dotted lines connect groups with approximately the same duration of smoking.

Apart from cigarette smoking, epidemiological data are available for certain other exposures:

For *asbestos*, the induction of mesothelioma appears to be independent of age at exposure, and, as mentioned before, asbestos appears to be responsible for most of

Fig. 4. Cumulative risk of dying of mesothelioma in the absence of other causes of death among North American insulation workers first exposed to asbestos at age 15–24 (– – –), 25–34 (——), or over 35 (. . .), plotted against age (upper graph) and against years since exposure (lower graph) From Peto *et al.*, 1982

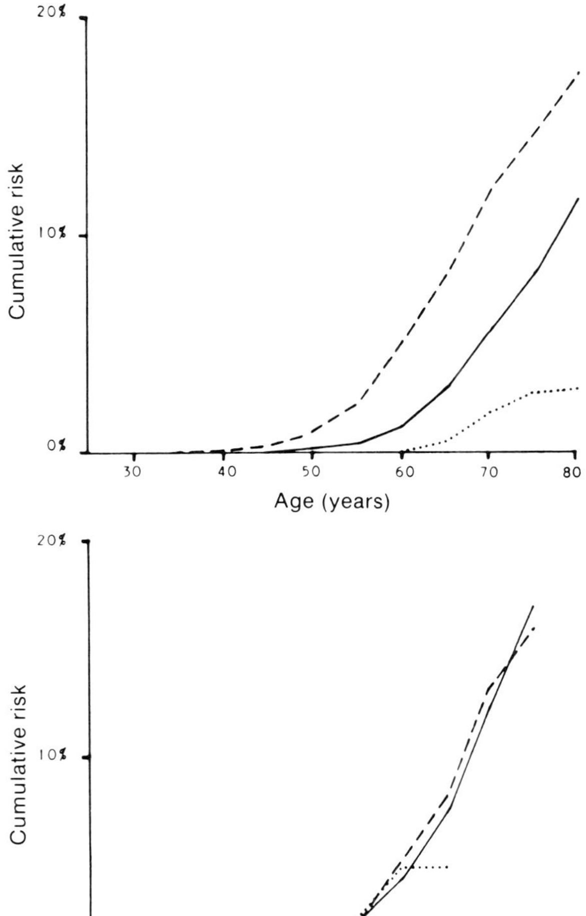


the early-stage events in mesothelioma induction (Fig. 4) (Peto *et al.*, 1982). By contrast, the excess risk of lung cancer among those exposed to asbestos rises rapidly with age at exposure, the relative risk varying only slightly with age (Table 2) (Selikoff *et al.*, 1973). Asbestos would, therefore, seem to play an important late-stage role in lung cancer induction.

The effect of age at exposure on excess risk of cancer following exposure to *ionizing radiation* is striking, the excess absolute risk rising rapidly with age at exposure for

Table 2. Expected and observed deaths from lung cancer among 17 800 asbestos insulation workers, 1 January 1967–31 December 1971; distribution by age at onset of exposure (from Selikoff *et al.*, 1973)

| Age at onset of exposure (years) | No. of deaths from lung cancer | | |
|---|---|---|---|
| | Expected[a] | Observed | Ratio |
| <25 | 18.19 | 102 | 5.61 |
| 25–34 | 15.20 | 66 | 4.34 |
| 35–44 | 8.78 | 38 | 4.33 |
| 45+ | 2.25 | 7 | 3.11 |

[a] Based upon age-specific death rate data from the US National Office of Vital Statistics. Rates for 1968–1971 were extrapolated from rates for 1961–1967.

Table 3. Lung cancer risks associated with exposure to arsenic: effect of age at first employment (from Brown & Chu, 1982)

| Age at initial employment (years) | Person-years at risk | Adjusted excess mortality rate/$10^{-3}$ population |
|---|---|---|
| <20 | 62 854 | 3.1 |
| 20–29 | 73 610 | 4.2 |
| 30–39 | 35 290 | 11.3 |
| 40–49 | 18 663 | 21.6 |
| 50+ | 6 932 | 27.5 |

most sites and the relative risk remaining roughly constant (Advisory Committee on the Biological Effects of Ionizing Radiations, 1980). Sites at which excess cancer risk does not follow this pattern include breast (Boice *et al.*, 1979) and thyroid (Advisory Committee on the Biological Effects of Ionizing Radiations, 1980). For leukaemia, the constancy of the relative risk is seen only in adult life, the effect of exposure in children being very much greater (Kato & Schull, 1982). This late-stage effect for ionizing radiation is surprising, given its ability to cause the type of genetic damage one would associate with early-stage events; this is discussed below.

The excess of lung cancer among people exposed to *arsenic* has been studied extensively in smelter workers in the USA. Absolute excess risk rises rapidly with age at first employment (see Table 3), although perhaps not as rapidly as is required for the relative excess to be the same at different ages; it is clear that the main effect of arsenic does not occur at an early stage (Brown & Chu, 1982; Lee-Feldstein, 1983).

Similar behaviour is seen for cancer of the nasal sinuses among people exposed to *nickel* compounds while working at a nickel smelter in South Wales, the absolute risk rising rapidly with increasing age at first employment (Table 4) (Doll *et al.*, 1970; Peto *et al.*, 1983). The effect of age at first exposure on excess risk for lung cancer among

Table 4. Number of men developing nasal-sinus cancer by age at first employment and number expected[a] after standardizing for year of employment and calendar year of observation (from Doll *et al.*, 1970)

| Age at first employment (years) | No. of men developing nasal sinus cancer | | Observed as proportion of expected |
|---|---|---|---|
| | Observed | Expected[a] | |
| Under 20 | 2 | 5.36 | 0.37 |
| 20–24 | 9 | 11.30 | 0.80 |
| 25–29 | 13 | 12.26 | 1.06 |
| 30–34 | 8 | 6.34 | 1.26 |
| 35 or over | 8 | 4.73 | 1.69 |
| All ages | 40 | 39.99 | – |

$\chi^2$ for trend = 5.12, n = 1, $P \simeq 0.03$
[a] If age at first employment had no effect on susceptibility to cancer induction

the same cohort is less clear, obscured perhaps by the rapidly changing rates in lung cancer in the general population during the extensive period of follow-up. It is possible, given results from Norway (Magnus *et al.*, 1982) suggesting that the excess risks associated with nickel and tobacco combine additively, that further analysis of these data using more complex statistical models (Thomas, 1981) will help to elucidate the picture, and that the nickel-associated risk combines additively with a rapidly increasing baseline risk.

Large excess risks for lung cancer have also been observed following exposure to *chloromethyl ethers* (Pasternack & Shore, 1981; Weiss, 1982) and to *chromium* compounds (Hayes, 1982). Explicit analysis of the epidemiological data do not appear to have been performed in terms of age at first exposure to either type of compound; however, in both cases, there are indications that lung tumours occur unusually early. Since, for given length of exposure, higher relative risks at a younger age would be consistent with absolute risks being independent of age, there is an indication that both exposures have early-stage effects.

(ii) *Time since exposure stopped*

The second main aspect of risk related to exposures of limited duration concerns the evolution of risk after exposure stops (Day & Brown, 1980). In practical terms, this evolution is of major importance, since it reflects the rapidity with which the benefits expected from intervention measures will be realized. One wants to know how soon risk falls after exposure stops.

Using, as before, the Armitage-Doll model, one can examine the predictions of multistage theory on the evolution of risk following removal of early-stage agents and of late-stage agents. We shall consider exposures that start at age $t_0$ and stop at age $t_1$. For agents affecting the first stage (taken as synonymous with early stage), the absolute excess risk after exposure stops is given by:

$$\text{excess risk at age t } \alpha \ (t-t_0)^{k-1} - (t-t_1)^{k-1}.$$

Fig. 5. Effect of stopping exposure at 20 years of age when carcinogenic exposure started at birth. Age-specific incidence (From Day & Brown, 1980)

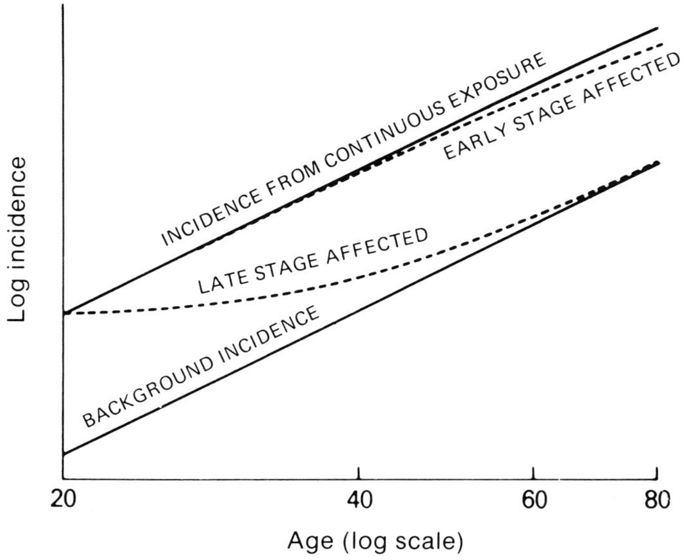


This expression indicates that excess risk will continue to rise almost as a function of $(t-t_0)^{k-1}$ for a considerable time after exposure. Typical curves are shown in Figure 5.

By contrast, if the penultimate stage is affected, the absolute excess cancer risk after exposure stops is given by:

$$\text{excess risk at age } t \ \alpha \ t_1^{k-1} - t_0^{k-1}.$$

This risk, as can be seen, is independent of t. That is, the absolute excess freezes at the value it had reached at the time exposure stopped. Since, for many tumours, risk will increase as $t^{k-1}$ increases, a constant absolute excess risk implies a rapidly decreasing relative risk. In the subsequent discussion, the distinction between constant absolute excess risk and decreasing relative excess risk needs to be borne in mind.

If the last stage is affected, then excess risk disappears as soon as exposure ceases. This is the behaviour one would expect in a single-stage process and it is perhaps the most convincing demonstration of the multistage nature of cancer induction that this sudden removal of excess is seldom observed. For almost all exposures, the continuation of some excess risk after exposure ceases suggests strongly that intermediate stages in cancer induction have been produced, with an irreversible tendency to manifest themselves in the future as the appearance of more cancers than would otherwise occur. The risk for endometrial cancer induced by exogenous oestrogens is the only well-documented occasion in cancer epidemiology where absolute excess risk disappears after exposure stops (Jick *et al.,* 1979, 1980), i.e., the only example, to date, of a *last*-stage agent.

For other agents, most of which were considered in the previous section, the distinction is made between early- and late-stage action, where 'late' corresponds to the penultimate stage (in the Armitage-Doll formulation) and not to the last stage.

The risk of lung cancer for ex-smokers has been particularly well documented (Doll & Peto, 1976). The evolution of incidence after stopping smoking corresponds well to a freezing of the absolute excess risk, with the relative risk falling rapidly towards unity (see Table 5). Thus, in terms of the effect of stopping exposure, the major effect of cigarette smoke is on late-stage events, in contrast to the conclusion drawn from the effect of age at starting to smoke.

By contrast, the effect of ionizing radiation leads to the opposite conclusion. Much of the evidence for the carcinogenic effect of ionizing radiation comes from short, or almost instantaneous, exposures, such as the atomic bomb explosions in Japan (Kato & Schull, 1982) and short courses of radiotherapy for a variety of malignant (Day & Boice, 1984) and non-malignant conditions (Smith & Doll, 1982). Except for leukaemia, and perhaps bone tumours, risk starts to rise ten or so years after exposure. In many studies (Beebe, 1982), although not all (Smith & Doll, 1982), the relative risk rises to a plateau at which it remains or even increases up to 30 years after exposure (Fig. 6). This behaviour is consistent only with a major early-stage effect, in contrast to what we saw earlier where the effect of age at exposure suggested a major role for late-stage effects.

For arsenic exposures, the conclusions based on risk after stopping exposure are more consistent with conclusions based on the effect of age at starting exposure. The risk of lung cancer among the Montana smelters exposed to arsenic, after the exposure stops, suggests a fall in the relative risk and fairly constant absolute excess risks (Brown & Chu, 1982). This effect is confined, however, to those aged over 55 years on leaving employment. The data on chloromethyl ethers are limited, but there is an indication that the excess relative risk remains high for 15 to 25 years after exposure (Table 6) (Pasternack & Shore, 1981).

Table 5. Evolution of mortality from lung cancer among ex-cigarette smokers (from Doll & Peto, 1976)

| Measurement | Years since smoking stopped | | | | |
|---|---|---|---|---|---|
| | 0 | <5 | 5–9 | 11–14 | >15 |
| No. of deaths among ex-smokers[a] | | 10 | 12 | 8 | 7 |
| No. of deaths as percent of no. expected among continuing smokers | 100 | 68 | 35 | 25 | 11 |
| No. of deaths divided by no. expected among lifelong nonsmokers | 15.8 | 10.7 | 5.9 | 4.7 | 2.0 |

[a] Excluding those who stopped smoking after developing lung cancer

Fig. 6. Observed to expected ratios of cancers at sites close to and at intermediate distance from the cervix, excluding uterine cancers, by time since diagnosis of cervical cancer for invasive cervical cancer patients treated with radiotherapy; 80% confidence intervals presented (From Day & Boice, 1984)

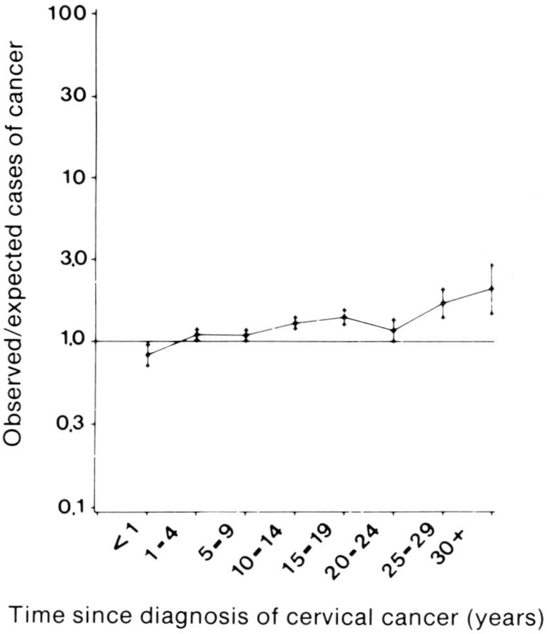


Table 6. Lung cancer mortality after exposure to chloromethyl ethers (from Pasternack & Shore, 1981)

| | Years since last exposure | | | | |
|---|---|---|---|---|---|
| | None | 1–4 | 5–9 | 10–14 | 15–25 |
| Observed deaths | 3 | 6 | 2 | 5 | 7 |
| Expected deaths | 3.8 | 3.2 | 3.5 | 6.4 | 6.0 |
| Relative risk[a] | 1.0 | 2.3 | 0.7 | 1.0 | 1.5 |

[a] Compared to a continuously exposed group

(iii) *Interpretation of time effects*

The results presented in the earlier sections of this paper indicate that a diversity of epidemiological observations can be interpreted in the framework of multistage models for cancer induction. It is clear, however, that some inconsistencies arise in these interpretations, with the same agent appearing to affect predominantly different stages on different occasions. Some of these inconsistencies arise because the environmental exposures under consideration consist of complex mixtures, different constituents of which may play a different role. Thus, cigarette smoke contains powerful genotoxic compounds capable of inducing early-stage events and other consituents with behaviour more like that of tumour promoters (Doll & Hill, 1964). Since most cases of lung cancer among smokers are due to cigarette smoke, it is hardly surprising if it provides the stimulus for most of the early- and of the late-stage events.

Other exposures, such as ionizing radiation, are not mixtures in this sense. However, it is becoming clear that agents that affect early stages may also play an important role in later stages as well, as demonstrated by the so-called initiation-promotion-initiation experiments (Scherer & Emmelot, 1983). Classification of an agent, in terms of its intrinsic characteristics, into 'early' or 'late' stage may not be meaningful. The characterization, using epidemiological data, is made in terms of whether, given other relevant exposures operating on the organ in question, the agent provides most of the early-stage stimuli and/or most of the late-stage stimuli. It is interesting in this respect that two sites, the breast and thyroid, where ionizing radiation appears to have primarily early-stage effects and contributes less at later stages, are both sites at which endogenous late-stage (hormonal) agents are of major importance.

## EPIDEMIOLOGY OF BREAST CANCER

As an illustration of many of the concepts outlined in the earlier sections, one can consider the relationship between several of the factors identified as influencing risk for breast cancer (Moolgavkar *et al.*, 1980; Pike *et al.*, 1983). The factors we consider are age, reproductive history including age at menarche and menopause, and exogenous oestrogens. Radiation has been discussed earlier.

(i) *Age*

Recent work has shown that most populations have very similar age incidence curves, if examined on a cohort basis rather than cross-sectionally. Typical shapes are shown in Figure 7. The curve rises rapidly at young ages, flattens out in the fifth and sixth decade of life, then continues to rise, although at a slower rate than at young ages.

(ii) *Age at first birth and parity*

A larger number of studies have shown an increasing risk with increasing age at first full-term pregnancy (MacMahon *et al.*, 1970). Some studies have shown, in addition, that further full-term pregnancies (Tulinius *et al.*, 1978) after the first confer additional protection.

Fig. 7. Shapes of age-specific incidence curves of breast cancer in females from different populations after adjustment for temporal trends, and shape of incidence curve generated by the model (parameters obtained from fit to Connecticut data)
All curves have been normalized, so that the sum of the rates over all age groups is the same. Note that incidence is given on a logarithmic scale. (From Moolgavkar *et al.*, 1980)

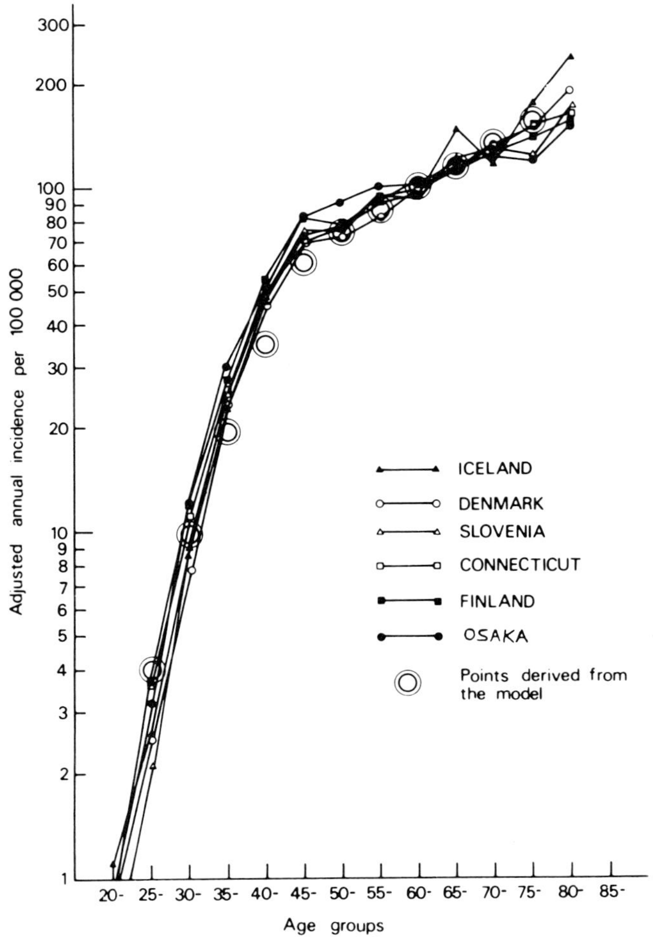


### (iii) *Age at menarche and menopause*

A consistent, if not very large, increase in risk with early menarche has been demonstrated regularly (Tulinius *et al.*, 1978). Of perhaps greater interest is the indication of a strong correlation between average age at menarche in a cohort of women and their overall risk for breast cancer. Late age at menopause increases risk to some degree, but early oopharectomy has a strong protective effect (MacMahon *et al.*, 1973).

(iv) *Exogenous oestrogens*

The effect on breast cancer risk of taking replacement oestrogens at the menopause is much less marked than the effect on risk of endometrial cancer, and several early studies showed no increase in risk. Recent, more rigorous cohort studies have shown that risk is increased, but only 10 to 15 years after beginning administration, and at most by a factor of two (Hoover *et al.*, 1976).

In addition, early induced cessation of ovarian function has a major effect on breast cancer risk. When women are treated by radiotherapy for cancer of the cervix, the ovaries would usually receive a radiation dose sufficient to inactivate them. For women under forty years of age at the time of irradiation, the effect on subsequent breast cancer risk is large (Table 7).

Most of this epidemiological behaviour can be described simply in terms of a multistage development of breast cancer, in which

(a) early-stage events begin to occur to an appreciable extent only around the time of menarche;

(b) the changes occurring in breast tissue during a full-term pregnancy render it less susceptible to early-stage events; and

(c) late-stage events are largely dependent on ovarian function and occur with greatly reduced frequency after cessation of ovarian function.

The type of age curve one would expect from such a model process is shown in Figure 7, and the predicted effect of age at first full-term pregnancy on subsequent

Table 7. Risk for breast cancer following irradiation of the ovaries (from Day & Boice, 1984)

A. By age at irradiation

| Age (years) | Observed cases | Expected cases | Relative risk |
|---|---|---|---|
| 25–39 | 41 | 115.5 | 0.35 |
| 40–49 | 186 | 264.7 | 0.70 |
| 50–59 | 201 | 249.7 | 0.80 |
| 60–69 | 140 | 175.4 | 0.80 |
| 70+ | 70 | 85.5 | 0.82 |

B. Among women aged less than 40 years at irradiation

| Breast cancer cases | Time since irradiation (years) | | | | | | |
|---|---|---|---|---|---|---|---|
| | <1 | 1–4 | 5–9 | 10–14 | 15–19 | 20+ | Total |
| Observed | 2 | 9 | 9 | 13 | 5 | 3 | 41 |
| Expected | 3.98 | 18.1 | 29.1 | 28.9 | 18.9 | 16.5 | 115.4 |
| Relative risk | 0.51 | 0.50 | 0.31 | 0.45 | 0.26 | 0.18 | 0.36 |

Fig. 8. Observed risks for women of different ages at first full-term pregnancy relative to first full-term pregnancy at age 20 (●), compared with predictions from the model (○) (From Day, 1982)

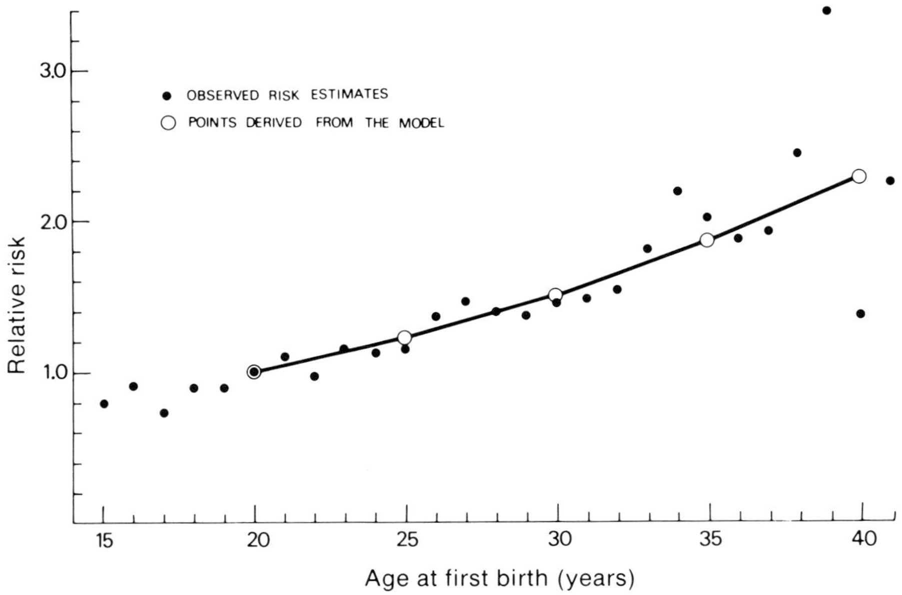


breast cancer risk is shown, compared to the observed risks, in Figure 8. The effect of age at menarche can be predicted roughly in terms of time since menarche raised to the fourth power, up to menopause, and increasing slowly thereafter. The risk of breast cancer associated with menarche at less than 12 years of age, relative to menarche at the age of 16 years or more is, for a woman aged 50, $(38/33)^4 = 1.76$, which corresponds well with observation (Tulinius *et al.*, 1978).

The effect on breast cancer risk of eliminating ovarian function (as shown in Table 7) is very similar to the effect on lung cancer risk of stopping smoking (seen in Table 5), particularly with regard to the evolution of the diminished risk with time since exposure ceased.

The effect of oestrogen replacement therapy at menopause might be expected to retard the turning over of the age-incidence curve. If (see Fig. 7) the turning over were retarded by 10 to 15 years, an increase risk of about two fold might be expected, corresponding to what is seen after 10 to 15 years' use of exogenous oestrogens.

As a final remark, increased risk has recently been reported in connection with exposure to radiation before the age of menarche. This suggests that early-stage events can occur at that age. The assumption made above that most early-stage events take place at or after menarche refers to 'spontaneously' occurring early-stage events, which would therefore appear to be ovarian-dependent.

## REFERENCES

Advisory Committee on the Biological Effects of Ionizing Radiations (1980) *The Effects on Populations of Exposure to Low Levels of Ionizing Radiation,* Washington DC, National Academy of Sciences

Armitage, P. & Doll, R. (1961) A two-stage theory of carcinogenesis in relation to the age distribution of human cancer. *Br. J. Cancer,* ***11,*** 161–169

Beebe, G.W. (1982) *Assessment of health risks from exposure to ionizing radiation.* In: Prentice, R.L. & Whittemore, A.S., eds, *Environmental Epidemiology: Risk Assessment,* Philadelphia, Society for Industrial and Applied Mathematics, pp. 3–21

Boice, J.D., Jr, Land, C.E., Shore, R.E., Norman, J.E. & Tokunaga, M. (1979) Risk of breast cancer following low-dose radiation exposure. *Radiology,* ***131,*** 589–597

Boyle, P., Day, N.E. & Magnus, K. (1983) Mathematical modelling of malignant melanoma in Norway, 1953–1978. *Am. J. Epidemiol.* (in press)

Brown, C.C. & Chu, K.C. (1982) *Approaches to epidemiological analysis of prospective and retrospective studies: example of lung cancer and exposure to arsenic.* In: Prentice, R.L. & Whittemore, A.S., eds, *Environmental Epidemiology: Risk Assessment,* Philadelphia, Society for Industrial and Applied Mathematics, pp. 94–106

Cook, P.J., Doll, R. & Fellingham, S.A. (1969) A mathematical model for the age distribution of cancer in man. *Int. J. Cancer,* ***4,*** 93–112

Day, N.E. (1982) *Epidemiological evidence of promoting effects – the example of breast cancer.* In: Hecker, E., Fusenig, N., Marks, F. & Kunz, W., eds, *Cocarcinogenesis and the Biological Effects of Tumor Promoters,* New York, Raven Press, pp. 183–199

Day, N.E. (1983) *Radiation and multi-stage carcinogenesis.* In: Boice, J.D., Jr & Fraumeni, J.F., Jr, eds, *Radiation Carcinogenesis: Epidemiology and Biological Significance,* New York, Raven Press, pp. 437–443

Day, N.E. & Boice, J.D., Jr (1984) *Summary chapter.* In: Boice, J.D., Jr & Day, N.E., eds, *Second Cancer in Relation to Radiation Treatment for Cervical Cancer: Results of a Cancer Registry Collaboration* (*IARC Scientific Publications No. 52*), Lyon, International Agency for Research on Cancer

Day, N.E. & Brown, C.C. (1980) Multistage models and primary prevention of cancer. *J. natl Cancer Inst.,* ***64,*** 977–989

Doll, R. (1971) The age distribution of cancer: implications for models of carcinogenesis. *J. R. Stat. Soc., A,* ***134,*** 133–155

Doll, R. & Hill, A.B. (1964) Mortality in relation to smoking: ten years' observations of British doctors. *Br. med. J.,* ***ii,*** 1460–1467

Doll, R. & Peto, J. (1976) Mortality in relation to smoking: 20 years' observations on male British doctors. *Br. med. J.,* ***ii,*** 1525–1536

Doll, R., Morgan, L.G. & Speizer, F.E. (1970) Cancers of the lung and nasal sinuses in nickel workers. *Br. J. Cancer,* ***24,*** 623–632

Hayes, R.B. (1982) *Carcinogenic effect of chromium.* In: Langard, S., ed., *Biological and Environmental Aspects of Chromium,* Amsterdam, Elsevier Biomedical Press, pp. 221–247

Hoover, R., Gray, L.A., Cole, P. & MacMahon, B. (1976) Menopausal estrogens and breast cancer. *New Engl. J. Med.*, ***295***, 401–405

Jick, H., Watkins, R.N., Hunter, J.R., Dinan, B.J., Madsen, S., Rothman, K.J. & Walker, A.M. (1979) Replacement estrogens and endometrial cancer. *New Engl. J. Med.*, ***300***, 218–222

Jick, H., Walker, A.M. & Rothman, K.J. (1980) The epidemic of endometrial cancer: a commentary. *Am. J. publ. Health*, ***70***, 264–267

Kahn, H.A. (1966) The Dorn study of smoking and mortality among US veterans. Report on eight and one-half years of observation. *Natl Cancer Inst. Monogr.*, ***42***, 1–125

Kato, H. & Schull, W.J. (1982) Studies on the mortality of A-bomb survivors. 7. Mortality, 1950–1978. Part I. Cancer mortality. *Radiat. Res.*, ***90***, 395–432

Lee-Feldstein, A. (1983) Arsenic and respiratory cancer in humans: follow-up of copper smelter employees in Montana. *J. natl Cancer Inst.*, ***70***, 601–610

MacMahon, B., Cole, P., Lin, T.M., Lowe, C.R., Mirra, A.P., Ravnihar, B., Salber, E.J., Valaoras, V.G. & Yuasa, S. (1970) Age at first birth and breast cancer risk. *Bull. World Health Organ.*, ***43***, 209–221

MacMahon, B., Cole, P. & Brown, J. (1973) Etiology of human breast cancer: a review. *J. natl Cancer Inst.*, ***50***, 21–42

Magnus, K., Andersen, A. & Høgetveit, A.C. (1982) Cancer of respiratory organs among workers at a nickel refinery in Norway. *Int. J. Cancer*, ***30***, 681–685

Moolgavkar, S.H. & Venzon, D.J. (1979) Two-event models for carcinogenesis: incidence curves for childhood and adult tumors. *Math. Biosci.*, ***47***, 55–77

Moolgavkar, S.H., Day, N.E. & Stevens, R.G. (1980) Two-stage model for carcinogenesis: epidemiology of breast cancer in females. *J. natl Cancer Inst.*, ***65***, 559–569

Pasternack, B.S. & Shore, R.E. (1981) *Lung cancer following exposure to chloromethyl ethers*. In: Chwat, M. & Dror, K., eds, *Proceedings of the International Conference on Critical Current Issues in Environmental Health Hazards, Tel-Aviv, Israel, 4–7 March 1979*, pp. 76–85

Peto, J., Seidman, H. & Selikoff, I.J. (1982) Mesothelioma mortality in asbestos workers: implications for models of carcinogenesis and risk assessment. *Br. J. Cancer*, ***45***, 124

Peto, J., Cuckle, H., Doll, R., Hermon, C. & Morgan, L.G. (1983) *Respiratory cancer mortality of Welsh nickel refinery workers*. In: Sunderman, F.W., Jr, ed.-in-chief, *Nickel in the Human Environment*, (*IARC Scientific Publications No. 53*), Lyon, International Agency for Research on Cancer (in press)

Peto, R., Roe, F.J.C., Lee, P.N., Levy, L. & Clack, J. (1975) Cancer and ageing in mice and men. *Br. J. Cancer*, ***32***, 411–426

Pike, M.C., Krailo, M.D., Henderson, B.E., Casagrande, J.T. & Hoel, D.G. (1983) 'Hormonal' risk factors, 'breast tissue age' and the age-incidence of breast cancer. *Nature*, ***303***, 767–769

Selikoff, I.J., Hammond, E.C. & Seidman, H. (1973) *Cancer risk of insulation workers in the United States*. In: Bogovski, P., Gilson, J.C., Timbrell, V. & Wagner, J.C., eds, *Biological Effects of Asbestos* (*IARC Scientific Publications No. 8*), Lyon, International Agency for Research on Cancer, pp. 209–216

Shanmugaratnam, K., Lee, H.P. & Day, N.E., eds (1983) *Cancer Registration in Singapore* (*IARC Scientific Publications No. 48*), Lyon, International Agency for Research on Cancer

Smith, P.G. & Doll, R. (1982) Mortality among patients with ankylosing spondylitis after a single treatment course with X rays. *Br. med. J.*, ***284***, 449–460

Thomas, D.C. (1981) General relative risk models for failure time and matched case-control studies. *Biometrics*, ***37***, 673–686

Tulinius, H., Day, N.E., Johannesson, G., Bjarnason, O. & Gonzalez, M. (1978) Reproductive factors and risk for breast cancer in Iceland. *Int. J. Cancer*, ***21***, 724–730

Waterhouse, J., Muir, C., Shanmugaratnam, K. & Powell, J., eds (1982) *Cancer Incidence in Five Continents, Volume IV* (*IARC Scientific Publications No. 42*), Lyon, International Agency for Research on Cancer

Weiss, W. (1982) Epidemic curve of respiratory cancer due to chloromethyl ethers. *J. natl Cancer Inst.*, ***69***, 1265–1270

# EARLY- AND LATE-STAGE CARCINOGENESIS IN MOUSE SKIN AND IN MAN

J. PETO

*Division of Epidemiology Institute of Cancer Research, Clifton Avenue, Sutton, Surrey SM2 5PX, UK*

## INTRODUCTION

The aim of this paper is to explain the epidemiologist's definitions of early- and late-stage carcinogenesis, and to discuss their connection with initiation and promotion as observed in the laboratory. There are good reasons for avoiding more specific terms, as it is still not possible to classify agents as first-, third- or last-stage carcinogens with much confidence; but the lack of a more detailed nomenclature has engendered a good deal of confusion, and a reasonable balance must be struck between scientific rigour and constructive speculation. There are striking similarities between the model of carcinogenesis that is now emerging in the laboratory and the 'multi-stage' model that epidemiologists have developed, but these models have arisen quite independently, and, with the possible exception of initiation, it is not clear which experimental phenomena correspond to the superficially analogous processes that the epidemiologist postulates but cannot observe directly.

The initiation/promotion phenomenon, in which agent A followed by agent B causes a high tumour incidence, but agent B followed by agent A does not, has never been observed directly in human carcinogenesis, and the epidemiologist classifies carcinogens chiefly on the basis of the pattern of excess cancer incidence caused by beginning or ceasing exposure at different ages. If there is a long delay between starting or stopping exposure and any resulting change in cancer incidence, and the excess risk is independent of age at exposure, the agent is regarded as an early-stage carcinogen. If the effect of starting or stopping exposure appears more quickly, and the excess risk increases with increasing age at exposure, a late-stage effect is assumed. There may, in fact, be quite a close connection between these seemingly arbitrary definitions and the simple initiation/promotion concept, but it cannot be explained without first outlining the multi-stage model.

## EPIDEMIOLOGY AND THE MULTI-STAGE MODEL

According to the simplest multi-stage model, a normal cell must undergo an ordered (or at least partially ordered) sequence of changes to become the seed of a proliferating malignant tumour, and the background rate at which each successive change occurs remains roughly constant throughout adult life, unless some endogenous or external influence alters it. (There are probably several modifying effects in this process, of which the most important may be the proliferation of partially transformed cells; but, for the moment, these can be ignored. For a more detailed discussion of multi-stage models, see Day, this volume; Peto, 1977; Doll, 1978; and Day & Brown, 1980). If the successive changes are extremely rare events, the number of unaltered cells will remain almost constant, and the number that have undergone the first K changes will be roughly proportional to the Kth power of time. In a 'natural' carcinogenic process, the successive changes occur at a constant rate throughout life, and the number of Kth-stage cells will thus be proportional to the Kth power of age. When continuous application of an initiating carcinogen begins the process, however, this number will be proportional to the Kth power of duration of exposure to the agent, irrespective of age at first exposure.

The predictions of this simple model account, at least qualitatively, for many observations on human cancer rates. The incidence of cancer will be proportional to the number of cells that have undergone all but the last change, and should therefore rise as the (N–1)th power of age or duration of carcinogenic exposure, where N is the number of stages. Many epithelial cancer rates exhibit such age or time dependence;

Fig. 1. Cumulative mesothelioma mortality (in the absence of other causes of death) among North American insulation workers first exposed to asbestos at age 15–24 (– – –), 25–34 (—), 35 or more (...) years
From Peto *et al.* (1982)

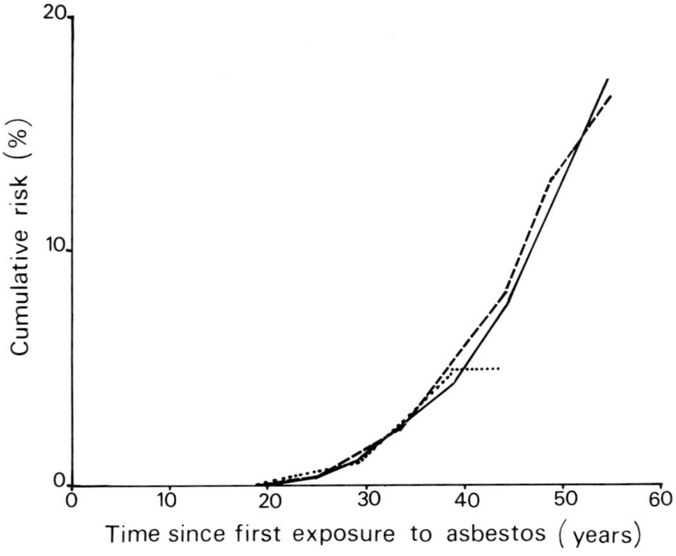

Fig. 2. Excess mortality from cancers of heavily irradiated sites other than leukaemia among patients with ankylosing spondylitis, by age at irradiation
From Smith & Doll (1982)

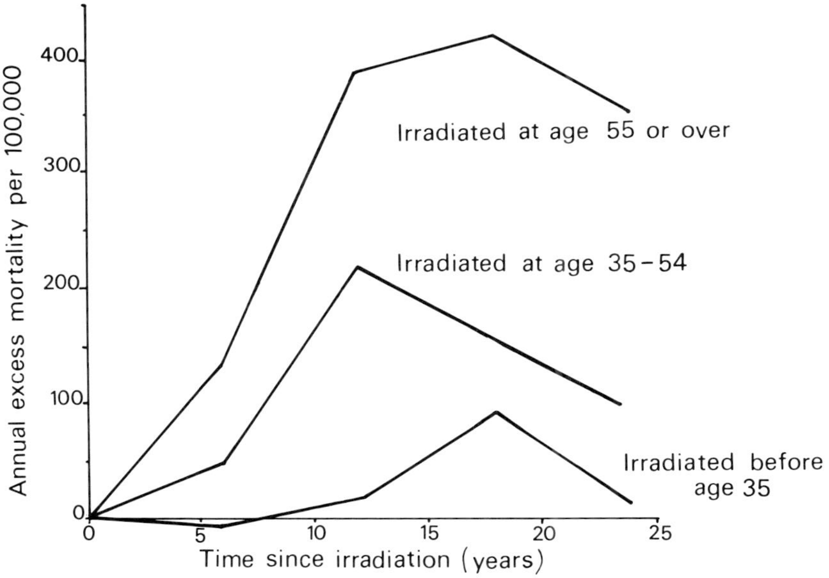


the incidence of lung cancer, for example, is proportional to the fourth or fifth power of duration of smoking in continuing smokers, and to a similar power of age in non-smokers (Doll, 1978). (This does not, in fact, constitute strong evidence that there are approximately five or six stages in bronchial carcinogenesis, since several factors, including genetic heterogeneity, selective proliferation and diagnostic delay, may alter the observed power of time.) Exposure to an initiator, an agent that acts at the first stage, will cause a subsequent incidence pattern that will be independent of age at first exposure; but later stage agents that act on the steadily increasing number of partially transformed cells will cause a greater increase in cancer risk when exposure occurs at older ages, since the target cell population will then be greater. Mesothelioma thus appears to be initiated by exposure to asbestos (Fig. 1; Peto *et al.,* 1982), while ionizing radiation seems to act primarily at a later stage or stages in most irradiated organs (Fig. 2; Smith & Doll, 1982). Agents that affect different stages in the process will act synergistically, causing an increase in risk approximately proportional to the product rather than the sum of their separate effects. A well-known example of such synergism is the combined effect of asbestos and cigarette smoking in causing lung cancer. Extension of the model to include hormone-related changes in the cellular activity of breast tissue provides a simple explanation of the age-distribution and major risk factors for breast cancer (Pike *et al.,* 1983).

## EXTENSIONS OF THE MULTI-STAGE MODEL

According to the simple multi-stage model outlined above:

1. Carcinogenesis involves a small number of discrete heritable changes, which are so rare that most cells are never affected.
2. Somatic processes such as central growth control or 'ageing' are irrelevant.
3. At least some of the stages must occur in a fixed sequence.
4. Nearly all cancers are monoclonal.
5. The probability that a cell will undergo any particular change during a fixed interval remains roughly constant throughout adult life unless the cell's environment is altered, as in female sex-specific organs at menopause or menarche, or by exposure to an external carcinogen.

There are exceptions to many, and perhaps all, of these generalizations, but they do not greatly alter the qualitative predictions or explanatory power of the model. An interesting example is the observation that exposure of C3H 10T ½ cells to X-rays produces a dose-related increase in susceptibility to subsequent transformation in virtually all irradiated cells. This effect appears to be due to an increase in the risk of a subsequent rare genetic event (Kennedy *et al.*, 1984), and even this fundamental change in the model therefore serves to extend rather than to challenge its generality. The multi-stage model should thus be regarded as a useful conceptual framework rather than a falsifiable scientific theory, and the proper role of such speculative models is to make scientists suspicious of counter-examples, but not unwilling to countenance them. Thus, for example, the suggestion that the simultaneous diagnosis of retinoblastoma in both eyes may be due to a host factor (Matsunaga, 1979 and this volume) constitutes a major extension of the model, and should therefore not be accepted, at least for the time being, as well established, particularly as the two-stage model for retinoblastoma proposed by Knudson (1971) now has strong experimental support (Cavenee *et al.*, 1983). Inclusion of the effect suggested by Matsunaga would not, however, necessarily alter the major predictions of Knudson's model.

## PENULTIMATE-STAGE CARCINOGENESIS

Contrary to popular belief, the excess incidence of lung cancer does not fall substantially when smoking stops, but remains more or less constant. A 70-year-old ex-smoker who stopped smoking at age 50 will therefore run roughly the same excess risk of developing lung cancer between the ages of 70 and 75 as a delayed result of his previous smoking as he did between 50 and 55 (Doll, 1978). (The long-term incidence pattern among ex-smokers has not yet been determined very precisely, but this is a reasonable interpretation of the data so far available.) A simple and plausible explanation of this observation is that smoking, as well as initiating the carcinogenic process, accelerates the penultimate stage, and after stopping smoking the number of cells in an ex-smoker's bronchial epithelium that require only one further change to begin malignant proliferation remains roughly constant for the remainder of his life.

## LAST-STAGE CARCINOGENESIS

Smoking does not seem to affect the last stage in bronchial carcinogenesis, for, if it did, the probability that 'last-stage' cells would undergo this final step would fall when smoking ceased, and cancer incidence would be significantly reduced. The only human carcinogens that have been shown to produce abrupt changes in cancer incidence when exposure begins or ceases are immunosuppressive therapy and hormone replacement therapy. Immunosuppressive drugs increase the incidence of Epstein-Barr virus-associated lymphomas, Kaposi's sarcoma, hepatoma, and certain skin cancers, particularly the squamous-cell type (Kinlen *et al.*, 1983). Evidence of a viral etiology has emerged for each of these tumours since the original observation that they can be caused by immunosuppression, and it is now reasonable to speculate that only (and perhaps all) virally induced tumours are strongly affected by the immune system. It remains to be seen whether viruses are involved in the development of the soft-tissue tumours that are also caused by immunosuppression. (Observations on immunosuppressed patients are also consistent with an excess of cervical cancer, but this is difficult to interpret, as such patients are carefully observed, and cervical carcinoma *in situ* is under-reported in the general population.) The incidence of endometrial cancer falls abruptly when post-menopausal hormone replacement therapy is withdrawn, but this may merely reflect a reduction in the cellular activity of the target tissue.

## THE PROGRESSIVE EVOLUTION OF INITIATED CELLS

The epidemiologist usually compares cancer incidence in people exposed to an agent with the 'normal' incidence in those who are not, and even in exposed individuals the risk is usually very much lower than that observed in the laboratory. Cigarette smoking takes about 50 years to cause cancer in 10% of smokers, for example. Experiments large enough to measure the natural incidence of cancer in animals are rarely conducted, however, and the experimenter can measure the incidence of tumours with any precision only in heavily exposed animals. This difference leads to the apparent contradiction that 'late-stage' carcinogenesis in man is characterized by an increase in susceptibility with increasing age, whereas with 7,12-dimethylbenz[*a*]anthracene (DMBA) initiation followed by promotion with 12-*O*-tetradecanoyl-13-phorbol acetate (TPA) produces a somewhat lower tumour yield when promotion is applied after a long delay rather than immediately (Stenback *et al.*, 1981). This may be, as those authors suggested, because older mice are less responsive to TPA; but the observation does still rather suggest that the number of initiated cells susceptible to promotion does not increase much, if at all, with the passage of time. The simplest explanation of these data in animals is that the main effect of TPA is to promote the second stage of tumorigenesis. The fact that the effect of TPA does not increase with time since initiation suggests that initiated cells do not proliferate, and that they do not have to undergo a second rate-limiting process to become susceptible to the effects of TPA. The initiating effect of DMBA is presumably so much greater than the spontaneous initiation rate in untreated animals that the subsequent effect of spontaneous initiation in DMBA-treated animals is relatively negligible, and the age dependence of 'late-stage' carcinogenesis in man, which according to the multi-stage model is due to the increase in number or further progression of initiated cells, cannot be detected.

This raises a further semantic point that conceals an important difference of perspective between epidemiologists and experimentalists. It is said that promotion alone cannot cause cancer, and hence the term 'complete carcinogen' has been coined to describe agents that can. The experimentalist is, however, accustomed to experiments in which a high proportion of animals develop tumours – indeed, many experimental treatments are distinguished more by the number of tumours per animal than by the proportion of animals affected, as the majority of animals develop at least one. If the multi-stage model is correct, however, any agent that affects any stage in carcinogenesis will cause some increase in the natural background cancer rate. A large experiment might be required to study the age dependence of tumour incidence caused by TPA alone, for example; but such small effects may provide some of the most informative clues to etiology, as they reflect the interaction of carcinogens with the natural process of carcinogenesis, which is swamped in most experimental protocols.

## PRECURSOR LESIONS AND CANCER IN ANIMALS AND MAN

The incidence patterns of both papillomas and carcinomas produced by chronic low-dose treatment with an initiator such as DMBA are quite different from those caused by initiation with DMBA followed by continuous promotion with TPA. In a typical experiment (Verma *et al.*, 1982), the initiation-promotion protocol caused a high incidence of papillomas within less than 10 weeks, and carcinomas did not appear until about 30 weeks later; but chronic DMBA treatment produced a lower incidence of papillomas, most of which appeared after 15 weeks, and carcinomas developed soon afterwards. At least two quite different types of papilloma probably occur in such experiments. Papilloma incidence following DMBA initiation and continuous promotion with either TPA (Burns *et al.*, 1978) or bromomethyl benzanthracene (Scribner *et al.*, 1983) is high initially, but few new tumours appear between about 15 weeks and 25 weeks, and many of the early tumours regress during this period even when TPA is applied continuously (Burns *et al.*, 1978). New papillomas begin to appear subsequently, however, and these late tumours are less likely to regress than the earlier ones, and may be particularly liable to malignant conversion. Differences between the patterns of papilloma and carcinoma incidence produced by different protocols may thus reflect differential effects on papillomas of different types, which in turn have differing susceptibilities to malignant transformation. A recent study suggests that papillomas caused by prolonged treatment with a mutagen are more often polyclonal than those induced by initiation and promotion (Reddy & Fialkow, 1983).

It is not clear that the second stage in promotion, the stimulation of the growth of reversible papillomas, bears any direct relation to carcinogenesis. The first stage in promotion, which is achieved quickly and perhaps irreversibly by TPA, may make initiated cells susceptible both to the effects of stimulation by agents such as mezerein

(Slaga *et al.,* 1980) and phorbol retinoate acetate (Furstenberger *et al.,* 1981) to develop into papillomas, and to a separate (third) change in the multi-stage evolution of carcinoma. The most direct evidence that papilloma growth does not necessarily increase the risk of carcinoma is the observation that fluocinolone acetonide can, in certain protocols, produce a large reduction in papilloma incidence without altering carcinoma incidence (Scribner *et al.,* 1983).

Whether the stem cells of the 'dependent' papillomas that grow or regress when mezerein or phorbol retinoate acetate is applied or withdrawn are precursors of carcinoma, or merely markers for the existence of cells of a different type that are also produced by first-stage promotion, could perhaps be answered directly by interrupting treatment and marking their position. The suggestion that autonomous (non-dependent) papillomas are the principle targets of further evolution to malignancy, and that they appear later than dependent papillomas (Scribner *et al.,* 1983) might also be tested by marking papillomas, observing which ones regress when promotion is interrupted, and then resuming promotion or applying an initiator. Such studies of the evolution of individual tumours were first conducted more than 40 years ago (Rous & Kidd, 1941), and it seems odd that this powerful method of distinguishing parallel and sequential processes is now rarely used.

Many human cancers are also associated both with benign lesions that are probably direct precursors of malignancy and with others that may be caused by some of the same agents but are 'terminally benign'. For example:

1. Benign breast disease can apparently be subdivided into types that are predictive of increased breast cancer risk and those that are not; and some, but not all, of the epidemiological correlates of breast cancer are predictive of benign breast disease (Ernster, 1981).

2. Colon cancer often (but not always) arises in an adenomatous polyp; but hyperplastic colonic polyps do not appear to be precursors of carcinoma, and their prevalence in different populations is less closely correlated with colon cancer incidence than that of the adenomatous type (Correa & Haenszel, 1978).

3. The prevalence of hyperplastic lesions in the bronchi of American smokers fell by an order of magnitude between 1955 and 1977, due perhaps to the concomitant reduction in average tar levels of American cigarettes (Auerbach *et al.,* 1979), yet the incidence of lung cancer doubled over this period. More detailed classification of these lesions might help to resolve this apparent contradiction, and the ability to subdivide and characterize separate stages in experimental promotion in respiratory-tract epithelium (Nettesheim *et al.,* this volume) could thus prove directly relevant to a better understanding of bronchial carcinogenesis in man.

## CARCINOGENS THAT ACT BOTH EARLY AND LATE

Just as some papillomas are precursors of malignancy and some are not, carcinomas that arise from pre-existing papillomas should be distinguished from those that do not. In this connection, an interesting contrast that appears to have passed unnoticed is the apparently marked difference between the late effects of urethane and DMBA after initiation and promotion. Treatment with urethane

Table 1. Synergism of 7,12-dimethylbenz[*a*]anthracene (DMBA) initiation, 12-*O*-tetradecanoyl-13-phorbol acetate (TPA) promotion and intraperitoneal urethane in causing malignant skin tumours in mice. Stage I: one application of 100 μg DMBA, or acetone. Stage II: 3.1 μg TPA, or acetone, twice-weekly for 15 weeks. Stage III: repeated twice-weekly intraperitoneal injections of 8 mg urethane, or water, from week 20 (Roe *et al.*, 1972)

| Treatment | | | No. of mice alive at 20 weeks | Observed no. with malignant skin tumours | Expected no. with malignant skin tumours[a] |
|---|---|---|---|---|---|
| Stage I | Stage II | Stage III | | | |
| DMBA | TPA | Urethane | 58 | 16 | 10.2 |
| DMBA | TPA | Water | 60 | 10 | 15.8 |
| Acetone | TPA | Urethane | 29 | 0 | – |
| DMBA | Acetone | Urethane | 56 | 0 | – |

[a] Mantel-Haenszel expected numbers, comparing first two groups ($p < 0.03$)

following DMBA initiation and TPA promotion produces a marked increase in carcinoma incidence (Table 1; Roe *et al.*, 1972). The effect is synergistic with both initiation and promotion, as omission of either DMBA or TPA reduced carcinoma incidence almost to zero in this experiment; and omission of urethane halved the excess carcinoma incidence, but did not alter its temporal pattern. These observations suggest that urethane increases the background rate of a third or later stage in skin carcinogenesis. In contrast, Shubik (1950) found that the carcinoma incidence caused by DMBA initiation followed by twice-weekly DMBA was not increased by the addition of twice-weekly croton oil, although the number of regressing or stationary papillomas was doubled (Table 2). Shubik's results thus suggest that DMBA does not convert the papillomas caused by DMBA initiation and TPA promotion to malignancy; for such a mechanism should imply a synergistic effect of late mutagenic treatment with both DMBA initiation and TPA promotion such as that observed for urethane by Roe *et al.* (1972). Urethane is an unusual initiator in several respects: it is a very weak 'complete carcinogen' in mouse skin, it does not cause hyperplasia, and its initiating action is strongly potentiated by pretreatment with croton oil (Hennings *et al.*, 1969).

Table 2. Repeated application of croton oil to 7,12-dimethylbenz[*a*]anthracene (DMBA)-initiated mice treated with repeated DMBA increased the papilloma yield, but not the number of malignant tumours (Shubik, 1950)

| Treatment | No. of survivors at time of first tumour | No. of malignant tumours | Total no. of tumours |
|---|---|---|---|
| One application of 1.5% DMBA, then, after 3 weeks, 0.1% DMBA twice weekly | 26 | 21 | 90 |
| One application of 1.5% DMBA, then mixture of 0.1% DMBA and 5% croton oil twice weekly | 30 | 19 | 143 |

These experiments suggest that there may be two quite independent pathways to carcinogenesis involving late-stage mutagenesis – one dependent on TPA promotion, and one not. Yuspa and his colleagues (Yuspa *et al.*, this volume; Hennings *et al.*, 1983) treated SENCAR mice with DMBA (stage I) followed by 10 weeks' promotion with TPA (stage II), which produced over 30 papillomas per mouse. This protocol was followed by 30 weeks' treatment with *N*-methyl-*N'*-nitro-*N*-nitrosoguanidine, 4-nitroquinoline oxide or urethane (stage III), all of which produced a higher carcinoma incidence than TPA or acetone given at stage III. These authors inferred that malignant conversion of the papillomas induced by initiation and promotion is a general property of mutagenic initiators. Control groups in which stage-II promotion was omitted were not included, however, and it is not clear that the incidence of malignant tumours would have been much lower in the animals treated with 4-nitroquinoline oxide or *N*-methyl-*N'*-nitro-*N*-nitrosoguanidine if the TPA had been omitted from the protocol. Moreover, the carcinomas were not shown to have arisen in pre-existing papillomas in these experiments. Even for urethane, which does act synergistically with both initiation and promotion, there could be a parallel pathway to malignancy that is TPA dependent in which TPA-induced papilloma formation is not an intermediate step. The meaning of a 'conversion rate' calculated by dividing the total number of malignant tumours by the total number of papillomas (Hennings *et al.*, 1983) is therefore not clear.

Various human carcinogens also appear to act at more than one stage in carcinogenesis, although the analogy with the observation in the laboratory that both 'initiators' and 'promotors' can act at two or more separate stages in tumorigenesis may be superficial. There is strong evidence that cigarette smoke acts both early and late in the production of lung cancer, although this may merely reflect the separate effects of different constituents; asbestos appears to initiate mesothelioma but to act at a later stage in causing lung cancer (Peto *et al.*, 1982); and the pattern of cancer incidence in early nickel refinery workers suggests an early effect for lung cancer but a late effect for nasal sinus cancer (Peto *et al.*, 1984).

## FURTHER EXAMPLES

The following examples illustrate a few ways in which the perspective provided by the multi-stage model could influence the planning and interpretation of animal experiments.

### *Age-related effects*

According to the multi-stage model, carcinogens for which the effect increases with age at exposure act on cells that are already partially transformed as a result of the natural evolution to malignancy that occurs, at however low a level, in the absence of any carcinogen. The mechanisms of experimental carcinogenesis may not be similar to those of 'natural' carcinogenesis in either animals or humans, and it would be reassuring to have some confirmation, however indirect, that the processes are related. It is therefore surprising, at least to epidemiologists, that the effect of age at exposure

Fig. 3. Relative incidences of malignant tumours (●) and of all tumours (○) in mice during the 23 weeks following initiation with 7,12-dimethylbenz[*a*]anthracene without subsequent promotion The incidence of malignancy (based on only 14 tumours) appears to be strongly age-related. From Stenback *et al.* (1981)

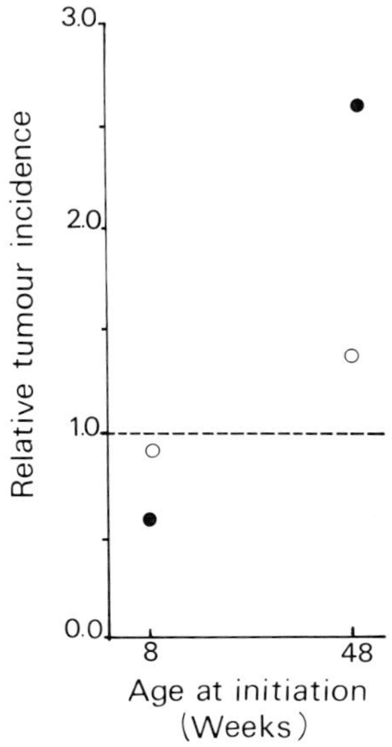


is so rarely investigated in the laboratory. For example, the application of TPA to untreated mice at different ages would give a low yield of carcinomas and papillomas, but in a large enough experiment both should show a marked (and possibly linear) increase with age at exposure if changes analogous to the initiating effects of DMBA occur in natural carcinogenesis. Similarly, the suggestion that mutagenic initiators also act at a third or later stage in carcinoma induction implies that the incidence of carcinomas produced by brief initiation without promotion might be roughly proportional to the second or higher power of age at exposure when mice are treated at different ages. The resulting incidence of papillomas should be almost independent of age at exposure, however, as initiating mutagens seem likely to act principally at the first stage in their production. Such an experiment has in fact been performed with DMBA, although not for this purpose, and the results, although of only marginal significance, appear to show both these effects (Fig. 3; Stenback *et al.,* 1981). This experiment might be worth repeating on a larger scale with various mutagens.

The prediction that continuous exposure to initiators should cause an increase in cancer risk, independent of age at first exposure, has already been confirmed by an experiment in which mice were treated continuously with benzo[*a*]pyrene starting at different ages (Peto *et al.,* 1975).

*Dose-response*

According to the multi-stage model, the dose-response for an agent acting at two stages should be roughly quadratic. Thus, for example, the suggestion that some mutagens act both early and late in carcinogenesis is further supported by the observation of Lee and O'Neill (1971) that tumour incidence in mice treated continuously with benzo[*a*]pyrene was roughly proportional to the square of dose. Similarly, the inference that cigarette smoking acts both early and late in bronchial carcinogenesis is reinforced by the dose-response, which shows significant upward curvature (Doll, 1978).

In relation to a model in which initiators act at one stage in papilloma production but at three stages in carcinoma production, it was recently stated that 'repeated doses of initiator ... should not change the ratio of papilloma incidence to carcinoma incidence.' (Scribner *et al.*, 1983). In fact, in such a model the dose-response for chronic initiation should be roughly linear for papillomas and cubic for carcinomas, and the ratio of carcinomas to papillomas should increase with both dose and duration of initiation.

*Temporal patterns*

In initiation/promotion protocols, 'dependent' papillomas that regress when TPA is withdrawn appear abruptly, the incidence of 'independent' or 'autonomous' papillomas seems initially to be roughly constant, and carcinoma incidence increases with time. Most experiments are conducted with small numbers of mice exposed to such high doses that random error and saturation effects make formal model-fitting difficult, and the effects of tumour promotion do not appear to be as regular as those of continuous initiation; but these temporal patterns suggest different numbers of stages in the production of these three tumour types. If the times of first appearance and malignant conversion of individual 'dependent' and 'independent' tumours were recorded, the sequence of different stages in promotion and late mutagenesis, and their relevance to carcinogenesis, could be studied more precisely, both by statistical modelling and by direct observation. In particular, the effect of second-stage promotion on carcinogenesis could be studied in a protocol of DMBA initiation, two weeks' TPA promotion, about 20 weeks' treatment with mezerein, and prolonged interperitoneal administration of urethane. Omission of the mezerein in such a protocol would certainly reduce the papilloma yield, but might not greatly alter the incidence of malignant tumours. Until the role of 'promotion' in animal carcinogenesis has been more clearly defined, it will be difficult to assess its relevance to human malignancy.

## REFERENCES

Auerbach, O., Hammond, E.C. & Garfinkel, L. (1979) Changes in bronchial epithelium in relation to cigarette smoking, 1955–1960 vs. 1970–1977. *New Engl. J. Med.*, ***300***, 381–386

Burns, F.J., Vanderlaan, M., Snyder, E. & Albert, R.E. (1978) *Induction and progression kinetics of mouse skin papillomas*. In: Slaga, T.J., Sivak, A. & Boutwell, R.K., eds, *Carcinogenesis – A Comprehensive Survey*, Vol. 2, *Mechanisms of Tumour Promotion and Cocarcinogenesis*, New York, Raven Press, pp. 91–96

Cavenee, W.K., Dryja, T.P., Phillips, R.A., Benedict, W.F., Godbout, R., Gallie, B.L., Murphree, A.L., Strong, L.C. & White, R.L. (1983) Expression of recessive alleles by chromosomal mechanisms in retinoblastoma. *Nature,* **305,** 779–784

Correa, P. & Haenszel, W. (1978) The epidemiology of large-bowel cancer. *Adv. Cancer Res.,* **26,** 1–141

Day, N.E. & Brown, C.C. (1980) Multistage models and primary prevention of cancer. *J. natl Cancer Inst.,* **64,** 977–989

Doll, R. (1978) An epidemiological perspective of the biology of cancer. *Cancer Res.,* **38,** 3573–3583

Ernster, V.L. (1981) The epidemiology of benign breast disease. *Epidemiol. Rev.,* **3,** 184–202

Furstenberger, G., Berry, D.L., Sorg, R. & Marks, R. (1981) Skin tumor promotion by phorbol esters is a two-stage process. *Proc. natl Acad. Sci. USA,* **78,** 7722–7726

Hennings, H., Bowden, G.T. & Boutwell, R.K. (1969) The effect of croton oil pretreatment on skin tumor initiation in mice. *Cancer Res.,* **29,** 1773–1780

Hennings, H., Shores, R., Wenk, M.L., Spangler, E.F., Tarone, R. & Yuspa, S.H. (1983) Malignant conversion of mouse skin tumours is increased by tumour initiators and unaffected by tumour promoters. *Nature,* **304,** 67–69

Kennedy, A.R., Cairns, J. & Little, J.B. (1984) Timing of the steps in transformation of C3H 10T½ cells by X-irradiation. *Nature,* **307,** 85–86

Kinlen, L., Doll, R. & Peto, J. (1983) The incidence of tumours in human transplant recipients. *Transplant Proc.,* **15,** 1039–1042

Knudson, A.G. (1971) Mutation and cancer: statistical study of retinoblastoma. *Proc. natl Acad. Sci. USA,* **68,** 820–823

Lee, P.N. & O'Neill, J.A. (1971) The effect both of time and dose applied on tumour incidence rates in benzopyrene skin painting experiments. *Br. J. Cancer,* **25,** 759–770

Matsunaga, E. (1979) Hereditary retinoblastoma: host resistance and age at onset. *J. natl Cancer Inst.,* **63,** 933–939

Peto, J., Seidman, H. & Selikoff, I.J. (1982) Mesothelioma mortality in asbestos workers: implications for models of carcinogenesis and risk assessment. *Br. J. Cancer,* **45,** 124–135

Peto, J., Cuckle, H., Doll, R., Hermon, C. & Morgan, L.G. (1984) *Respiratory cancer mortality of Welsh nickel refinery workers.* In: Sunderman, F.W., Jr, ed.-in-chief, *Nickel in the Human Environment (IARC Scientific Publications No. 53),* Lyon, International Agency for Research on Cancer (in press)

Peto, R. (1977) Epidemiology, multistage models and short-term mutagenicity tests. *Cold Spring Harbor Conf. Cell Proliferation,* **4,** 1403–1428

Peto, R., Roe, F.J.C., Lee, P.N., Levy, L. & Clack, J. (1975) Cancer and ageing in mice and men. *Br. J. Cancer,* **32,** 411–426

Pike, M.C., Krailo, M.D., Henderson, B.E., Casagrande, J.T. & Hoel, D.G. (1983) 'Hormonal' risk factors, 'breast tissue age' and the age-incidence of breast cancer. *Nature,* **303,** 767–770

Reddy, A.L. & Fialkow, P.J. (1983) Papillomas induced by initiation-promotion differ from those induced by carcinogen alone. *Nature,* **304,** 69–71

Roe, F.J.C., Carter, R.L., Michley, B.C.V., Peto, R. & Hecker, E. (1972) On the persistence of tumour initiation and the acceleration of tumour progression in mouse skin tumorigenesis. *Int. J. Cancer,* ***9,*** 264–273

Rous, P. & Kidd, J.G. (1941) Conditional neoplasms and subthreshold neoplastic states. *J. exp. Med.,* ***73,*** 365–389

Scribner, J.D., Scribner, N.K., McKnight, B. & Mottet, N.K. (1983) Evidence for a new model of tumour progression from carcinogenesis and tumour promotion studies with 7-bromomethylbenz(a)anthracene. *Cancer Res.,* ***43,*** 2034–2041

Shubik, P. (1950) The growth potentialities of induced skin tumours in mice. The effects of different methods of chemical carcinogenesis. *Cancer Res.,* ***10,*** 713–717

Slaga, T.J., Fischer, S.M., Nelson, K. & Gleason, G.L. (1980) Studies on the mechanism of skin tumour promotion: Evidence for several stages in promotion. *Proc. natl Acad. Sci. USA,* ***77,*** 3659–3663

Smith, P.G. & Doll, R. (1982) Mortality among patients with ankylosing spondylitis after a single treatment course with X-rays. *Br. med. J.,* ***284,*** 449–460

Stenback, F., Peto, R. & Shubik, P. (1981) Initiation and promotion at different ages and doses in 2 200 mice. II. Decrease in promotion by TPA with ageing. *Br. J. Cancer,* ***44,*** 15–23

Verman, A.K., Conrad, E.A. & Boutwell, R.K. (1982) Differential effects of retinoic acid and 7,8-benzoflavone on the induction of mouse skin tumours by the complete carcinogenesis process and by the initiation-promotion regimen. *Cancer Res.,* ***42,*** 3519–3525

# MULTISTAGE AND MULTIFACTORIAL CARCINOGENESIS IN HEREDITARY TUMOURS, WITH SPECIAL REFERENCE TO RETINOBLASTOMA

E. MATSUNAGA

*Department of Human Genetics, National Institute of Genetics, Mishima, 411 Japan*

## INTRODUCTION

The multistage model of carcinogenesis, as implied by the common pathological observation of progression to cancer through a papilloma and supported by laboratory evidence for separate roles of initiators and promoters, has been successfully used as a framework to interpret epidemiological data on common cancers the incidence of which increases rapidly with age (e.g., Day & Brown, 1980). The model is also compatible with clinical observations for certain dominantly inherited tumours such as retinoblastoma, Wilms' tumour and thyroid medullary cancer, and for polyposis coli, which, with the passage of time, almost inevitably develops into cancer. These neoplasms also occur more frequently in persons who do not have the gene. If mutation, whether germinal or somatic, is the first step in carcinogenesis, then carriers of the germinal mutation should tend to develop the malignancy earlier, and often from multiple foci in the same tissue, than persons not carrying the gene. This is indeed the case with the above-mentioned tumours (Table 1) and probably also with other dominantly inherited tumours (Knudson, 1973). Ashley (1969) analysed age-specific prevalence data for colonic cancer in polyposis patients and suggested that the effect of the gene is to reduce by one or two the number of 'hits' necessary in the intestinal mucosal cells before neoplasia can develop, but that the development of cancer in these polyps is dependent on external factors of the same type as in the case of colonic cancer in persons not affected with polyposis.

The principal theme of this Symposium has been the nature of individual steps of carcinogenesis and the factors that promote or suppress them. Therefore, I shall review some of the recent studies on the genetics and genesis of retinoblastoma, because it is a cancer to which the multistage model may be applied in its simplest form.

Table 1. Average age at onset, diagnosis or death of patients with certain neoplasms: Comparison of hereditary and nonhereditary forms

| Neoplasm (No. of cases) | Average age at | Reference |
|---|---|---|
| *Retinoblastoma* | *Diagnosis* | |
| Familial bilateral (30) | 10 months | |
| Familial unilateral (19) | 19 months | Matsunaga (1976) |
| Sporadic unilateral (24) | 28 months | |
| *Wilms' tumour* | *Diagnosis* | |
| Familial bilateral (11) | 21 months | |
| Familial unilateral (42) | 32 months | Matsunaga (1981) |
| Sporadic unilateral (63) | 46 months | |
| *Thyroid medullary cancer* | *Onset* | |
| Familial bilateral (20) | 36 years | Jackson *et al.* (1979) |
| Sporadic unilateral (22) | 52 years | |
| *Intestinal cancer* | *Death from cancer* | |
| Familial polyposis (86) | 42 years | Dukes (1952) |
| General population | 68 years | |

## PRIMARY GENETIC CHANGE IN RETINOBLASTOMA

Retinoblastoma occurs at a rate of one per approximately 20 000 newborns. Although the age at risk of children extends up to seven years or more, that is, long after embryonic retinal cells have ceased to divide, a significant proportion of patients with this tumour are diagnosed shortly after birth. This finding indicates that tumours can be induced during the later fetal period, and that it involves a minimal number of carcinogenic steps.

Etiologically, retinoblastoma may be classified according to three distinct types, although tumours of each type cannot be distinguished histologically. Tumours of the first type, which represent about 35% of all retinoblastomas, are due to a dominant mutation with incomplete penetrance and variable expressivity. The locus of this mutation has been assigned to the q14 region on chromosome 13, and it is closely linked to esterase D (EsD) (Sparkes *et al.*, 1983). A gene carrier may be unilaterally or bilaterally affected, or he may remain unaffected.

The second type, which constitutes a minority of all tumours, is associated with a constitutional chromosomal deletion of 13q14, resulting in 50% of EsD activity in normal cells of the patients (Sparkes *et al.*, 1980). Expression of this type is also bilateral or unilateral, and it is usually accompanied by developmental retardation and other congenital abnormalities, depending upon the extent of deletion involving 13q14. Although most of these cases occur sporadically, familial cases have been reported in which the deletion seen in the patients was transmitted from a balanced insertional translocation carried by an unaffected parent (Strong *et al.*, 1981). In these cases, the apparent lack of penetrance in the parent is due to a chromosomal mechanism.

The third type, most of which are sporadic unilateral but not bilateral cases, is generally believed to be due to a somatic mutation of the same nature as the germinal one. That this is indeed the case was suggested recently by Godbout *et al.* (1983), who examined electrophoretic variants of EsD in tumour cells of four sporadic unilateral cases who were heterozygous for EsD and found, in two of them, only one EsD variant in the tumour cells. This finding implies that somatic inactivation of genes on 13q14 is responsible for the genesis of a nonheritable tumour.

Although, at present, the fraction of the deletion type appears to be no larger than 5%, examination of EsD activity is likely to show a much higher frequency of patients with a minute constitutional deletion or inactivation of the DNA segment involving the retinoblastoma locus (Benedict *et al.*, 1983). The question arises as to whether or not the 'dominant mutation' for retinoblastoma is also a nonfunctional genetic change (amorph) equivalent to the deletion type. There is some evidence that the nature of the mutant gene differs essentially from that of deletion of 13q14. In a study of cultured skin fibroblasts from patients with retinoblastoma, Sasaki (1982) found frequent occurrence of non-constitutional chromosomal rearrangements (reciprocal translocations and inversions) in samples from patients of the dominant mutation type but not in those from patients of the deletion type. In addition, fibroblasts from patients of the dominant type showed abnormally high susceptibility to transformation by murine sarcoma virus, whereas those from patients of the deletion type were as sensitive as normal controls (Miyaki *et al.*, 1983). Furthermore, the carcinogenic potential of deletion of 13q14 seems to be significantly lower than that of the dominant mutation, as inferred from the decreased proportion of bilateral disease among the patients (Table 2). If this is true, there must be an appreciable fraction of persons who are hemizygous for the chromosome region of 13q14 but who would not develop a tumour (Matsunaga, 1980a). This prediction could be tested by routine screening of EsD activity in children with retinoblastoma and of their parents.

Table 2. Distribution of unilaterally and bilaterally affected persons among reported cases of 13q− retinoblastoma (modified from Matsunaga, 1983)

| | No. of cases | | |
|---|---|---|---|
| | Unilateral | Bilateral | Total |
| Cases with 13q− | 25 | 32 | 57 |
| Expected number[a] | 9.7 | 47.3 | 57 |

[a] $\chi^2 = 29.1$ for 1 degree of freedom, $p < 0.001$. Expected number is based on the estimated ratio (0.17:0.83) of unilateral to bilateral disease among all sporadic cases that are heritable.

## MULTIFACTORIAL CARCINOGENESIS

Incomplete penetrance and variable expressivity of the dominant mutation or deletion of 13q14 means that the primary genetic change alone is not always sufficient to develop retinoblastoma in children at risk. Two lines of evidence show that both environmental and genetic factors can modify expression of the primary genetic change. First, there are occasional case reports of discordant pairs of identical twins with retinoblastoma. In a literature survey by Warburg (1974), while complete concordance was common (9/17 pairs), there were also incompletely concordant (5/17) and completely discordant (3/17) pairs. Of the three completely discordant pairs, one twin was unilaterally affected and his retinoblastoma was probably due to somatic mutation; one unaffected twin died at the age of three months; and in the third pair, one twin developed bilateral retinoblastoma at the age of two and one-half years, while the other remained unaffected during a four-year clinical observation period (Kanter & Harris, 1964). Although such case reports are highly selected, it is clear that some unknown environmental factors are responsible, to some extent, for incomplete penetrance and variable expression in the gene carriers.

Participation of genetic factors was demonstrated by analysis of family data on inherited cases of retinoblastoma, which showed that not only the segregation ratio of affected children but also the degree of expressivity, as measured by the proportion of bilaterally affected children and their age at diagnosis, varied consistently with expressivity in carrier parents (Matsunaga, 1978, 1979).

Such a correlation can be ascribed formally to a variety of mechanisms, including multiple alleles, modifier genes, chromosomal mechanisms and maternal effect. The existence of multiple alleles with different expressivity can be ruled out because all three phenotypes—unaffected, unilaterally and bilaterally affected—can occur among members of the same family who share the identical mutant gene. As mentioned earlier, chromosomal rearrangement in a balanced state may explain apparent non-expression in carriers in certain families. However, most patients with familial retinoblastoma do not show the developmental retardation usually seen in the cases associated with 13q–, so that the fraction of familial cases of the deletion type seems to be small. Even if a minute chromosome deletion not detectable by current cytogenetic techniques existed in some patients, it is difficult to account for the reduced penetrance and expressivity in offspring of *affected* individuals by chromosomal mechanisms.

The question of possible maternal effect is pertinent, because tumour formation can be induced in the intrauterine stage. Thus, transplacental factors, such as maternal immunoglobulins and viral infection, may modify the degree of expressivity. Should this be the case, the proportion of bilateral disease in the affected children would differ according to the sex of the carrier parents. However, analysis of relevant family data did not reveal such a difference (Matsunaga, 1982a).

We proposed therefore, that host resistance or suppressor genes at other loci play an important role in the development of hereditary retinoblastoma, i.e., unaffected carriers are inherently resistant to tumour formation, patients with bilateral disease are the most susceptible and hereditary unilateral cases are the intermediate form. In view of the fact that ophthalmoscopic examination reveals no abnormality in the retinae of most unaffected carriers, the suppressor genes appear to be involved mainly with the process of malignant transformation of embryonic retinal cells that are already mutated or 'initiated', although the progression phase may also be modified by genetic factors, as suggested by infrequent spontaneous regression of bilateral retinoblastoma (Boniuk & Girard, 1969; Morris & Lapiana, 1974).

Table 3 was constructed after analysing over 200 families in which two or more cases of retinoblastoma had been reported (Matsunaga, 1978). Since host resistance is controlled by genetic and environmental factors, the distribution of the three phenotypes is likely to follow a multifactorial model of inheritance with two thresholds. Assuming a normal distribution of host resistance, the distance between the thresholds is expected to be constant for different groups of children who received the gene, provided that the underlying scale is the same. If $T_1$ is the threshold beyond which neither eye is affected and $T_2$ that below which both eyes are affected, for children with unaffected carrier parents, the deviation of $T_1$ from the population mean in terms of the standard deviation unit is 0.305, corresponding to the proportion

Table 3. Distribution of unaffected, unilaterally and bilaterally affected children who inherited the gene for retinoblastoma (Matsunaga, 1978)

| Expressivity of carrier parents | Distribution of children who inherited the gene | | | |
|---|---|---|---|---|
| | Unaffected | Unilateral | Bilateral | Total |
| Unaffected | 0.38 | 0.28 | 0.34 | 1.00 |
| Unilateral | 0.16 | 0.20 | 0.64 | 1.00 |
| Bilateral | 0.02 | 0.10 | 0.88 | 1.00 |

of unaffected carriers (38%); that of $T_2$ is $-0.412$, corresponding to the proportion of bilaterally affected (34%), giving 0.717 for $T_1$–$T_2$. For children with unilaterally affected parents, $T_1$–$T_2$ is 0.636; and for those with bilaterally affected parents, it is 0.879. Thus, the three estimates for $T_1$–$T_2$ are similar, suggesting that host resistance is a multifactorial trait. In view of the marked shift in the proportion of the three phenotypes among carrier children according to parental expressivity, it can be hypothesized that host resistance is determined largely by genetic factors. In fact, heritability was estimated at about 90%. The number of genes involved seems to be small.

Knudson (1971) advanced a two-mutation model, according to which the eyes acquire tumours independently. If the number of tumours formed in the gene carriers follows a Poisson distribution, as assumed by Knudson, then the square of the proportion of unilaterally affected should be equal to four times the product of the proportion of unaffected and that of bilaterally affected. A simple calculation using the data given in Table 3 shows a deviation from this expectation by a factor of seven to ten. However, we cannot conclude from this calculation that the second hit is *not* a somatic mutation. Bonaïti-Pellié and Briard-Guillemot (1981) proposed that the rate of somatic mutation itself could be partly determined by genes. If this is the case, it may be difficult to distinguish the model from that of host resistance.

Nevertheless, there is evidence that the host resistance genes are tissue-specific. As is well known, survivors of the heritable form of retinoblastoma are prone to developing second primary tumours, mainly osteosarcoma, not only in the area of irradiation but also outside this zone (Sagerman *et al.*, 1969; Jensen & Miller, 1971).

In light of this finding, Kitchin and Ellsworth (1974) argued that the increased risk of second primary tumours is a pleiotropic effect of the retinoblastoma gene. In fact, nonradiogenic osteosarcoma occurs not infrequently even in gene carriers who did not develop retinoblastoma (Gordon, 1974). We collected from the literature 26 cases of nonradiogenic osteosarcoma in patients with retinoblastoma and in their close relatives and found that their distribution agreed with the expectation that the risk of nonradiogenic osteosarcoma did not differ by phenotype with respect to retinoblastoma (Matsunaga, 1980b). Therefore, susceptibility to malignant transformation of retinal cells is not correlated with that of bone cells in gene carriers.

The risk of gene carriers of incurring nonradiogenic osteosarcoma was estimated to be 1.2%, which should be considered a minimal value but which is about 230 times that in the general population (Matsunaga, 1980b). Of the 26 who developed nonradiogenic osteosarcoma, two were siblings both of whom had survived bilateral retinoblastoma (Schimke *et al.*, 1974), suggesting that susceptibility to second primary tumours is also a multifactorial trait with a threshold. The heritability was estimated to be 71% (Matsunaga, 1980b), which implies that inherited tissue susceptibility plays an important role in the development of osteosarcoma, as is true for the development of retinoblastoma. This conclusion is supported by the occasional familial occurrence of osteosarcoma (Epstein *et al.*, 1970).

The risk of radiogenic osteosarcoma in gene carriers could be approximately 4%, depending upon the dose of radiation (Sagerman *et al.*, 1969). The increased risk may be a consequence of induction of somatic mutations in the tissue-specific suppressor system. The number of genes in the system is probably small; if the number of induced mutations accumulated in the cell at risk exceeds a certain threshold, malignant transformation would follow. The number of induced mutations required to exceed the threshold may differ from individual to individual according to the number of mutant genes that have been inherited *via* the germinal lines. This interpretation is compatible with the wide range of latent periods (4–30 years, with a mean of 11 years) observed for radiation-induced second primary tumours in retinoblastoma patients (Sagerman *et al.*, 1969).

## NATURE OF THE PRESUMED SECOND HIT

At the cellular level, malignant transformation is a rare event, even in carriers of the retinoblastoma gene. There are two different views concerning the nature of the presumed second hit responsible for this transformation: Knudson (1978) regards it as a somatic mutation, probably of the same type as the first hit that occurs in the homologous chromosome, while we argued that it is rather a host-dependent error in differentiation (Matsunaga, 1979).

Evidence supporting the first view has been obtained recently in studies of EsD activity of normal and tumour cells from patients with retinoblastoma. Benedict *et al.* (1983) reported that in a bilaterally affected patient whose normal cells showed 50% EsD activity but no detectable deletion of 13q14, tumour cells were missing one chromosome 13 and showed no EsD activity. The second hit in this patient therefore appeared to be absence of the homologous chromosome. This finding led the authors to propose that the retinoblastoma gene is recessive at the cellular level. However, further studies are needed to generalize this idea, because random karyotypic change occurs with progression of a tumour. More recently, Godbout *et al.* (1983) found only one electrophoretic variant of EsD in tumour cells from two patients with bilateral retinoblastoma who were heterozygous for EsD; analysis of chromosomes of the tumours failed to reveal deletion of 13q14. This finding indicates somatic inactivation of genes in the q14 region of one of the two chromosomes 13, but, unfortunately, it was not possible to decide whether the inactivation had occurred on the chromosome carrying the mutant gene or on the homologous chromosome carrying the normal allele. If the latter is the case, then it would mean that the second somatic event is indeed a mutation and hence the retinoblastoma gene is recessive at the cellular level. If the former is the case, it may be difficult to determine whether the inactivation of linked genes such as EsD was a result of a new mutation or of an epigenetic change secondary to the original germline mutation.

Our argument was based on the clinical observation of apparently almost synchronous appearance of bilateral tumours in persons considered to be most susceptible to tumour formation. The degree of synchrony was measured in terms of correlation with respect to age at diagnosis in the right and left eyes; it was as high as 0.82, after removal of bias due to the fact that the diagnosis for each eye was never independent. If the eyes acquire tumours independently, then, because the ages at risk are distributed over several years after birth, the correlation would not be so high. The high correlation can easily be explained by assuming that the second hit is an error in differentiation, because differentiation in the development of a paired organ is usually synchronous. The error could be suppressed completely in the most resistant group, which would remain unaffected, but it could not be suppressed completely in the less resistant group. The liability of a mutant cell to such an error at a given stage of development is largely controlled by tissue-specific suppressor genes, although it may decline with age as a consequence of developmental maturity of target cells (Matsunaga, 1979).

The almost synchronous appearance of tumours in the most susceptible group of gene carriers is a phenomenon that also seems to apply to a single eye. In unilateral cases, the tumour is usually too far advanced when the diagnosis is made to allow discrimination of multifocal tumours, although this is often possible in the less advanced eye of a bilaterally affected patient. For example, Figure 1 shows five tumours that are clearly separated, three of which appear to be almost equal in size. Here again, since differentiation is usually synchronous in a group of cells within a developing organ, this finding can be explained by assuming that all retinal cells in one eye are equally liable to an error in differentiation at the same stage of development. However, the argument is based on circumstantial evidence, and it is difficult to prove it by laboratory studies, because the basic mechanism of differentiation is still poorly understood and no animal model is available.

Finally, the almost synchronous appearance of multiple tumours might be reconciled with the somatic mutation model if it is assumed that the primary genetic change generates an abnormally high frequency of somatic mutations. Sasaki (1982) found that non-constitutional chromosomal rearrangements occur frequently in cultured skin fibroblasts from patients with hereditary retinoblastoma but not in

Fig. 1. Multiple tumours in the eye of a patient with bilateral retinoblastoma
Reproduced, with permission, from Takagi & Ikui, 1977

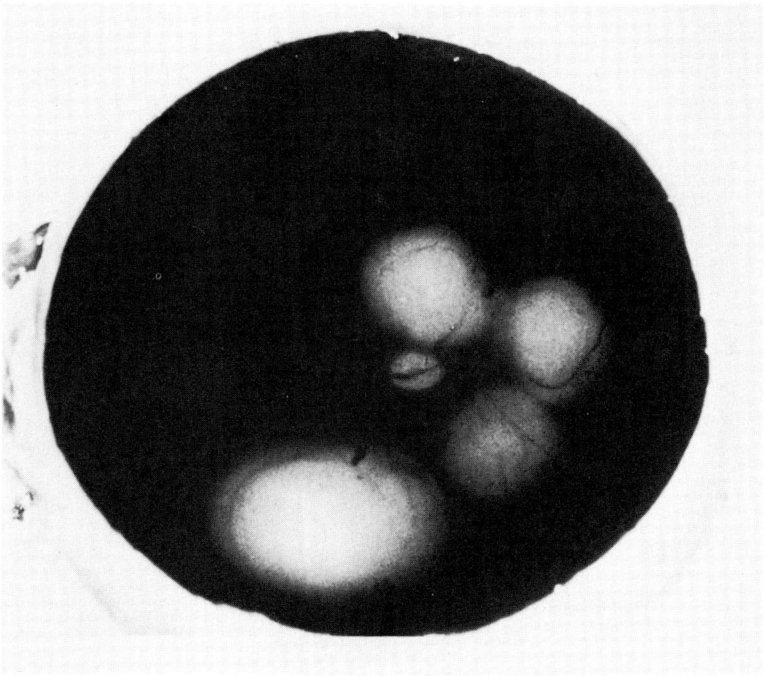

those from patients with 13q–. In most patients with 13q– who developed bilateral retinoblastoma, however, the disease was already bilateral when the diagnosis was first made in either eye (Matsunaga, 1980a). Therefore, if deletion of 13q14 has no mutation-like effect, it seems difficult to interpret this observation in terms of the somatic mutation model. In this connection, it may be argued that if tumours in the gene carriers could be induced by a somatic mutation at a very early stage of retinal development, the simultaneous occurrence of bilateral tumours in both eyes could be expected. If this were the case, then, assuming equal rate of tumour growth, the age at initial diagnosis should tend to be lower in patients with tumours of the same Reese group (Reese, 1976) in both eyes than in those with tumours of different Reese group or with sequentially bilateral cases. However, this was not observed (Matsunaga, 1982b).

## CONCLUSION

The multistage model of carcinogenesis is compatible with the clinical observation of heritable neoplasms that are characterized by earlier onset and, often, multiple primaries in the same tissue, in contrast to nonheritable neoplasms of the same kind.

Review of recent studies on retinoblastoma suggests that the primary genetic change responsible for this tumour, whether of the heritable or nonheritable form, is either a dominant mutation at the locus on the chromosomal region of 13q14 or deletion (or inactivation) of that region, although the nature of the respective change may be distinct. Even if one of these two changes is present in retinoblasts or osteoblasts, tissue-specific modifier genes at other loci, together with some unknown environmental factors, can suppress malignant transformation of the cells. The nature of the presumed second hit may be a somatic genetic change of the same type as the first one that occurs in the homologous chromosome; an alternative is a possible epigenetic change resulting in a differentiation error. Further studies are needed to provide a definite answer for this critical issue.

## ACKNOWLEDGEMENT

This paper, contribution number 1514 from the National Institute of Genetics, was supported partly by a grant-in-aid from the Ministry of Education, Science, and Culture, Japan.

Note added in proof: Cavenee *et al.*, (1983, *Nature*, ***305***, 779–784) and Dryja *et al.* (1984, *New Engl. J. Med.*, ***310***, 550–553) have reported the frequent occurrence of homozygosity for large portions of 13q in retinoblastomas and that the homozygosity can be brought about by a variety of mechanisms, including mitotic nondisjunction and mitotic recombination.

## REFERENCES

Ashley, D.J.B. (1969) Colonic cancer arising in polyposis coli. *J. med. Genet.*, ***6***, 376–378

Benedict, W.F., Murphree, A.L., Banerjee, A., Spina, C.A., Sparkes, M.C. & Sparkes, R.S. (1983) Patient with 13 chromosome deletion: Evidence that the retinoblastoma gene is a recessive cancer gene. *Science*, ***219***, 973–975

Bonaïti-Pellié, C. & Briard-Guillemot, M.L. (1981) Segregation analysis in hereditary retinoblastoma. *Human Genet.*, ***57***, 411–419

Boniuk, M. & Girard, L.J. (1969) Spontaneous regression of bilateral retinoblastoma. *Trans. Am. Acad. Ophthalmol. Otolaryngol.*, ***73***, 194–198

Day, N.E. & Brown, C.C. (1980) Multistage models and primary prevention of cancer. *J. natl Cancer Inst.*, ***64***, 977–989

Dukes, C.E. (1952) Familial intestinal polyposis. *Ann. Eugen.*, ***17***, 1–29

Epstein, L.I., Bixler, D. & Bennett, J.E. (1970) An incident of familial cancer, including 3 cases of osteosarcoma. *Cancer*, ***25***, 889–891

Godbout, R., Dryja, T.P., Squire, J., Gallie, B.L. & Phillips, R.A. (1983) Somatic inactivation of genes on chromosome 13 is a common event in retinoblastoma. *Nature*, ***304***, 451–453

Gordon, H. (1974) *Family studies in retinoblastoma.* In: Bergsma, D., Rimoin, D.L., Schimke, R.N. & Paul, N.W., eds, *Medical Genetics Today,* Baltimore, Johns Hopkins University Press, pp. 185–190

Jackson, C.E., Block, M.A., Greenawald, K.A. & Tashjian, A.H., Jr (1979) The two-mutational-event theory in medullary thyroid cancer. *Am. J. human Genet.,* ***31,*** 704–710

Jensen, R.D. & Miller, R.W. (1971) Retinoblastoma: Epidemiologic characteristics. *New Engl. J. Med.,* ***285,*** 307–311

Kanter, Y.C. & Harris, J.E. (1964) Retinoblastoma occurring in one of a pair of identical twins. *Arch. Ophthalmol.,* ***72,*** 783–787

Kitchin, F.D. & Ellsworth, R.M. (1974) Pleiotropic effects of the gene for retinoblastoma. *J. med. Genet.,* ***11,*** 244–246

Knudson, A.G., Jr (1971) Mutation and cancer: Statistical study of retinoblastoma. *Proc. natl Acad. Sci. USA,* ***68,*** 820–823

Knudson, A.G., Jr (1973) Mutation and human cancer. *Adv. Cancer Res.,* ***17,*** 317–352

Knudson, A.G., Jr (1978) Retinoblastoma: A prototypic hereditary neoplasm. *Semin. Oncol.,* ***5,*** 57–60

Matsunaga, E. (1976) Hereditary retinoblastoma: Penetrance, expressivity and age of onset. *Human Genet.,* ***33,*** 1–15

Matsunaga, E. (1978) Hereditary retinoblastoma: Delayed mutation or host resistance? *Am. J. human Genet.,* ***30,*** 406–424

Matsunaga, E. (1979) Hereditary retinoblastoma: Host resistance and age at onset. *J. natl Cancer Inst.,* ***63,*** 933–939

Matsunaga, E. (1980a) Retinoblastoma: Host resistance and 13q– chromosome deletion. *Human Genet.,* ***56,*** 53–58

Matsunaga, E. (1980b) Hereditary retinoblastoma: Host resistance and second primary tumors. *J. natl Cancer Inst.,* ***65,*** 47–51

Matsunaga, E. (1981) Genetics of Wilms' tumor. *Human Genet.,* ***57,*** 231–246

Matsunaga, E. (1982a) Hereditary retinoblastoma: Lack of maternal effect. *Human Genet.,* ***62,*** 124–128

Matsunaga, E. (1982b) Almost synchronous appearance of bilateral retinoblastomas. *Am. J. med. Genet.,* ***11,*** 485–487

Matsunaga, E. (1983) Retinoblastoma: A model for the study of carcinogenesis in humans. *Jpn. J. human Genet.,* ***28,*** 57–71

Miyaki, M., Akamatsu, N., Ono, T. & Sasaki, M.S. (1983) Susceptibility of skin fibroblasts from patients with retinoblastoma to transformation by murine sarcoma virus. *Cancer Lett.,* ***18,*** 137–142

Morris, W.E. & Lapiana, F.G. (1974) Spontaneous regression of bilateral multifocal retinoblastoma with preservation of normal visual acuity. *Ann. Ophthalmol.,* ***6,*** 1192–1194

Reese, A.B. (1976) *Tumors of the Eye,* 3rd ed., New York, Harper & Row

Sagerman, R.H., Cassady, J.R., Tretter, P. & Ellsworth, R.M. (1969) Radiation induced neoplasia following external beam therapy for children with retinoblastoma. *Am. J. Roentgenol.,* ***105,*** 529–535

Sasaki, M.S. (1982) Dominantly expressed procancer mutations and induction of chromosome rearrangements. *Prog. Mutat. Res.*, ***4***, 75–84

Schimke, R.N., Lowman, J.T. & Cowan, G.A. (1974) Retinoblastoma and osteogenic sarcoma in siblings. *Cancer*, ***34***, 2077–2079

Sparkes, R.S., Sparkes, M.C., Wilson, M.G., Towner, J.W., Benedict, W., Murphree, A.L. & Yunis, J.J. (1980) Regional assignment of genes for human esterase D and retinoblastoma to chromosome band 13q14. *Science*, ***208***, 1042–1044

Sparkes, R.S., Murphree, A.L., Lingua, R.W., Sparkes, M.C., Field, L.L., Funderburk, S.J. & Benedict, W.F. (1983) Gene for hereditary retinoblastoma assigned to human chromosome 13 by linkage to esterase D. *Science*, ***219***, 971–973

Strong, L.C., Riccardi, V.M., Ferrell, R.E. & Sparkes, R.S. (1981) Familial retinoblastoma and chromosome 13 deletion transmitted via an insertional translocation. *Science*, ***213***, 1501–1503

Takagi, I. & Ikui, H. (1977) *Eye tumors*. In: Majima, K., ed., *Genetics of Eye Diseases*, Tokyo, Igaku Shoin, pp. 192–209 (in Japanese)

Warburg, M. (1974) *Retinoblastoma*. In: Goldberg, M.F., ed., *Genetic and Metabolic Eye Disease*, Boston, Little, Brown & Co., pp. 447–461

# OESTROGENS AND THE ETIOLOGY AND CLINICAL COURSE OF BREAST CANCER

R.D. BULBROOK, J.W. MOORE, D.Y. WANG & G.M.G. CLARK
*Imperial Cancer Research Fund, Department of Clinical Endocrinology, Lincoln's Inn Fields, London, UK*

## INTRODUCTION

There is a considerable amount of indirect evidence that the oestrogenic hormones are of cardinal importance in the etiology and clinical course of breast cancer. The paradox is that efforts to obtain direct evidence for their involvement have led to equivocal results. It might have been expected that analytical methods for the measurement of oestrogens in urine and blood (which became available from 1955 onwards) would have led to a clear definition of the role of the oestrogens in human carcinogenesis. This has not been the case, but there now appears to be sufficient new evidence that goes a long way towards explaining the discrepancies between epidemiological and analytical work.

In this commentary, the indirect evidence will be examined briefly, prior to a consideration of discordant results obtained in earlier studies in which direct measurements of oestrogenic status were used. Finally, the possibility is discussed that new work on the biological availability of the oestrogens might bring all the results into harmony.

## INDIRECT EVIDENCE

### *Age-specific and cohort-corrected incidence curves: mathematical models*

There is a linear relationship between logarithms of death rates and age for a wide range of cancers, with the notable exception of breast cancer. Instead of an uninterrupted rise in incidence with age, with incidence related to a sixth or seventh power function of age, breast cancer incidence increases steadily until the menopause and then inflects (Clemmensen's hook). In most Western countries, the inflexion is

Fig. 1. Oestrogen action and extended model of Moolgavkar *et al.* (1980)
N, normal cell; D, dead cell; I, intermediate cell; T, transformed cell; $\alpha$, cell proliferation rate; $\beta$, cell death rate; $\mu$, transition probability; $\Rightarrow$, oestrogen-responsive pathway

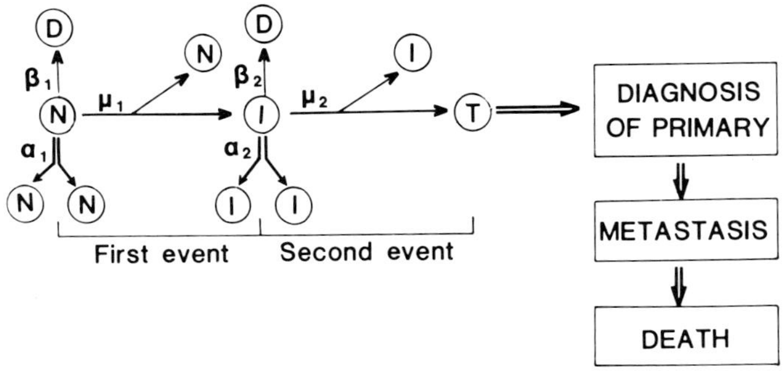


followed by a further rise in incidence, but at a somewhat slower rate. In countries with relatively low incidences, such as Finland, Yugoslavia and Japan, a fall in incidence rates is seen after the menopause.

Armitage and Doll (1957) proposed a two-stage theory of carcinogenesis. They postulated that the first stage resulted in a precancerous clone of cells which had a slight selective advantage over surrounding unaffected cells. Although their model closely predicted the observed incidence rates of cancers of several sites, it did not do so for breast cancer. In order to accommodate this uncomfortable fact, a further postulate was proposed: that for breast cancer the selective advantage was hormonally dependent.

More recently, Moolgavkar *et al.* (1980) have extended the two-stage model of Armitage and Doll. They have attempted to overcome the defect present in the earlier model – that no allowance was made for the growth of target tissue and for the shedding and replenishment of epithelial cells. They postulated that carcinogenesis is the end result of two discrete and irreversible events in the target tissue and that each event occurred during a single cell division. Their model (with some modifications) is shown in Figure 1. A normal cell can divide at a rate $\alpha_1$ or die at rate $\beta_1$; it could also undergo a transition with a probability of $\mu_1$. Transition of a normal cell would produce an intermediate cell with corresponding rates of proliferation and death ($\alpha_2$ and $\beta_2$). The intermediate cell could also undergo another transition (probability $\mu_2$) to yield a cancer cell.

The implications of this model are as follows: if $\alpha_1 = \beta_1$ then there is no net growth. If $\alpha_1 > \beta_1$ or $\alpha_1 - \beta_1 > 0$, then there is growth, or, conversely, $\alpha_1 < \beta_1$ or $\alpha_1 - \beta_1 < 0$, a reduction in target tissue. Similarly, the total number of intermediate cells is also governed by the magnitude of $\alpha_2 - \beta_2$, which in turn is related to the incidence of cancer.

The model was tested using breast cancer incidence data from Connecticut, Denmark, Japan, Iceland, Finland and Slovenia. However, instead of using cross-sectional age-specific incidences, which are strongly influenced by temporal trends in cancer incidence, Moolgavkar and his colleagues (1980) used statistically adjusted data to obtain age-incidence curves free of distortion due to such changes. The curves obtained were very close to those predicted for countries with both high and low incidences of breast cancer.

The model can be used to explain changes in risk due to age at birth of first child, age at menarche and age at menopause. It is also implicit that any factor which increases either $\alpha_1 - \beta_1$ or $\alpha_2 - \beta_2$ will also increase breast cancer incidence.

There are five phases in the extended model in which oestrogenic activity may play a decisive role. The first two phases concern the growth rates of the normal and first-hit cell pools ($\alpha_1$ and $\alpha_2$). The third phase of oestrogen action involves the time period between transformation and diagnosis. The time between diagnosis (in the majority of patients with local, operable disease) and the appearance of metastases would be the fourth area of oestrogen action. Finally, even in the relatively short period between overt metastatic disease and death, powerful effects of alteration of oestrogenic status can be demonstrated.

On the basis of the concept that oestrogenic action 'explains' the model (just as the model 'explains' incidence and fatality curves), the epidemiological evidence might now be examined.

### *Age at menarche and menopause*

The earlier the age at menarche, the higher is the risk of breast cancer (Kelsey, 1979). During the menstrual cycle, parenchymal proliferation occurs with epithelial budding; it is induced by oestrogens secreted by the ovary. At the end of the cycle, there is some regression of these structures, but the new oestrogenic stimulus of the next cycle leads to a slight net increase in mammary development. This process continues throughout some 20 years of reproductive life, unless interrupted by pregnancy (Vorherr, 1974). Thus, an earlier age at menarche could be expected to have two effects; first, it increases the cell pool at risk and, second, it increases the length of time of exposure of these cells. These effects are largely brought about by oestrogens.

The role of progesterone at this early stage in breast development is not clear. One of the main planks in the Sherman-Korenman hypothesis of 1974 (which gives progesterone a dominant role as a modifier of oestrogenic action) was the observation that post-menarchical menstrual cycles may be anovulatory or there may be a deficient production of progesterone in the luteal phase for several years. Thus, early menarche would lead to unopposed oestrogen action on tissue which – if ionizing radiation is an example – is particularly susceptible to carcinogenesis.

This thesis hardly seems tenable in the light of new findings that the earlier the menarche, the sooner regular ovulatory cycles are established (Wallace *et al.*, 1978), and ovulation is related to time from menarche, not age at menarche (Brown, 1981). Furthermore, as far as progestational stimuli are concerned, there is a striking finding by Pike and his colleagues (1983) that long-term use of oral contraceptives in young women (before the age 25 years) carries a substantial risk of breast cancer and that this is highly correlated with the progestin 'potency' of the pill. They speculate that the oestrogen-progestin mixture may stimulate the mitotic activity of breast tissue.

As far as the menopause is concerned, much the same arguments apply as for early menarche. Late menopause and, hence, prolonged exposure to oestrogens (which are not always opposed by progesterone in the decade before the menopause) is associated with high risk (Kelsey, 1979). If incidence is related to a power function of the time of exposure to oestrogens, then small changes in age at menarche and menopause would have a marked effect on incidence. This is precisely what the epidemiological data show.

*Artificial menopause*

The most compelling evidence for a predominant role for the ovarian steroids comes from studies of the effects of oophorectomy or radiation castration on subsequent incidence of breast cancer. The effects are dramatic, and, even up to age 40, cessation of ovarian function leads to a diminution in incidence of some 75% (Feinleib, 1968). It has been pointed out that women with diseases that make them candidates for an artificial menopause are completely atypical of the normal population and may be a sub-set with a low risk of breast cancer. This does not appear to be true, since Japanese women who were aged 40–49 when they were exposed to radiation from the atomic bombs show no dose-related increase in breast cancer, in contrast to all other cohorts (Tokunaga *et al.*, 1979). The explanation appears to be that ovarian function was diminished or abolished in the 40–49-year-old group.

Intuitively, the effects of oophorectomy might be expected to act on the growth rates of intermediate cells ($\alpha_2$) or in the period between transformation and diagnosis.

*Early age at birth of first child*

Two important rate constants in the model of Moolgavkar *et al.* (1980) relate to losses from the cell pool because of cell death or terminal differentiation ($\beta_1$, $\beta_2$). Recently, Russo *et al.* (1982) have quantitated breast epithelial cell numbers in the rat and have shown that pregnancy brings about permanent structural changes in the breast which effectively reduce the cell pool at risk of carcinogenesis. They point out that tumours in women almost certainly originate in terminal ducts and/or intralobular terminal ducts and that these structures disappear when pregnancy and lactation induce full differentiation. Of the several explanations offered for the protective effects of early and repeated pregnancies (which include hypotheses about the type of women who become pregnant early in life; changes in immunological function; permanent changes in endocrine function even when menstruation is resumed after pregnancy), the mechanism proposed by Russo *et al.* (1982) is the most persuasive: early pregnancy protects by removing cells at risk because of differentiation and by causing permanent loss of cells following parturition and lactation.

*Administration of oestrogens*

Doubts are sometimes expressed about the power of the oestrogens in the control of human mammary carcinogenesis, because of the weak and inconstant effects on incidence when oestrogens are given for menopausal symptoms. It has to be borne in mind that, in the majority of cases, menopausal involution of the breast may be well advanced, with almost complete disappearance of alveolar-lobular structures, with a considerable increase in connective tissue, resulting in only a rudimentary ductal system. Complete carcinogens, initiators and promoters (and the oestrogens) need target cells to act upon.

The most convincing data come from the work of Hoover and his colleagues (1976), who found a small time-dependent and dose-dependent increase in incidence which did not become significant until a decade of treatment had elapsed.

### *Treatment of the disease*

Discussion of etiological factors in breast cancer is often kept separate from considerations of what happens when the disease is diagnosed. Epidemiologists hand the problem over, as it were, to clinicians and resume their search for determinants of risk. But it is quite clear that malignant breast cells retain many of the characteristics of their normal progenitors. One of these is a dependency on hormonal stimuli for growth, in at least a third of the patients. Suffice it to say that measures such as oophorectomy and radiation-induced menopause, adrenalectomy, hypophysectomy, and the administration of anti-oestrogenic compounds can lead to massive tumour-cell death even in advanced disease, and can lead to a significant prolongation of disease-free interval and survival if anti-oestrogenic treatment is used as adjuvant therapy (see, for example, Meakin *et al.,* 1979; Baum *et al.,* 1983).

It follows that the model of Moolgavkar *et al.* (1980) can be extended to include two more phases in which the oestrogens are important factors. In addition to their influence on the size of the normal cell pool (and the rate constant $\alpha_1$), and on the size of the first-hit cell pool (rate constant $\alpha_2$), they determine the time at which the transformed cells become clinically apparent. If this period could be prolonged by deliberate intervention, a normal life span might be achieved in spite of the fact that the tumour had not been eradicated. The model could also be extended to include the period between diagnosis and metastasis, another phase where anti-oestrogenic treatment is effective.

## ANALYTICAL RESULTS

### *Urinary oestrogens and total blood oestradiol*

Indirect evidence from mathematical models and from epidemiological studies clearly implicates oestrogens as prime factors in the etiology of breast cancer. It might, therefore, have been expected that the introduction of analytical methods for the determination of oestrogens in urine and blood (Brown, 1955; Korenman *et al.,* 1969) would have led to the discovery of an unequivocal link between oestrogen status and risk. In fact, analytical case-control studies have led to a good deal of confusion, since, in many instances, normal levels have been found, and the same thing has happened in work on high-risk groups (Bulbrook *et al.*, 1978). No consistent pattern has emerged (for review, see Shore *et al.*, 1983).

A comparison of urinary and plasma oestrogens in normal British and Japanese women was carried out by Bulbrook *et al.* (1976). They found virtually identical levels of oestradiol in the blood and of oestrone, oestradiol and oestriol in the urine, in young girls and in pre-menopausal, menopausal and post-menopausal women and concluded that oestrogenic status did not account for the eight-fold difference in incidence in the two races.

*Progesterone, androgens and prolactin*

These largely negative findings led to a number of hypotheses, which still envisage a central role for the oestrogens but which seek to reconcile apparently normal oestrogenic status with an enhanced oestrogenic stimulation to the breast. For example, Sherman and Korenman (1974) have proposed that risk is mediated by the levels of progesterone, which would 'oppose' oestrogen action. Bulbrook *et al.* (1971) have shown that urinary androgen metabolite levels are subnormal in pre-cancer cases; a highly speculative interpretation of these results would be that net oestrogenic stimulation is enhanced by diminution of oestrogenic antagonists. It has yet to be shown that such women have sub-normal amounts of the precursors of these urinary steroids in their blood, although some case-control studies suggest that this is so (Wang *et al.*, 1979; Zumoff, 1981). Considerable attention has been paid to the role of prolactin, since it is clear that many murine mammary carcinomas can be induced by, or are dependent on, this hormone. There is some tentative evidence that high levels of prolactin are associated with increased risk in post-menopausal women (Kwa *et al.*, 1981). Finally, it has been suggested that breast tissue in some women is hypersensitive to oestrogen. In these cases, a 'normal' blood level of oestrogen would still be related to enhanced risk.

All these factors may well be important as determinants of risk, but it now seems to us that a more simple explanation is available: that previous measurements of oestrogenic status have not taken into account the fact that blood oestrogens are largely protein-bound and that this binding modifies their biological activity.

## PROTEIN BINDING OF BLOOD OESTRADIOL

*Protein-bound oestradiol in case-control studies*

The development of centrifugal ultrafiltration-dialysis by Hammond *et al.* (1980) made it possible to measure three oestradiol fractions in blood: free oestradiol (E2) (i.e., not bound to protein), albumin-bound E2 and E2 bound to sex-hormone binding globulin (SHBG). The balance of the evidence is that only the first two fractions are biologically active; these have been termed 'available E2' by Siiteri *et al.* (1981). In normal women, between 45–65% of blood E2 is in the available E2 compartment.

Siiteri *et al.* (1981) found a remarkable difference between controls and women with breast cancer. All but one of the controls had free E2 levels below 2%, whereas all but three of the cancer cases had free E2 levels above 2%. The percentage of free E2 was highly correlated with SHBG capacity.

Moore and his colleagues (1982) confirmed these results in Siiteri's own laboratory and showed that in a well-characterized group of women with breast cancer (Stage II), age- and weight-matched with controls, the free E2 fraction was elevated compared with that of normal women, in the presence of normal SHBG capacity.

The increased amounts of free E2 in patients with breast cancer would be consistent with the finding that such women have a higher metabolic clearance rate for E2 than do normal women (Kirschner *et al.*, 1978; James *et al.*, 1982).

The evidence obtained so far from case-control studies clearly shows that women with breast cancer are exposed to significantly higher levels of biologically available E2 than women without the disease.

*Available E2 and geographical variation*

We have described above our failure to find significant differences in the plasma total E2 levels in British and Japanese women, in spite of an eight-fold difference in risk of breast cancer. When this work was repeated with the new E2 assay system, it was shown that in normal Japanese women a significantly larger proportion of E2 is bound to SHBG than in British women (Moore *et al.*, 1983). These authors suggest that this result provides a logical explanation of the difference in incidence rates in the two countries.

*Free E2 in pre-cancer cases*

The evidence cited above, that the serum transport of oestrogens is a critical factor as far as geographical risk of breast cancer is concerned, and the evidence that in Caucasian women a greater percentage of blood E2 is in the available fraction is strongly supportive of the thesis that a hyperoestrogenic stimulus is a prime factor in the etiology of human breast cancer. Definitive evidence for this proposition can come only from prospective studies designed to investigate oestrogenic status before the disease becomes manifest.

Since 1977, blood has been collected from 4 000 normal women living in the Island of Guernsey, and serum has been prepared and stored at $-20$ °C. Serum samples were available for oestrogen assay from 13 women whose breast cancers were either found at a subsequent mammographic screening or which developed after screening. Controls were selected for these pre-cancer cases, matched only for menopausal status and age. Free E2 was then measured. The results are shown in Figure 2. It is quite apparent that the pre-cancer cases have free E2 fractions that are at the top of, or near the top of, the control range. This is the first direct evidence that women who develop breast cancer are subjected to a hyperoestrogenic stimulus before the disease develops.

Quite obviously, these results are preliminary: more pre-cancer cases are required, and the albumin and SHBG fractions must be measured. Nevertheless, they fit well with the general thesis that oestrogens are of paramount importance in the biology of breast cancer.

Fig. 2. Non-protein bound (free) oestradiol ($E_2$) in women who subsequently developed breast cancer The black circles denote pre-cancer cases: the white circles, matched controls. The significance of the finding was tested by the method of Cuzick described by Kwa *et al.* (1981); Z = 4.9; $p < 0.00005$.

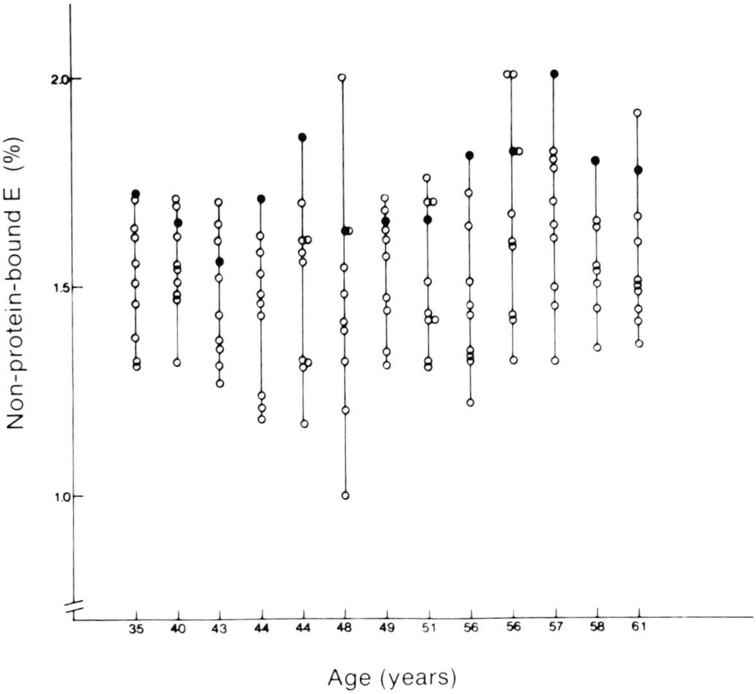


*Mechanisms*

The question now arises as to the reason for the increase in available blood E2 in women at risk or women with breast cancer. The first and most likely cause would be a decreased SHBG capacity, but this turns out to be not so (Siiteri *et al.*, 1981; James *et al.*, 1981; Moore *et al.*, 1983). There is unanimity that the capacity of the protein (as measured with a 5α-dihydrotestosterone probe) is normal.

A second and attractive explanation would be that, as available E2 increases with increasing weight, the high proportion of biologically active oestrogen simply reflects a degree of obesity in women at high risk. Once again, this is not the case. For example, James *et al.* (1981) and Moore *et al.* (1982) found that the free fraction was elevated in their cases even when the controls were carefully matched for weight. Moore *et al.* (1983) compared availability in Japanese and British women of equal weight and found that the latter still had a greater proportion of available E2 in their blood.

This is not to say that obesity is unimportant as a risk factor. It is well established that there is increased adrenal secretion of androstenedione in obese women, and the peripheral conversion of androstenedione to oestrone is also increased (Siiteri *et al.*,

1981). These effects are exacerbated by the low SHBG capacity associated with obesity.

Thus, obese women are hyperoestrogenic, and this would account for the relation between weight and risk of breast cancer. But our results show that high-risk women who are of normal weight are also exposed to an increased oestrogenic stimulus, and this is not mediated by decreased SHBG capacity.

These results lead to the third thesis: the high level of available E2 is due to substances in the blood that alter protein binding. Siiteri *et al.* (1981) have suggested that these may be plasma lipids. If this were so, it might link the high risk associated with dietary intake of fats to a hormonal mechanism. There are already some strong leads that this is so. For example, Armstrong and his colleagues (1981) showed that vegetarian post-menopausal women had lower urinary oestrogen levels, lower plasma prolactin levels and higher SHBG titres, the latter being highly correlated with high-density lipoprotein cholesterol. Prolactin levels rise with increasing daily intake of total fat, oleic acid and linoleic acid. Plasma oestradiol and oestriol levels are significantly related to dietary linoleic acid and protein intake in pre-menopausal Seventh-day Adventist vegetarian women (Shultz & Leklem, 1983).

## CONCLUSIONS

If the promise of the early results of assays of free and protein-bound oestrogens can be confirmed generally, there would exist a central mechanism that would bring many strands of evidence into a harmonious picture. For example, risk in Caucasian women may be proportional to the amount of biologically active oestrogen in the blood. Geographical risk may be explicable in terms of protein binding of oestrogen and, hence, biological availability. Risk associated with various diets may be due to effects on the amount of oestrogen secreted and the proportion that is bound to proteins. A great deal more experimental data are required, but the new findings, indicating the importance of protein binding of steroids, point to the possibility that the factors that influence risk of breast cancer in women are not very dissimilar to those which influence risk in rats and mice.

## ACKNOWLEDGEMENTS

The authors wish to express their gratitude to Mr J.L. Hayward, FRCS and Dr R.R. Millis.

## REFERENCES

Armitage, P. & Doll, R. (1957) A two-stage theory of carcinogenesis in relation to the age distribution of human cancer. *Br. J. Cancer*, ***11***, 161–169

Armstrong, B.K., Brown, J.B., Clarke, H.T., Crooke, D.K., Hahnel, R., Masarei, J.R. & Ratajczak, T. (1981) Diet and reproductive hormones: A study of vegetarian and non-vegetarian postmenopausal women. *J. natl Cancer Inst.*, ***67***, 761–767

Baum, M., Brinkley, D.M., Dossett, J.A., McPherson, K., Patterson, J.S., Rubens, R.D., Smiddy, F.G., Stoll, B.A., Wilson, A., Lea, J.C., Richards, S. & Ellis, S.H. (1983) Nolvadex Adjuvant Trial Organisation – Controlled Trial of tamoxifen as adjuvant agent in management of early breast cancer. *Lancet*, ***i***, 257–260

Brown, J.B. (1955) A chemical method for the determination of oestriol, oestrone and oestradiol in human urine. *Biochem. J.*, ***60***, 185–193

Brown, J.B. (1981) *A study of ovarian function during theelarche, menarche and menopause and after childbirth.* In: Pike, M.C., Siiteri, P.K. & Welsch, C.W., eds, *Hormones and Breast Cancer (Banbury Report No. 8)* Cold Spring Harbor, NY, Cold Spring Harbor Laboratory, pp. 33–56

Bulbrook, R.D., Hayward, J.L. & Spicer, C.C. (1971) Relation between urinary androgens and corticoid excretion and subsequent breast cancer. *Lancet*, ***ii***, 395–398

Bulbrook, R.D., Swain, M.C., Wang, D.Y., Hayward, J.L., Kumaoka, S., Abe, O. & Utsunomiya, J. (1976) Plasma estradiol-17β, oestrone and progesterone and their urinary metabolites in normal British and Japanese women. *Eur. J. Cancer*, ***12***, 725–735

Bulbrook, R.D., Moore, J.W., Clark, G.M.G., Wang, D.Y., Tong, D. & Hayward, J.L. (1978) Plasma oestradiol and progesterone levels in women with varying degrees of risk of breast cancer. *Eur. J. Cancer*, ***14***, 1369–1375

Feinleib, M. (1968) Breast cancer and artificial menopause. A cohort study. *J. natl Cancer Inst.*, ***41***, 315–329

Hammond, G.L., Nisker, J.A., Jones, L.A. & Siiteri, P.K. (1980) Estimation of the percent free steroid in undiluted serum by centrifugal ultrafiltration dialysis. *J. biol. Chem.*, ***255***, 5023–5026

Hoover, R., Gray, L.A., Cole, P. & MacMahon, B. (1976) Menopausal estrogens and breast cancer. *New Engl. J. Med.*, ***295***, 401–405

James, V.H.T., Reed, M.J. & Folkerd, E.J. (1981) Studies of oestrogen metabolism in postmenopausal women with cancer. *J. Steroid Biochem.*, ***15***, 235–246

James, V.H.T., Folkerd, E.J., Bonney, R.C., Beranek, P.A. & Reed, M.J. (1982) Factors influencing oestrogen production and metabolism in post-menopausal women with endocrine cancer. *J. endocrinol. Invest.*, ***5***, 335–345

Kelsey, J.L. (1979) A review of the epidemiology of human breast cancer. *Epidemiol. Rev.*, ***1***, 74–109

Kirschner, M.A., Cohen, F.B. & Ryan, C. (1978) Androgen-estrogen production rates in postmenopausal women with breast cancer. *Cancer Res.*, ***38***, 4029–4035

Korenman, S.G., Perrin, L.E. & McCallum, T.P. (1969) A radio-ligand binding assay system for estradiol measurement in human plasma. *J. clin. Endocrinol. Metab.*, ***29***, 879–883

Kwa, H.G., Cleton, F., Wang, D.Y., Bulbrook, R.D., Bulstrode, J.C., Hayward, J.L., Millis, R.R. & Cuzick, J. (1981) A prospective study of plasma prolactin levels and subsequent risk of breast cancer. *Int. J. Cancer*, ***28***, 673–676

Meakin, J.W., Allt, W.E.C., Beale, F.A., Brown, T.C., Bush, R.S., Clark, R.M., Fitzpatrick, P.J., Hawkins, N.V., Jenkin, R.D.T., Pringle, J.F., Reid, J.G., Rider, W.D., Hayward, J.L. & Bulbrook, R.D. (1979) Ovarian irradiation and prednisolone following surgery and radiotherapy for carcinoma of the breast. *Can. med. Assoc. J.*, ***120***, 1221–1229

Moolgavkar, S.H., Day, N.E. & Stevens, R.G. (1980) Two-stage model for carcinogenesis. Epidemiology of breast cancer in females. *J. natl Cancer Inst.*, ***65***, 559–569

Moore, J.W., Clark, G.M.G., Bulbrook, R.D., Hayward, J.L., Murai, J.T., Hammond, G.L. & Siiteri, P.K. (1982) Serum concentrations of total and non-protein-bound oestradiol in patients with breast cancer and in normal controls. *Int. J. Cancer*, ***29***, 17–21

Moore, J.W., Clark, G.M.G., Takatani, O., Wakabayashi, Y., Hayward, J.L. & Bulbrook, R.D. (1983) Distribution of estradiol in the serum of normal British and Japanese women. *J. natl Cancer Inst.*, ***71***, 749–754

Pike, M.C., Henderson, B.E., Krailo, M.D., Duke, A. & Roy, S. (1983) Breast cancer in young women and use of oral contraceptives: Effect of formulation and age at use. *Lancet*, ***ii***, 926–930

Russo, J., Tay, L.K. & Russo, H. (1982) Differentiation of the mammary gland and susceptibility to carcinogenesis. *Breast Cancer Res. Treat.*, ***2***, 5–73

Sherman, B.M. & Korenman, S.G. (1974) Inadequate corpus luteum function: a pathophysiological interpretation of human breast cancer epidemiology. *Cancer*, ***33***, 1306–1312

Shore, R.E., Pasternak, B.S., Bulbrook, R.D., Moseson, M., Kwa, H.G., Wang, D.Y., Moore, J.W. & Strax, P. (1983) *Endocrine and environmental factors in breast cancer. The case for prospective studies.* In: Bulbrook, R.D. & Taylor, D.J., eds, *Commentaries in Research on Breast Disease*, New York, Alan Liss & Co. (in press)

Shultz, T.D. & Leklem, J.E. (1983) Nutrient intake and hormonal status of pre-menopausal vegetarian Seventh-day Adventists. *Nutrit. Cancer*, ***4***, 247–259

Siiteri, P.K., Hammond, G.L. & Nisker, J.A. (1981) *Increased availability of serum estrogens in breast cancer: A new hypothesis.* In: Pike, M.C., Siiteri, P.K. & Welsch, C.W., eds, *Hormones and Breast Cancer (Banbury Report No. 8)*, Cold Spring Harbor, NY, Cold Spring Harbor Laboratory, pp. 87–106

Tokunaga, M., Norman, J.E. & Asano, S.M. (1979) Malignant breast tumours among atomic bomb survivors, Hiroshima and Nagasaki, 1950–1974. *J. natl Cancer Inst.*, ***62***, 1347–1359

Vorherr, H. (1974) *The Breast*, New York, Academic Press, pp. 1–18

Wallace, R.B., Sherman, B.M., Bean, J.A., Leeper, J.P. & Treloar, A.E. (1978) Menstrual cycle patterns and breast cancer risk factors. *Cancer Res.*, ***38***, 4021–4024

Wang, D.Y., Moore, J.W., Thomas, B.S., Bulbrook, R.D., Hoare, S.A., Tong, D. & Hayward, J.L. (1979) Plasma and urinary androgens in women with varying degrees of risk of breast cancer. *Eur. J. Cancer*, ***15***, 1269–1274

Zumoff, B. (1981) *Abnormal plasma hormone levels in women with breast cancer.* In: Pike, M.C., Siiteri, P.K. & Welsch, C.W., eds, *Hormones and Breast Cancer (Banbury Report No. 8)*, Cold Spring Harbor, NY, Cold Spring Harbor Laboratory, pp. 143–166

# EXPERIMENTAL MODELS TO STUDY ETIOLOGICAL FACTORS IN MULTI-STAGE CARCINOGENESIS

# DRUGS, FOOD ADDITIVES AND NATURAL PRODUCTS AS PROMOTERS IN RAT URINARY BLADDER CARCINOGENESIS

N. ITO, S. FUKUSHIMA, T. SHIRAI, A. HAGIWARA & K. IMAIDA

*First Department of Pathology, Nagoya City University, Medical School, Nagoya, Japan*

## SUMMARY

The promoting effects of various chemicals on urinary bladder carcinogenesis in rats initiated with *N*-butyl-*N*-(4-hydroxybutyl)nitrosamine (BBN) were studied. Male Fischer 344 rats were given BBN at 0.01% or 0.05% in their drinking-water for four weeks. One of the following chemicals was then administered in the diet for 32 or 34 weeks: acetazolamide, allopurinol, phenobarbital, phenacetin, *ortho*-phenylphenol, sodium *ortho*-phenylphenate, diphenyl, sodium L-ascorbate, butylated hydroxyanisole, butylated hydroxytoluene, sodium saccharin, aspartame, sodium cyclamate, stevioside, DL-tryptophan, quercetin, caffeine, nicotine and hippuric acid.

Phenacetin, sodium *ortho*-phenylphenate, sodium L-ascorbate and butylated hydroxyanisole were significant promoters of urinary bladder neoplasia in rats initiated with BBN. Sodium saccharin, diphenyl, butylated hydroxytoluene, allopurinol, and DL-tryptophan caused moderate or slight promotion of neoplastic changes in the experimental animals. No change in tumour yield was observed after administration of the other chemicals.

## INTRODUCTION

The two-stage process of chemical carcinogenesis, initiation and promotion, was first proposed on the basis of the mouse skin model (Berenblum & Shubik, 1947). It is now the accepted process of chemical carcinogenesis in many organs (Peraino *et al.*, 1971; Narisawa *et al.*, 1974; Goerttler *et al.*, 1979; Ito *et al.*, 1980; Slaga *et al.*, 1981; Imaida *et al.*, 1983a). A two-stage process in urinary bladder carcinogenesis has been demonstrated in rats treated with carcinogen and then with saccharin, cyclamate or DL-tryptophan (Ito *et al.*, 1973; Hicks *et al.*, 1973, 1975; Cohen *et al.*, 1979; Fukushima *et al.*, 1981; Cohen *et al.*, 1982; Fukushima *et al.*, 1983a, b). A high proportion of human cancers has been attributed to environmental factors such as chemicals, drugs, food additives and natural products (Clayson & Cooper, 1970; Sugimura, 1979). When given experimentally, some compounds present in our environment induce urinary bladder cancer (Pamukcu *et al.*, 1980; Hiraga & Fujii, 1981; Hirono *et al.*, 1981). Therefore, evaluation of the promoting activities of these compounds, in urinary bladder carcinogenesis, for example, is particularly worthwhile.

Preneoplastic lesions during rat urinary bladder carcinogenesis have been the object of many reports (Ito *et al.*, 1969; Cohen *et al.*, 1976; Fukushima *et al.*, 1982a). There is strong evidence of correlation between papillary or nodular (PN) hyperplasia and the eventual development of urinary bladder cancer. Thus, the preneoplastic lesion of the rat urinary bladder, PN hyperplasia, may be used as a marker to study the two-stage process of urinary bladder carcinogenesis (Nakanishi *et al.*, 1980; Fukushima *et al.*, 1983b; Ito *et al.*, 1983a,b).

In the present investigation, we examined the promoting effects of various chemicals, such as drugs, food additives and natural products, on urinary bladder carcinogenesis in rats initiated with *N*-butyl-*N*-(4-hydroxybutyl)nitrosamine (BBN). Effects were evaluated by measuring the formation of PN hyperplasia (preneoplastic lesions), papillomas or carcinomas of the urinary bladder.

## MATERIALS AND METHODS

### *Animals and experimental design*

Six-week-old male Fischer 344 rats (Charles River Japan, Inc, Kanagawa, Japan) were used. Each group consisted of 20 to 30 rats, which were administered 0.01% or 0.05% BBN in the drinking-water for four weeks and were then given test compounds in the basal diet (Oriental M) or in the drinking-water for 32 or 34 weeks. Controls receiving only the carcinogen and controls receiving only one of the test substances were also included. Diets or water containing test compounds were prepared freshly once a week. The concentrations administered of the 19 test chemicals are shown in Table 1.

After sacrifice of the animals, the urinary bladders were processed by inflation and immersion in fixative. The bladders were then divided sagitally and, under a dissecting microscope, each half was cut into four strips. Sections were taken and stained with haematoxylin and eosin. The lesions were counted under a light microscope; the total length of the basement membrane under analysis was measured with a colour video image processor; and the incidence of lesions was expressed in terms of number of lesions per 10 cm of basement membrane.

## RESULTS

### *Sodium L-ascorbate* (Imaida *et al.*, 1982)

The histopathological findings in the urinary bladder of rats treated with sodium L-ascorbate are summarized in Table 2. The incidences of PN hyperplasia, papilloma

Table 1. Investigation of potential promotion of rat urinary bladder carcinogenesis: substances tested and promoting activity

| Chemical tested | Usual source of human exposure | Concentration tested (%) | Promoting activity[a] |
|---|---|---|---|
| DL-tryptophan | natural product | 5.0 | + |
| Quercetin | natural product | 5.0 | − |
| Caffeine | natural product | 0.1 | − |
| Nicotine | natural product | 0.0025 | − |
| Hippuric acid | natural product | 5.0 | − |
| Sodium L-ascorbate | food additive, drug | 5.0 | + + + |
| Butylated hydroxyanisole | food additive | 2.0 | + + + |
| Butylated hydroxytoluene | food additive | 1.0 | + + |
| Sodium saccharin | food additive | 5.0 | + + |
| Aspartame | food additive | 5.0 | − |
| Sodium cyclamate | food additive | 2.5 | − |
| Stevioside | food additive | 5.0 | − |
| Acetazolamide | drug | 0.35 | − |
| Allopurinol | drug | 0.02 | + |
| Phenobarbital | drug | 0.05 | − |
| Phenacetin | drug | 2.5 | + + + |
| *ortho*-Phenylphenol | drug | 2.0 | − |
| Sodium *ortho*-phenylphenate | drug | 2.0 | + + + |
| Diphenyl | drug | 0.5 | + + |

[a] + + +, strong; + +, moderate; +, weak; −, none

and cancer were significantly greater after administration of the higher dose of BBN followed by 5.0% sodium L-ascorbate, than after administration of BBN alone. Moreover, quantitative analysis of the lesions showed that the number of PN hyperplasias, papillomas and cancers per 10 cm basement membrane was also increased significantly. The lower dose of sodium L-ascorbate did not appear to increase the occurrence of bladder lesions in rats pretreated with BBN.

*Butylated hydroxyanisole (BHA) and butylated hydroxytoluene (BHT)* (Fukushima *et al.*, 1982)

The incidences of lesions of the urinary bladder in rats initiated with BBN and then exposed to BHA and BHT are shown in Table 3. Rats given 0.05% BBN followed by 2% BHA had a greater incidence of tumours of the urinary bladder than those in the carcinogen control group. Also, the number of papillomas and cancers per 10 cm basement membrane was increased significantly in comparison with that of the control. The incidence of cancer increased moderately after BHT treatment, showing a significant difference from that of the carcinogen control group. The number of PN hyperplasias was also elevated in the groups treated with 0.01% BBN followed by BHA or BHT. No histopathological change in the urinary bladder of rats given BHA or BHT alone was observed.

Table 2. Histological findings in the urinary bladders of rats initiated with *N*-butyl-*N*-(4-hydroxybutyl)nitrosamine (BBN) and then treated with sodium L-ascorbate (ascorbate)

| Treatment | | No. of rats | Papillary or nodular hyperplastic lesions | | Papilloma | | Cancer | |
|---|---|---|---|---|---|---|---|---|
| BBN | Ascorbate | | Incidence (%) | No.[a] | Incidence (%) | No.[a] | Incidence (%) | No.[a] |
| 0.01 | 5.0 | 20 | 17 (85)** | 4.9 ± 5.7** | 12 (60) | 1.1 ± 1.2 | 0 – | 0 |
| 0.01 | 1.0 | 20 | 10 (50) | 1.1 ± 1.3 | 9 (45) | 0.8 ± 1.3 | 0 – | 0 |
| 0.01 | – | 20 | 8 (40) | 0.5 ± 0.6 | 5 (25) | 0.5 ± 1.0 | 0 – | 0 |
| 0.05 | 5.0 | 25 | 25 (100)*** | 7.0 ± 3.0*** | 23 (92)*** | 3.1 ± 1.6*** | 24 (96)*** | 1.4 ± 0.7*** |
| 0.05 | 1.0 | 29 | 11 (37.9) | 0.6 ± 1.0 | 12 (41.4) | 0.4 ± 0.6 | 0 – | 0 |
| 0.05 | – | 30 | 8 (26.7) | 0.3 ± 0.5 | 12 (40) | 0.5 ± 0.5 | 1 (3.3) | 0.0 ± 0.2 |
| – | 5.0 | 20 | 0 – | 0 | 0 – | 0 | 0 – | 0 |

[a] Per 10 cm basement membrane; mean ± SD
Significantly different from carcinogen control at **, $p < 0.01$; ***, $p < 0.001$

Table 3. Histological findings in the urinary bladders of rats initiated with *N*-butyl-*N*-(4-hydroxybutyl)nitrosamine (BBN) and then treated with butylated hydroxyanisole (BHA) or butylated hydroxytoluene (BHT)

| Treatment | | No. of rats | Papillary or nodular hyperplastic lesions | | Papilloma | | Cancer | |
|---|---|---|---|---|---|---|---|---|
| BBN | Ascorbate | | Incidence (%) | No.[a] | Incidence (%) | No.[a] | Incidence (%) | No.[a] |
| 0.05 | BHA | 25 | 25 (100) | 4.3 ± 2.7*** | 22 (88.0)*** | 2.0 ± 1.4*** | 19 (76.0)*** | 0.8 ± 0.7** |
| 0.05 | BHT | 24 | 23 (95.8) | 4.0 ± 1.9*** | 17 (70.8)** | 0.9 ± 0.8* | 13 (54.2)* | 0.4 ± 0.6 |
| 0.05 | – | 26 | 24 (92.3) | 2.0 ± 0.8 | 11 (42.3) | 0.4 ± 0.6 | 5 (19.2) | 0.2 ± 0.4 |
| 0.01 | BHA | 25 | 24 (96.0)* | 3.0 ± 2.3*** | 11 (44.0) | 0.7 ± 1.3 | 5 (20.0) | 0.1 ± 0.3 |
| 0.01 | BHT | 22 | 20 (90.9)* | 2.0 ± 1.2** | 3 (13.6) | 0.1 ± 0.3 | 1 (4.5) | 0.0 ± 0.0 |
| 0.01 | – | 24 | 15 (62.5) | 1.1 ± 1.0 | 7 (29.2) | 0.2 ± 0.5 | 2 (8.3) | 0.1 ± 0.2 |
| – | BHA | 25 | 0 – | 0 | 0 – | 0 | 0 – | 0 |
| – | BHT | 25 | 0 – | 0 | 0 – | 0 | 0 – | 0 |
| – | – | 19 | 0 – | 0 | 0 – | 0 | 0 – | 0 |

[a] Per 10 cm basement membrane; mean ± SD
Significantly different from the carcinogen control at *, $p < 0.05$; **, $p < 0.01$; ***, $p < 0.001$

Table 4. Histological findings in the urinary bladders of rats initiated with *N*-butyl-*N*-(4-hydroxybutyl)nitrosamine (BBN) and then treated with sodium *ortho*-phenylphenate (OPP-Na) or *ortho*-phenylphenol (OPP)

| Treatment | | No. of rats | Papillary or nodular hyperplasia | | Papilloma | | Cancer | |
|---|---|---|---|---|---|---|---|---|
| BBN (%) | Chemical | | Incidence (%) | No.[a] | Incidence (%) | No.[a] | Incidence (%) | No.[a] |
| 0.01 | OPP-Na | 28 | 28 (100)*** | 5.8 ± 4.1*** | 9 (32.1) | 0.4 ± 0.7 | 2 (7.1) | 0.1 ± 0.2 |
| 0.01 | – | 30 | 14 (46.7) | 0.5 ± 0.6 | 8 (26.7) | 0.2 ± 0.4 | 1 (3.3) | 0.0 ± 0.1 |
| – | OPP-Na | 29 | 25 (86.2) | 4.4 ± 4.7 | 5 (17.2) | 0.2 ± 0.3 | 0 – | 0 |
| 0.05 | OPP-Na | 30 | 29 (96.7)*** | 18.7 ± 10.8*** | 30 (100)*** | 4.1 ± 1.7*** | 27 (90)*** | 1.4 ± 0.9 |
| 0.05 | OPP | 30 | 17 (56.7) | 0.9 ± 1.0 | 11 (36.7) | 0.3 ± 0.5 | 6 (20) | 0.2 ± 0.3 |
| 0.05 | – | 30 | 13 (43.3) | 0.7 ± 1.1 | 7 (23.3) | 0.3 ± 0.5 | 2 (6.7) | 0.1 ± 0.3 |
| – | OPP-Na | 15 | 14 (93.3) | 5.6 ± 4.0 | 2 (13.3) | 0.1 ± 0.3 | 1 (6.7) | 0.1 ± 0.2 |
| – | OPP | 14 | 0 – | 0 | 0 – | 0 | 0 – | 0 |

[a] Per 10 cm basement membrane; mean ± SD
Significantly different from carcinogen control at ***, $p < 0.001$

*Sodium* ortho-*phenylphenate (OPP-Na) and* ortho-*phenylphenol (OPP)* (Fukushima *et al.,* 1982)

The histological findings in bladders of rats treated with BBN followed by OPP-Na and OPP are shown in Table 4. The incidences of PH hyperplasia, papilloma and cancer were significantly higher in the BBN group exposed subsequently to 2% OPP-Na. Although there was no remarkable change in the urinary bladders of BBN-initiated rats treated with OPP alone, one cancer was observed after OPP-Na administration.

*Others* (Nakanishi *et al.,* 1978, 1980; Hagiwara *et al.,* 1981; Fukushima *et al.,* 1983b)

The potentials of all the chemicals tested to promote BBN-initiated urinary bladder lesions are shown in Table 1. Phenacetin had a strong promoting activity; sodium saccharin, DL-tryptophan, allopurinol and diphenyl showed moderate or weak promoting activity; whereas quercetin, caffeine, nicotine, hippuric acid, aspartame, sodium cyclamate, stevioside, acetazolamide, phenobarbital and *ortho*-phenylphenol had no promoting activity.

## DISCUSSION

The two-stage process of chemical carcinogenesis – initiation and promotion – has been demonstrated in many organs, including the urinary bladder (Miyata *et al.,* 1981; Oyasu *et al.,* 1981). BBN is a potent, complete carcinogen for the urinary bladder. When given for too short a period or at a dose too low for tumour induction, its initiating activity can be promoted by substances such as sodium saccharin. Our model for evaluating chemicals as bladder promoters is based on initiation by BBN for four weeks followed by continuous administration of the test chemical for 32 or 36 weeks (Nakanishi *et al.,* 1978, 1980; Ito *et al.,* 1982, 1983a,b; Fukushima *et al.,* 1983b; Imaida *et al.,* 1983a).

In the present study, it was shown that the drugs, phenacetin, OPP-Na, allopurinol and diphenyl, the food additives, sodium L-ascorbate, BHA, BHT and sodium saccharin and DL-tryptophan, a natural product, had promoting activity for bladder carcinogenesis. The drugs, acetazolamide, phenobarbital and OPP, the food additives, aspartame, sodium cyclamate and stevioside, and the natural products, quercetin, caffeine, nicotine and hippuric acid had no promoting activity when given at maximum tolerable doses to the animals.

The underlying mechanism of these promoting activities is unknown. Recently, however, we measured the membrane potentials of the bladder epithelium in rats treated with BBN and saccharin. The effect of BBN on increasing membrane potential was clearly dose-dependent, but only the highest dose level of saccharin caused a significant increase in the potential compared with the effect observed in the control group (Imaida *et al.,* 1983b). These findings suggest that one result of the treatment may be inactivation of the sodium pump located in the apical membrane. It has been suggested that bladder cancers may be induced by the formation of stones in the urinary bladder (Clayson & Cooper, 1970; Flakes & Clayson, 1975). In our previous studies, however, no correlation was found between the number of crystals in the urine sediment, the urinary osmolality and the occurrence of neoplastic lesions in rat experimental models using BBN (Fukushima *et al.*, 1983b).

The present results show that various environmental chemicals may promote development of urinary bladder cancers. This fact is relevant not only to detection of environmental risk factors for humans but also to future research directed at the mechanisms underlying the neoplastic process.

## ACKNOWLEDGEMENTS

This work was supported by Grants-in-Aid for Cancer Research from the Ministry of Education Science and Culture of Japan, the Ministry of Health and Welfare of Japan, the Japan Tobacco and Salt Public Corporation, the Society for Promotion of Pathology of Nagoya, and the Experimental Pathological Research Association.

## REFERENCES

Berenblum, O. & Shubik, P.A. (1947) A new, quantitative approach to the study of the stages of chemical carcinogenesis in the mouse skin. *Br. J. Cancer,* ***1,*** 383–391

Cohen, S.M., Jacobs, J.B., Arai, M., Johansson, S. & Friedell, G.H. (1976) Early lesions in experimental bladder cancer: Experimental design and light microscopic findings. *Cancer Res.,* ***36,*** 2508–2511

Cohen, S.M., Arai, M., Jacobs, J.B. & Friedell, G.H. (1979) Promoting effect of saccharin and DL-tryptophan in urinary bladder carcinogenesis. *Cancer Res.,* ***39,*** 1207–1215

Cohen, S.M., Murasaki, G., Fukushima, S. & Greenfield, R.E. (1982) Effect of regenerative hyperplasia on the urinary bladder: Carcinogenicity of sodium saccharin and *N*-[4-(5-nitro-2-furyl)-2-thiazolyl]formamide. *Cancer Res.,* ***42,*** 65–71

Clayson, D.B. & Cooper, E.H. (1970) Cancer of the urinary tract. *Adv. Cancer Res.,* ***13,*** 271–381

Flakes, A. & Clayson, D.B. (1975) The influence of ammonium chloride on the induction of bladder tumors by 4-ethylsulphonylnaphthalene-1-sulphonamide. *Br. J. Cancer,* ***31,*** 585–587

Fujii, T. & Hiraga, K. (1982) Induction of tumors of urinary bladder in male F344 rats by dietary administration of *o*-phenylphenol. *Proc. Jpan. Cancer Assoc.,* ***41,*** 16

Fukushima, S., Friedell, G.H., Jacobs, J.B. & Cohen, S.M. (1981) Effect of L-tryptophan and sodium saccharin on urinary tract carcinogenesis initiated by *N*-[4-(5-nitro-2-furyl)-2-thiazolyl]formamide. *Cancer Res.,* ***41,*** 3100–3103

Fukushima, S., Murasaki, G., Hirose, M., Nakanishi, K., Hasegawa, R. & Ito, N. (1982) Histopathological analysis of preneoplastic changes during *N*-butyl-*N*-(4-hydroxybutyl)nitrosamine-induced urinary bladder carcinogenesis in rats. *Acta pathol. jpn.,* ***32,*** 243–250

Fukushima, S., Arai, M., Nakanowatari, J., Hibino, T., Okuda, M. & Ito, N. (1983a) Differences in susceptibility to sodium saccharin among various strains of rats and other animal species. *Gann, **74,*** 8–20

Fukushima, S., Hagiwara, A., Ogiso, T., Shibata, M. & Ito, N. (1983b) Promoting effects of various chemicals in rat urinary bladder carcinogenesis initiated by *N*-butyl-*N*-(4-hydroxybutyl)amine. *Food Chem. Toxicol., **21,*** 59–68

Goerttler, K., Loehrke, H., Schweizer, J. & Hesse, B. (1979) Systemic two-stage carcinogenesis in the epithelium of the forestomach of mice using 7,12-dimethylbenz(*a*)anthracene as initiator and the phorbol ester 12-*o*-tetradecanoylphorbol-13-acetate as promoter. *Cancer Res., **39,*** 1293–1297

Hagiwara, A., Fukushima, S., Ogiso, T., Nakanishi, K. & Ito, N. (1981) Effects of various chemicals on rat bladder carcinogenesis initiated by BBN. *Proc. Jpn. Cancer Assoc., **40,*** 51

Hicks, R.M., Wakefield, J.StJ. & Chowaniec, J. (1973) Co-carcinogenic action of saccharin in the chemical induction of bladder cancer. *Nature, **243,*** 347–349

Hicks, R.M., Wakefield, J.StJ. & Chowaniec, J. (1975) Evaluation of a new model to detect bladder carcinogens or co-carcinogens; results obtained with saccharin, cyclamate and cyclophosphamide. *Chem.-biol. Interact., **11,*** 225–233

Hiraga, K. & Fujii, T. (1981) Induction of tumors of the urinary system in F344 rats by dietary administration of sodium *o*-phenylphenate. *Food Cosmet. Toxicol., **19,*** 303–310

Hirono, I., Ueno, I., Hosaka, S., Takanashi, H., Matsushima, T., Sugimura, T. & Natori, S. (1981) Carcinogenicity examination of quercetin and rutin in ACI rats. *Cancer Lett., **13,*** 15–21

Imaida, K., Fukushima, S., Shirai, T., Hagiwara, A., Kitaori, M. & Ito, N. (1982) Promoting activities of antioxidants – BHA, BHT and L-ascorbate – in urinary bladder and liver of F344 rats. *Proc. Jpn. Cancer Assoc., **41,*** 79

Imaida, K., Ohshima, M., Fukushima, S., Ito, N. & Hotta, K. (1983a) Promoting activities of butylated hydroxyanisole and butylated hydroxytoluene on 2-stage urinary bladder carcinogenes and inhibition of γ-glutamyl transpeptidase-positive foci in the liver of rats. *Carcinogenesis, **4,*** 895–899

Imaida, K., Fukushima, S., Shirai, T., Ohatani, M., Nakanishi, K. & Ito, N. (1983b) Membrane potentials of urinary bladder epithelium in F344 rats treated with *N*-butyl-*N*-(4-hydroxybutyl)nitrosamine or sodium saccharin. *Carcinogenesis, **4,*** 659–661

Ito, N., Hiasa, Y., Tamai, A., Okajima, E. & Kitamura, H. (1969) Histogenesis of urinary bladder tumors induced by *N*-butyl-*N*-(4-hydroxybutyl)nitrosamine in rats. *Gann, **60,*** 401–410

Ito, N., Matayoski, K., Arai, M., Yoshioka, Y., Kamamoto, Y., Makiura, S. & Sugihara, S. (1973) Effect of various factors on induction of urinary bladder tumors in animals by *N*-butyl-*N*-(4-hydroxybutyl)nitrosamine. *Gann, **64,*** 151–159

Ito, N., Tatematsu, M., Nakanishi, K., Hasegawa, R., Takano, T., Imaida, K. & Ogiso, T. (1980) The effects of various chemicals on the development of hyperplastic liver nodules in hepatectomized rats treated with *N*-nitrosodiethylamine or *N*-2-fluorenylacetamide. *Gann, **71,*** 832–842

Ito, N., Nakanishi, K., Fukushima, H., Tsuda, H. & Shirai, T. (1982) *Promoting and inhibiting factors on liver and urinary bladder carcinogenesis in rats*. In: Pani, P., Feo, F. & Columbano, A., eds, *Recent Trends in Chemical Carcinogenesis*, ESA, Cagliari, pp. 199–213

Ito, N., Fukushima, S., Shirai, T., Nakanishi, K., Hasegawa, R. & Imaida, K. (1983a) Modifying factors in urinary bladder carcinogenesis. *Environ. Health Perspect.*, ***49***, 217–222

Ito, N., Fukushima, S., Shirai, T. & Nakanishi, K. (1983b) Effects of promoters on *N*-butyl-*N*-(4-hydroxybutyl)nitrosamine-induced urinary bladder carcinogenesis in the rat. *Environ. Health Perspect.*, ***4***, 895–899

Miyata, Y., Babaya, K. & Oyasu, R. (1981) Carcinogenesis in heterotopically transplanted urinary bladder by *N*-methyl-*N*-nitrosourea: a model for initiation and promotion. *Carcinogenesis*, ***2***, 495–497

Nakanishi, K., Fukushima, S., Shibata, M., Shirai, T., Ogiso, T. & Ito, N. (1978) Effect of phenacetin and caffeine in the urinary bladder of rats treated with *N*-butyl-*N*-(4-hydroxybutyl)nitrosamine. *Gann*, ***69***, 395–400

Nakanishi, K., Hagiwara, A., Shibata, M., Imaida, K., Tatematsu, M. & Ito, N. (1980) Dose-response of saccharin in induction of urinary bladder hyperplasias in Fischer 344 rats pretreated with *N*-butyl-*N*-(4-hydroxybutyl)nitrosamine. *J. natl Cancer Inst.*, ***65***, 1005–1010

Narisawa, T., Magadia, N.E., Weisburger, J.H. & Wynder, E.L. (1974) Promoting effect of bile acids on colon carcinogenesis after intrarectal instillation of *N*-methyl-*N*′-nitro-*N*-nitrosoguanidine in rats. *J. natl Cancer Inst.*, ***53***, 1093–1097

Oyasu, R., Hirao, Y. & Izumi, K. (1981) Enhancement by urine of urinary bladder carcinogenesis. *Cancer Res.*, ***41***, 478–481

Pamukcu, A.M., Yalciner, S., Hatcher, J.F. & Bryan, G.T. (1980) Quercetin, a rat intestinal and bladder carcinogen present in bracken fern (*Pteridium aquilium*). *Cancer Res.*, ***40***, 3468–3472

Peraino, C., Fry, J.M. & Staffeldt, E. (1971) Reduction and enhancement by phenobarbital or hepatocarcinogenesis induced in the rat by 2-acetyl-aminofluorene. *Cancer Res.*, ***31***, 1506–1512

Sugimura, T. (1979) *Naturally occurring genotoxic carcinogens*. In: Miller, E.C., Miller, J.A., Hirono, I., Sugimura, T. & Takayama, S., eds, *Naturally Occurring Carcinogens – Mutagens and Modulators of Carcinogenesis*, Tokyo, Japan Scientific Society Press/Baltimore, University Park Press, pp. 241–261

# 5-AZACYTIDINE. PROMOTING ACTIVITY FOR RAT HEPATOCELLULAR CARCINOMA

B.I. CARR, J.G. REILLY & A.D. RIGGS

*Departments of Medical Oncology and Molecular Biology*
*City of Hope National Medical Center*
*Duarte, CA 91010, USA*

## INTRODUCTION

Of the four DNA bases, cytidine is the only one which undergoes post-transcriptional modification, forming a methyl derivative. This modification occurs at the cytosine-guanine (CG) junction, and it affects about 3% of cytidine bases. Recent evidence shows that gene activity is regulated, at least in part, by the degree of gene methylation (Riggs & Jones, 1983). Thus, a decrease in gene methylation would lead to an increase in transcription, which in turn would produce an increase in protein synthesis. There is a change in the overall level of gene activation in tumorigenesis, and, in general, there is an increase in gene activity. Several carcinogens have been shown to cause a decrease in DNA methyl content *in vitro* (Wilson & Jones, 1983) and *in vivo* (Lapeyre & Becker, 1979), and some tumours have been shown to have an increased expression of certain oncogenes (see reviews: Anon., 1982; Temin, 1983; Weinberg, 1983). Specifically, a decrease in the level of methylation of both oncogenes and normal genes is observed (Feinberg & Vogelstein, 1983). This is to be expected if the amount of methylation is a controlling factor in gene expression.

An increase in the expression of certain important genes during carcinogenesis is thus controlled by the level of methylation. In light of this observation, we proposed that an agent that directly causes undermethylation of genes might be a carcinogen. We designed experiments to test this hypothesis. The compound 5-azacytidine was chosen for testing because it is an analogue of cytidine and it is known to interfere with the methylation of newly-synthesized DNA cytidine.

## MATERIALS AND METHODS

Male Fischer rats weighing 160–180 g were kept in a small animal facility and fed a basal chow with access to water *ad libitum*. They were housed in metal-bottomed

Table 1. Experimental regimens for testing hepatocarcinogenicity of 5-azacytidine

| Regimen | Property examined | No. of rats with hepatocellular carcinoma |
|---|---|---|
| 1. Partial hepatectomy and 5-azacytidine injections followed by phenobarbital feeding for 12 months | Initiation | 0/12 |
| 2. 5-Azacytidine injection followed 2 weeks later by dietary *N*-2-acetylaminofluorene for 2 weeks and partial hepatectomy | Initiation | 0/12 |
| 3. Partial hepatectomy and 50 mg/kg *N*-nitrosodiethylamine followed by 10 mg/kg 5-azacytidine twice weekly i.p. | Promotion | 8/10 |
| 4. 5-Azacytidine, 10 mg/kg, twice weekly, i.p. | Complete carcinogenesis | 0/12 |
| 5. Partial hepatectomy and 5-azacytidine, 10 mg/kg once only, i.p. | 5-Azacytidine control | 0/6 |
| 6. Partial hepatectomy and *N*-nitrosodiethylamine 50 mg/kg, once only, i.p. | *N*-Nitrosodiethyl-amine control | 0/6 |
| 7. No chemical or procedure administered | Age control | 0/12 |

cages and kept on a 12-hourly light cycle. After 12 months on various regimens (Table 1), the rats were sacrificed by exsanguination under light ether anaesthesia. Their livers were fixed in formalin, stained with haematoxylin and eosin and subjected to histological examination. The groups of rats were scored according to the number of hepatocellular carcinomas.

## RESULTS

Two regimens were used to study tumour initiation. In the first, 10 mg/kg body weight 5-azacytidine were given 18 h after partial hepatectomy, following the procedure of Pitot *et al.* (1978), and then 0.05% phenobarbital (w/w) was incorporated in the diet. The second regimen for testing initiation was that described by Solt and Farber (1976): a single dose of 20 mg/kg body weight 5-azacytidine was given by intraperitoneal injection in saline, and two weeks later *N*-2-acetylaminofluorene was fed for a period of two weeks; during this period, a partial hepatectomy was performed. The purpose of feeding *N*-2-acetylaminofluorene and a partial hepatectomy was to select for the growth of the initiated cells. Regimen 3 was designed to evaluate the promoting action of 5-azacytidine: a single initiating dose of 50 mg/kg body weight *N*-nitrosodiethylamine was given intraperitoneally 18 h after partial hepatectomy, followed by twice weekly intraperitoneal administration of 5-azacytidine in saline. In view of the fact that the solution of 5-azacytidine is relatively unstable, it was made freshly and injected immediately each time.

Twelve months after the start of the experiment, all rats were examined by laparotomy for hepatocellular carcinomas. Tumours were found only in those on experimental regimen 3, which was designed to test for possible promoting activity of 5-azacytidine. All the animals in this group were sacrificed and their livers subjected to histological examination to confirm the presence of malignant tumours. All macroscopic tumours observed were found to be hepatocellular carcinomas. The livers of animals on all other regimens were histologically normal.

## DISCUSSION

To our knowledge, this is the first report of a tumour-promoting action of 5-azacytidine. It appeared to have promoting action only in the liver. Regimens 1 and 2 were designed to test for initiating action of chemicals in experimental hepatocarcinogenesis. Initiating agents are thought to act by inducing mutation-like changes. The results of our experiments thus provide possible evidence against a mutation-like effect of 5-azacytidine, at least in rat liver, since no tumour was seen after chronic administration of 5-azacytidine without prior administration of the initiating carcinogen *N*-nitrosodiethylamine. The mechanism by which 5-azacytidine exerts its promotion-like action in the liver is not yet clear. Most promoters are thought to act neither by a direct interaction with DNA nor as mutagens. If 5-azacytidine exerts its promotion-like activity *via* an undermethylation of DNA, this would be compatible with a non-mutational activity, since cytidine undermethylation can be considered an epigenetic alteration.

The interpretation of these experiments as being indicative of a tumour-promoting activity for 5-azacytidine is somewhat clouded by the results of later experiments. Twelve of 18 rats that were treated subsequently only with 5-azacytidine for 18 months developed a variety of tumours in other organs, and hepatocellular carcinomas or nodules were never observed. Thus, for organs other than the liver, 5-azacytidine can act as a complete carcinogen (unpublished data).

It would appear that, in the experiments described here, 5-azacytidine exerted its activity in producing hepatocellular carcinomas either as a tumour promotor or as a syncarcinogen with *N*-nitrosodiethylamine. According to the former interpretation, 5-azacytidine would be a complete carcinogen for one organ but only a tumour promotor for another, namely the liver.

## REFERENCES

Anon. (1982) Oncogenes in solid tumours. *Nature*, ***300***, 477

Feinberg, A.P. & Vogelstein, B. (1983) Hypomethylation of rat oncogenes in primary human cancers. *Biochem. biophys. Res. Commun.*, ***111***, 47–54

Lapeyre, J.N. & Becker, F.F. (1979) 5-Methylcytosine content of nuclear DNA during chemical hepatocarcinogenesis and in carcinomas which result. *Biochem. biophys. Res. Commun.*, ***87***, 698–705

Pitot, H.C., Barsness, L., Goldsworthy, T. & Kitagawa, T. (1978) Biochemical characterization of stages of hepatocarcinogenesis after a single dose of diethylnitrosamine. *Nature*, ***271***, 456–477

Riggs, A.D. & Jones, P.A. (1983) 5-Methyl cytosine, gene regulation and cancer. *Adv. Cancer Res.*, ***40***, 1–30

Solt, D. & Farber, E. (1976) New principle for the analysis of chemical carcinogenesis. *Nature,* ***263,*** 701–703

Temin, H.M. (1983) We still don't understand cancer. *Nature,* ***302,*** 656

Weinberg, R.A. (1983) Alteration of the genomes of tumor cells. *Cancer,* ***52,*** 1971–1975

Wilson, V.L. & Jones, P.A. (1983) Inhibition of DNA methylation by chemical carcinogens *in vitro*. *Cell,* ***32,*** 239–246

# INFLUENCE OF ETHYL ALCOHOL ON CARCINOGENESIS INDUCED WITH *N*-NITROSODIETHYLAMINE


L. GRICIŪTĖ

*Oncological Institute of Ministry of Health of the Lithuanian SSR, Vilnius, Lithuanian SSR, USSR*

M. CASTEGNARO & J.-C. BÉRÉZIAT

*International Agency for Research on Cancer, 150 cours Albert Thomas, 69372 Lyon Cedex 08, France*


## INTRODUCTION

Between 20% and 50% of apple brandy samples analysed in the IARC analytical laboratory contained *N*-nitrosodimethylamine (NDMA), *N*-nitrosodiethylamine (NDEA) and *N*-nitrosodi-*n*-propylamine (NDPA) (Tuyns *et al.*, 1980). In view of the fact that the levels of these nitrosamines were low, their role in the development of endemic oesophageal cancer in the north-west of France seemed doubtful. These compounds may be important if ethanol increases the carcinogenic activity of the *N*-nitrosamines in alcoholic beverages.

Some experimental data indicate that the carcinogenicity of NDEA, *N*-nitrosopiperidine and *N*-nitrosopyrrolidine is increased by ethanol (Gibel, 1967; McCoy *et al.*, 1982). However, results obtained by other investigators with the same or other nitrosamines have been contradictory (Schmähl *et al.*, 1965; Schmähl, 1976; McCoy *et al.*, 1982; Gurkalo & Zabezhinsky, 1982).

In two previous papers, we demonstrated that ethanol, used as a solvent, increased the carcinogenic activity of NDMA and NDPA (Griciūtė *et al.*, 1981, 1982). This paper describes experiments in which NDEA was administered in the same way as in the two previous studies.

## MATERIALS AND METHODS

Two-hundred-and-eight male and female C57B1 mice, eight weeks old, bred in the IARC animal house, were separated into three groups. The following treatments were given by gastric intubations: Group I, 0.2 mL 40% ethanol:water solution containing 0.03 mg NDEA; Group II, 0.2 mL tap-water, containing 0.03 mg NDEA; and Group III, 0.2 mL 40% ethanol:water solution. Mice were treated twice a week for 50 weeks. The total dose of NDEA given to groups I and II was 3 mg; and the total amount of 40% ethanol:water solution administered to groups I and III was 20 mL. The animals were kept in Macrolon N III cages under normal laboratory conditions, maintained on Aliment-Extra-Labo-Bisquits and given water *ad libitum*.

Seventy-eight weeks after the beginning of the experiment, all mice still alive were sacrificed. Necropsy was performed on all animals that were killed or found dead. Lungs, oesophagus, stomach, spleen, liver, kidney, adrenals, brain and some other organs (when pathological changes were noted macroscopically) were fixed in 10% formalin and embedded in paraffin; sections were stained with haematoxylin and eosin and were examined histologically.

## RESULTS

Tumour morbidity was high both in group I (NDEA/ethanol) and group II (NDEA/water). There was no difference in the percentage of animals with tumours or in the average number of tumours per animal. The numbers of animals with multiple tumours were almost the same in the two groups. The most frequently observed tumours were those of the forestomach, which are obviously attributable to NDEA, lymphosarcomas, which are peculiar to the colony of mice used, and pulmonary adenomas. Hepatomas, as well as other tumours, occurred less frequently (Table 1).

Tumour morbidity was lowest in group III (ethanol); however, with the exception of forestomach cancer, the same kinds of tumours were observed in this group, but at lower incidence. The most striking difference in tumour morbidity between groups I and II was in the number of forestomach cancers: in 34% of males and 57% of females given NDEA in ethanolic solution, but in only 10% of males and 9% of females given NDEA in water solution (Table 2). Several papillomas, but only one cancer, were observed in the oesophagus. All forestomach cancers in group I were spinocellular with or without keratinization. In group II, one adenocarcinoma and one combined spinocellular cancer and adenocarcinoma were observed. In both males and females of group I, 40% of forestomach cancers metastasized to the lungs, liver and some other organs. No metastasizing forestomach cancer was observed in group II. The first forestomach cancer was detected in group I at the 39th week and in group II at the 46th week. The average age of mice with oesophageal cancer was 64 weeks for those in group I and 68 weeks for those in group II.

There was no difference in frequency or number of pulmonary adenomas in the two groups given NDEA, but both lymphomas and hepatomas were seen more frequently in group II (NDEA/water).

Several other malignant tumours (tracheal, skin, nasal fossa cancer) were seen in group I, but in group II only a few benign tumours (haemangioma, papillomas) were observed.

Table 1. Tumour morbidity in animals treated with *N*-nitrosodiethylamine (NDEA), with or without ethanol, or with ethanol alone

| Treatment group | | No. of animals | | Animals with tumours (%) | Average no. of tumours | Animal with multiple tumours (%) | Oesophagus/ forestomach | | Lymphomas | Pulmonary adenomas | Hepatomas | Other | |
|---|---|---|---|---|---|---|---|---|---|---|---|---|---|
| | | Initial | Effective | | | | Benign No. (%) | Malignant No. (%) | No. (%) | No. (%) | No. (%) | Benign No. (%) | Malignant No. (%) |
| I. NDEA/ ethanol | M | 38 | 38 | 37 (97) | 2.1 | 27 (71) | 14 (37) | 13 (34) | 8 (21) | 31 (81) | 4 (10) | 1 (3) | 7 (18) |
| | F | 32 | 31 | 31 (100) | 1.8 | 18 (58) | 7 (23) | 19 (61) | 13 (42) | 15 (48) | 2 (6) | – | 2 (6) |
| | Total | 70 | 69 | 68 (98) | 2.0 | 45 (65) | 21 (30) | 32 (46) | 21 (30) | 46 (67) | 6 (9) | 1 (1) | 9 (13) |
| II. NDEA/ water | M | 38 | 38 | 37 (97) | 2.0 | 22 (58) | 18 (47) | 4 (10) | 21 (55) | 27 (71) | 6 (16) | 2 (5) | – |
| | F | 32 | 32 | 31 (97) | 2.2 | 25 (78) | 13 (41) | 3 (9) | 24 (75) | 21 (66) | 9 (28) | 1 (3) | – |
| | Total | 70 | 70 | 68 (97) | 2.1 | 47 (67) | 31 (44) | 7 (10) | 45 (64) | 48 (69) | 15 (21) | 3 (4) | – |
| III. Ethanol | M | 36 | 36 | 13 (36) | 0.34 | 0 (0) | 1 (3) | – | 6 (17) | 2 (6) | 1 (3) | 3 (8) | – |
| | F | 32 | 32 | 8 (25) | 0.26 | 1 (3) | 2 (6) | – | 7 (22) | 2 (6) | – | – | – |
| | Total | 68 | 68 | 21 (31) | 0.3 | 1 (1.5) | 3 (4) | – | 13 (19) | 4 (6) | 1 (1.5) | 3 (4) | – |

Table 2. Observed and expected numbers of animals with forestomach cancer after treatment with *N*-nitrosodiethylamine (NDEA) in ethanol or in water

| Sex | Age (weeks) | Group I NDEA in ethanol | | | Group II NDEA in water | | |
|---|---|---|---|---|---|---|---|
| | | No. of animals | No. in which tumours observed | No. in which tumours expected | No. of animals | No. in which tumours observed | No. in which tumours expected |
| Males | 49 | 38 | 1 | 1.0 | 38 | 1 | 1 |
| | 50–59 | | | | | | |
| | 60–69 | 33 | 5 | 2.3 | 38 | 0 | 2.7 |
| | 70 + | 26 | 7 | 4.3 | 35 | 3 | 5.7 |
| | Total | | 13 | 7.6 | | 4 | 9.4 |
| Females | 49 | 32 | 3 | 1.5 | 32 | 0 | 1.5 |
| | 50–59 | 30 | 2 | 1.0 | 32 | 0 | 1.0 |
| | 60–69 | 22 | 8 | 3.7 | 31 | 1 | 5.3 |
| | 70 + | 16 | 6 | 2.8 | 29 | 2 | 5.2 |
| | Total | | 19 | 9.0 | | 3 | 13.0 |
| Total males & females | | | 32 | 16.6 | | 7 | 22.4 |

## DISCUSSION AND CONCLUSIONS

In this experiment, ethanol used as a solvent for NDEA enhanced the development of two kinds of tumour: forestomach cancers and 'other' malignant tumours. Thus, ethanol modified the carcinogenicity of NDEA in the same way as that of NDPA, the other oesophagotropic nitrosamine. In our previous experiment with NDPA, ethanol increased the number of forestomach tumours; more became malignant, and almost 50% metastasized to other organs (Griciūtė *et al.*, 1982). In the present study, the total number of oesophagus/forestomach tumours was not very different in the two groups given NDEA (Table 1): 53 in group I and 38 in group II. However, many more of those in group I were malignant and 40% metastasized. Ethanol, therefore, precipitated progression of malignant tumours, and the oesophagus/forestomach was the main target organ for NDEA.

At the same time, morbidity from lymphomas and hepatomas was reduced by the presence of ethanol. This phenomenon had been observed by other investigators (Schmähl *et al.*, 1965; Gurkalo & Zabezhinsky, 1982). No influence on the occurrence of pulmonary adenomas was observed.

It is evident that ethanol, even if used in the same way, modifies in different ways the carcinogenic activity of various nitrosamines. In addition, its influence on different organs is not the same. Further work is necessary to determine all the possible modifying effects of ethanol, as well as its underlying mechanism of action. However, the fact that ethanol, when used as a solvent, enhances the carcinogenic activity of oesophagotropic nitrosamines, suggests that it may play an important role in human cancer development.

## REFERENCES

Gibel, W. (1967) Experimentelle Untersuchungen zur Synkarzinogenese beim Ösophaguskarzinom. *Arch. Geschwulstforsch.*, ***30***, 181–189

Griciūtė, L., Castegnaro, M. & Béréziat, J.-C. (1981) Influence of ethyl alcohol on carcinogenesis with *N*-nitrosodimethylamine. *Cancer Lett.*, ***13***, 345–352

Griciūtė, L., Castegnaro, M. & Béréziat, J.-C. (1982) *Influence of ethyl alcohol on the carcinogenic activity of* N-*nitrosodi*-n-*propylamine*. In: Bartsch, H., O'Neill, I.K., Castegnaro, M. & Okada, M., eds, N-*Nitroso Compounds: Occurrence and Biological Effects* (*IARC Scientific Publications No. 41*), Lyon, International Agency for Research on Cancer, pp. 643–648

Gurkalo, V.K. & Zabezhinsky, M.A. (1982) Modifying effect of clondine, caffeine and ethanol on *N*-nitrosodiethylamine-induced carcinogenesis (in Russian). *Exp. Onkol.*, ***4***, 25–29

McCoy, G.D., Katayama, S., Young, R., Wyatt, M. & Hecht, S. (1982) *Influence of chronic ethanol consumption on the metabolism and carcinogenicity of tobacco related nitrosamines*. In. Bartsch, H., O'Neill, I.K., Castegnaro, M. & Okada, M., eds, N-*Nitroso Compounds. Occurrence and Biological Effects* (*IARC Scientific Publications No. 41*), Lyon, International Agency for Research on Cancer, pp. 635–642

Schmähl, D. (1976) Investigations on oesophageal carcinogenicity by methyl-phenyl-nitrosamine and ethyl alcohol in rats. *Cancer Lett.*, ***1***, 215–218

Schmähl, D., Thomas, C., Sattler, W. & Scheld, G.F. (1965) Experimentelle Untersuchungen zur Syncarcinogenese. III. Versuch zur Krebserzeugung bei Ratten bei gleichzeitiger Gabe von Diathylnitrosamin und Tetrachlorkohlenstoff bzw. Äthylalkohol, zugleich ein experimenteller Beitrag zur Frage der Alkoholcirrhose. *Z. Krebsforsch.*, ***66***, 526–532

Tuyns, A.J., Castegnaro, M., Toussaint, G., Walker, E.A., Griciūtė, L.L., La Talaer, J.Y., Loquet, C., Guerain, J. & Drilleau, J.F. (1980) Recherches concernant les facteurs étiologiques du cancer de l'oesophage dans l'Ouest de la France. *Bull. Cancer*, ***67***, 2–28

# ETIOLOGY OF HUMAN MULTI-STAGE CARCINOGENESIS

# INITIATION AND PROMOTION ACTIONS OF ULTRAVIOLET RADIATION ON MALIGNANT MELANOMA

J. M. ELWOOD

*University of Nottingham, Queen's Medical Centre, Nottingham, UK*

## ANIMAL DATA ON NON-MELANOMA SKIN CANCER

Carcinomas and sarcomas in animals can be produced relatively easily by ultraviolet radiation (UVR), and they have been studied extensively and quantitatively. Even for the non-melanoma skin cancers (NMSC), a single or short exposure to UVR will not produce tumours; a considerable dose over a protracted period seems necessary, with the minimum recorded latent period from first exposure in mouse skin experiments being 74 days (Blum, 1959). Tumour production after a single exposure has been seen: papillomas arose at the edge of an area of mouse skin severely traumatized by UVR (Harber & Forbes, 1974). The yield from an UVR exposure can be increased by subsequent application of croton oil, which must be acting as a promoter, as its application alone produces no tumours (Epstein & Roth, 1968) and can also be increased by heat, humidity and wind (National Research Council, 1982). Tumours have been produced using UVR of wavelengths up to the UVB range (280–320 nm); the addition of UVA (above 320 nm) increases the yield, while a similar dose of UVA alone produced no tumour (Urbach *et al.*, 1974). For a given total dose of UVR (intensity × time of exposure), tumour yield is greater if the dose is given in many repeated portions, e.g., daily fractionation, rather than in more intensive exposures less frequently, although comparisons between continuous and intermediate dosage have given different results in different species (National Research Council, 1982).

Thus, in animals, non-melanoma tumours can be produced by UVR, particularly UVB, acting as an initiator (shown by the yield after UVB exposure plus a chemical promoter); but UVB and the longer wavelength UVA can also have a promoter effect. The initiator action seems most likely to be due to the action of UVR on DNA, and it seems probable that the action spectra for DNA damage and carcinogenesis are similar, and that the action spectra for erythema production are similar but not identical (National Research Council, 1979b). Comparison of the action spectra and

Fig. 1. Action spectra for DNA damage and for erythema production, and solar spectrum at earth's surface, calculated for Gainsville, Florida
From National Research Council (1979b)

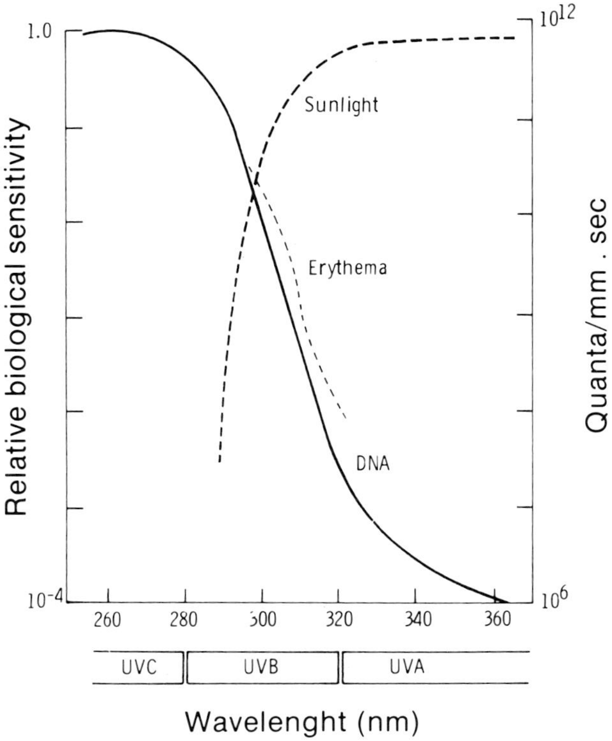


the absorption spectra of solar UV by atmospheric ozone shows that the UVB range, 280 to 320 nm, is the important one: shorter wavelength UVC is absorbed by ozone, and longer wavelength UVA has only a weak DNA damaging effect (Fig. 1).

*Immunological promoter actions of UVR*

Fisher and Kripke (1977) studied the growth of tumours induced by 16 weeks of UV irradiation in a donor mouse and then transferred as a skin graft to syngeneic recipient mice that had been irradiated with X-rays and then given lymphoid tissue either from UV-irradiated mice or from non-irradiated mice (Table 1). The yield of tumours was greater if the lymphoid tissue came from UV-irradiated mice. Similar results were obtained using a spontaneous B16 melanoma, but not with other tumours (Kripke, 1979). These workers interpret this as a 'pseudo-promoter' effect, and later investigation has suggested that it operates through the induction by UVR of suppressor T lymphocytes (Fisher & Kripke, 1978). Thus, UVR can produce an immunological repression which allows greater growth of independently initiated tumours. UVR is unique as a carcinogen in its action in suppressing the immune response to tumours it produces.

Table 1. Summary of experiments on immunosuppression effect of ultraviolet irradiation (UVR) (from Fisher & Kripke, 1977)[a]

| Pretreatment of recipients | Treatment of lymphoid donor mice | |
|---|---|---|
| | None | UV |
| X-irradiation | 13/18 | 0/17 |
| UV-irradiation | 0/10 | – |
| X plus UV | 0/19 | 1/17 |

[a] A UV-induced fibrosarcoma was transplanted into recipient syngeneic mice, which had had pretreatment and cell transfer of lymphoid tissue from donor mice. Number of rejected tumours and total number of tumours transplanted shown.

## EXPERIMENTAL WORK ON MELANOMA

There is much less experimental work available specifically on melanoma, and, with one exception, to be described, the application of UVR in the many experiments which have been done on rodents has not produced melanomas. Melanoma in guinea-pigs has been produced by chronic topical application of 7,12-dimethylbenz[*a*]anthracene (DMBA) and in hamsters by neonatal administration of urethane (Vesselinovitch *et al.*, 1970; Clark *et al.*, 1976).

Kripke (1979) reported that a melanoma developed in one mouse used in experimental work with UVR. This mouse was given ten one-hour exposures to UVR of 280–340 nm wavelengths, followed by twice weekly applications of croton oil, and a black lesion occurred in a pigmented area after 92 weeks. This tumour was transplanted and evaluated for the presence of melanin and the presence of typical melanosomes on electron microscopy. It appeared to be a true malignant melanoma. Apparently, this work has not been repeated.

Non-invasive dermal melanocytic tumours which resemble blue naevi have been produced primarily in hamsters and pigmented mice following the application of chemical carcinogens. Epstein *et al.* (1967) found that repeated exposures of these naevi to UVR below 320 nm led to the production of large invasive tumours containing melanin, while earlier work attempting traumatic malignant transformation was unsuccessful. They interpret these results as being the only experimental work demonstrating UVR to be an initiator of a melanoma; but, as it is based on irradiation of exisiting naevi, it is disputable whether this is truly an initiation effect.

Four mechanisms by which UVR may produce melanoma can be considered (Kripke, 1979):

1. Direct initiation of melanoma; there is no animal model for this.
2. Initiation of tumours which require additional promotion before expression; there

is no clearly reproducible evidence from animal work on melanoma produced by this mechanism. Kripke has reported the one instance of a melanoma arising in a mouse after UVR followed by croton oil treatments.

3. UV acting as a promoter on cells already initiated. The work of Epstein *et al.* (1967) on UVR applied to naevi that had been produced by DMBA may fall in this category, rather than being an example of initiation by UVR.

4. Indirect promotion action of UV *via* an immunological suppressor action or by some biochemical action, as demonstrated by the experiment on B16 melanoma. This mechanism implies that the promotion action of UVR is not confined to initiated melanocytes exposed directly to the UVR, but includes effects on unexposed cells.

*Effects of UVR on melanocytes*

Blog and Szabo (1979a,b, 1982) have studied changes in melanocyte number, estimated after treatment with DOPA, and structure in mouse tail skin exposed to UV and to chemicals. Irradiation with UVB alone produced an increase in the number of melanocytes, which also became larger and more irregular, while UVA alone produced no change. However, UVA plus 8-methoxypsoralen (the 'PUVA' regime used in the treatment of psoriasis), DMBA alone or with UVB produced similar changes. Although no tumour was produced, this experiment suggests that the short-term effects of UVB and DMBA on melanocytes are similar; and, although UVA produces no effects on its own, it produces effects similar to those of UVB if combined with psoralen.

## EPIDEMIOLOGICAL DATA

It is not possible to distinguish directly between promotion and initiation actions of UVR on the basis of current human data. However, one can postulate that one model of a UVR effect that is consistent with the extensive animal data for NMSC is a linear positive relationship of risk to cumulative lifetime dose of UV or solar radiation. This predicts that the incidence of skin tumours should be related positively to (1) increasing age; (2) residence at low latitudes; (3), for a given latitude, residence at high altitude and in places with sunny and unpolluted atmospheric conditions; (4) outdoor exposure, such as occupation or long lasting and regular recreational or vacation activities, and a male excess from occupational exposure; (5) exposure due to habits of wearing clothing, hats and hair; (6) physiological and anatomical features that affect the absorption of UVR, such as skin pigmentation and thickness.

The epidemiological features of NMSC fit this model well, showing a linear log-log incidence-age curve with a slope that is similar to that of other epithelial tumours, an increased incidence at lower latitudes for a given type of population, a strong association with outdoor employment, and associations with light skin and hair colour, and with Celtic ancestery within Caucasian populations (National Research Council, 1982). The latitude association can be replaced by a clear association with measured UVR, obtained in the US for several locations using Robertson-Berger meters, although the association between latitude and UVR is so close that it cannot be shown clearly that the association with UVR is stronger than that with latitude (National Research Council, 1982). A latitude gradient for NMSC in blacks in the US has been reported (Scott & Fraumeni, 1982). US incidence data show a male excess of 1.6:1 for basal cancer and 2.7:1 for squamous-cell cancer (Scotto & Fraumeni, 1982). The site distribution gives strong evidence that the solar effects are localized to the skin exposed, as it follows closely that expected from exposure patterns. There is little evidence available on altitude and associations with local climate. There is also little information on time trends, as incidence data are unlikely to be consistent and mortality data are affected by treatment effects. Incidence rates show a slight rise in the US between the 2nd and 3rd National Surveys (Scotto & Fraumeni, 1982).

### *Epidemiology of cutaneous melanoma*

The features of lentigo maligna melanoma (LMM) have been described consistently in clinical series, and these show that LMM occurs at older ages and on exposed sites; a convincing case can be made that LMM may be similar in etiology to NMSC (National Research Council, 1979b; Lee, 1982). However, larger data sets often do not separate LMM. LMM accounts for six to ten percent of all cutaneous melanomas, but for about 50 percent of melanomas of the head and neck region, so differences between head and neck melanoma and melanoma of other sites can be expected (Clark & Mihm, 1969; McGovern *et al.*, 1980).

*Geography:* Melanoma incidence and mortality rise with decreasing latitude in large areas with similar populations, such as the US and Canada, Australia, England and Wales, and Scandinavia (Elwood *et al.*, 1974; Lee, 1982). The proportional increase with latitude is similar to that of NMSC, and the slopes of regressions of incidence against solar UV measurements in eight areas of the US are similar for melanoma and for basal-cell cancer (National Research Council, 1982). The change in rate with latitude is greater for females.

This findings alone contributes little to understanding the mechanism. A short-term promotion effect alone might be expected to allow migration to weaken the latitude gradient; and melanoma death rates in Florida, for example, are 20 percent below those expected on the basis of latitude alone, while death rates from NMSC are 40 percent below the expected figure (Elwood *et al.*, 1974). This could reflect a migration effect, or social and medical care factors. The proportion of LMM or of head and neck melanoma does not appear to vary with latitude (Lee, 1982); but if LMM is related to cumulative dose and other types to recent dosage, it does not follow that the proportion of LMM will change.

In Israel and Queensland, Australia, residents of coastal areas have higher rates than inland residents, which could be due to either climatic or behavioural differences (Anaise *et al.*, 1978; Beral, personal communication).

*Migrant studies:* These should be very helpful. A short-term promoting action of UV alone should mean that incidence rates of lifetime residents in high-incidence areas should be similar to those of migrants of perhaps five to ten years' standing, although this assumes that the occupation and recreational exposure to sunlight in the host country are similar in both groups. Data from Australia, Israel and

Fig. 2. Annual incidence rate, age-standardized, for melanoma during the period 1960–1972 in Israel by date of immigration
From Anaise *et al.* (1978)

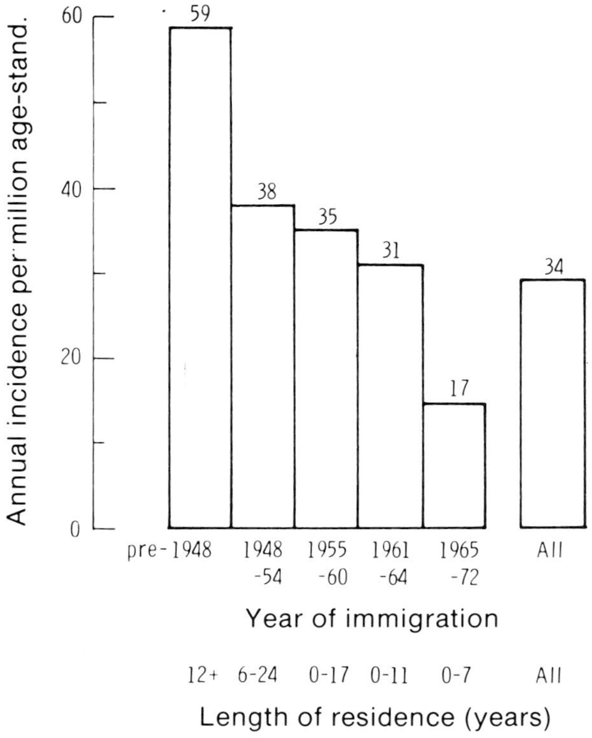


California indicate that this is not true, since the locally born population has higher rates (Anaise *et al.,* 1978; Holman *et al.,* 1980; McMichael & Bonett, 1981; Dobson & Leeder, 1982; National Research Council, 1982).

Dobson and Leeder (1982) showed that Australian residents who are migrants from the UK and have lived in Australia for less than 24 years have melanoma mortality rates similar to those of the population of England and Wales, while increases were seen in those who had lived in Australia longer, irrespective of age at death. The cut-off at 24 years was arbitrary, and more detailed information was not available. In particular, we do not know the actual distribution of times of residence of the group who were resident in Australia less than 24 years. In Israel, Anaise *et al.* (1978) compared melanoma incidence by year of immigration for patients diagnosed in 1960 to 1972 (Fig. 2). There is an approximate doubling of risk for those who immigrated since 1965 and in 1961 to 1964, suggesting a fairly short-term effect of recent immigration; thereafter, there is a further gradual increase and a sharp jump in risk for those who were resident in 1947 and so may have been born in Israel. These data

Fig. 3. Standardized mortality ratio from melanoma during three peri-censal periods combined (1949–1953, 1959–1963, 1970–1972), in England and Wales, by social class for men (●), and by husband's social class for married women (○)
From Lee & Strickland (1980)

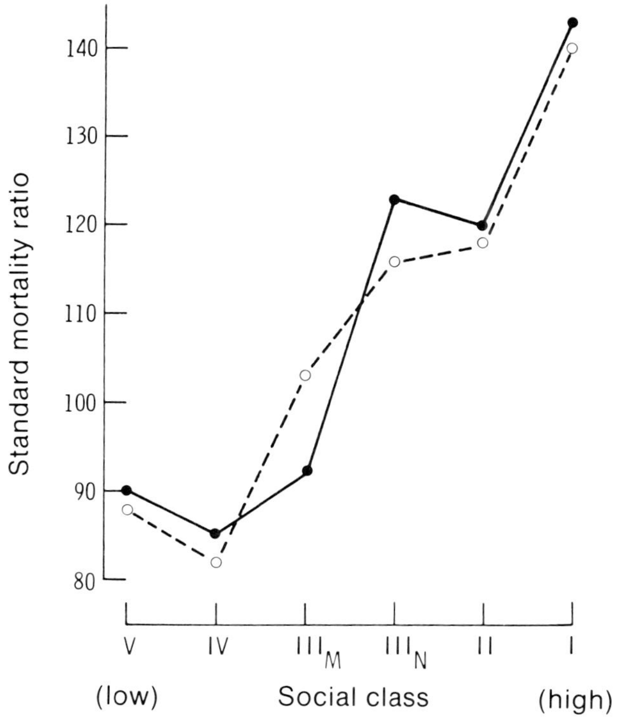


alone would be consistent with both a short-term effect and either a long-term effect or critical events occurring in early life. Data from Hawaii shows higher rates in immigrants (Hinds & Kolonel, 1980) – could a more intense dedication to sun exposure in middle or later life overcome a weaker exposure earlier?

*Occupation and social class:* NMSC shows clear associations with outdoor occupations and with lower socio-economic status (SES) (National Research Council, 1982). Melanoma shows neither (Fig. 3). A strong positive association with high SES is seen, and within a given SES group there is no association with outdoor occupation in studies in the US, UK and Australia (Holman *et al.*, 1980a; Lee & Strickland, 1980; Lee, 1982); in fact, a slightly higher rate is seen with indoor employment, although this may still be due to residual SES differences. In contrast, kibbutz workers in Israel show a three-fold excess incidence compared to city dwellers (Anaise *et al.*, 1978), but there is a need for an analysis that accounts for any social, ethnic and immigration differences. The high SES association, seen best in the UK data, may relate to recreational and vacation habits; it is perhaps surprising that it is as marked in data for 1949–1953 from the UK as in 1969–1971 data (Lee & Strickland, 1980).

Fig. 4. Annual incidence rates per million, age standardized, from melanoma in Connecticut by year, site and sex, 1935–1939 to 1968–1972
——, male; – – –, female. From Elwood & Lee (1975)

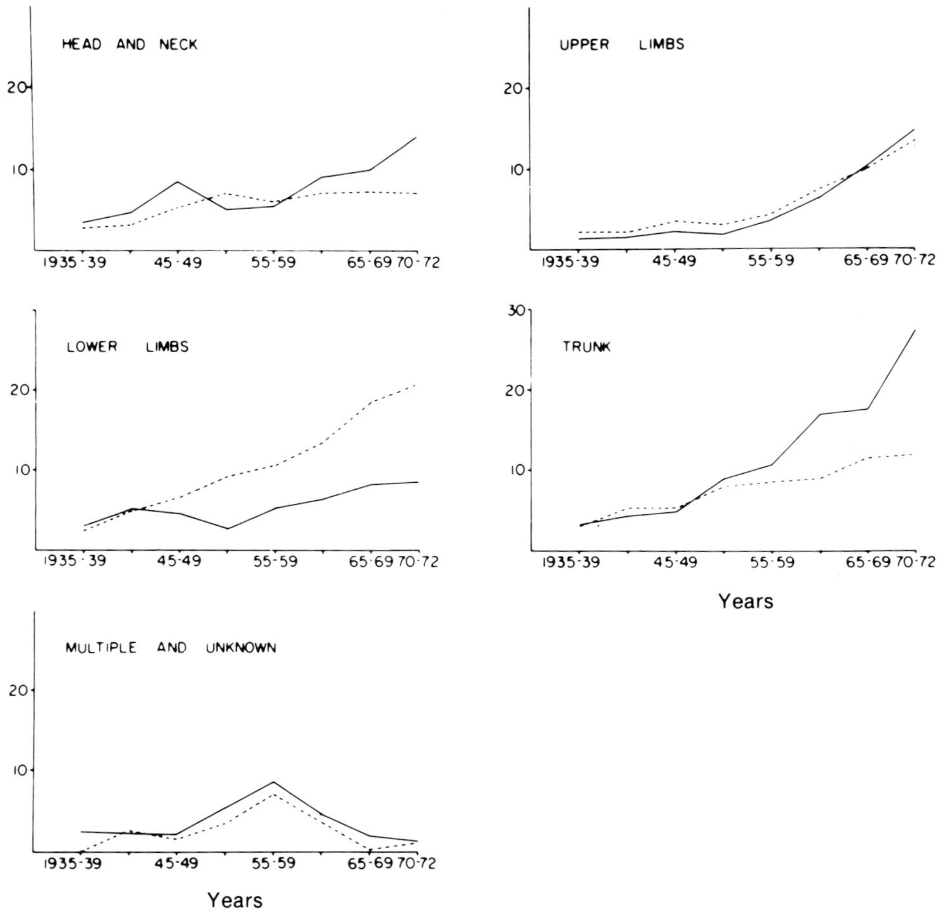


One would expect a higher proportion of LMM or head and neck tumours in outdoor workers and in the lower SES groups. McCarthy *et al.* (1980) found a lower proportion of superficial spreading melanoma (SSM) in the lower SES groups in Sydney, Australia; and, in the UK a specific association of head and neck tumours with outdoor employment has been noted (Beral & Robinson, 1981).

*Age, time and site:* The age and time associations show that melanoma is quite different from NMSC, demonstrating a marked cohort-related increase, and, as a result, a relatively flat age-incidence curve for a given time period (Elwood & Lee, 1974, 1975; Lee, 1982). Head and neck melanoma shows the least evidence for the cohort increase, and melanoma of the foot also shows little evidence of an increase.

Fig. 5. Site distribution of a continuous clinical series of 281 superficial spreading or nodular melanomas, British Columbia, Canada, 1976–1979
From Elwood & Gallagher (1983)

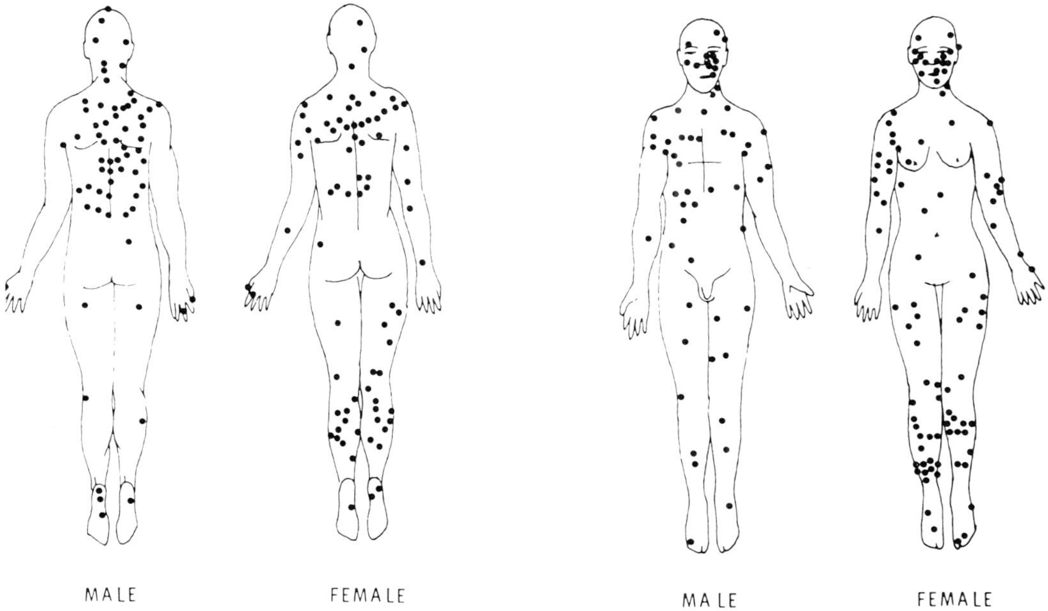


The increase has been due mainly to tumours of the trunk and limbs, and particularly of the trunk in men and of the lower limbs in women (Elwood & Lee, 1975; Magnus, 1977). Thus, a comparison of recent data with those for 1935–1944 from Connecticut shows a major change in the site and sex distribution of melanoma (Elwood & Lee, 1975) (Fig. 4). More detailed site studies on clinical series show that the excess of male trunk lesions is on the back, and that of female lower limb lesions is on the leg between mid-calf and ankle (Clark & Mihm, 1969; Lee, 1982; Elwood & Gallagher, 1983) (Fig. 5).

Thus, the increases over time in totally exposed sites (head and neck) and in relatively unexposed sites (feet) have been small and similar in both sexes, although there has been a definite increase even in these sites. The much larger increases have been at sites where it seems likely that changes in clothing habits have resulted in much more regular exposure. For example, old-fashioned stocking material worn by women in Europe and North America up to the time of World War II transmitted only about 10–30 percent of solar UVR, while nylon transmits 70 percent (National Research Council, 1979a). Death rates for lower limb melanoma in the UK (Fig. 6) begin to increase with the cohort born in 1903 (aged 40 or so when nylons became available in 1940 to 1945), and the increase ceased for those born around 1923 (aged 20 or so in 1940–1945) (Elwood & Lee, 1975). One might expect a later trend in eastern

Fig. 6. Mortality rates from melanoma of the lower limb in women, England and Wales, 1958–1962 and 1968–1972, by age, shown as cross-sectional (left) and as birth cohort (right) analyses Median year of birth shown for each cohort. From Elwood & Lee (1975)

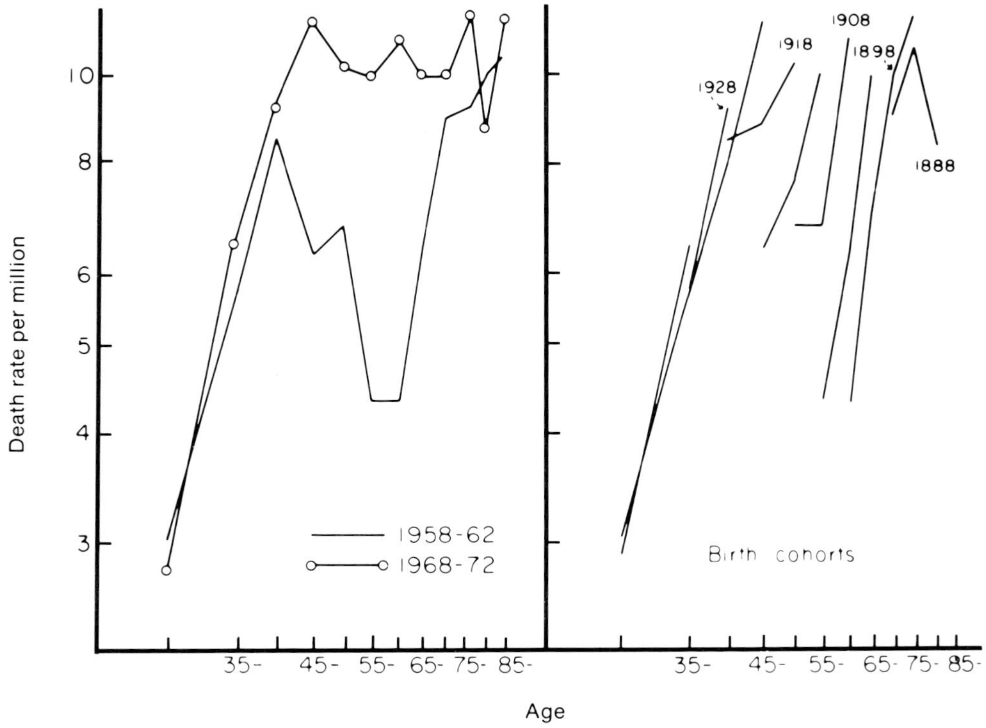


Europe. On the basis of similar reasoning, the trend for more melanomas on men's backs would be expected to relate to the increasing social acceptability of going shirtless to work or for recreation, although no abrupt change could be predicted. Australian melanoma rates (all sites) began to increase for cohorts born around 1865, and it has been suggested that this is linked to the emergence of an Australian middle class who could and would choose to expose themselves selectively through recreational pursuits to sunlight, in contrast to the previous aristocracy who would avoid exposure to sunlight for reasons of fashion, and to the earlier poorer classes who had no choice but to accept long, continuous solar exposure (Holman *et al.*, 1980b). Studies of US, Canadian and UK data are consistent with increases starting somewhat later, which might indicate a similar theme of the emergence of a choice of recreational or vacational exposure (Lee, 1982).

The UK data for lower limb tumours in women show that the trend occurs in birth cohorts rather than as a sudden jump in rates at all ages after 1940–1945, and suggests that a relatively long-term or cumulative effect is involved rather than only a short-term effect; the other cohort data, for all sites, would be consistent with this.

Current data thus show that a high proportion of melanomas occurs on body sites that are intermittently and seasonally exposed. However, the incidence rates per unit area of skin are still highest on the exposed sites – the face or head and neck (Magnus, 1981; Elwood & Gallagher, 1983). Irrespective of the personal environment created by an individual, cumulative exposure to UVR at intermittently exposed sites will never exceed that at totally exposed sites. If the incidence rates per unit area were the same, or were higher for intermittently exposed sites, it could mean that intermittent exposure is more carcinogenic than continuous exposure for a given total dose. Data from Canada for young adults do suggest that the rates may be similar for exposed and intermittently exposed sites (Elwood & Gallagher, 1983) (Table 2). An alternative explanation is that the incidence-dose curve flattens at higher dosages, so that with recent exposure patterns the dose is sufficient to reach maximal levels even on intermittently exposed skin; also, it may be necessary to take skin pigmentation, thickness and melanocyte density into account.

Table 2. Estimated annual incidence rates per 100 000 population from melanoma, British Columbia, Canada, 1976–1979, per unit area of skin, by age and by site grouping

| Site group[a] | Incidence rates[b] 15–34 | 35–49 | 50+ | All ages |
|---|---|---|---|---|
| Exposed | 1.8 (10) | 6.3 (11) | 20.6 (20) | 8.8 |
| Intermittently exposed | 2.8 (69) | 9.2 (73) | 16.1 (70) | 8.5 |
| Unexposed | 0.9 (8) | 3.1 (9) | 6.9 (11) | 3.3 |
| All sites | 2.2 (87) | 7.4 (93) | 14.6 (101) | 7.2 |

[a]Exposed, face, neck, scalp, hand; intermittently exposed, upper arm, back, thigh, leg, forearm, male chest; unexposed, abdomen, foot, female chest

[b]Cases per 100 000 population per year per unit area of skin, and numbers of patients (in parentheses), by age

From Elwood & Gallagher (1983)

These secular trends are, therefore, consistent with an overall model of intermittent UVR exposure related to recreational and vacation exposure, and to clothing habits, and suggest that the critical exposures are those which occur fairly early in life – in childhood, adolescence or early adulthood. If these events act as initiators, increased exposure to recreational sunlight at those ages would be expected to be accompanied by a higher risk throughout later life, manifesting itself from the ages of 30 or so upwards. If the effect of vacation and recreational exposure was primarily that of a promoter, one might expect to see in cohort data some fall off in incidence rate beyond the age of perhaps 40 to 50, particularly in societies such as that of the UK where recreational exposure tends to be curtailed in middle age. This hypothesis might not apply in societies such as that of Australia or of the southern states of the US. Information from Norway does suggest this type of age trend for tumours of the trunk in men and the lower limbs in women, but more data are required to make a definitive conclusion (Magnus, 1981).

## HOST FACTORS

### *Sun tolerance and sunburn*

Analytical studies and clinical investigations are now giving fairly consistent evidence that melanoma patients are intolerant to the sun, tending to burn easily and tan poorly. This has been shown with test doses of UV in studies by Everett (Everett *et al.*, 1960) and by Beitner (1981). Klepp and Magnus (1979) found that melanoma patients tolerated the sun less well than controls and freckled more easily. Beitner classified cases by skin type, and found that a higher proportion of melanoma patients had skin types 1 or 2, defined respectively as 'always burn, never tan' and 'always burn, sometimes tan'. He had only five patients with LMM in his group, and it is interesting that these had the more resistant skin types 3 and 4. Beral *et al.* (1983) showed that their patients tended to burn or freckle after exposure to sunlight and had an above-average number of naevi. Adam *et al.* (1981) found that their cases tended to burn easily. MacKie and Aitchison (1982) found no association with skin reaction to sun, but a positive association with a history of severe sunburn.

The Western Canada Melanoma Study ascertained all residents in the four western provinces of Canada who were newly diagnosed with cutaneous melanoma over a two-year period during 1979 to 1981, and an age-, sex- and province-matched comparison series of subjects was obtained by random sampling from the general population. Preliminary analysis on 595 subjects with SSM or NM and their controls shows significant associations with a tendency to burn easily and tan poorly on sun exposure, and also with a history of severe sunburn and with severe or frequent sunburns in childhood (Elwood *et al.*, 1984 and unpublished data).

Evidence is also accumulating that melanoma patients tend to have fair skin, light-coloured hair and blue eyes, and these features are presumably closely associated to sun intolerance (Adam *et al.*, 1981; Beral *et al.*, 1983; Elwood *et al.*, 1984).

### *Melanoma and naevi*

It may be essential to understand the relationship of melanoma to pre-existing pigmented lesions – naevi, moles or freckles – to understand the pathogenesis of melanoma. Beral *et al.* (1983) found that women with melanoma had more naevi than women being compared, and both her study and that of Klepp and Magnus (1979) report that melanoma patients freckle more easily after exposure to sunlight. The data of the Western Canada Melanoma Study (Elwood *et al.*, 1984) show a strong association with intensity of freckling in childhood.

Nicholls has reported that the prevalences of freckles, of moles and of birthmarks in individuals are correlated positively, and that freckles are more common in individuals with red hair, perhaps being linked by a single gene (Nicholls, 1968). He also showed that the prevalence of pigmented moles varies by age, being rare before puberty, peaking at ages 15–25 with prevalences of over 25–40 per subject, and then decreasing with age (Nicholls, 1973; Lee, 1982). Thus, if melanoma occurrence is related to effects on naevi, effects in the age range 15–25 may be particularly important.

Fig. 7. A model for the pathogenesis of cutaneous melanoma

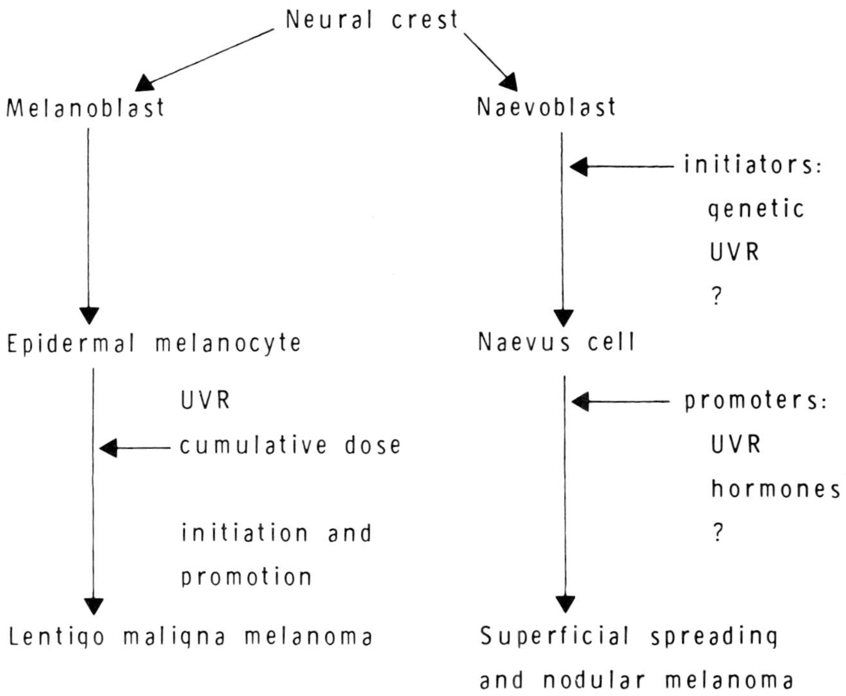


Histological evidence of a pre-existing naevus was found in about 50 percent of a series of early and borderline lesions and in only approximately 25 percent of a clinical series of melanomas (McGovern, 1976; Sagebiel, 1979), suggesting that the evidence of the naevus diminishes over time. Evidence of a naevus is found less frequently in cases of LMM (Rippey & Whiting, 1977; Heenan & Holman, 1982), which may suggest a different origin. However, this finding would also be expected because of the long clinical histories characteristics of LMM.

Many years ago, Bloch distinguished 'naevoid' and 'non-naevoid' melanoma, and recently Mishima (1960, 1967) has shown that the ultrastructure of LMM is similar to that of normal melanocytes while the ultrastructure of other melanomas (NM and SSM) is similar to that of naevus cells. MacKie (1982) has postulated that naevoblasts give rise to naevus cells and also to NM and SSM, while melanoblasts give rise to melanocytes and hence LMM, as well as to the rarer pigmented naevi.

Nicholls (1973) regards naevi as clones of cells that have been mutated by initiators, which may include radiation, including UVR, chemicals, viruses and genetic predisposition. Thus, UVR may act as a promoter on these initiated cells.

The differences in structure between LMM and other melanomas, shown by Mishima, can be used with the differences in epidemiology to suggest a model for pathogenesis (Fig. 7).

LMM may result from long-term exposure of melanocytes in the basal layer of the epidermis to UVR. Its etiology is therefore similar to that of non-melanoma skin cancer, showing a similar relationship to total lifetime UVR dosage, and a site distribution consistent with a direct association to sunlight exposure. In contrast, SSM and NM may arise after promotion, after exposure to UVR and perhaps also to other agents, of initiated naevus cells. Accordingly, persons with more naevi, or with naevi that are more sensitive to sunlight, are at higher risk; this may be the explanation of the associations with skin type and colouration. As the main effect of UVR is to promote, relatively short-term effects may be apparent, although UVR exposure in adolescence and early adult life may be particularly important because of the higher frequency of naevi at those ages. A diminution of a promoting action of solar UVR by pigment or other changes associated with tanning and outdoor acclimatization may explain the lack of an association with outdoor occupation. Moreover, the similarity of the site distribution of melanoma between places at different latitudes and between persons of different skin types indicates that the promoting activity of UVR may not be a direct effect of irradiation, but may be indirect – the unspecified 'solar circulating factor' suggested by Lee and Merrill (1970) – perhaps relating to the immunosuppressive action of UVR seen in animal experiments.

*UVR and melanoma: nature of the relationship*

The relationship between NMSC and LMM and UVR may be a simple one of risk being proportional to total lifetime dosage. The etiology of other types of cutaneous melanoma is clearly different, as shown by the lack of association with outdoor exposure.

A predominant relationship of intense sun exposure to unacclimatized skin is one of the possibilities. Such a relationship would explain the lack of association with outdoor occupation, as outdoor workers develop a permanent protective tan. High-risk patients are indoor workers who receive heavy sun exposure during an occasional holiday abroad or recreational activity. One could predict that the regular recreational sun-seeker who has a year-round tan, perhaps maintained by sunlamps, would not be at as high a risk as the annual holidaymaker. Direct evidence on these issues is still sparse. In Norway, Klepp and Magnus (1979), in a relatively small study, found that melanoma patients said they liked sunbathing less than did controls. In spite of this, the patients worked outdoors more, more often went to southern Europe for sunbathing, and more often used sun lotions, although none of these associations was significant. Adam *et al.* (1981) in the UK found no difference in time spent outdoors during work or leisure, but found that patients more often reported deliberate tanning of the legs or trunk and an interest in tanning on holidays, and an increased frequency of sunlamp usage. Beral *et al.* (1983) in Australia found no association with outdoor sports in general, nor with sunburn or blistering, but their data relating to early ages has some suggestion of a slight increase for those who were frequently out of doors. However, those who as children were usually covered up when outdoors had a higher risk of melanoma.

A modification of this hypothesis is to emphasize the role of sunburn rather than only exposure, to fit the quite strong associations seen with sun intolerance. Canadian data (Elwood *et al.*, unpublished data) and the study of MacKie and Aitchison (1982) in Scotland show an association with sunburn history. It may be possible in further work to estimate induction period from such an event.

Perhaps it is not the type as much as the timing of exposure that matters. Exposure in adolescence or early adult life, when the prevalence of naevi is maximal, may be particularly important. Paffenbarger *et al.* (1978) found that, in Harvard alumni, outdoor employment before college was associated with a four-fold excess of melanoma later, although there is no information on later outdoor exposures. Further data from migrant studies could clarify this point. An apparently specific relationship to sun exposure in early life may come about because self selection for sun exposure or avoidance may be less marked then than in adult life, and so the expected negative correlation between sun sensitivity and sun exposure may be less strong.

Most of the observations on melanoma risk factors are consistent with both short and long latency. Because people who prefer outdoor activity and sunbathing are likely to do so throughout life, it will be difficult to estimate latent period from analytical studies. The secular trends noted above argue against a very short latent period. Data on short-term (one- to three year) correlations between melanoma incidence rates and sunspot activity or particularly sunny summers have been published, and are intriguing although hardly unequivocal. Viola and Houghton (1982) have shown that in Connecticut, New York State, Alberta and Saskatchewan there appears to be an increased melanoma incidence about two years after long-term sunspot activity. An association was seen in Finland with a one-year lag, but no association was seen in Norway. Viola and Houghton argue that years of maximum sunspot activity are years of decreased atmospheric ozone level and, therefore, of increased solar UV radiation, particularly in areas close to the poles. In the UK, Swerdlow (1979) has suggested that higher incidence rates of melanoma occur about two years after particularly good summers. In terms of season, a summer peak in diagnosis of melanomas in women on the upper and lower limbs and under age 54 were seen in the southern states of the US; a similar but non-significant trend was seen for tumours of the upper limb in men (Scotto & Nam, 1980). In Hawaii, a seasonal summer peak is seen, but it is for a different set of tumours: predominantly head and neck and lower limb tumours in people over 50 (Hinds *et al.*, 1981). A summer peak has also been seen in Sweden (Malec & Eklund, 1978). These effects could be due to awareness rather than incidence of the tumour, and one might expect an incidence effect to require at least a few weeks' latency; the US summer peak is almost exactly at mid-summer, which suggests an awareness effect or a remarkably specific role of first exposure in early summer.

If UV causes melanoma, does it act directly on exposed cells or systemically? Information on the site distribution of melanoma is still sparse, but the available data show that there are low rates on unexposed skin and perhaps similar rates on intermittently and on constantly exposed skin. However, there seem to be no major differences in site distribution between areas of differing incidence rate, so both direct and systemic effects may be involved. The lack of geographical or secular trends for melanoma of the eye argues against a systemic effect of UV common to all melanocytes. Some other factors may be systemic, for example, the Scandinavian countries have relatively high rates of both cutaneous and of ocular melanoma (Lee, 1982).

## INITIATION *VERSUS* PROMOTION

A promoter action of UVR seems likely on the basis of animal work and of the increased melanoma incidence in xeroderma pigmentosa patients and in psoriasis patients treated with PUVA (National Research Council, 1982). The young, and decreasing, age distribution of melanoma patients and the rapid secular trends seem in keeping with a promoter action. If so, what is the initiator? It may be that, as with NMSC, UVR is both initiator and promoter. The initiator action may be associated with traumatic sunburn in childhood or adolescence, or it may be related to the production of naevi at those ages, while continued further bursts of UVR may have a promoting action on them. Another possible set of initiators are genetic factors linking naevi and pigmentation characteristics, and those acting in familial cases. Ionizing radiation and chemical initiators are clearly of concern, but little evidence is available; a postulated cluster of melanoma cases in workers exposed to nuclear radiation is under investigation (Lee, 1982). Canadian data show no association of melanoma with smoking or with several aspects of diet (Elwood *et al.*, unpublished data). Other promoters, such as hormones, may also be involved (Lee, 1982).

## CONCLUSIONS

The descriptive, epidemiological features of melanoma show enough differences from those of other skin cancer to argue that a simple cumulative dose hypothesis, which would be consistent with an initiation effect, followed by a later promotion action of UVR, while applicable for NMSC, is not likely to be applicable to melanoma. The one proviso in this statement is that, on the basis of the limited data available, LMM appears to be similar in its epidemiology to NMSC.

The geographical variation for melanoma is similar to that of NMSC. However, in contrast, there is no clear association with outdoor exposure, and a strong increase in risk with higher socio-economic status is observed. Some preliminary data from case-control studies suggest that melanoma patients have a poor tanning ability and tend to sunburn. To date, the published material shows no consistent, direct relationship with recreational exposure. If persons whose jobs involve constant occupational exposure either tend to protect themselves if they have sensitive skin, or to acclimatize themselves, the high-risk individual may be the person with naturally sensitive skin, who tends to burn rather than to tan on solar exposure, and who exposes himself to considerable amounts of ultraviolet in the form of short, intermittent exposure of untanned skin. This hypothesis could be consistent with the time trends, and, in particular, with the fact that the time trend has been most marked for body sites for which such intermittent exposure is highly likely, such as the male trunk and the female lower limb, whereas for sites where exposure has always been constant, such as the face, there has not been such a marked trend.

Thus, the importance of short-term, intermittent exposure may be equal to or greater than that of chronic exposure. The evidence is divided as to whether this is a short- or long-term phenomenon with regard to latency. The seasonal data, and the evidence for short-term time trends, would suggest a short-term effect with a latent period ranging from one month or two to a few years. However, the possibility that the seasonal variation simply reflects bias in recognition and diagnosis cannot be excluded. Also, the short-term time associations are not consistent among populations, and the difficult problem of multiple statistical testing in terms of the various latent periods is encountered.

Migration data suggest that people who migrate early in life have higher risks than more recent immigrants, indicating a long-term component. Therefore, it seems unlikely that the role of UVR is restricted to that of a short-term promoter. Some of the findings of recent studies suggest that exposure to sunlight in adolescence or early adulthood may be more important than exposure later; UVR may be acting here either as an initiator, or as a promoter of cells in naevi.

Although the evidence supporting a role for UVR in the causation of melanoma is now strong, we need to understand the interrelationships between host factors, such as skin type and exposure, to the environmental agent, the latent period involved, whether the effects are local or systemic, and to what extent other causal agents are involved. Epidemiological, clinical, animal and in-vitro observations will undoubtedly add much to our knowledge in the next few years.

## ACKNOWLEDGEMENT

The Western Canada Melanoma Study is supported by grants from the National Cancer Institute of Canada, from Health and Welfare Canada and from the Alberta Heritage Fund.

## REFERENCES

Adam, S.A., Sheaves, J.K. Wright, N.H., Mosser, G., Harris, R.W. & Vessey, M.P. (1981) A case-control study of the possible association between oral contraceptives and malignant melanoma. *Br. J. Cancer*, ***44***, 45–50

Anaise, D., Steinitz, R. & Ben Hur, N. (1978) Solar radiation: a possible etiological factor in malignant melanoma in Israel: a retrospective study (1960–72). *Cancer*, ***42***, 299–304

Beitner, H., Ringborn, U., Wennersten, G. & Lagerlöf, B. (1981) Further evidence for increased light sensitivity in patients with malignant melanoma. *Br. J. Dermatol.*, ***104***, 289–294

Beral, V. & Robinson, N. (1981) The relationship of malignant melanoma, basal and squamous skin cancers to indoor and outdoor work. *Br. J. Cancer*, ***44***, 886–891

Beral, V., Evans, S., Shaw, H. & Milton, G. (1983) Cutaneous factors related to the risk of malignant melanoma. *Br. J. Dermatol.* (in press)

Blog, F.B. & Szabo, G. (1979a) The effects of psoralen and UVA (PUVA) on epidermal melanocytes of the tail in C57BL mice. *J. invest. Dermatol.*, ***73***, 533–537

Blog, F.B. & Szabo, G. (1979b) The effects of UVB and 7,12-dimethylbenz(*a*)anthracene (DMBA) on epidermal melanocytes of the tail in C57BL mice. *J. invest. Dermatol.*, ***73***, 538–544

Blum, H.F. (1959) *Carcinogenesis by Ultraviolet Light*, Princeton, NJ, Princeton University Press

Clark, W.H. & Mihm, M.C. (1969) Lentigo maligna and lentigo-maligna melanoma. *Am. J. Pathol.*, ***55***, 39–67

Clark, W.H., Jr, Min, B.H. & Kligman, L.H. (1976) The developmental biology of induced malignant melanoma in guinea pigs and a comparison with other neoplastic systems. *Cancer Res.*, ***36***, 4079–4091

Dobson, A.J. & Leeder, S.R. (1982) Mortality from malignant melanoma in Australia: effects due to country of birth. *Int. J. Epidemiol.*, ***11***, 207–211

Elwood, J.M. & Gallagher, R.P. (1983) Site distribution of malignant melanoma. *Can. med. Assoc. J.*, ***128***, 1400–1404

Elwood, J.M. & Lee, J.A.H. (1974) Trends in mortality from primary tumours of skin in Canada. *Can. med. Assoc. J.*, ***110***, 913–915

Elwood, J.M. & Lee, J.A.H. (1975) Recent data on the epidemiology of malignant melanoma. *Semin. Oncol.*, ***2***, 149–154

Elwood, J.M., Lee, J.A.H., Walter, S.D., Mo, T. & Green, A.E.S. (1974) Relationship of melanoma and other skin cancer mortality to latitude and ultraviolet radiation in the United States and Canada. *Int. J. Epidemiol.*, ***3***, 325–332

Elwood, J.M., Gallagher, R.P., Hill, G.B., Spinelli, J.J., Pearson, J.C.G. & Threlfall, W. (1984) Pigmentation and skin reaction to sun as risk factors for cutaneous melanoma: Western Canada Melanoma Study. *Br. med. J.*, ***288***, 99–102

Epstein, J.H. & Roth, H.L. (1968) Experimental ultraviolet light carcinogenesis: a study of croton oil promoting effects. *J. invest. Dermatol.*, ***50***, 387–389

Epstein, J.H., Epstein, W.L. & Nakai, T. (1967) Production of melanomas from DMBA induced blue nevi in hairless mice with ultraviolet light. *J. natl Cancer Inst.*, ***38***, 19–30

Everett, M.A., Bell, R. & Hagans, J.A. (1960) Melanogenesis and skin carcinoma. *Arch. Dermatol.*, ***82***, 110–114

Fisher, M.S. & Kripke, M.L. (1977) Systemic alteration induced in mice by ultraviolet light irradiation and its relationship to ultraviolet carcinogenesis. *Proc. natl Acad. Sci. USA*, ***74***, 1688–1692

Fisher, M.S. & Kripke, M.L. (1978) Further studies on the tumor-specific suppressor cells induced by ultraviolet radiation. *J. Immunol.*, ***121***, 1139–1144

Harber, L.C. & Forbes, P.D. (1974) In: Urbach, E., Epstein, J.H. & Forbes, P.D. *Ultraviolet carcinogenesis: experimental, global, and genetic aspects.* In: Pathak, M.A., Harber, L.C., Seiji, M., Kukita, A. & Fitzpatrick, T.B., eds, *Sunlight and Man: Normal and Abnormal Photobiologic Responses,* Tokyo, University of Tokyo Press

Heenan, P.J. & Holman, C.D.J. (1982) A histological comparison of cutaneous malignant melanoma between the Oxford Region and Western Australia. *Histopathology,* **6,** 703–716

Hinds, M.W. & Kolonel, L.N. (1980) Malignant melanoma of the skin in Hawaii, 1960–77. *Cancer,* **45,** 811–817

Hinds, M.W., Lee, J. & Kolonel, L.N. (1981) Seasonal patterns of skin melanoma incidence in Hawaii. *Am. J. public Health,* **71,** 496–499

Holman, C.D.J., Mulroney, C.D. & Armstrong, B.K. (1980a) Epidemiology of preinvasive and invasive malignant melanoma in Western Australia. *Int. J. Cancer,* **25,** 317–323

Holman, C.D.J., James, I.R., Gattey, P.H. & Armstrong, B.K. (1980b) An analysis of trends in mortality from malignant melanoma of the skin in Australia. *Int. J. Cancer,* **26,** 703–709

Klepp, O. & Magnus, K. (1979) Some environmental and bodily characteristics of melanoma patients. A case-control study. *Int. J. Cancer,* **23,** 482–486

Kripke, M.L. (1979) Speculations on the role of ultraviolet radiation in the development of malignant melanoma. *J. natl Cancer Inst.,* **63,** 541–545

Lee, J.A.H. (1982) Melanoma and exposure to sunlight. *Epidemiol Rev.,* **4,** 110–132

Lee, J.A.H. & Merrill, J.M. (1970) Sunlight and the aetiology of malignant melanoma: a synthesis. *Med. J. Aust.,* **2,** 846–851

Lee, J.A.H. & Strickland, D. (1980) Malignant melanoma: social status and outdoor work. *Br. J. Cancer,* **41,** 757–763

MacKie, R.M. (1982) *The biology of malignant melanoma. The pathology of cutaneous malignant melanoma.* In: Jarrett, A., ed., *The Physiology and Pathophysiology of the Skin,* Vol. 7, London, Academic Press, pp. 2180–2203

MacKie, R.M. & Aitchison, T. (1982) Severe sunburn and subsequent risk of primary cutaneous malignant melanoma in Scotland. *Br. J. Cancer,* **46,** 955–960

Magnus, K. (1977) Incidence of malignant melanoma of the skin in five Nordic countries: significance of solar radiation. *Int. J. Cancer,* **20,** 477–485

Magnus, K. (1981) Habits of sun exposure and risk of malignant melanoma: an analysis of incidence rates in Norway 1955–77 by cohort, sex, age and primary site. *Cancer,* **48,** 2329–2335

Malec, E. & Eklund, G. (1978) The changing incidence of malignant melanoma of the skin in Sweden, 1959–1968. *Scand. J. Plast. Reconstr. Surg.,* **12,** 19–27

McCarthy, W.H., Black, A.L. & Milton, G.W. (1980) Melanoma in New South Wales. *Cancer,* **46,** 427–432

McGovern, V.J. (1976) *Malignant Melanoma: Clinical and Histological Diagnosis,* New York, John Wiley & Sons, pp. 47–48

McGovern, V.J., Shaw, H.M., Milton, G.W. & Farago, G.A. (1980) Is malignant melanoma arising in a Hutchinson's melanotic freckle a separate disease entity? *Histopathology,* **4,** 235–242

McMichael, A.J. & Bonett, A. (1981) Cancer profiles of British and southern-European migrants. *Med. J. Aust.*, ***1***, 229–232

Mishima, Y. (1960) Melanosis circumscripta praecancerosa (Dubreuilh). A non-nevoid premelanoma distinct from junction nevus. *J. invest. Dermatol.*, ***34***, 361–375

Mishima, Y. (1967) Melanocytic and nevocytic malignant melanomas: cellular and sub-cellular differentiation. *Cancer*, ***20***, 632–649

National Research Council (1979a) *Protection against Depletion of Stratospheric Ozone by Chlorofluorocarbons*, Washington DC, National Academy of Sciences, pp. 74–105

National Research Council (1979b) *Protection against Depletion of Stratospheric Ozone by Chlorofluorocarbons*, Washington DC, National Academy of Sciences, pp. 335–341

National Research Council (1982) *Causes and Effects of Stratospheric Ozone Reduction: An Update (Report of the Commission on Natural Resources)*, Washington DC, National Academy Press

Nicholls, E.M. (1968) Genetic susceptibility and somatic mutation in the production of freckles, birthmarks and moles. *Lancet*, ***i***, 71–73

Nicholls, E.M. (1973) Development and elimination of pigmented moles and the anatomical distribution of primary malignant melanoma. *Cancer*, ***32***, 191–195

Paffenbarger, R.S., Wing, A.L. & Hyde, R.T. (1978) Characteristics in youth predictive of adult-onset malignant lymphomas, melanomas and leukemias: brief communication. *J. natl Cancer Inst.*, ***60***, 89–92

Rippey, J.J. & Whiting, D.A. (1977) Moles and melanomas. *Lancet*, ***ii***, 137

Sagebiel, R.W. (1979) Histopathology of borderline and early malignant melanomas. *Am. J. Surg. Pathol.*, ***3***, 543–552

Scotto, J. & Nam, J. (1980) Skin melanoma and seasonal patterns. *Am. J. Epidemiol.*, ***111***, 309–314

Scotto, J. & Fraumeni, J.F., Jr (1982) *Skin (other than melanoma)*. In: Schottenfeld, D. & Fraumeni, J.F., Jr, eds, *Cancer Epidemiology and Prevention*, Philadelphia, W.B. Saunders Co., pp. 996–1011

Swerdlow, A.J. (1979) Incidence of malignant melanoma of the skin in England and Wales and its relationship to sunshine. *Br. med. J.*, ***ii***, 1324–1327

Szabo, G., Blog, F.B. & Kornhauser, A. (1982) Toxic effect of ultraviolet light on melanocytes: use of animal models in pigment research. *J. natl Cancer Inst.*, ***69***, 245–250

Urbach, F., Epstein, J.H. & Forbes, P.D. (1974) *Ultraviolet carcinogenesis: experimental, global, and genetic aspects*. In: Pathak, M.A., Harber, L.C., Seiji, M., Kukita, A. & Fitzpatrick, T.B., eds, *Sunlight and Man: Normal and Abnormal Photobiologic Responses*, Tokyo, University of Tokyo Press, pp. 259–283

Vesselinovitch, S.D., Mihailovich, N. & Richter, W.R. (1970) The induction of malignant melanomas in Syrian white hamster by neonatal exposure of urethan. *Cancer Res.*, ***30***, 2543–2547

Viola, M.V. & Houghton, A.N. (1982) Solar radiation and cutaneous melanoma. *Hosp. Pract.*, September, 97–106

# COCARCINOGENS OF THE TUMOUR-PROMOTER TYPE AS POTENTIAL RISK FACTORS OF CANCER IN MAN

## A first complete experimental analysis of an etiological model situation and some of its consequences

E. HECKER

*Institute of Biochemistry, German Cancer Research Center*
*6900 Heidelberg, Federal Republic of Germany*

## SUMMARY

The black and Creole population of the Caribbean island of Curaçao (Netherlands Antilles) is burdened by an exceedingly high rate of oesophageal cancer. As a part of the local diet, the fresh green leaves of the aromatic bush *Croton flavens* L., known locally as 'welensali', are used to prepare a 'bush tea' drunk commonly as a beverage. Additional habitual uses of the leaves and of other parts of the plant are widespread. Investigations of soluble extracts of roots and leaves of *welensali* and of *welensali* tea revealed the presence of a multitude of irritant '*welensali* factors', of which there are essentially two activity types, F and F′. F-types exhibit strong initiation (or tumour)-promoting activity on the back skin of the mouse, qualitatively and quantitatively comparable with that of the chemically related and well established promoter 12-*O*-tetradecanoyl-phorbol-13-acetate. F′-types are less active than the corresponding F-types, yet they are 'cryptic promoters' operationally. F- and F′-types are, respectively, diterpene di- and triesters, with polyfunctional tigliane structures, e.g., *welensali* factor $F_1$. Together, they comprise a minimum content of 0.32 and 0.04‰ in roots and fresh green leaves, respectively. *Welensali* tea contains two mixtures of F- and of F′-types, each comprising three *welensali* factors, irritant and promoting in mouse skin. The estimated total minimum content of *welensali* factors per cup of tea is 1.6 μg/L. The estimated content of *welensali* factors type F in one cup of *welensali* tea, (the preparation of *Croton flavens* most frequently consumed on Curaçao) is equivalent to more than 10 times the irritant dose 50 of the typical *welensali* promoter $F_1$ on the mouse ear. *Welensali* factors type F′ contained in one cup are approximately equivalent to the irritant dose 50 of the typical 'cryptic' *welensali* promoter $F_1$-20-decanoate. Therefore, the overall exposure of persons at risk on Curaçao exceeds that expected to maintain chronic irritation in the human oesophagus, which is considered an important element of *initiation/promotion*. After completion of chemical analyses, on the basis of epidemiological hints derived from the local situation, experimental evidence for the involvement in cancer associated with consumption of this plant also of *putative initiators* of the polycyclic aromatic hydrocarbon type is presented. Thus, for the first time in an epidemiologically established dietary cancer, chronic exposure to well-defined cocarcinogens of the promoter type is shown most likely to represent the principal carcinogenic risk involved ('cocarcinogen hypothesis'). This analysis may provide the scientific background for risk/benefit evaluations by local health authorities in taking measures of primary prevention. As an important goal for future developments, it is proposed to develop by mechanistic and epidemiological investigations criteria for classifying and grading carcinogenic risk factors – in terms of solitary carcinogens on the one hand, and cocarcinogens, non-carcinogenic amplifiers *per se* of carcinogenesis, on the other.

## INTRODUCTION

Numerous clinical, experimental and epidemiological investigations indicate that environmental risk factors play an important role as *causative agents* in the etiology of human cancer. In addition, such contributions from the *individual host* as genetic susceptibility and hormonal influences have also to be considered. Carcinogenesis represents, therefore, interactive systems of a considerable degree of complexity, involving exogenous and endogenous carcinogenic *risk factors* in both experimental animals and human beings (Hecker, 1981a,b). Assessment of exposure to carcinogenic risk factors is known to be extremely problematic, e.g., because the validity of extrapolations from the short-term in-vitro assays currently available remains doubtful, since these assays cannot in principle fully represent the responses of the whole mammalian or human organism. Therefore, meaningful progress in this area greatly depends upon (1) establishing tight links between areas of epidemiology of cancer in man and of toxicology in whole animal models, and (2) developing techniques for quantitating carcinogenic risk in both animal models and human beings.

To date, over 700 *solitary carcinogens* (for terminology used, see Hecker 1981a,b) have been detected as exogenous carcinogenic risk factors in animals. Of these, about 30 have also been identified as carcinogenic risk factors in the generation of human cancers by the International Agency for Research an Cancer (IARC; Tomatis *et al.*, 1978). For example, it is evident that certain solitary carcinogens are involved as principal carcinogenic risk factors in such typical human etiological model situations as occupational and iatrogenic exposures.

Solitary carcinogens exhibit more or less pronounced organotropy in *etiological investigations* using experimental dose/time-effect models of unifactorial carcinogenesis, as exemplified in Figure 1. As a working hypothesis, it was postulated that exposure of the host, even to a single, subcarcinogenic dose, i, of a solitary carcinogen (Fig. 1, line 1, 'initiation'), may produce in the cells of target tissue(s) not only certain important side-effects but also latent, irreversible lesions. During chronic

Fig. 1. Prototype experimental dose/time-effect model in unifactorial carcinogenesis ('solitary carcinogenesis')

Target tissue: e.g., mouse skin

Solitary carcinogen: e.g., 7,12-dimethylbenz[a] anthracene topically

Protocol: single subcarcinogenic doses, i( ), of solitary carcinogen (initiator), followed by multiple doses, i, of solitary carcinogen (total dose, $\Sigma$i)

| DOSE/TIME PROTOCOL | EFFECT (TUMOURS) | STAGE AND PRINCIPAL PROCESS OF CARCINOGENESIS |
|---|---|---|
| ● – – – – | 0 | 'INITIATION' |
| ● ●●●● | + | SOLITARY CARCINOGENESIS |

exposure, e.g., to repeated identical doses, i (Fig. 1), the lesions induced by the single doses, i, may add up to the manifestation of cancer within the lifespan of the host (Fig. 1). This unifactorial protocol verifies one principal process of carcinogenesis, i.e., *'solitary carcinogenesis'* (Hecker, 1976a–d, 1981b, 1984a,b).

*Phenomenologically,* the dose/time-effect relationships in solitary carcinogenesis can be described in mathematical terms, as pioneered by Druckrey and associates (e.g., Druckrey & Küpfmüller, 1948). The linear relationship of the logarithm of doses plotted against the logarithm of time of administration was briefly termed the 'log/log approach' (e.g., by Peto, 1977). This relationship has been established experimentally for many solitary carcinogens and for diverse organs (e.g., Druckrey, 1967). More recently, it was shown that the log/log approach is also valid for the early events in solitary liver carcinogenesis (e.g., Kunz *et al.* 1982, 1983; Vesselinovitch & Michailovich, 1983).

*Mechanistically,* initiation of normal cells of target tissues is postulated to be the key biological event in carcinogenesis. It is considered essentially irreversible. The ability to initiate carcinogenesis is probably a unique property of solitary carcinogens, be they of physical, chemical or viral nature. The up-dated interpretation of the 'somatic mutation' hypothesis, postulated long before (Bauer, 1928, 1963) the material substrate of the cellular genome – DNA – was identified, relates initiation to somatic mutation(s). However, the essentials of the ultimate biochemical or molecular mechanism(s) of initiation or of the 'important side effects' associated with solitary carcinogens (see above) and of their organotropy remain to be established.

It is now widely accepted that solitary carcinogens are the most critical yet *not the only class* of causative agents in the etiology of cancer. In the 1940s it was discovered that not only the ability to initiate target cells but also certain other toxicological qualities may be involved in carcinogenesis, related partly, perhaps, to the important side-effects of solitary carcinogens mentioned above (e.g., Boutwell, 1964). Non-classical qualities of this kind have, for example, been attributed to so-called

Fig. 2. Prototype experimental dose/time-effect models in multifactorial carcinogenesis ('cocarcinogenesis')

Target tissue: e.g., mouse skin

Solitary carcinogen (as initiator): e.g., 7,12-dimethylbenz[a] antracene topically or intragastrically

Cocarcinogen (as promoter): e.g., 12-0-tetradecanoylphorbol-13-acetate (TPA) topically

Protocol: single subcarcinogenic doses, i( ), of initiator, followed by multiple single doses, p( ), of promoter (total dose, $\Sigma p$)

| DOSE/TIME PROTOCOL | EFFECT (TUMOURS) | STAGE AND PRINCIPAL PROCESS OF COCARCINOGENESIS |
|---|---|---|
| ● — — — — | 0 | 'initiation' |
| — ○ ○ ○ ○ | 0 | 'promotion' |
| ● ○ ○ ○ ○ | + | 'initiation/promotion' |

Alternative protocol: Stimulated initiation/promotion (see text)

'cocarcinogens'. *Phenomenologically,* these entities 'amplify' carcinogenesis, although they are considered non-carcinogenic entities *per se*[1]. The existence of such compounds was indicated for the first time in combination experiments on the rabbit ear using Shope papilloma virus and coal-tar (Kidd & Rous, 1938) and, independently, in mouse skin using polycyclic aromatic hydrocarbons (PAH) and a non-carcinogenic fraction of coal-tar, creosote oil (Shear, 1938).

A prototype experimental dose/time-effect model for such multifactorial type carcinogenesis was developed essentially by Berenblum (1941a,b), Mottram (1944) and Berenblum and Shubik (1947), using as solitary carcinogen the PAH 7,12-dimethylbenz[*a*]anthracene (DMBA) and as cocarcinogen the skin irritant croton oil, the seed oil of the Euphorbiacea *Croton tiglium* L. In Figure 2 12-*O*-tetradecanoylphorbol-13-acetate (TPA) is used instead of the now obsolete cocarcinogen croton oil, of which it constitutes the major cocarcinogenic component (Hecker, 1968; Van Duuren, 1969). As depicted in line 2 of the figure, cocarcinogens are not expected to produce tumours on their own, even after chronic exposure of the target tissue (provided the target tissue is not predisposed by uncontrolled previous initiation

[1] The term 'cocarcinogen', previously introduced in the broadest possible sense (Shear, 1938; Berenblum 1941a,b), is now used by some researchers in a much more specific way for one of the principal protocols of cocarcinogenesis, i.e., for stimulated initiation/promotion (see bottom of Fig. 2 and text, below).

before the start of the cocarcinogen protocol). If a single subcarcinogenic dose, i, of a solitary carcinogen, such as DMBA, precedes the non-carcinogenic protocol of the cocarcinogen, tumours develop (see line 3, Fig. 2). This multifactorial protocol verifies another principal model of carcinogensis, i.e., *cocarcinogenesis,* in the form of one of the possible combinations of a solitary and a co-carcinogen (Hecker, 1976a–d, 1981b). Operationally, it is well known as 'initiation/promotion' and constitutes the most important, though not the only, principal protocol of cocarcinogenesis (see bottom, Fig. 2).

After croton oil was shown to function as *promoter* of initiation, it was found by others (e.g., Pound & Bell, 1962; Shinozuka & Ritchie, 1967) to possess in addition the ability to *stimulate* initiation, if administered within certain limits of time prior to the initiator (followed by the usual promotional regimen). (This alternative protocol of cocarcinogenesis and the corresponding principal process of multifactorial carcinogenesis, i.e., stimulated initiation/promotion, are mentioned at the bottom of Fig. 2.) While croton oil (and, in fact, also TPA) are complete promoters, it is important to note that stimulators of initiation in general may or may not be promoters (e.g., Van Duuren *et al.,* 1971, 1973).

Despite many etiological investigations, the concept of cocarcinogenesis, and particularly that of initiation/promotion, was not fully accepted for about 20 years. Some investigators even denied entirely the existence in carcinogenesis of 'non-classical' entities of this type (for reviews of arguments see Hecker, 1972, 1976a–d). In the last 20 years or so, the existence of *cocarcinogens* as another principal class of *well-defined* causative agents was finally established in etiological animal experiments and in mechanistic studies. This was accomplished both by chemical identification and by biological characterization of the highly irritant and initiation-promoting entities of croton oil, which up to then were unknown diterpene esters (e.g., Hecker, 1968; Van Duuren, 1969). The concept was further strengthened by the finding of various different diterpene ester structures with similar activities, either isolated from plant species or made by partial syntheses in order to answer specific mechanistic questions (e.g., Hecker, 1971, 1972, 1978; Evans & Soper, 1978; Hecker *et al.,* 1984).

The three principal parent diterpene structures that occur in any one of the presently-known polyfunctional diterpene esters comprise the tetracyclics tigliane (e.g., in phorbol esters such as TPA[1], Fig. 3), ingenane (e.g., in ingenol esters such as 3-hexadecanoylingenol, Fig. 3) and the tricyclic daphnane (e.g., in resiniferonol-derived orthoesters such as simplexin, Fig. 3, or mezerein).

The biological complexity of carcinogenesis in mouse skin may be separated operationally into the well-known sequence of three defined principal stages: initiation/promotion/progression (Fig. 4), by deliberate utilization in mouse skin of initiators such as DMBA or urethane followed by promoters of the diterpene ester type. Urethane may be used also as a 'progressor' (Roe *et al.,* 1972) within the promotional part of the protocol. Investigations carried out to date indicate that organotropy in initiation/promotion is determined both by the initiator and by the

[1] Some commercial suppliers and investigators assign the name 'phorbol-myristate-acetate', or PMA, to this promoter.

Fig. 3. Principal parent skeletons, tigliane, ingenane and daphnane, and corresponding prototype initiation promoters of mouse skin occurring in species of the plant families of Euphorbiaceae and Thymelaeceae

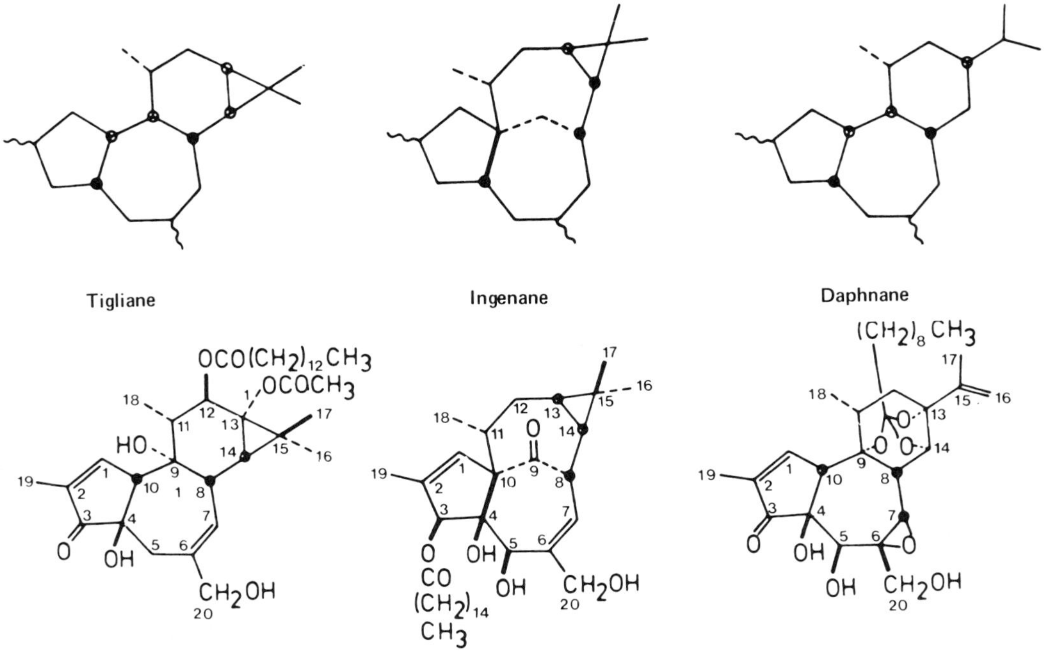


12-*O*-tetradecanoylphorbol-13-acetate (TPA)
from croton tiglium

3-*O*-hexadecanoylingenol
from euphorbia ingens
from euphorbia lathyris

Simplex
from pimelea simplex
from pimelea prostrata
Daphnopsis racemosa

Fig. 4. Experimental carcinogenesis: The three biologically defined stages at the cell level of initiation/promotion/progression of the back skin of the mouse
DMBA, 7,12-dimethylenz[*a*]anthracene. Results for urethane from Roe *et al.* (1972)

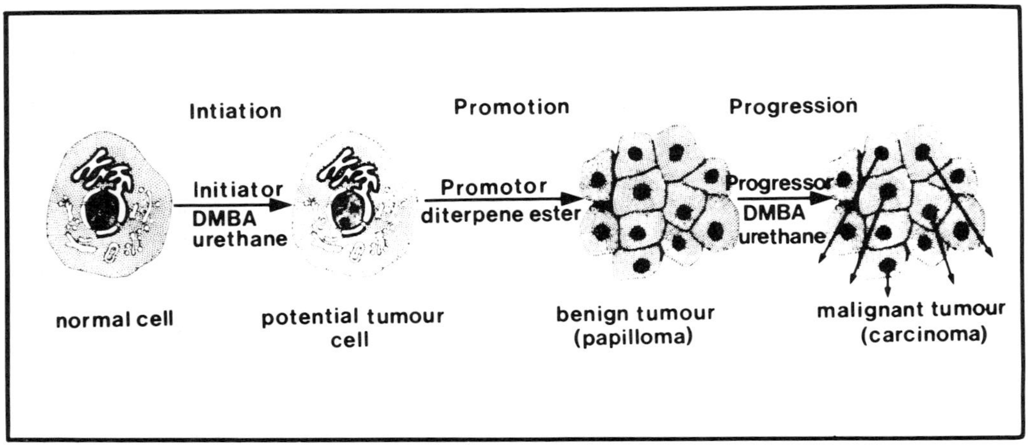

accessibility of initiated cells to promoters – at least in promoters of the diterpene ester type (for review, see Hecker 1981b). The biological and biochemical events evoked by diterpene ester type promoters are numerous, and the critical event for promotion remains unknown. By contrast with the actions of initiators, this event(s) is considered to be essentially reversible (e.g., Boutwell, 1964, 1974; Hecker, 1972, 1981b; see, however, Marks & Fürstenberger, this volume).

The issue of stages in carcinogenesis, as revealed experimentally (Figs 1, 2, 4), has also been elaborated for human cancers by the epidemiological approach in certain etiological model situations, e.g., 'lifestyle cancers' (see, for example, Peto, 1977; Higginson, 1979; Hirayama, 1981; Day, 1982). Altogether, the in-depth investigation of the new class of diterpene ester-type skin irritants and promoters has added a new dimension to the exploration of the etiology of cancer and to investigations of the mechanisms of carcinogenesis at the level of the tissue, the cell and the molecule (e.g., Hecker, 1972; Slaga *et al.*, 1978; Higginson, 1979; Hecker *et al.*, 1982 and this volume). The multistage concept of carcinogenesis is now fully accepted in cancer research. However, corresponding *complete experimental* analyses of etiological model situations of human cancer involving defined cocarcinogens, especially of the initiation-promoter type, have been lacking until recently (Hecker *et al.*, 1983).

## CANCER OF THE OESOPHAGUS ON THE CARIBBEAN ISLAND OF CURAÇAO AND ETIOLOGICAL HYPOTHESES

The incidence of oesophageal cancer varies considerably all over the world, as descriptive epidemiological investigations show (Waterhouse *et al.*, 1976). Regions with particularly high incidence rates are located, for example, in Japan, northern People's Republic of China, Islamic Republic of Iran, southern Africa, northern France, and in Central America, especially on the Caribbean island of Curaçao. The latter is an almost ideal etiological model situation for epidemiological investigations (Hartz, 1940, 1958; Eibergen, 1961; Morton, 1968a,b). From 1962 to 1973, autopsies carried out at St Elizabeth, the only hospital on Curaçao, revealed that the black/Creole and mostly poor population of the island suffers from the highest incidence rate of oesophageal cancer not only in the Caribbean region of Central America but also in the world (see Table 1). The sex ratio appears to be somewhat controversial (about 2:1, Table 1; or about 1:1, Eibergen, 1961; O'Gara, 1968). Follow-up data for 1974–1979 were presented recently (Freni & Freni-Titulaer, 1981), indicating a slight decrease in the incidence rates, while the sex ratio was claimed to remain essentially unchanged.

Analytical epidemiological investigations based on interviews with many individuals from the Netherlands Antilles and neighbouring regions (Morton 1968a, b) revealed that people on Curaçao commonly use preparations made from numerous local plants as beverages and medicines. In other areas of the region, both the habits of the Curaçao inhabitants and the high incidence rates of oesophageal cancer are uncommon.

The plant species used most frequently on Curaçao were identified, and unknown carcinogenic risk factors contained in some of these plants were considered to be

Table 1. Age-standardized annual incidence rates of oesophageal carcinoma in some regions of Central America related to 100 000 of the European and world population

| Region | Europe | | World | | References |
|---|---|---|---|---|---|
| | ♂ | ♀ | ♂ | ♀ | |
| Curaçao [a] | 32.3 | 19.4 | 21.2 | 12.9 | de Boer (1979) |
| Venezuela | | | | | |
| Caracas | – | – | – | – | Dunham & Bailar (1968) |
| Falcon, Coro [b] | | | | | Morton (1974) |
| Puerto Rico | 21.5 | 8.1 | 14.8 | 5.4 | Waterhouse *et al.* (1976) |
| Cuba | 8.7 | 3.7 | 5.7 | 2.4 | Waterhouse *et al.* (1976) |
| Jamaica | | | | | |
| Kingston | 13.4 | 6.6 | 9.1 | 4.7 | Waterhouse *et al.* (1976) |
| Brazil | | | | | |
| Recife | 7.2 | 2.5 | 5.2 | 1.6 | Waterhouse *et al.* (1976) |
| São Paulo | 18.9 | 3.2 | 13.1 | 2.2 | Waterhouse *et al.* (1976) |
| Chile | | | | | |
| Santiago | – | – | – | – | Dunham & Bailar (1968) |
| Colombia | | | | | |
| Cali | 4.3 | 2.0 | 2.8 | 1.3 | Waterhouse *et al.* (1976) |
| Bogota | – | – | – | – | Dunham & Bailar (1968) |
| New Mexico | | | | | |
| Spanish | 3.6 | 1.8 | 2.2 | 1.1 | Waterhouse *et al.* (1976) |
| Other white | 4.4 | 1.2 | 3.0 | 0.8 | Waterhouse *et al.* (1976) |
| Am. Indians | 1.8 | 0.0 | 1.4 | 0.0 | Waterhouse *et al.* (1976) |
| El Paso | | | | | |
| Spanish | 10.0 | 1.6 | 6.7 | 0.9 | Waterhouse *et al.* (1976) |
| Other white | 4.5 | 0.7 | 3.4 | 0.5 | Waterhouse *et al.* (1976) |

[a] Data refer to Netherlands Antilles (Aruba, Curaçao, Bonaire, St Maarten, Saba, St Eustatius) without Aruba and cover the period 1962–1973; 90% of the population of these islands live in Curaçao. Limited data for Aruba: in the period 1963–1966, 5 male and 2 female patients out of a population of about 60 000 had oesophageal carcinoma (Morton, 1968a).

[b] Approximately 15 oesophageal carcinoma in 28 months in a population of about 45 000

responsible for the high rate of oesophageal cancer. Extracts of the most frequently used plants were tested in experimental animals, and solitary carcinogenic activity was found to be associated with five species, namely *Heliotropum angiospermum, Annona muricata, Krameria ixina, Acacia villosa* and *Melochia tomentosa*. These findings were interpreted to support an etiological *hypothesis of solitary carcinogen* causation of oesophageal cancer on Curaçao (O'Gara, 1968; O'Gara *et al.*, 1971, 1974; Dunham *et al.*, 1974). More specifically, in the cases of the three botanically unrelated plant species, *Krameria ixina, Acacia villosa* and *Melochia tomentosa,* the content of condensed tannins was related to the high risk of oesophageal cancer on the island (Morton, 1970, 1972, 1979). So far, this hypothesis has not been substantiated further by rigorous identification of putative solitary carcinogens involved. An extract of *Krameria ixina,* which was found previously to exhibit solitary carcinogenic activity (see above), was negative in an assay for initiating activity in mouse skin using TPA as promoter (Adolf & Hecker, unpublished data).

However, two of the 23 plants most commonly uses on Curaçao are *Euphorbiaceae*, i.e., *Croton flavens* L. (*welensali*) and *Jatropha gossypifolia* L. ('bellyache bush') (Morton, 1968a,b, 1971, 1981). Many, though not all, of the species of this plant family are known to contain strong irritants that may be highly active as cocarcinogens, especially of the initiation-promotion type, on the back skin of mice (e.g., Hecker, 1981b and previous papers). A general correlation between chronic irritation (including inflammation) and cancer was pointed out at the beginning of this century by R. Virchow and is familiar to clinicians. Nowadays, it is accepted that the effect can be associated with cocarcinogens, and especially with initiation-promoters (e.g., Hecker, 1972, 1981b). In Curaçao, such a correlation is strongly supported by autopsies recorded at the local hospital: in patients above the age of 50 without manifested cancer, the oesophagus frequently showed severe chronic inflammation (Hartz, 1958). Furthermore, ingestion of preparations made from parts of the plants possessing solitary carcinogenic activity (Morton, 1974; Merino *et al.*, 1980) can also be correlated with 'initiation' of oesophageal tissue. Further, as a result of interviewing the population at risk, the hypothesis was put forward that in the past heavy contamination of the drinking-water of the island with petrol may have been a source of putative initiators (Morton, 1968b).

The local situation therefore implicates important elements of an etiological *hypothesis of cocarcinogen* causation of local oesophageal cancer (Morton, 1971; Hecker & Weber, 1977; Adolf *et al.*, 1983). This hypothesis suggests exposure of the group at risk to subcarcinogenic doses of solitary carcinogen(s) as 'initiator(s)' followed by irritant cocarcinogens, especially of the promoter type (Figs 2, 3): commonly-used preparations of parts of *welensali (Croton flavens* L) and/or of the 'bellyache bush' (*Jatropha gossypifolia* L.) may be the local sources of the cocarcinogens involved.

## DITERPENE ESTER IRRITANTS OF *WELENSALI* AS OESOPHAGEAL COCARCINOGENS OF THE PROMOTER TYPE

*Welensali* grows as a bush from two to six feet (0.6–1.8 m) in height, and is found in abundance on the Caribbean islands, as well as in southern Mexico and in northern parts of South America (Morton, 1971). On Curaçao, several parts of this plant are used so extensively in everyday life as to give rise to chronic human exposure: a 'bush tea' is prepared from the aromatic green leaves and the tips of twigs, as a free or inexpensive everyday beverage (Brenneker, 1961; Morton, 1968a), and the aromatic roots of the bush are chewed for their stimulating effect. Occasionally, the leaves of the bush are kept in the mouth as a counterirritant, are used as a detergent to clean ovens and dishes, and are also used as an insect repellent (Morton, 1971).

### *Detection and identification of irritant and promoting* 'welensali *factors' in roots and in fresh green leaves; estimation of content*

Extracts of roots and of fresh green leaves of the plant, when tested in the standardized assay for irritancy on the mouse ear (Hecker, 1971; Hecker & Schmidt,

Table 2. Typical soluble extracts of roots and leaves of *welensali*, their irritancy and the irritant *welensali* factors contained in the extracts[a]

| Typical extracts (signature and weight of sample) | Irritancy ($\mu g^{-1}$) | *Welensali* factors | | |
|---|---|---|---|---|
| | | Number | Minimum content (% by weight) | Activity type |
| Roots, methanol extract (meR II, 223 g) | 0.16 | 17 | 1.4 | F, F′ |
| Leaves, methanol extract (meL III, 1265 g) | 0.11 | 28 | 0.06 | F, F′, $F^{y}$ |
| TPA[b] (croton oil factor $A_1$) | 100 | – | – | F |

[a] Irritant activity was measured quantitatively on the mouse ear as irritant dose 50 ($ID_{50}^{24}$) in µg/ear and expressed as irritancy ($1/ID_{50}^{24}$) in $\mu g^{-1}$; the number of factors, their minimum contents and the type of irritant activity were determined with methods specifically developed

[b] 12-*O*-Tetradecanoylphorbol-13-acetate

1974), exhibit low but definite irritancy as compared with the classical irritant cocarcinogen and promoter TPA (croton oil factor $A_1$; see Table 2). Moreover, in the standardized assay for promoters on the back skin of NMRI mice (for experimental protocol, see Fig. 2), using DMBA as initiator (Hecker, 1971; Hecker & Schmidt, 1974), the extracts of roots and leaves exhibit definite promoting activity (Hecker & Weber, 1977; Lutz & Hecker, 1979). If assayed according to the two-stage protocol, but *without* initiator (see Fig. 2, line 2), the extracts did not evoke tumours (no solitary carcinogenic activity). Also, no solitary carcinogenic activity of *welensali* extracts was observed in assays using other protocols in mice, rats and hamsters (O'Gara, 1968; O'Gara *et al.*, 1971; Dunham *et al.*, 1974). Therefore, the promoting activity of the extracts may be attributed to irritant '*welensali* factors' (Hecker & Weber, 1977; Lutz & Hecker, 1979; Hecker *et al.*, 1983).

Assay-monitored systematic fractionation procedures were developed to isolate and identify the irritant and promoting factors in extracts of roots and fresh green leaves from *welensali*, as well as to estimate the amounts present (Hecker & Weber, 1977; Lutz & Hecker, 1979). All the fractions obtained were tested in the standard assay for irritation. The most plentiful active entities contained in the extracts, and hence in the roots and leaves, were isolated qualitatively, and the minimum content of active entities contained in the roots and leaves measured quantitatively. The individual systematic fractionation procedures comprised separation techniques such as counter-current distribution and chromatographic methods, including high-performance liquid chromatography. High-resolution spectroscopic methods (ultraviolet, infrared, $^1H$-nuclear magnetic resonance, mass) and derivatization were used mostly for complete identification of the pure irritants isolated (Hecker *et al.*, 1983).

A total of 17 irritant *welensali* factors of the diterpense ester type was found to be present in the methanol extract of roots; taken together, they represent a minimum content of 1.4% by weight of *welensali* factors in the extract (Table 2), i.e., of 0.32‰

Table 3. Structures and irritant activities of four typical *welensali* factors isolated from roots and leaves. *Welensali* factors $F_1$ and $F_2$ (activity type F) and their corresponding cryptic forms (activity type F′) as compared to 12-*O*-tetradecanoylphorbol-13-acetate (TPA)

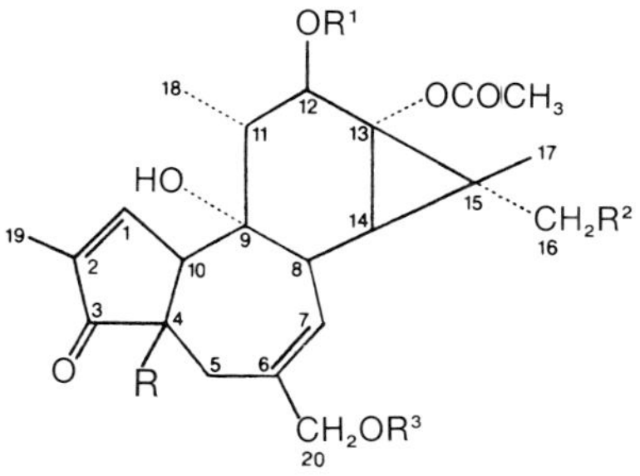


| Name *Welensali* factor, typical forms | Structures | | | | | Irritant activity | |
|---|---|---|---|---|---|---|---|
| | Ester of | *Welensali* factors | | | | Irritancy $(nmol^{-1})$ | Activity type |
| | | R | $R^1$ | $R^2$ | $R^3$ | | |
| $F_1$ | 16-Hydroxy- | HO- | $CH_3(CH_2)_{14}CO$- | HO- | H- | 30 | F |
| $F_1$-20-decanoate | phorbol | HO- | $CH_3(CH_2)_{14}CO$- | HO- | $CH_3(CH_2)_8CO$- | 9 | F′ |
| $F_2$ | 4-Deoxy-16- | H- | $CH_3(CH_2)_{14}CO$- | HO- | H- | 24 | F |
| $F_2$-20-octanoate | hydroxyphorbol | H- | $CH_3(CH_2)_{14}CO$- | HO- | $CH_3(CH_2)_6CO$- | 3 | F′ |
| TPA (croton oil factor $A_1$) | Phorbol | HO- | $CH_3(CH_2)_{12}CO$- | H- | H- | 63 | F |

of the roots. In the methanol extract of leaves, a total of 28 irritant *welensali* factors of the diterpene ester type was detected, representing together a minimum content of 0.06% by weight of the extract (Table 2), i.e., of 0.04‰ of the leaves. According to their irritancies, the *welensali* factors detected in roots and leaves may be classified into two (roots) and three (leaves) principal groups of irritant *activity types*, F, F′ and $F^y$ (see Table 2). Each of these groups comprises a variety of individual *welensali* factors – 17 altogether in roots and 28 in leaves. TPA, used for comparison, represents the activity type F (Table 2).

Some of the more typical and abundant *welensali* factors contained in roots and leaves are shown together with their structures in Table 3. *Welensali* factors $F_1$ and $F_2$ are 12,13-diesters of the polyfunctional diterpenes 16-hydroxy- and 4-deoxy-16-hydroxyphorbol, respectively, and represent activity type F of the *welensali* factors contained in roots and leaves (Table 3). Although they differ from TPA in chemical structure (see Fig. 3), $F_1$ and $F_2$ exhibit comparable, yet somewhat lower, activity than TPA as irritants (Table 3) and as promoters (Fig. 5). The activity type F′ is represented by corresponding 12,13,20-triesters, e.g., by $F_1$-20-decanoate and $F_2$-20-octanoate, respectively (Table 3). These types are less active as irritants (Table 3) and

Fig. 5. Cocarcinogenic (as initiation-promoting) activity of *welensali* factors $F_1$, $F_2$ and their 20-decanoates ('cryptic' promoters) in the standardized assay on back skin of NMRI mice, compared with croton oil factor $A_1$ 12-*O*-tetradecanoylphorbol-13-acetate (TPA)
*Initiator:* 7,12-dimethylbenz[*a*]anthracene (DMBA), i = 100 nmol, 28 females/group; *promoter:* $A_1$, $F_1$, $F_2$ and 20-decanoates, doses p as indicated.

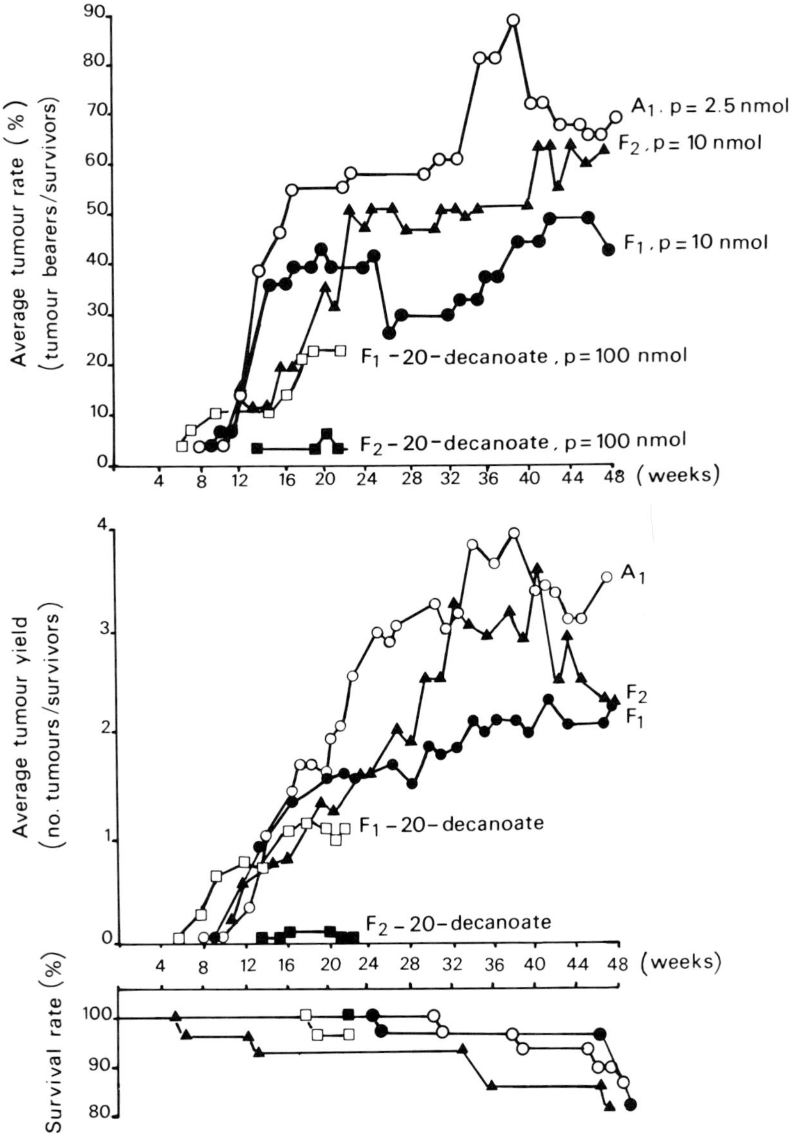


promoters (Fig. 5) than the corresponding *welensali* factors F; however, since they possess the 20-ester group, they may be converted to the corresponding highly active 12,13-diesters of the F-type by the action of tissue esterases or lipases, to yield *welensali* factors $F_1$ and $F_2$ ('metabolic activation'). The 12,13,20-triesters are therefore considered 'cryptic' irritants and promoters. As a potential source of highly active promoters, cryptic types deserve particular attention ('cryptic' cocarcinogenic risk factors, e.g., Hecker, 1981b). *Welensali* factors of the third activity type, $F^y$ (Table 2), were isolated only from leaves and in very low amounts. They were identified as weakly irritant 12,13,16-triesters of 16-hydroxyphorbol. It was impossible to investigate these factors much further (Hecker *et al.*, 1983) because of the very small quantities present.

When assayed for solitary carcinogenic activity in the promotional protocol on the back skin of mice *without* initiator (see Fig. 2, line 2), the mixtures containing preferentially *welensali* factors $F_1$ and $F_2$, as well as their corresponding cryptic types (Table 3), proved to be virtually inactive (Table 4) as compared to data in Figure 5.

Table 4. Assay for solitary carcinogenic activity of mixtures of typical activity type F-factors and F′-factors[a]

| Mixtures of typical *welensali* factors and -20-decanoates[b] (doses p in nmol)[c] | No. of tumours/survivors | | |
|---|---|---|---|
| | 12 weeks | 24 weeks | 48 weeks |
| $\overline{F}_1$ (p = 10) | 0/15 | 1/14 | 0/10 |
| $\overline{\overline{F}}_2$ (p = 10) | 0/14 | 0/14 | 1/13 |
| $\overline{F_1\text{-20-decanoate}}$ (p = 100) | 0/16 | 1/16 | 2/14 |
| $\overline{F_2\text{-20-decanoate}}$ (p = 100) | 0/16 | 0/16 | 0/12 |

[a] Standardized promotional protocol, NMRI mice without initiator, 15 or 16 females/group, doses p identical with those used in the full initiation/promotion protocol of corresponding pure factors and -20-decanoates, respectively
[b] Each mixture containing as the main component the factor indicated, besides minor components of same structural type
[c] Based upon molecular weight of factor indicated

### *Detection and identification of irritant and promoting* welensali *factors in* welensali *tea; estimation of content*

About 400 L of a concentrate of the preparation of *welensali* consumed most extensively on Curaçao, i.e., *welensali* tea, were prepared on the island according to the local recipe (Lutz, 1982). Instead of the usual amount (4 g) of fresh green leaves per cup (about 240 mL), ten times the amount of leaves was used. Of a typical 168-L batch (IIa) of the tea concentrate (corresponding to 1930 L of the tea as consumed on Curaçao), an extract in the form of the ethyl acetate fraction (efT IIa), was prepared (Hecker *et al.*, 1983). According to previous experience with the *welensali* factors contained in roots and leaves, this fraction was expected to contain all factors that could possibly be extracted from the leaves during preparation of the tea.

Two mixtures of *welensali* factors, representing activity types F and F′, were isolated from fraction efT IIa and also, consistently, from similar other fractions, by systematic assay-monitored fractionation (Hecker *et al.*, 1983). Each of the F- and

Table 5. Mixtures of *welensali* factors of activity types F and F′ contained in *welensali* tea and minimum content of one cup of *welensali* tea

| Mixture of *welensali* factors (composition) | Activity type | Minimum content of one cup of *welensali* tea[a] | | | | | |
|---|---|---|---|---|---|---|---|
| | | Determined | | | Estimated | | |
| | | absolute (μg) | sum | ratio | absolute (μg) | sum | ratio |
| $F_1$, $F_3$, $F_5$ | F | 0.06 | 0.75 | 0.5/1 | 0.27 | 1.6 | 2.2/1 |
| $F_1$-20-octanoate, $F_1$-20-decanoate, $F_3$-20-decanoate | F′ | 0.12 | | | 0.12 | | |

[a] One cup, ~240 mL

F′-type mixtures contained three *welensali* factors (Table 5): the *welensali* factor $F_1$ and the two structurally-related *welensali* factors $F_3$ and $F_5$ *(activity type F)*; the $F_1$-20-octanoate and the $F_1$- and $F_3$-20-decanoates *(activity types F′)*. Other factors, including *$F^y$ types,* which occur in leaves (see above), were not present in detectable amounts in the tea concentrate. Interestingly, all six *welensali* factors in the F- and F′-type mixtures isolated from the tea are esters of 16-hydroxyphorbol, whereas in leaves such esters are found in association also with esters of 4-deoxy-16-hydroxyphorbol (Table 3). In fact, esters of 16-hydroxyphorbol are more hydrophilic. During the isolation procedure they are also considered to be the more stable of the 28 *welensali* factors of leaves to heat and to oxygen exposure (see Table 2).

Quantitatively, in terms of minimum contents per cup of tea as consumed on Curaçao, the amount of activity type F mixture was 0.06 μg/cup, while that of activity type F′ mixture was 0.12 μg/cup. Taken together, the total minimum content of F- and F′-types in one cup is 0.75 μg/L (Table 5). It would be expected that the ratio of the minimum contents of the two principal activity types as determined for one cup of the tea (Table 5) and that determined for leaves (F:F′ = 2.2:1; Hecker *et al.*, 1983) should be approximately identical. In fact, the ratio F:F′ as determined for the tea is lower (Table 5, F:F′ = 0.5:1), indicating that isolation of the F-types starting with an aqueous extract of leaves such as tea is less efficient than starting with a methanol extract (see Table 2). In this context, it is interesting to note that the cryptic forms of *welensali* factors, the F′-types, are more stable than the corresponding F-types. Therefore, for a realistic estimation (Hecker *et al.*, 1983) of the minimum content of F-types in one cup of tea, the minimum content of F′-types may be taken as an internal standard to correct the ratio (F:F′ = 0.5:1) *determined* for the F:F′ ratio found in leaves (see Table 5). Hence the minimum content of F-types estimated to be present *in one cup of tea* as consumed on Curaçao is 0.27 μg of the mixture. Together with 0.12 μg of F′-types, the *estimated* total minimum content of *welensali* factors per cup of tea would be 1.6 μg/L (Table 5).

### *Detection and identification of putative initiators*

Experimental analysis was complemented by investigating *initiation* in the oesophagus, stimulated by findings of responsiveness of the oesophagus, e.g., of the rat, to promotion, indicated by a significant increase in $^{3}H$-thymidine incorporation following administration of croton oil (Mirvish *et al.*, 1979). In fact, in mice, the administration of a single small dose of DMBA by stomach tube followed by stomach intubations of the promoter TPA, according to the initiation/promotion protocol (Fig. 2), produced tumours of the forestomach (see Goerttler *et al.*, 1979). Similar initiation/promotion studies in rats, using *N*-methyl-*N′*-nitro-*N*-nitrosoguanidine as initiator and croton oil as promoter, revealed adenocarcinomas of the glandular stomach (Matsukura *et al.*, 1979). In-vitro experiments also provide evidence that PAH and nitrosamines act as initiators in oesophageal tissue (e.g., Cheng *et al.*, 1982). Taken together, these results show that the upper digestive tract of rats and mice is responsive to the initiation/promotion regimen. In addition, recent findings on the stimulation of latent genomes of certain DNA and RNA viruses by TPA and congeners (zur Hausen *et al.*, 1978, 1979; Ohigashi *et al.*, 1983; Wunderlich *et al.*, this volume; Amtmann *et al.*, 1983) and specifically by 12-*O*-hexadecanoyl-16-hydroxyphorbol-13-acetate, i.e., by *welensali* factor $F_1$ (Ito *et al.*, 1983), appear to support the possibility that latent viruses act as initiators (zur Hausen *et al.*, 1979; Hirayama & Ito, 1981), perhaps also of the oesophagus.

In the inhabitants of Curaçao, initiators similar to those demonstrated experimentally may be effective – for example, solitary carcinogenic PAH from the petrol-contaminated drinking-water (see above). Even if, from epidemiological data, PAH, nitroso compounds (e.g., Mahboubi & Aramesh, 1980) or viruses would seem to show no ability to induce oesophageal cancer as solitary carcinogens (see Fig. 1), this does not exclude the possibility of their acting as *initiators* of that target tissue in an initiation/promotion protocol (see Fig. 2).

## EXTRAPOLATION OF EXPERIMENTAL DATA TO HUMAN OESOPHAGEAL CANCER

The *welensali* factors of activity type F exhibit similar irritant and promoting activities in mouse skin; the same is true for the activity type F′ factors (Hecker & Weber, 1977; Lutz & Hecker, 1979; Lutz, 1982). Therefore, their estimated minimum contents contained in the tea (Table 5) may be represented in terms of biological activity by one of their prototypes, e.g., by the *welensali* factors $F_1$ or $F_1$-20-decanoate (for irritancy or irritant dose 50, see Table 3; for promoting activity, see Fig. 5). The estimated minimum content of the mixture of *welensali* factors type F in one cup of *welensali* tea (0.27 µg; Table 5) corresponds to 0.41 nmol $F_1$, and hence to *12 times the irritant dose 50 of* welensali *factor $F_1$* as determined on the mouse ear (Table 6). Similarly, the estimated minimum content of the mixture of *welensali* factors type F′ in one cup (0.12 µg) corresponds to 0.15 nmol $F_1$-20-decanoate, which is *1.4-times the irritant dose$_{50}$ of $F_1$-20-decanoate* (Table 6).

Table 6. Comparison of estimated minimum content of diterpene ester activity types F and F′ in one cup of *welensali* tea with irritant dose 50 of prototype *welensali* factors, the 16-hydroxyphorbol-12,13-di- and 12,13,16-triesters $F_1$ and $F_1$-20-decanoate, respectively

| Activity type | Estimated minimum content per cup | | Prototype factor | $ID_{50}^{24\,a}$ (nmol) | Ratio[b] |
|---|---|---|---|---|---|
| | (μg) | (nmol) | | | |
| F | 0.27 | 0.41 | $F_1$ | 0.033 | ~12:1 |
| F′ | 0.12 | 0.15 | $F_1$-20-decanoate | 0.11 | ~1.4:1 |

[a] Per mouse ear
[b] Estimated minimum contents of factors type F and F′ in nmol $F_1$ and $F_1$-20-decanoate, respectively, to irritant dose 50 of corresponding prototype factor

If the initiated tissues exposed to *welensali* factors, i.e., mouse epidermis, and that exposed in the human situation, i.e., oesophageal epidermis, were similarly responsive to exposure to putative initiators and to irritant diterpene esters shown to be present in the tea as well as in parts of *welensali* plants utilized otherwise, the data presented suggest that daily consumption of only *one* cup of *welensali* tea would suffice to provide the oesophagus with a substantial basal dose of promoter. This dose is already far in excess of that required to induce irritation of the mouse ear (Table 6); in the promotional protocol on the back skin of the mouse (Fig. 5), this amount is lower than the promoting dose p administered *twice weekly*. In Curaçao, the basal dose contained in one cup of tea may be considerably exceeded (Brennecker, 1961; Morton, 1971). Less regular consumption of other parts of *welensali* plants (see above), together with the medicinal uses of the 'bellyache bush' (Adolf *et al.*, 1983), may additionally increase the basal dose of promoter. Thus, for persons at risk in Curaçao, when dose, frequency and duration of exposure to diterpene ester type promoters are taken into account, an etiological situation of cocarcinogenesis in terms of initiation/promotion, as well as, perhaps, of stimulated initiation/promotion (see Fig. 2), is very likely to exist. The experimental results presented support an etiological *cocarcinogen hypothesis* in which diterpene ester-type cocarcinogens are the *principal etiological risk factors*. An etiology of the initiation/promotion type involving other, quite different 'local' promoters (Hirayama & Ito, 1981) is suggested by incomplete epidemiological and/or experimental data for high-incidence areas of oesophageal cancer both in Japan (Hirayama, 1981) and in northern China (Cheng *et al.*, 1982).

As a concluding step in the scientific evaluation of the problem of Curaçao, it might appear desirable to investigate the etiological cocarcinogen hypothesis by prospective epidemiological research. The installation of a cancer registry on the island (reported by Freni & Freni-Titulaer, 1981) may be of great help in achieving this goal. However, before the final results of expensive and time-consuming investigations of this kind become available, the evidence presented here might be considered by local health authorities to be sufficient for making immediate risk/benefit evaluations followed by *appropriate action* to prevent future exposure to the incriminated plant preparations.

Recent epidemiological evidence already indicates that in both males and females incidence rates of oesophageal cancer are declining (Freni & Freni-Titulaer, 1981). In support of the conclusions drawn from the experimental evaluation, this may be attributed to a failure among the younger generations on the island to adopt old-fashioned customs such as the preferential use of plant preparations, especially the drinking of *welensali* tea and other common utilizations of plant materials, and their replacement by habits considered more fashionable (Hecker *et al.*, 1983).

## GENERAL CONCLUSIONS

The employment of experimental dose/time-effect models (Figs 1, 2) to mimic the principal etiologies of human cancer helps to clarify the major carcinogenic risk factors and the pattern of exposure involved. However, in such models the complex reality of everyday human life is intentionally oversimplified. The diversity of individuals and of their personal habits make it highly unlikely that just one initiator and one promoter, i.e., a 'pure and simple' pattern of combined exposure used in corresponding experimental models, will prevail consistently (e.g., Hecker, 1981a). The experimental evidence presented here is not intended to exclude the possibility that under local conditions on Curaçao, risk factors other than the principal initiator(s) and promoter(s) suggested, such as condensed tannins (see above), excessive consumption of alcohol (e.g., Tuyns *et al.*, 1979) and/or cigarettes (Wynder & Hoffmann, 1979), consumption of hot food (e.g., Eps, 1970) and nutritional deficiencies (e.g., Wynder *et al.*, 1957), may not also contribute to the high risk of oesophageal cancer. Furthermore, in the various other high-risk areas of oesophageal cancer of the world (e.g., Table 1), depending on local life style, quite different 'local' risk factors and/or different combination patterns of exposure may be operative.

In a number of recent experimental investigations, the existence of a variety of structurally different cocarcinogens for several target tissues has come to light experimentally (for recent data, see this entire volume and Hecker *et al.*, 1982), in addition to the irritant polyfunctional diterpenes (Hecker, 1981b). The results of such investigations may be generalized to suggest that, in the etiology of human cancer, besides solitary carcinogens, physicochemically well-defined cocarcinogens of whatever origin and nature have to be considered as risk factors. As compared with solitary carcinogens – *the* classical *first-order carcinogenic risk factors* – for theoretical reasons and with the intention of grading the risk of cancer, cocarcinogens may be postulated to be *second-order carcinogenic risk factors* (Hecker, 1976a–d, 1978, 1981a,b, 1984a,b). As a consequence of the progress made in basic scientific knowledge regarding etiologies and mechanisms of carcinogenesis, such grading may allow for *more refined risk/benefit* evaluations (Hecker, 1981b; Marshall, 1982; Hecker 1984a,b) in the future. The refinement intended for theoretical reasons may be helpful in practice in finding a scientifically more appropriate balance between an over-protective legislation aiming at absolute safety (which in fact cannot be accomplished) and an all-permissive absence of restriction – both of which are disadvantageous to the individual. However, at the present stage of research, it is considered premature to materialize such grading in preventive legislation on the basis of putative mechanistic categories, such as, e.g., genotoxic–non-genotoxic (e.g., Marshall, 1982), for which neither sufficient experimental evidence nor criteria for evaluating results of short-term assays are presently available (IARC, 1983; Hecker, this volume, Concluding Remarks).

Finally, it appears important to point out to the public that in both principal classes of defined carcinogenic risk factors – solitary and cocarcinogens – the most active entities known, the *aflatoxins* produced by moulds, as well as the *diterpene ester-type promoters* produced by many, but not all, Euphorbiaceae and Thymelaeaceae species, are of *plant origin*. Therefore, the presence in the human environment of 'natural' carcinogenic risk factors certainly cannot be neglected. Nevertheless, it some societies it appears fashionable to incriminate solely and collectively our technological civilization for pollution of the human environment with 'anthropogenic' carcinogenic risk factors. The truth is, however, that *carcinogenic risk factors of whatever origin* – 'God-made' or 'man-made' – *must be detected and identified* in order to prevent or at least to control human exposure. Our technological civilization is surely capable of identifying the hazards and of providing the necessary techniques of prevention.

## ACKNOWLEDGEMENTS

Generous financial support of the *welensali* project in its many stages by the Wilhelm- and Maria-Meyenburg-Stiftung, Heidelberg-Leimen, is gratefully acknowledged. I thank Dr B. Sorg and Apotheker R. Schmidt for critical discussions during preparation of the manuscript.

## REFERENCES

Adolf, W., Opferkuch, H.J. & Hecker, E. (1983) Irritant phorbol-derivatives from four Jatropha species. *Phytochemistry*, **23**, 129–132

Amtmann, E., Volm, M. & Wayss, K. (1983) *Synergism between latent papilloma-virus genomes and a tumor promoter in the rodent* Mastomys natalensis. In: *Abstracts of International Symposium: Role of Co-carcinogens and Promoters in Human and Experimental Carcinogenesis, 16–18 May, Budapest, Hungary*, p. 1

Bauer, K.H. (1928) *Mutationstheorie der Geschwulstentstehung*, Berlin, Springer

Bauer, K.H. (1963) *Das Krebsproblem*, 2. Aufl., Berlin, Springer

Berenblum, I. (1941a) The cocarcinogenic action of croton resin. *Cancer Res.*, **1**, 44–48

Berenblum, I. (1941b) The mechanism of carcinogenesis. A study of significance of cocarcinogenic action and related phenomena. *Cancer Res.*, **1**, 383–391

Berenblum, I. & Shubik, P. (1947) A new quantitative approach to the study of the stages of chemical carcinogenesis in the mouse skin. *Br. J. Cancer*, **1**, 383–391

de Boer, S.Y. (1979) *Frequentie van Kanker van Mond-tong-Pharynx-Slokdarm en de Nederlandse Antillen*. Dissertation (Landslaboratorium voor de Volkszondheid, Afdeling Pathologisch anatomisches Laboratorium Curacao, Niederländische Antillen)

Boutwell, R.K. (1964) Some biological aspects of skin carcinogenesis. *Progr. exp. Tumor Res.*, ***4***, 207–250

Boutwell, R.K. (1974) The function and mechanism of promoters of carcinogenesis. *CRC crit. Rev. Toxicol.*, **2**, 419–443

Brenneker, P. (1961) *Jerba: Kruiden van Curacao en hun gebruik*, Curaçao, Boekhandel St Augustinus, p. 67

Cheng, J.S., Sala, M., Li, M.H. & Chouroulinkov, I. (1982) *Esophageal cancer in Linxian County, China: A possible etiology and mechanism (initiation and promotion)*. In: Hecker, E., Fusenig, N.E., Kunz, W., Marks, F. & Thielmann, H.W., eds, *Carcinogenesis – A Comprehensive Survey*, Vol. 7, *Cocarcinogenesis and the Biological Effects of Tumour Promoters*, New York, Raven Press, pp. 167–174

Day, N.E. (1982) *Epidemiological evidence of promoting effects – the example of breast cancer*. In: Hecker, E., Fusenig, N.E., Kunz, W., Marks, F. & Thielmann, H.W., eds, *Carcinogenesis — A Comprehensive Survey*, Vol. 7, *Cocarcinogenesis and the Biological Effects of Tumour Promoters*, New York, Raven Press, pp. 183–199

Druckrey, H. (1967) *Quantitative aspects in chemical carcinogenesis*. In: Truhaut, R., ed., *Potential Carcinogenic Hazards from Drugs (UICC Monographs Series, Vol. 7)*, Berlin, Springer, pp. 60–77

Druckrey, H. & Küpfmüller, K. (1948) *Dosis und Wirkung*, Aulendorf, Editio Canctor KG

Dunham, L.J. & Bailar, J.C. (1968) World maps of cancer mortality rates and frequency ratios. *J. natl Cancer Inst.*, ***41***, 155–203

Dunham, L.J., Sheets, R.H. & Morton, J.F. (1974) Proliferative lesions in cheek pouch and esophagus of hamsters treated with plants from Curaçao, Netherlands Antilles. *J. natl Cancer Inst.*, ***53***, 1259–1269

Eibergen, R. (1961) *Kanker op Curaçao*, Groningen, J.B. Wolters, p. 134

Eps, L.W. (1970) *Esophageal Cancer*, Curaçao, St Elisabeth Hospital Medical Library

Evans, F.J. & Soper, C.J. (1978) The tigliane, daphnane and ingenane diterpenes, their chemistry, distribution and biological activities. *Lloydia*, ***41***, 193–233

Freni, S.C. & Freni-Titulaer, L.W.J. (1981) Cancer incidence in the Netherland Antilles. A survey covering the period 1968–1979. *Cancer*, ***48***, 2535–2541

Goerttler, K., Loehrke, H., Schweizer, J. & Hesse, B. (1979) Systemic two-stage carcinogenesis in the epithelium of the forestomach of mice using 7,12-dimethylbenz(*a*)anthracene as initiator and the phorbol ester 12-*O*-tetradecanoylphorbol-13-acetate as promoter. *Cancer Res.*, ***39***, 1292–1297

Hartz, P.H. (1940) The incidence of malignant tumors in unselected autopsy material at Curaçao, Netherlands West Indies. *Am. J. Cancer*, ***40***, 355–358

Hartz, P.H. (1958) The incidence of carcinoma of the esophagus in the Caribbean region and in Venezuela, compared with that of gastric cancer. *Acta unio int. cancrum*, ***14***, 548–553

zur Hausen, H., O'Neill, F.B., Freese, U.K. & Hecker, E. (1978) Persisting oncogenic herpesvirus induced by the tumor promoter TPA. *Nature*, ***272***, 373–374

zur Hausen, H., Bornkamm, G.W., Schmidt, R. & Hecker, E. (1979) Tumor initiators and promoters in the induction of Epstein-Barr virus. *Proc. natl Acad. Sci. USA*, ***76***, 782–785

Hecker, E. (1968) Cocarcinogenic principles from the seed oil of *Croton tiglium* L. and from other Euphorbiaceae. *Cancer Res.*, ***28***, 2338–2349 [see also *Planta Med.* (Suppl.) (1968), pp. 24–45]

Hecker, E. (1971) Isolation and characterization of the cocarcinogenic principles from croton oil. *Meth. Cancer Res.*, ***6***, 439–484

Hecker, E. (1972) Aktuelle Probleme der Krebsentstehung. *Z. Krebsforsch.*, ***78***, 99–122

Hecker, E. (1976a) Definitions and terminology in cancer (tumor) etiology – an analysis aiming at proposals for a current internationally standardized terminology. *Int. J. Cancer*, ***18***, 122–129

Hecker, E. (1976b) Definitions and terminology in cancer (tumor) etiology – an analysis aiming at proposals for a current internationally standardized terminology. *Z. Krebsforsch.*, ***86***, 219–230

Hecker, E. (1976c) Definitions and terminology in cancer (tumor) etiology – an analysis aiming at proposals for a current internationally standardized terminology. *Gann*, ***67***, 471–481

Hecker, E. (1976d) Definitions and terminology in cancer (tumor) etiology – an analysis aiming at proposals for a current internationally standardized terminology. *Bull. World Health Organ.*, ***54***, 1–10

Hecker, E. (1978) *Structure-activity relationships in diterpene esters irritant and cocarcinogenic to mouse skin.* In: Slaga, T.J., Sivak, A. & Boutwell, R.K., eds, *Carcinogenesis — A Comprehensive Survey,* Vol. 2, *Mechanisms of Tumor Promotion and Cocarcinogenesis,* New York, Raven Press, pp. 11–48

Hecker, E. (1981a) Prototype processes as experimental models in multifactorial carcinogenesis. *J. Cancer Res. clin. Oncol.*, ***99***, A29

Hecker, E. (1981b) Cocarcinogenesis and tumor promoters of the diterpene ester type as possible carcinogenic risk factors. *J. Cancer Res. clin. Oncol.*, ***99***, 103–124

Hecker, E. (1984a) Co-carcinogens of the initiation-(or tumor) promoter type as environmental risk factors of cancer in man — experimental analysis of an etiological model situation of life style cancer and current problems of assessment of cancer risk in multifactorial carcinogenesis. *Acta pharmacol. toxikol.*, Suppl. (in press)

Hecker, E. (1984b) *Multifaktorielle und Mehrstufen-Karzinogenese – Ätiologische und experimentelle Modelle sowie aktuelle Schlüsselprobleme für die Bewertung von Krebsrisikofaktoren der Umwelt, Eröffnungsvortrag Expertengespräch 'Tumorpromotoren: Erkennung, Wirkungsmechanismen und Bedeutung'.* In: *Bundesgesundheitsamt, Max-von-Pettenkofer-Institut, 6–7 February 1984* (in press)

Hecker, E. & Schmidt, R. (1974) Phorbolesters – the irritants and cocarcinogens of *Croton tiglium* L. *Progr. Chem. Org. Nat. Prod.*, ***31***, 377–467

Hecker, E. & Weber, J. (1977) *Cocarcinogens from* Croton flavens *L. and the high incidence of esophageal cancer in Curaçao.* In: *Abstracts of the 7th International Symposium on the Biological Characterization of Human Tumors, Budapest, 13–15 April, 1977,* p. 52 (see also *Experientia (Basel)*, ***34***, 679–682 (1978)

Hecker, E., Fusenig, N.E., Kunz, W., Marks, F. & Thielmann, H.W. eds (1982) *Carcinogenesis – A Comprehensive Survey,* Vol. 7, *Cocarcinogenesis and Biological Effects of Tumor Promoters,* New York, Raven Press

Hecker, E., Lutz, D., Weber, J., Goerttler, K. & Morton, J.F. (1983) *Multistage tumor development in the human esophagus – the first identification of cocarcinogens of the tumor promoter type as principal carcinogenic risk factors in a local life style cancer*. In: *13th International Cancer Congress, Part B, Biology of Cancer (1)*, New York, Alan R. Liss Inc, pp. 219–238

Hecker, E., Adolf, W., Hergenhahn, M., Schmidt, R. & Sorg, B. (1984) *Keynote lecture: Irritant diterpene ester promoters of mouse skin: Contributions to etiologies of environmental cancer and to biochemical mechanisms of carcinogenesis*. In: Fujiki, H., Hecker, E., Moore, R.E., Sugimura, T. & Weinstein, I.B., eds, *Cellular Interactions by Environmental Tumor Promoters*, Tokyo, Japan Scientific Society Press; Utrecht, VNU Science Press, pp. 3–36

Higginson, J. (1979) *Environmental carcinogenesis: A global perspective*. In: Emmelot, P. & Kriek, E., eds, *Environmental Carcinogenesis: Occurrence, Risk Evaluation and Mechanisms*, Amsterdam, Elsevier/North-Holland Biomedical Press, pp. 9–24

Hirayama, T. (1981) Operational epidemiology of cancer. *J. Cancer Res. clin. Oncol.*, ***99***, 15–28

Hirayama, T. & Ito, Y. (1981) A new view of etiology of nasopharyngeal carcinoma. *Prev. Med.*, ***10***, 614–622

IARC (1983) *Approaches to Classifying Chemical Carcinogens According to Mechanism of Action (IARC Internal Technical Report, No 83/001)*, Lyon, International Agency for Research on Cancer

Ito, Y., Yanase, S., Tokuda, H., Kishishita, M., Ohigashi, H., Hirota, M. & Koshimizu, K. (1983) Epstein-Barr virus activation by Jung oil, extracts of *Aleurites fordii* and its diterpene ester 12-*O*-hexadecanoyl-16-hydroxyphorbol-13-acetate. *Cancer Lett.*, ***18***, 87–95

Kidd, J.G. & Rous, P. (1983) The carcinogenic effect of a papilloma virus on the tarred skin of rabbits. *J. exp. Med.*, ***68***, 529–562

Kunz, H.W., Schaude, G., Schwarz, M. & Tennekes, H. (1982) *Quantitative aspects of drug-mediated tumour promotion in liver and its toxicological implications*. In: Hecker, E., Fusenig, N.E., Kunz, W., Marks, F. & Thielmann, H. W., eds, *Carcinogenesis — A Comprehensive Survey*, Vol. 7, *Cocarcinogenesis and Biological Effects of Tumor Promoters*, New York, Raven Press, pp. 111–125

Kunz, H.W., Tennekes, H.A., Port, R.E., Schwarz, M., Lorke, D. & Schaude, G. (1983) Quantitative aspects of carcinogenesis and tumor promotion in liver. *Environ. Health Perspect.*, ***50***, 113–122

Lutz, D. (1982) *Vorkommen von cocarcinogenen Diterpenestern in 'Welensali'* (Croton flavens *L.) sowie in dem auf Curaçao gebräuchlichen Welensali-Tee*, Thesis, University of Heidelberg

Lutz, D. & Hecker, E. (1979) *Esophageal cancer on Curaçao – further new tumor-promoters from* Croton flavens *L.* In: *Abstracts of the 8th International Symposium on the Biological Characterization of Human Tumors, 8–11 May, Athens, Greece*

Mahboubi, E.O. & Aramesh, B. (1980) Epidemiology of esophageal cancer in Iran, with special reference to nutritional and cultural aspects. *Prev. Med.*, ***9***, 613–621

Marshall, E. (1982) EPA's high risk carcinogen policy. *Science*, ***218***, 975–978

Matsukura, N., Kawachi, T., Sano, R., Sasajima, K. & Sugimura, T. (1979) Promoting action of croton oil on gastrocarcinogenesis by *N*-methyl-*N*-nitro-*N*-nitroso-guanidine. *J. Cancer Res. clin. Oncol.,* ***93,*** 323–327

Merino, F., Zaisman, I., Grand, R., Lopez, V., Amesty, C., Garnica, H., Montserrat, R., Palao, R., Bonstein, M., Lugo, J.A., Boada, P.P. & Serrano, M.C. (1980) Cancer gastrico en el Estado Falcon: epidemiologia, immunologia y pesquisa. *Acta oncol. Venezolana,* ***13,*** 219–286

Mirvish, S.S., Rose, E.F. & Sutherland, D.M. (1979) Studies on the esophagus. II. Enhancement of $^3$H-thymidine incorporation in the rat esophagus by *Bidens pilosa* and croton oil. *Cancer Lett.,* ***6,*** 159–165

Morton, J.F. (1968a) A survey of medicinal plants of Curaçao. *Econ. Bot.,* ***22,*** 87–102

Morton, J.F. (1968b) Plants associated with esophageal cancer cases in Curaçao. *Cancer Res.,* ***28,*** 2268–2271

Morton, J.F. (1970) Tentative correlations of plant usage and esophageal cancer zones. *Econ. Bot.,* ***24,*** 217–226

Morton, J.F. (1971) Welensali *(Croton flavens):* Folk uses and properties. *Econ. Bot.,* ***25,*** 457–463

Morton, J.F. (1972) Further associations of plant tannins and human cancer. Q. J. Crude Drug Res., ***12,*** 1829–1841

Morton, J.F. (1974) Folk remedy plants and esophageal cancer in Coro, Venezuela. *Morris Arboretum Bull.,* ***25,*** 24–34

Morton, J.F. (1979) *Plant tannins and esophageal cancer.* In: *Proceedings of the 10th International Conference on Toxicology and Occupational Medicine,* Amsterdam, Elsevier/North-Holland, pp. 129–137

Morton, J.F. (1981) *Atlas of Medicinal Plants of Middle America,* Springfield, IL, Charles C. Thomas

Mottram, J.C. (1944) A developing factor in blastogenesis. *J. Pathol. Bacteriol.,* ***56,*** 181–187

O'Gara, R.W. (1968) Biologic screening of selected plant material for carcinogens. *Cancer Res.,* ***28,*** 2272–2275

O'Gara, R.W., Lee, C. & Morton, J.F. (1971) Carcinogenicity of extracts of selected plants from Curaçao after oral and subcutaneous administration to rodents. *J. natl Cancer Inst.,* ***46,*** 1131–1137

O'Gara, R.W., Lee, C.W., Morton, J.F., Kapadia, G.J. & Dunham, L.J. (1974) Sarcoma induced in rats by extracts of plants and by fractionated extracts of *Krameria ixina. J. natl Cancer Inst.,* ***52,*** 445–448

Ohigashi, H., Ohtsuka, T., Hirota, M., Koshimzu, K., Tokuda, H. & Ito, Y. (1983) Tigliane type diterpene esters with Epstein-Barr virus inducing activity from *Sapium sebiferum. Agric. biol. Chem.,* ***47,*** 1617–1622

Peto, R. (1977) *Epidemiology, multistage models, and short term mutagenicity tests.* In: Hiatt, H.H., Watson, J.D. & Winsten, J.A., eds, *Origins of Human Cancer,* Cold Spring Harbor, NY, Cold Spring Harbor Laboratory, pp. 1403–1428

Pound, A.W. & Bell, J.R. (1962) The influence of croton oil stimulation on tumor initiation by urethane in mice. *Br. J. Cancer,* ***16,*** 690–695

Roe, F.J.C., Carter, R.J., Mitchley, B.C.V., Peto, R. & Hecker, E. (1972) On the persistence of tumor initiation and the acceleration of tumor progression in mouse skin tumorigenesis. *Int. J. Cancer*, ***9***, 264–273

Shear, M.J. (1938) Studies on carcinogenesis. V. Methyl-derivatives of 1,2-benzanthracene. *Am. J. Cancer*, ***33***, 499–537 (see, especially, p. 532)

Shinozuka, H. & Ritchie, A.C. (1967) Pretreatment with croton oil, DNA synthesis and carcinogenesis by carcinogen followed by croton oil. *Int. J. Cancer*, ***2***, 77–84

Slaga, T.J., Sivak, A. & Boutwell, R.K., eds (1978) *Carcinogenesis — A Comprehensive Survey*, Vol. 2, *Mechanisms of Tumor Promotion and Cocarcinogenesis*, New York, Raven Press

Tomatis, L., Agthe, C., Bartsch, H., Huff, J., Montesano, R., Saracci, R., Walker, E. & Wilbourn, J. (1978) Evaluation of the carcinogenicity of chemicals. A review on the monograph program of the International Agency for Research on Cancer 1971 to 1977. *Cancer Res.*, ***38***, 877–885

Tuyns, A.J., Pequignot, G. & Abbalucci, J.S. (1979) Oesophageal cancer and alcohol consumption: importance of type of beverage. *Int. J. Cancer*, ***23***, 443–447

Van Duuren, B.L. (1969) Tumor promoting agents in two stage carcinogenesis. *Progr. exp. Tumor Res.*, ***11***, 31–68

Van Duuren, B.L., Blazej, T., Goldschmidt, B.M., Katz, C., Melchione, S. & Sivak, A. (1971) Cocarcinogenesis, studies on mouse skin and inhibition of tumor induction. *J. natl Cancer Inst.*, ***46***, 1039–1044

Van Duuren, B.L., Katz, C. & Goldschmidt, B.M. (1973) Cocarcinogenic agents in tobacco carcinogenesis. *J. natl Cancer Inst.*, ***51***, 703–705

Vesselinovitch, S.D. & Mihailovich, N. (1983) Kinetics of diethylnitrosamine-hepatocarcinogenesis in the infant mouse. *Cancer Res.*, ***43***, (in press)

Waterhouse, J., Muir, C., Correa, P. & Powell, J., eds (1976) *Cancer Incidence in Five Continents, Vol. III (IARC Scientific Publications No. 15)*, Lyon, International Agency for Research on Cancer

Wynder, E.L. & Hoffmann, D.H. (1979) Tobacco and health: A societal challenge. *New Engl. J. Med.*, ***300***, 894–903

Wynder, E.L., Hultberg, S., Jacobson, F. & Bross, I.J. (1957) Environmental factors in cancer of the upper alimentary tract. *Cancer*, ***10***, 470–487

# AGRICULTURALLY-RELATED CARCINOGENIC RISK

M. BÖRZSÖNYI, G. TÖRÖK, A. PINTÉR & A. SURJÁN
*National Institute of Hygiene, Budapest, Hungary*

## SUMMARY

Although all people are exposed throughout life to pesticides (during manufacture and use, in the environment, *via* the food chain), with the exception of vinyl chloride and the arsenic compounds, no human carcinogen pesticide is known. In experimental animals and short-term tests, however, many pesticides have proved to be carcinogenic or genotoxic.

In order to elucidate possible modes of action related to genotoxicity (short-term tests) and carcinogenicity, data on 83 pesticides were analysed. A definitive promoter effect was demonstrated for five compounds, and a suspected promoter effect could be attributed to 16 compounds. Almost all were organohalogens.

Ethylenthiourea and aminotriazole are also carcinogens, which induce tumours through hormonal imbalance. Ethylenthiourea is the degradation product and metabolite of certain ethylene-bisdithiocarbamate pesticides. Chlorphenol and chlorophenoxyacetic acid-type pesticides contain 2,3,7,8-tetrachlorodibenzo-*para*-dioxin (TCDD) as a contaminant. TCDD has definite promoter action.

Seventeen tumorigenic pesticides could be regarded as genotoxic, and similar activity could be suspected in three other carcinogenic pesticides. Many pesticides contain *N*-nitroso impurities in various amounts. Nitrosation of the original pesticide or its derivative, such as dialkylamines, alkyl-arylamines, methyleneimines, gives rise to the formation of *N*-nitroso compounds. Amides containing secondary amines, such as ethylcarbamate and alkylurea, could be nitrosated *in vivo* and *in vitro*. Most nitrosated pesticides are strong genotoxic carcinogens.

## INTRODUCTION

Pesticides are the most widely used chemicals in agriculture. They are being applied in increasing amounts, and a large number of people risk contamination during their manufacture and application as well as through the food chain (Moses, 1980).

In estimating the potential human carcinogenic risk one must consider the quantity of pesticides, their stability, appearance in food, metabolism in plants and animals, chemical interactions with other environmental pollutants, and genotoxicity (short-term effect). Several pesticides and metabolites cross the placental barrier and are excreted in milk; therefore, they present a life-long risk of exposure to human beings (McEven & Stephenson, 1979).

In order to establish the possible hazard to man, we attempted to evaluate pesticides according to their activity in short-term tests and their carcinogenicity. Furthermore, compounds inactive in short-term tests may yield strong genotoxic carcinogens during their manufacture and/or in the environment. In estimating human risk, this factor should be given serious consideration.

## MATERIALS AND METHODS

In evaluating the pesticides, the following main sources were used: *The Pesticide Manual* (Worthing, 1979) (chemical structure, use), *IARC Monographs* Vols 1–29 (IARC, 1972–1982) (short-term effects and carcinogenicity) and Chu *et al.* (1981) (carcinogenicity).

The pesticides were grouped according to their chemical structure as follows: organohalogens, organophosphates, carbamates and other pesticides. Four endpoints were considered in evaluating the short-term effects (Table 1), based on suggestions

Table 1. Short term tests for evaluation of genotoxicity[a, b]

| |
|---|
| DNA damage, repair and recombination |
| Preferential killing or growth inhibition of repair-deficient bacteria |
| Prophage induction |
| Mitotic recombination and/or gene conversion in yeast |
| DNA binding *in vitro* and *in vivo* |
| DNA breakage *in vitro* and *in vivo* |
| Unscheduled DNA synthesis in mammalian cells and in rodents |
| Sister chromatid exchange in mammalian cells and in mammals |
| Gene mutation |
| Reverse and forward mutation in bacteria |
| Reverse and forward mutation in fungi |
| Sex-linked recessive lethal mutations in *Drosophila melanogaster* |
| Forward mutations in mammalian cells |
| Specific locus mutations in mice |
| Chromosomal mutation |
| Heritable chromosomal damages in *Drosophila melanogaster* |
| Chromosomal aberrations in mammals and in cultured mammalian cells |
| Micronuclei in rodent bone-marrow cells |
| Dominant lethal mutations in rodents |
| Heritable translocations in rodents |
| Mammalian cell transformation |
| Morphological transformation |
| Colony formation in soft agar |

[a] Modified from: US Environmental Protection Agency (1978); IARC (1982)
[b] For the definition of 'genotoxicity' used in this report, see 'Materials and Methods'.

of the IARC (1982) and the US Environmental Protection Agency (1978). In establishing carcinogenicity, data published by IARC (1972–1982) were accepted. If no such data were available, we tried to follow the criteria published in the *IARC Monographs*. Judgements as to fulfillment of the various criteria (classification of short-term tests, importance of a test within its group, estimation of the relationship between chemical structure and biological activity) were somewhat arbitrary and by no means free of subjectivity.

Pesticides were regarded as definitive or proven promoters if negative or equivocally negative data from a short-term test were available and a successful two-stage experiment had been carried out, whether or not they induced tumours when applied at a maximum tolerable dose over a long period of time. There is no known promoter which would not have proved to be at least a weak carcinogen.

Tumorigenic pesticides that were found to give negative or equivocally negative results in short-term tests and which had a chemical structure similar to those of definite promoters but which had not been subjected to two-stage experiments, were considered suspected promoters.

A potential promoting effect was anticipated for a pesticide on the basis of its chemical structure and biological activity when no data on activity in the short-term tests considered or on carcinogenicity were available.

Tumorigenic pesticides giving positive or equivocally positive results in short-term tests were considered to be genotoxic carcinogens. Of the short-term tests considered, cell transformation is not usually regarded as a test of 'genotoxicity', but in this report, the term 'genotoxic' is used only operationally and refers also to results from tests for cell transformation. In the absence of results in short-term tests or when equivocal results were obtained, carcinogenic pesticides with chemical structures similar to those of proven genotoxic carcinogens were considered suspected genotoxic carcinogens.

The possibility of a pure initiating effect was considered for pesticides when a long-term effect could not be evaluated as positive, when the chemical structure was similar to that of proven genotoxic carcinogens, and when positive or equivocally positive results had been obtained in short-term tests.

With regard to the nitrosation of pesticides, their grouping was based on the chemical structure of the *N*-nitroso derivatives (dialkyl-, alkylaryl, cyclic nitrosamines and nitrosamides).

## DISCUSSION

*Halogenated hydrocarbons* (Table 2)

*Haloalkanes and haloalkenes:* Carbon tetrachloride gives negative results in short-term tests; however, *in vivo,* it induces liver tumours in mice and rats. Its promoting and carcinogenic effect has also been demonstrated in rats and mice, particularly in the induction of liver tumours. These effects are thought to be due to its hepatotoxic activity and consequent cell proliferation (Pound & McGuire, 1978).

Table 2. Genotoxicity[a] and carcinogenicity of halogenated hydrocarbon pesticides

| Pesticide | Use | Short term effect[b] | | | | | Animal carcinogenicity (IARC evaluation) | Comment[c] | References |
|---|---|---|---|---|---|---|---|---|---|
| | | D | M | C | T | IARC evaluation | | | |
| *Alkanes and alkenes* | | | | | | | | | |
| Carbon tetrachloride | Insecticide | − | ∓ | − | | I | S | P | IARC (1972–1982a,b); Pound & McGuire (1978) |
| Chloroform | Insecticide | − | ∓ | − | ± | I | S | SP | IARC (1972–1982a,b) |
| Hexachloroethane | In formulations | | | | | | L | ND | IARC (1972–1982a) |
| 1,1,2,2-Tetrachloroethane | Insecticide | + | + | | | (L) | L | GC | IARC (1972–1982a) |
| Vinyl chloride | Propellant | + | ± | ± | | S | S | GC(HC) | IARC (1972–1982a,b) |
| Ethylene dibromide | Insecticide | + | + | + | | S | S | GC | IARC (1972–1982a,b) |
| Ethylene dichloride | Insecticide | − | + | ∓ | | (I) | S | SGC | IARC (1972–1982a) |
| Tetrachloroethylene | Insecticide | − | ∓ | − | | I | L | SP | IARC (1972–1982a,b) |
| 1,1,1-Trichloroethane | In formulations | | + | | | (I) | I | ND | IARC (1972–1982a) |
| 1,2-Dibromo-3-chloro-propane | Insecticide | | + | + | | (L) | S | GC | IARC (1972–1982a) |
| Hexachlorobutadiene | Fungicide | | + | | | (I) | L | ND | IARC (1972–1982a) |
| *Cyclohexanes* | | | | | | | | | |
| α– Hexachlorocyclohexane | Insecticide | − | − | | | I | S | P | IARC (1972–1982a,b); Moriya *et al.* (1983) |
| β– Hexachlorocyclohexane | Insecticide | − | − | + | | I | L | SP | IARC (1972–1982a,b); Kawachi *et al.* (1980) |
| γ– Hexachlorocyclohexane (lindane) | Insecticide | ∓ | − | ∓ | | I | S | SP | Fahrig (1974); IARC (1972–1982a,b); Kawachi *et al.* (1980) |
| Technical hexachloro-cyclohexane | Insecticide | − | − | | | I | S | SP | IARC (1972–1982a,b) |
| *Benzenes* | | | | | | | | | |
| Hexachlorobenzene | Fungicide | | − | − | | (I) | S | SP | IARC Monographs (1972–1982) |
| Quintozene | Fungicide | − | - | | | (I) | (L) | ND | Chu *et al.*, 1981; Fahrig, 1974; IARC Monographs 1972–1982; Moriya *et al.*, 1983 |
| Pentachlorophenol | Herbicide, fungicide | + | ∓ | ∓ | | I | I | ND | Fahrig, 1974; IARC Monographs 1972–1982; IARC Monographs Suppl. 4, 1982; Moriya *et al.*, 1983 |

| | | | | | | | | | |
|---|---|---|---|---|---|---|---|---|---|
| 2,4,6-Trichlorophenol | Insecticide | | | | | | S | ND | IARC Monographs 1972–1982; IARC Monographs Suppl. 4, 1982 |
| *Toluenes* | | | | | | | | | |
| Benzyl chloride | Herbicide | + | + | ∓ | + | S | L | GC | IARC Monographs 1972–1982; IARC Monographs Suppl. 4, 1982 |
| Benzal chloride | Herbicide | + | + | | | L | L | GC | IARC Monographs 1972–1982; IARC Monographs Suppl. 4, 1982 |
| Benzotrichloride | Herbicide | + | + | | | L | S | GC | IARC Monographs 1972–1982; IARC Monographs Suppl. 4, 1982 |
| Benzoyl chloride | Herbicide | – | – | | | I | I | ND | IARC Monographs 1972–1982; IARC Monographs Suppl. 4, 1982 |
| Trifluralin | Herbicide | ∓ | – | | | (I) | (L) | SP | Carere & Morpurgo, 1981; Chu *et al.*, 1981; Moriya *et al.*, 1983 |
| *DDT group* | | | | | | | | | |
| *p,p′*-DDT | Insecticide | – | ∓ | ∓ | | I | S | P | Fahrig, 1974; IARC Monographs 1972–1982; IARC Monographs Suppl. 4, 1982 |
| *p,p′*-TDE (DDD) | Insecticide | – | ∓ | | | (I) | (L) | SP | Fahrig, 1974; IARC Monographs 1972–1982; Moriya *et al.*, 1983 |
| *p,p′*-DDE | Insecticide | – | – | | | (I) | (L) | SP | Fahrig, 1974; IARC Monographs 1972–1982; Moriya *et al.*, 1983 |
| Chlorobenzilate | Insecticide | – | – | | | (I) | (S) | SP | Fahrig, 1974; IARC Monographs 1972–1982; Moriya *et al.*, 1983 |
| Methoxychlor | Insecticide | | – | ∓ | | (I) | I | ND | IARC Monographs 1972–1982 |
| Perthane (Ethylan) | Insecticide | | | | | | (I) | ND | Chu *et al.*, 1981 |
| Dicofol (Kelthane) | Insecticide | – | – | ± | | (I) | (L) | SP | Chu *et al.*, 1981; Kawachi *et al.*, 1980 |
| *Terpenes and related pesticides* | | | | | | | | | |
| Aldrin | Insecticide | ∓ | – | ± | | I | L | SP | IARC Monographs 1972–1982; IARC Monographs Suppl. 4, 1982 |
| Dieldrin | Insecticide | ∓ | ∓ | ∓ | – | I | L | SP | IARC Monographs 1972–1982; IARC Monographs Suppl. 4, 1982 |
| Endrin | Insecticide | – | – | | | (I) | I | P? | Fahrig, 1974; IARC Monographs 1972–1982 |
| Chlordane | Insecticide | ∓ | ∓ | – | | I | L | SP | Gentile *et al.*, 1982; IARC Monographs 1972–1982; IARC Monographs Suppl. 4, 1982 |

Table 2. (Continued)

| Pesticide | Use | Short term effect[b] | | | | | Animal carcinogenicity (IARC evaluation) | Comment[c] | References |
|---|---|---|---|---|---|---|---|---|---|
| | | D | M | C | T | IARC evaluation | | | |
| Heptachlor | Insecticide | $\mp$ | – | $\pm$ | | I | L | SP | Gentile *et al.*, 1982; IARC Monographs 1972–1982; IARC Monographs Suppl. 4, 1982 |
| Endosulfan | Insecticide | – | – | | | (I) | (I) | ND | Chu *et al.*, 1981; Fahrig, 1974 |
| Mirex | Insecticide | | | – | | (I) | S | P? | IARC Monographs 1972–1982 |
| Chlordecone (Kepone) | Insecticide | | | – | | (I) | S | P? | IARC Monographs 1972–1982 |
| Toxaphene (Camphechlor) | Insecticide | | + | $\pm$ | | (L) | S | ND | IARC Monographs 1972–1982 |
| Strobane | Insecticide | | | | | | I | ND | IARC Monographs 1972–1982 |
| *Miscellaneous organohalogen pesticides* | | | | | | | | | |
| Biphenyls (PCBs) | Insecticide | $\mp$ | $\mp$ | – | | I | S | P | IARC Monographs 1972–1982; IARC Monographs Suppl. 4, 1982; Kawachi *et al.*, 1980 |
| Hexachlorophene | Fungicide | | – | – | | (I) | I | ND | IARC Monographs 1971–1982 |
| Nitrofen | Herbicide | | + | | | | (S) | ND | Chu *et al.*, 1981; Moriya *et al.*, 1983 |
| Chloramben | Herbicide | | | | | | (L) | ND | Chu *et al.*, 1981 |
| Captan | Fungicide | + | $\pm$ | $\mp$ | | (L) | (L) | GC | Carere & Morpurgo, 1981; Chu *et al.*, 1981; Fahrig, Kawachi *et al.*, 1980; Moriya *et al.*, 1983 |
| Folpet | Fungicide | + | $\pm$ | – | | (L) | (I) | | Fahrig, 1974; Kada *et al.*, 1980; Moriya *et al.*, 1983 |
| TCDD | Impurity | | $\mp$ | $\mp$ | | I | S | P | IARC Monographs 1972–1982; IARC Monographs Suppl. 4, 1982 |
| 2,4,5-T | Herbicide | – | $\mp$ | – | | I | I | P? | IARC Monographs 1972–1982; IARC Monographs Suppl. 4, 1982 |
| 2,4-D | Herbicide | $\mp$ | $\mp$ | $\mp$ | | I | I | P? | IARC Monographs 1972–1982; IARC Monographs Suppl. 4, 1982 |
| Bis(2-chloroethyl)ether | Insecticide | | | | | | L | ND | IARC Monographs 1972–1982 |

[a] For the definition of 'genotoxicity' used in this report, see 'Materials and Methods'.
[b] D, DNA damage, repair and recombination; M, gene mutation; C, chromosomal mutation; T, mammalian cell transformation; +, positive; –, negative; $\pm$, equivocally positive; $\mp$, equivocally negative; S, sufficient evidence; L, limited evidence; I, inadequate data; indications in parentheses represent our opinion, based on IARC criteria
[c] GC, genotoxic carcinogen; SGC, suspected genotoxic carcinogen; P, promoter; SP, suspected promoter; ND, insufficient data

The biological activities of chloroform and tetrachloroethylene are similar to those of carbon tetrachloride; however, data from two-stage experiments are not available.

Other partially halogenated hydrocarbons, as well as the unsaturated aliphatic hydrocarbons, are either proven or suspected genotoxic carcinogens.

*Hexachlorocyclohexanes:* Of the eight known isomers, the γ-isomer (lindane) has the greater insecticidal activity. The isomers cause neither DNA damage nor gene mutation, and their ability to induce chromosome mutation is questionable. All isomers were found to induce liver tumours in mice, and the α-isomer proved to be an effective promoter in rat liver initiation by *N*-nitrosodiethylamine.

*Chlorinated benzenes:* Hexachlorobenzene is inactive in short-term tests but induces liver tumours in rats and mice. It was found to be hepatoxic and to induce various hepatic mixed-function oxidases.

The pentachloronitrobenzene (quintozene) is hepatocarcinogenic in mice; but in all short-term tests carried out up to now, it was found to be negative. An initiating effect was described in mouse skin, but because of the lack of an appropriate control group, the experiment could not be evaluated.

The results of experiments with chlorophenols could not be interpreted, because the samples were contaminated with polychlorinated dibenzo-*para*-dioxins and dibenzofurans.

*Halogenated toluenes:* Except for the unstable benzoyl chloride, the chlorinated toluene pesticides are genotoxic carcinogens which induce primarily local tumours. Benzoyl chloride was also found to cause a slight increase in local tumours in two mouse experiments.

Trifluralin, which is inactive in short-term tests, was shown to induce liver tumours in female mice. An increase in lung and forestomach tumours was also described (Chu *et al.*, 1981).

*DDT group:* DDT is hepatocarcinogenic in mice; experiments in rats gave mostly negative results, but some hepatocarcinogenicity has been described. DDT is not genotoxic. It proved to be an effective promoter in rat liver after initiation with *N*-nitrosodiethylamine (Peraino *et al.*, 1975).

Two of its metabolites (TDE and DDE), chlorobenzilate and difocol, cause liver tumours in mice and are therefore considered suspected promoters.

Carcinogenicity studies of methoxychlor and perthane gave essentially negative results. Short-term tests of methoxychlor proved to be negative.

*Chlorinated terpenes and related insecticides:* Compounds in this group are characterized by hepatotoxicity, enzyme-inducing activity and hepatocarcinogenicity in mice. Carcinogenicity studies in rats gave mostly negative results. Some of these compounds were shown to induce liver and thyroid gland tumours.

Except for toxaphene, all of these proved to be inactive in short-term tests. However, most of them are suspected of having a promoting action.

Aldrin is metabolized to dieldrin *in vivo*. Dieldrin is a stereoisomer of endrin. Technically pure chlordane always contains heptachlor impurities and *vice versa*. Chlordecone is a degradation product of Mirex.

*Miscellaneous organohalogen pesticides:* The polychlorinated biphenyl group consists of a mixture of biphenyls chlorinated to different extents. The characteristics of this group are as follows: hepatotoxicity, enzyme-inducing activity, as well as induction of benign and malignant liver tumours in rats and mice. No activity in short-term tests was demonstrated. Of these compounds, Kanechlor-400 (Kimura *et al.,* 1976), Kanechlor-500 (Nishizumi, 1976) and Arochlor 1254 (Preston *et al.,* 1981) were found to have promoting effects in rat liver.

2,3,7,8-Tetrachlorodibenzo-*para*-dioxin (TCDD) may be present as a contaminant in 2,4,5-trichlorophenoxy acetic acid, chlorophenol and hexachlorophene pesticides. This compound is a potent enzyme inducer. It is hepatotoxic and, in addition to liver tumours in mice and rats, it causes epithelial tumours of the lung and other organs in rats. Equivocally negative results were obtained in short-term tests. In mouse skin experiments, no promoting effect was found (after initiation with 7,12-dimethylbenz[*a*]anthracene), but a weak initiating activity (after promotion with 12-*O*-tetradecansylphorbol-13-acetate) could be demonstrated. In a rat liver experiment (partial hepatectomy followed by initiation with *N*-nitrosodiethylamine 24 h later), TCDD proved to be a strong promoter (Pitot *et al.,* 1980).

TCDD was found to bind to cellular macromolecules, including DNA, in rat liver, but this binding was lower by several orders of magnitude than the binding observed with most carcinogens (Poland & Glover, 1979).

Chlorophenoxyacetic acids (2,4-D, 2,4,5-T) proved to be negative or equivocally negative when evaluated in short-term tests. Their carcinogenicity has not been proven. They are hepatotoxic in rats, and they cause proliferation of peroxisomes in hamster liver.

Captan and Folpet were found to have DNA-damaging and mutagenic effects in prokaryotic and eukaryotic microorganisms. However, no such effect was demonstrated in *Drosophila melanogaster* or rodents. Captan was shown to induce tumours of the duodenum in mice.

*Organophosphate pesticides* (Table 3)

The nature of the biological activities of organophosphate insecticides is controversial. Although positive results have been obtained in short-term tests, long-term carcinogenicity studies gave mostly negative results. This fact could be explained by the strong toxicity and rapid breakdown of these pesticides.

Dichlorvos, a typical representative of this group, alkylates cellular macromolecules, including DNA, *in vivo.* Its DNA-damaging and mutagenic action could be detected in microorganisms much more readily than in higher organisms, presumably because of its strong reactivity (IARC, 1972–1982; Kawachi *et al.,* 1980; Carere & Morpurgo, 1981). In one experiment, dichlorvos was found to induce focal hyperplasia, as well as benign and malignant epithelial tumours of the oesophagus in some mice (National Cancer Institute, 1977).

A definite opinion cannot as yet be made as to the carcinogenicity of the organophosphate esters. Two-stage type experiments would be desirable to study the possible initiating effect of these compounds.

*Carbamate pesticides* (Table 4)

Dimethylcarbamoylchloride, a direct-acting acylating agent, is a genotoxic carcinogen. The dialkyl-dithiocarbamate pesticides, Ziram, Ferbam, ethyl selenac,

Table 3. Genotoxicity[a] and carcinogenicity of organophosphate insecticides

| Pesticide | Use | Short term effect[b] | | | | | Animal carcinogenicity (IARC evaluation) | Comment[c] | References |
|---|---|---|---|---|---|---|---|---|---|
| | | D | M | C | T | IARC evaluation | | | |
| Dichlorvos | Insecticide | + | ± | ∓ | | (I) | I | IC? | Carere & Morpurgo, 1981; IARC Monographs 1972–1982; IARC Monographs Suppl. 4, 1982 |
| Tetrachlorvinphos | Insecticide | ± | − | | | (I) | (L) | SGC | Carere & Morpurgo, 1981; Chu *et al.*, 1981; Moriya *et al.*, 1983 |
| Phosphamidon | Insecticide | | | | | | (I) | ND | Chu *et al.*, 1981 |
| Parathion-methyl | Insecticide | ± | ± | | | (L) | (I) | IC? | Carere & Morpurgo, 1981; Chu *et al.*, 1981; Fahrig, 1974; Sobti *et al.*, 1982 |
| Parathion | Insecticide | ± | − | | | (I) | (I) | ND | Chu *et al.*, 1981; Fahrig, 1974; Sobti *et al.*, 1982 |
| Dimethoate | Insecticide | + | + | ± | | (S) | (I) | IC? | Chu *et al.*, 1981; Fahrig, 1974; Kawachi *et al.*, 1980; Moriya *et al.*, 1983; Sobti *et al.*, 1982 |
| Trichlorphon | Insecticide | + | + | + | | (S) | | IC? | Carere & Morpurgo, 1981; Kawachi *et al.*, 1980; Moriya *et al.*, 1983 |

[a] For the definition of 'genotoxicity' used in this report, see 'Materials and Methods'.
[b] D, DNA damage, repair and recombination; M, gene mutation; C, chromosomal mutation; T, mammalian cell transformation; +, positive; −, negative; ±, equivocally positive; ∓, equivocally negative; S, sufficient evidence; L, limited evidence; I, inadequate data; indications in parentheses represent our opinion, based on IARC criteria
[c] GC, genotoxic carcinogen; SGC, suspected genotoxic carcinogen; P, promoter; SP, suspected promoter; ND, insufficient data

Table 4. Genotoxicity[a] and carcinogenicity of carbamate pesticides

| Pesticide | Use | Short term effect[b] | | | | | Animal carcinogenicity (IARC evaluation) | Comment[c] | References |
|---|---|---|---|---|---|---|---|---|---|
| | | D | M | C | T | IARC evaluation | | | |
| Dimethylcarbamoyl chloride | Intermediate | ± | ± | ± | + | S | S | GC | IARC Monographs 1972–1982; IARC Monographs Suppl. 4, 1982 |
| Ziram | Fungicide | ± | ± | + | | (L) | I | IC? | Fahrig, 1974; IARC Monographs 1972–1982; Kada *et al.*, 1980; Moriya *et al.*, 1983 |
| Ferbam | Fungicide | + | + | | | (L) | I | IC? | IARC Monographs 1972–1982; Kada *et al.*, 1980 |
| Ethyl selenac | Fungicide | | | | | | I | IC? | IARC Monographs 1972–1982 |
| Bis(2-hydroxyethyl)-dithiocarbamic acid K salt | Fungicide | | | | | | S | SGC | IARC Monographs 1972–1982 |
| Zineb | Fungicide | | − | + | | (I) | I | | IARC Monographs 1972–1982; Moriya *et al.*, 1983 |
| Maneb | Fungicide | + | − | ± | | (I) | I | | IARC Monographs 1972–1982; Kawachi *et al.*, 1980 |
| Ethylenethiourea | Metabolite and degradation product | ∓ | ∓ | − | + | L | S | | IARC Monographs 1972–1982; IARC Monographs Suppl. 4, 1982; Kada *et al.*, 1980; Moriya *et al.*, 1983 |
| Chlorpropham | Herbicide | | ∓ | | | (I) | I | ND | IARC Monographs 1972–1982; Moriya *et al.*, 1983 |
| Propham | Herbicide | | − | | | (I) | IC | GC(IC) | IARC Monographs 1972–1982 |
| Di-allate | Herbicide | ± | ± | | | (L) | L | GC | Carere & Morpurgo, 1981; IARC Monographs 1972–1982 |
| Pebulate | Herbicide | | | | | (L) | L | ND | |
| Thiram | Fungicide | + | + | ± | | (S) | I | IC? | IARC Monographs 1972–1982; Kawachi *et al.*, 1980; Moriya *et al.*, 1983 |
| Sulfallate | Herbicide | + | + | | | (S) | (S) | GC | Carere & Morpurgo, 1981; Chu *et al.*, 1981 |
| Zectran | Insecticide | | + | | | (I) | I | ND | IARC Monographs 1972–1982 |
| Carbaryl | Insecticide | − | ∓ | | | (I) | I | ND | Fahrig, 1974; IARC Monographs 1972–1982; Moriya *et al.*, 1983 |

[a] For the definition of 'genotoxicity' used in this report, see 'Materials and Methods'.
[b] D, DNA damage, repair and recombination; M, gene mutation; C, chromosomal mutation; T, mammalian cell transformation; +, positive; −, negative; ±, equivocally positive; ∓, equivocally negative; S, sufficient evidence; L, limited evidence; I, inadequate data; indications in parentheses represent our opinion, based on IARC criteria
[c] GC, genotoxic carcinogen; SGC, suspected genotoxic carcinogen; P, promoter; SP, suspected promoter; ND, insufficient data

Table 5. Genotoxicity[a] and carcinogenicity of other pesticides

| Pesticide | Use | Short term effect[b] | | | | | Animal carcinogenicity (IARC evaluation) | Comment[c] | References |
|---|---|---|---|---|---|---|---|---|---|
| | | D | M | C | T | IARC evaluation | | | |
| Inorganic arsenic compounds | Insecticide | + | ∓ | ± | + | L | I(HC) | GC | IARC Monographs 1972–1982; IARC Monographs Suppl. 4, 1982 |
| Formaldehyde | Fungicide | + | ± | ∓ | ± | S | S | GC | IARC Monographs 1972–1982; IARC Monographs Suppl. 4, 1982 |
| Ethylene oxide | Insecticide | + | + | + | | S | L | GC | IARC Monographs 1972–1982; IARC Monographs Suppl. 4, 1982 |
| β– Propiolactone | Disinfectant | + | + | ± | | (S) | S | GC | IARC Monographs 1972–1982; Kawachi *et al.*, 1980 |
| *N*-(2-Hydroxyethyl)-hydrazine | Herbicide | + | + | | | (L) | L | GC | Innes *et al.*, 1969; Kada *et al.*, 1980; Moriya *et al.*, 1983 |
| Aminotriazole | Herbicide | ± | ∓ | ∓ | + | I | S | | Carere & Morpurgo, 1981; IARC Monographs 1972–1982; IARC Monographs Suppl. 4, 1982; Moriya *et al.*, 1983 |
| Monuron | Herbicide | | − | | | | (I) | ND | IARC Monographs 1972–1982; Kada *et al.*, 1980 |
| Di(2-ethylhexyl)phthalate | In formulations | ∓ | − | ∓ | | (I) | S | SP | IARC Monographs 1972–1982; Kawachi *et al.*, 1980 |
| Aramite | Insecticide | | | | | | S | ND | IARC Monographs 1972–1982 |

[a] For the definition of 'genotoxicity' used in this report, see 'Materials and Methods'.
[b] D, DNA damage, repair and recombination; M, gene mutation; C, chromosomal mutation; T, mammalian cell transformation; +, positive; −, negative; ±, equivocally positive; ∓, equivocally negative; S, sufficient evidence; L, limited evidence; I, inadequate data; indications in parentheses represent our opinion, based on IARC criteria
[c] GC, genotoxic carcinogen; SGC, suspected genotoxic carcinogen; P, promoter; SP, suspected promoter; ND, insufficient data

Thiram, bis(2-hydroxyethyl)dithiocarbamic acid, were tested. Only bis(2-hydroxyethyl)dithiocarbamic acid proved to be carcinogenic. Ziram, Ferbam and Thiram gave positive results in short-term tests. Therefore it would be worthwhile to investigate these compounds in two-stage experiments for possible initiating effects.

Ethylenethiourea induces tumours of the thyroid gland and liver, and its tumorigenic activity is thought to be connected with mechanisms perhaps related to hormonal imbalance (see also Amitrol, below). One should bear in mind that ethylenethiourea (ETU) is the major breakdown product and metabolite of Zineb and Maneb.

Propham and Chlorpropham, when tested in two-stage experiments, proved to be potent initiators (after croton oil promotion), but the results obtained with Chlorpropham could not be reproduced.

*Other pesticides* (Table 5)

On the basis of short-term experiments and long-term studies, formaldehyde, ethylene oxide, β-propiolactone and *N*-(2-hydroxyethyl)hydrazine can be considered genotoxic carcinogens.

In-vivo studies of the inorganic arsenic compounds, generally considered as human carcinogens, gave mostly negative results. In recent years, however, positive data have been published. Ivankovic *et al.* (1979) reported the induction of lung tumours in rats after a single intratracheal instillation of a calcium arsenate-containing pesticide. We found that arsenic trioxide, when administered pre- and postnatally, induced lung adenomas in mice (Rudnai & Börzsönyi, 1980).

Aminotriazole (Amitrol) has biological activities similar to those of ETU. It gave equivocal results in short-term tests and induced tumours of the thyroid gland and the liver. Its tumour-inducing ability may perhaps be explained by its antithyroid effect and hormonal imbalance.

Di(2-ethylhexyl)phthalate proved to be negative in short-term tests. However, *in vivo,* it causes proliferation of peroxisomes in rat liver. It also induced liver tumours in rat and mice.

Hepatic peroxisome proliferators cause hepatomegaly and increase DNA synthesis and cell proliferation without previous cell necrosis (Reddy *et al.,* 1980). Some of these compounds were found to be efficient promoters after initiation by *N*-nitrosodiethylamine (Reddy & Rao, 1978).

Six groups of pesticides could be differentiated on the basis of their proven or suspected mode of action (see Tables 6 & 7). Sufficient data could not be obtained for 24 out of 83 compounds. Twenty-nine pesticides proved to be definite or suspected genotoxic carcinogens. Their chemical structures are heterogeneous: carbamates, organophosphates and haloalkanes, haloalkenes, halogenated toluenes.

Twenty-six pesticides with carcinogenic activity were inactive in short-term tests. Most of these compounds are insecticides and they are almost exclusively halogenated hydrocarbons, haloalkanes, polychlorinated biphenyls, benzenes, cyclohexanes, dibenzodioxins, terpenes and related pesticides and members of the DDT group.

Hormonal imbalance is thought to be the mechanism of tumour formation in the case of aminotriazole and ETU (antithyroidal-agents).

Table 6. Grouping of pesticides on the basis of their proven or suspected mode of action: carcinogens inactive in short-term tests[a]

| Promoters | Suspected promoters | Promoters? |
|---|---|---|
| Haloalkanes and haloalkenes | | |
| Carbon tetrachloride (S) | Chloroform (S) | |
| | Tetrachloroethylene (L) | |
| Hexachlorocyclohexanes (HCH) | | |
| α-HCH (S) | β-HCH (L) | |
| | Lindane (S) | |
| | BHC (S) | |
| Chlorinated benzenes | | |
| | Hexachlorobenzene (S) | |
| Halogenated toluenes | | |
| | Trifluralin (L) | |
| DDT group | | |
| DDT (S) | TDE (L) | |
| | DDE (L) | |
| | Chlorobenzilate (S) | |
| | Dicofol (L) | |
| Polychlorinated terpenes and related compounds | | |
| | Aldrin (L) | Endrin (I) |
| | Dieldrin (L) | Mirex (S) |
| | Chlordane (L) | Chlordecone (S) |
| | Heptachlor (L) | |
| Miscellaneous organohalogens | | |
| PCBs (S) | | 2,4,5-T (I) |
| TCDD (S) | | 2,4-D (I) |
| Other compounds | | |
| | Di(2-ethylhexyl)phthalate (S) | |

[a] Symbols in parentheses: evaluation of animal carcinogenicity based on criteria of IARC; see Table 2 for abbreviations

## N-*Nitroso derivatives of pesticides*

Nitrogen-containing pesticides could, theoretically, be nitrosated during their manufacture, in the environment and *in vivo* in man and animals. This process may be hazardous to man, because the non-carcinogenic or weakly carcinogenic pesticides could be converted to strongly genotoxic carcinogens. It is known that about 80% of *N*-nitroso compounds are mutagens and carcinogens (Montesano & Bartsch, 1976; Börzsönyi *et al.*, 1981a). For instance, mutagenicity studies of ETU in micro-organisms showed equivocal results, and tests in higher organisms and mammalian cells were negative, except for cell transformations. However, both simultaneous treatment with ETU and sodium nitrite (nitrosating agent) and application of *N*-ethyl-*N*-nitrosourea (ENU) resulted in point and chromosomal mutations.

Both ETU and ENU are carcinogenic in mice, but ENU induces benign and malignant lung tumours and lymphomas at doses several orders of magnitude lower than those required with ETU (Innes *et al.*, 1969; Moriya *et al.*, 1979).

Table 7. Grouping of pesticides on the basis of their proven or suspected mode of action: genotoxic[a] carcinogens[b]

| Genotoxic carcinogens | Suspected genotoxic carcinogens | Pure initiators? |
|---|---|---|
| Haloalkanes and haloalkenes | | |
| Vinyl chloride (S) | Ethylene dichloride (S) | |
| Tetrachloroethane (L) | | |
| Ethylene dibromide (S) | | |
| Dibromochloropropane (S) | | |
| Halogenated toluenes | | |
| Benzyl chloride (L) | | |
| Benzal chloride (L) | | |
| Benzotrichloride (S) | | |
| Miscellaneous organohalogens | | |
| Captan (L) | | Folpet (I) |
| Organophosphates | | |
| | Tetrachlorvinphos (L) | Dichlorvos (I) |
| | | Parathion-methyl (I) |
| | | Dimethoate (I) |
| | | Trichlorphon |
| Carbamates | | |
| Dimethylcarbamoyl chloride (S) | Bis(2-hydroxyethyl)dithiocarbamic acid K salt (S) | Ziram (I) |
| Propham (IC) | | Ferbam (I) |
| Diallate (L) | | Ethyl selenac (I) |
| Sulfallate (S) | | Thiram (I) |
| Other compounds | | |
| Inorganic arsenic compounds (I/HC) | | |
| Formaldehyde (S) | | |
| Ethylene oxide (L) | | |
| β-Propriolactone (S) | | |
| *N*-(2-Hydroxyethyl)-hydrazine (L) | | |

[a]For the definition of 'genotoxic' used in this report, see 'Materials and Methods'.
[b]Symbols in parentheses: evaluation of animal carcinogenicity based on criteria of IARC; see Table 2 for abbreviations

Pesticides that contain nitroso impurities, either in technical or formulated products, are particularly dangerous. Nitroso products can be demonstrated in pesticides containing secondary and tertiary amines, as well as in dimethylamine salt and quaternary salt pesticides, and in *N*-alkylamides, carbamates and ureas. The chemical structures of these compounds are shown in Tables 8–11.

The dialkylnitrosamine-yielding pesticides are shown in Table 8. These nitroso compounds are among the most potent animal carcinogens known. Some pesticides contain preformed nitroso impurities, the highest concentration being found in dinitro-aniline-type herbicides, which contain a tertiary amino group.

Alkyl-aryl-nitrosamines are often found in aminotriazine and dinitroaniline herbicides, which have nitrosatable secondary amine groups (Table 9). Carcinogenicity data on these compounds are not available.

Pesticides that contain mostly tertiary amines can give rise to cyclic nitrosamines, and the yield of nitrosation is fairly high. The methylene, imine, piperazine and

Table 8. Pesticides containing dialkyl nitrosamine impurities

*Dithiocarbamates*

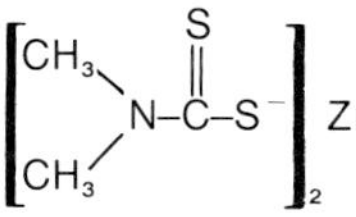

Ziram

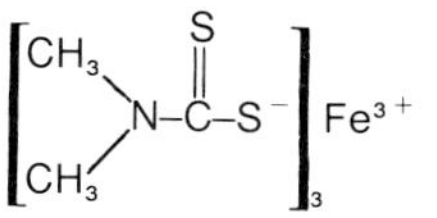

Ferbam

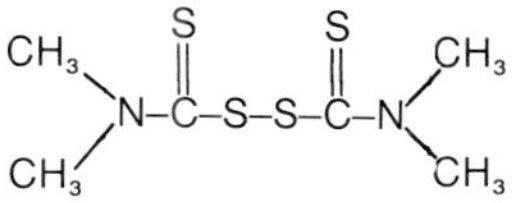

Thiram

*N*-Nitrosodimethylamine impurity in Ziram[a,b], Ferbam[b,c], Thiram[b,d] (1.2 mg/kg)

*Dimethylamine salts of chlorophenoxycarbonic acids*

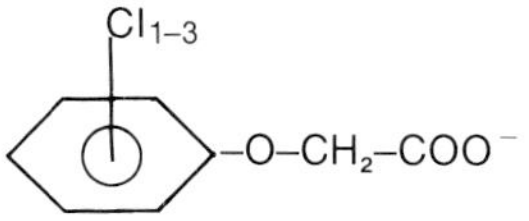

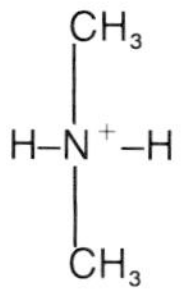

*N*-Nitrosodimethylamine impurity in 2,4-D[b], 2,4-DB[b], MCPA[b], MCPP[b](H) (0.2–14 mg/kg)

*Dinitroanilines*

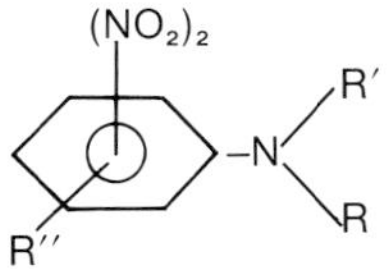

*N*-Nitrosoethylbutylamine[b], *N*-nitrosodiethylamine[b], *N*-nitrosodipropylamine[b] impurity in herbicides, 0.5–153 mg/kg

[a] Eisenbrand *et al.* (1975a)
[b] Zweig *et al.* (1980)
[c] Eisenbrand *et al.* (1974)
[d] Egert & Greim (1976b)

morpholine pesticides are important representatives of these compounds. Cyclic nitrosamines are proven carcinogens (Table 10).

All nitrosamides obtained from secondary amines, found in carbamate-, guanidine- and amide-type pesticides, are direct mutagens and strong carcinogens. This finding was substantiated by in-vitro and in-vivo experiments (Table 11).

Samples of various pesticides were shown to contain *N*-nitroso contaminants in quantities ranging from > 1 mg to > 200 mg/kg.

In earlier experiments, we found that an antioxidant, MTDQ-DA, similar to vitamin C, reduced significantly the nitrosation of morpholine (by at least

Table 9. Pesticides containing preformed alkyl nitrosamines

| | |
|---|---|
| Aminotriazines | |
| 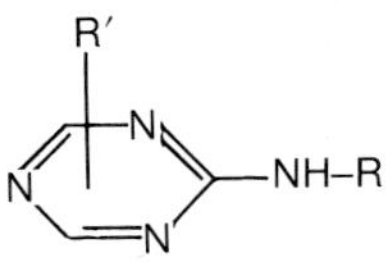 | Nitrosated herbicide (Ametryn, Atrazine, Prometrin[c], Simazin[b]) impurities, about 1 mg/kg |
| Dinitroanilines | |
| 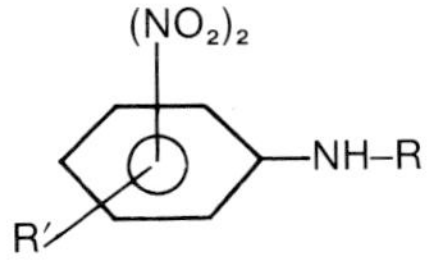 | Nitrosated herbicide impurities, 25–430 mg/kg in Butralin[a,b] and Pendimethalin[a,b] |

[a] Bontoyan *et al.* (1979)
[b] Zweig *et al.* (1980)
[c] Egert & Greim (1976a)

Table 10. Nitrosatable cyclic nitrosamines

| | |
|---|---|
| *Methyleneimines* | |
| 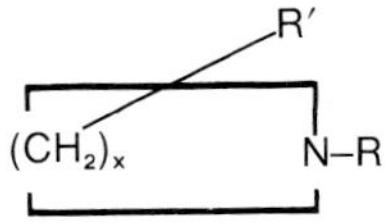 | Nitrosamine derivatives: *N*-nitrosopyrrolidine[e], *N*-nitropiperidine, *N'*-nitrosonornicotine[d] |
| *Piperazines* | |
| 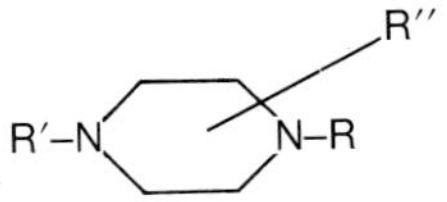 | Nitrosamine derivatives: *N*-nitrosomonopiperazine, *N*-nitrosodipiperazine |
| *Morpholines* | |
| 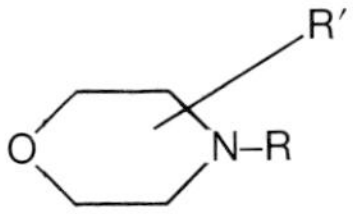 (Dodemorph, Tridemorph, Tifenmorph, Trimorphamid[a]) | Nitrosamine derivatives: *N*-nitrosomorpholine[c], 2,6-methyl-*N*-nitrosomorpholine |

[a] Börzsönyi *et al.* (1980a)
[b] Börzsönyi *et al.* (1980b)
[c] Börzsönyi *et al.* (1982)
[d] Hoffmann *et al.* (1980)
[e] Eisenbrand *et al.* (1974)

Table 11. Nitrosatable pesticides (precursors of nitrosamides)

| | |
|---|---|
| Carbamates | |
| 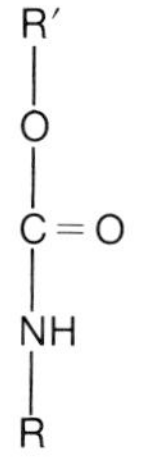 | Can be nitrosated in the presence of nitrosating agent (e.g., Aldicarb[e], Benomyl[f], Dioxacarb[e], Propoxur[d])<br><br>Nitroso derivatives are mutagenic and carcinogenic (e.g., Aldicarb[c], Bux Ten[c], Carbaryl[b,c,d], Landrin[c], Methomyl[c]) |
| Ureas | |
| 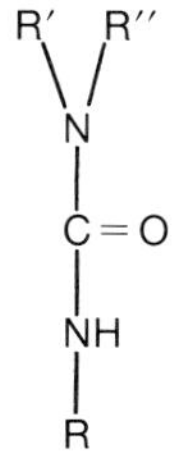 | Nitrosated derivatives are mutagenic (Tribunil[g]) and carcinogenic (Benzthiazuron[a], ethylenethiourea[e]) |
| Guanidines | |
| 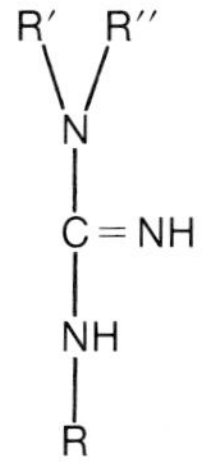 | Can be nitrosated and form mutagenic and carcinogenic compounds (Dodine[a]) |
| Amides | |
| 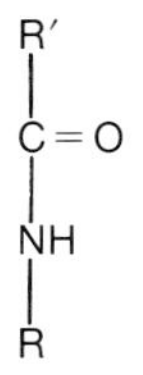 | Can be nitrosated and form mutagenic derivatives (Dimethoate[e], Mecarbam) |

[a] Egert & Greim (1976a)
[b] Eisenbrand *et al.* (1975)
[c] Lijinsky & Schmähl (1978)
[d] Uchiyama *et al.* (1975)
[e] Seiler (1977)
[f] Börzsönyi & Pintér (1977)
[g] Börzsönyi (1981)

Table 12. Inhibition of nitrosation of morpholine with an antioxidant, MTDQ-DA, in rats

| MTDQ-DA (mg/kg) | Morpholine hydrochloride (mg/kg) | Sodium nitrite (mg/kg) | Yield (%) of *N*-nitrosomorpholine in gastric content[a] | SGPT (IU)[b] | Necrosis in liver[b] |
|---|---|---|---|---|---|
| – | 1 000 | 125 | 2.72 | 618.6 | + |
| 500 | 1 000 | 125 | 0.1 | 20.6 | – |
| 500 | – | – | ND | 17.6 | – |
| – | 1 000 | – | ND | 15.7 | – |
| – | – | 125 | ND | 13.3 | – |

Influence of MTDQ-DA on induction of ATPase-deficient foci induced by *N*-nitrosomorpholine formed *in vivo*

| Initiation | | | Promotion[c] | Enzyme altered foci/cm² in liver[d] |
|---|---|---|---|---|
| MTDQ-DA (mg/kg) | Morpholine hydrochloride (mg/kg) | Sodium nitrite (mg/kg) | Phenobarbital in diet (%) | |
| – | 1 000 | 125 | 0.05 | 16.28 |
| 500 | 1 000 | 125 | 0.05 | 12.32 |
| 500 | – | 125 | 0.05 | 1.24 |

[a] Two-hour incubation
[b] Serum glutamate-pyruvate transaminase; animals sacrified 48 h after i.g. treatment
[c] Feeding started 2 months after initiation and lasted for 6 months
[d] Animals killed at end of 8th month

one-twentieth) (Börzsönyi *et al.*, 1981b). The *N*-nitrosomorpholine formed in this experiment was not hepatotoxic in rats. When phenobarbital promotion was added to the treatment protocol, MTDQ-DA did not decrease significantly the number of enzyme-deficient foci (Table 12). This result supports earlier observations that there is no threshold for initiators. It also indicates that trace amounts of *N*-nitroso contamination, present in pesticides, might be potential initiators.

The purpose of this survey is to point out factors that may be potential hazards to humans. Of course, this does not mean that pesticides should be banned. But we should encourage further experimental and epidemiological studies, because 'the civilisation without agricultural chemicals would soon revert to a condition where malnutrition and infectious diseases would replace cancer as leading causes of death' (Burchfield & Storrs, 1977).

## REFERENCES

Bontoyan, W.R., Law, M.W. & Wright, D.P., Jr (1979) Nitrosamines in agricultural and home-use pesticides. *J. Agric. Food Chem.*, **27**, 631–635

Börzsönyi, M. (1981) *Formation of Carcinogenic* N-*Nitroso Compounds from Precursors*, Postdoctoral Thesis, Budapest (in Hungarian)

Börzsönyi, M. & Pintér, A. (1977) The carcinogenicity of *N*-nitroso compounds formed endogenously in mice from benzimidazole carbamate pesticides. *Neoplasma*, ***24***, 119–122

Börzsönyi, M. Surján, A., Pintér, A., Török, G., Csík, M., Tamás, J., Fetter, J. & Ferenc, A. (1980a) *Endogenous formation of* N-*nitrosomorpholine from a new fungicide*. In: Walker, E.A., Castegnaro, M., Griciute, L. & Börzsönyi, M., eds, N-*Nitroso Compounds: Analysis, Formation and Occurrence (IARC Scientific Publications No. 31)*, Lyon, International Agency for Research on Cancer, pp. 677–683

Börzsönyi, M., Török, G., Pintér, A., Surján, A., Nádasdi, L. & Roller, P.P. (1980b) Carcinogenic effect of dinitrosopiperazine in adult Swiss mice and after transplacental or translactational exposure. *Cancer Res.*, ***40***, 2925–2927

Börzsönyi, M., Török, G., Pintér, A., Surján, A. & Csík, M. (1981a) *Mutagenicity and carcinogenicity of environmental* N-*nitroso compounds (NNOS)*. In: *11th Annual Meeting on Environmental Mugagenesis, 6–11 July, Budapest, Hungary*

Börzsönyi, M., Török, G., Surján, A., Challis, B.C. & Bär, V. (1981b) Protective effect of a new antioxidant on acute hepatotoxicity caused by morpholine plus nitrite in rats. *Toxicol. Lett.*, ***7***, 285–288

Börzsönyi, M., Török, G., Pintér, A., Surján, A., Csík, M. & Bär, V. (1982) *Inhibition by an antioxidant of the carcinogenic effect of nitrosomorpholine formed* in vivo. In: Bartsch, H., O'Neill, I.K., Castegnaro, M. & Okada, M., eds, N-*Nitroso Compounds: Occurrence and Biological Effects (IARC Scientific Publications No. 41)*, Lyon, International Agency for Research on Cancer, pp. 659–664

Burchfield, H.P. & Storrs, E.E. (1977) *Organohalogen carcinogens*. In: Kraybill, H.F. & Mehlman, M.A., eds, *Environmental Cancer Advances in Modern Toxicology*, Vol. 3, Washington DC, Hemisphere Publishing Corp., pp. 319–372

Carere, A. & Morpurgo, G. (1981) Comparison of the mutagenic activity of pesticides *in vitro* in various short term assays. *Prog. Mutat. Res.*, ***2***, 87–104

Chu, K.C., Cueto, C. & Ward, J.M. (1981) Factors in the evaluation of 200 National Cancer Institute carcinogen bioassays. *J. Toxicol. environ. Health*, ***8***, 251–280

Egert, G. & Greim, H. (1976a) Formation of mutagenic *N*-nitroso compounds from the pesticides Prometryne, Dodine and Carbaryl in the presence of nitrite at pH 1. *Mutat. Res.*, ***37***, 179–186

Egert, G. & Greim, H. (1976b) Formation of dimethylnitrosamine from pesticides carrying methylated tertiary aminogroups in the presence of nitrite at pH 3. *Food Cosmet. Toxicol.*, ***14***, 193–195

Eisenbrand, G., Ungerer, O. & Preussmann, R. (1974) Rapid formation of carcinogenic *N*-nitrosamines by interaction of nitrite with fungicides derived from dithiocarbamic acid *in vitro* under simulated gastric condition and *in vivo* in the rat stomach. *Food Cosmet. Toxicol.*, ***12***, 229–232

Eisenbrand, G., Ungerer, O. & Preussmann, R. (1975a) *Formation of* N-*nitroso compounds from agricultural chemicals and nitrite*. In: Bogovski, P. & Walker, E.A., eds, N-*Nitroso Compounds in the Environment (IARC Scientific Publications No. 9)*, Lyon, International Agency for Research on Cancer, pp. 71–74

Eisenbrand, G., Ungerer, O. & Preussmann, R. (1975b) The reaction of nitrite with pesticides. II. Formation, chemical properties, and carcinogenic activity of the *N*-nitroso derivative of *N*-methyl-1-naphthyl carbamate (Carbaryl). *Food Cosmet. Toxicol.,* ***13,*** 365–367

Environmental Protection Agency (1978) Pesticide programs, proposed guidelines for registering pesticides in the US hazard evaluation: Humans and domestic animals. *Fed. Regist.,* ***43,*** 37388–37394

Fahrig, R. (1974) *Comparative mutagenicity studies with pesticides.* In: Montesano, R. & Tomatis, L., eds, *Chemical Carcinogenesis Essays (IARC Scientific Publications No. 10),* Lyon, International Agency for Research on Cancer, pp. 161–181

Gentile, J.M., Gentile, G.J., Bultman, J., Sechriest, R., Wagner, E.D. & Plewa, M.J. (1982) An evaluation of the genotoxic properties of insecticides following plant and animal activation. *Mutat. Res.,* ***101,*** 19–29

Hoffmann, D., Adams, J.D., Piade, J.J. & Hecht, S.S. (1980) *Chemical studies on tobacco smoke. LXVIII. Analysis of volatile and tobacco-specific nitrosamines in tobacco products.* In: Walker, E.A., Castegnaro, M., Griciute, L. & Börzsönyi, M., eds, N-*Nitroso Compounds: Analysis, Formation and Occurrence (IARC Scientific Publications No. 31),* Lyon, International Agency for Research on Cancer, pp. 507–516

IARC (1972–1982) *IARC Monographs on the Evaluation of the Carcinogenic Risk of Chemicals to Humans,* Vols 1–29, Lyon, International Agency for Research on Cancer

IARC (1982) *IARC Monographs on the Evaluation of the Carcinogenic Risk of Chemicals to Humans,* Supplement 4, *Chemicals, Industrial Processes and Industries Associated with Cancer in Humans (IARC Monographs, Volume 1 to 29),* Lyon, International Agency for Research on Cancer

Innes, J.R.M., Ulland, B.M., Marion, G., Valerio, L., Petrucelli, L., Fischbein, L., Hart, E.R., Pallotta, A.J., Batles, R.R., Falk, H.I., Gart, J.J., Klein, M., Mitchell, I. & Peters, J. (1969) Bioassay of pesticides and industrial chemicals for tumorigenicity in mice: a preliminary note. *J. natl Cancer Inst.,* ***42,*** 1101–1114

Ivankovic, S., Eisenbrand, G. & Preussmann, R. (1979) Lung carcinoma induction in BD rats after a single intratracheal instillation of an arsenic-containing pesticide mixture formerly used in vineyards. *Int. J. Cancer,* ***24,*** 786–788

Kada, T., Hirano, K. & Shirasu, Y. (1980) *Screening of environmental mutagens by the rec-assay system with* Bacillus subtilis. In: de Serres, F.J. & Hollaender, A., eds, *Chemical Mutagens,* Vol. 6, New York, Plenum Press, pp. 149–173

Kawachi, T., Yahagi, T., Kada, T., Tazima, Y., Ishidate, M., Sasaki, M. & Sugiyama, T. (1980) *Cooperative programme on short-term assays for carcinogenicity in Japan.* In: Montesano, R., Bartsch, H. & Tomatis, L., eds, *Molecular and Cellular Aspects of Carcinogen Screening Tests (IARC Scientific Publications No. 27),* Lyon, International Agency for Research on Cancer, pp. 323–330

Kimura, N.T., Kanematsu, T. & Baba, T. (1976) Polychlorinated biphenyls as a promotor in experimental hepatocarcinogenesis in rats. *Z. Krebsforsch.,* ***87,*** 257–266

Lijinsky, W. & Schmähl, D. (1978) Carcinogenicity of *N*-nitroso derivatives of *N*-methylcarbamate insecticides in rats. *Ecotoxicol. environ. Saf.*, ***2***, 413–419

McEven, F.L. & Stephenson, G.R. (1979) *The Use and Significance of Pesticides in the Environment,* New York, John Wiley & Sons, pp. 453–465

Montesano, R. & Bartsch, H. (1976) Mutagenic and carcinogenic *N*-nitroso compounds. Possible environmental hazards. *Mutat. Res.*, ***32***, 179–228

Moriyama, M., Mitsumor, K., Kato, K., Miyazwa, T. & Shirasu, Y. (1979) Carcinogenicity of *N*-nitroso ethylenethiourea in female mice. *Cancer Lett.*, ***7***, 339–342

Moriya, M., Ohta, T., Watanabe, K., Miyazawa, T., Kato, K. & Shirasu, Y. (1983) Further mutagenicity studies on pesticides in bacterial reversion assay systems. *Mutat. Res.*, ***116***, 185–216

Moses, M. & Maxey-Rosenau, J. (1980) *Pesticides.* In: Last, J.M., ed., *Public Health and Preventive Medicine,* New York, Appleton-Century-Crofts, pp. 731–749

National Cancer Institute (1977) *Bioassay of Dichlorvos for Possible Carcinogenicity (Carcinogenesis Technical Report Series, No. 10; DHEW Publication No. (NIH) 77–810),* Washington DC, US Government Printing Office

Nishizumi, M. (1976) Enhancement of diethylnitrosamine hepatocarcinogenesis in rats by exposure to polychlorinated biphenyls or phenobarbital. *Cancer Lett.*, ***2***, 11–16

Peraino, C., Fry, R.J.-M., Staffeldt, E. & Christopher, J.P. (1975) Comparative enhancing effects of phenobarbital, amobarbital, diphenylhydantoin and dichlorodiphenyltrichloroethane on 2-acetylaminofluorene-induced hepatic tumorigenesis in rat. *Cancer Res.*, ***35***, 2884–2890

Pitot, H.C., Goldsworthy, T., Campbell, H.A. & Poland, A. (1980) Quantitative evaluation of the promotion by 2,3,7,8-tetrachlorodibenzo-*p*-dioxin of hepatocarcinogenesis from diethylnitrosamine. *Cancer Res.*, ***40***, 3616–3620

Poland, A. & Glover, E. (1979) An estimate of the maximum *in vivo* covalent binding of 2,3,7,8-tetrachlorodibenzo-*p*-dioxin to rat liver protein, ribosomal RNS, and DNA. *Cancer Res.*, ***39***, 3341–3344

Pound, A.W. & McGuire, L.J. (1978) Influence of repeated liver regeneration on hepatic carcinogenesis by diethylnitrosamine in mice. *Br. J. Cancer*, ***37***, 595–602

Preston, B.D., van Miller, J.P., Moore, R.W. & Allen, J.R. (1981) Promoting effects of polychlorinated biphenyls (Aroclor 1254) and polychlorinated dibenzofuran-free Aroclor 1254 on diethylnitrosamine-induced tumorigenesis in the rat. *J. natl Cancer Inst.*, ***66***, 509–515

Reddy, J.K. & Rao, M.S. (1978) Enhancement by WY-14,643, a hepatic peroxisome proliferator, of diethylnitrosamine-initiated hepatic tumorigenesis in the rat. *Br. J. Cancer*, ***38***, 537–543

Reddy, J.K., Azarnoff, D.L. & Hignite, C.E. (1980) Hypolipodaemic hepatic peroxisome proliferators from a novel class of chemical carcinogens. *Nature*, ***283***, 397–398

Rudnai, P. & Börzsönyi, M. (1980) Carcinogenic effect of arsenic trioxide in transplacentally and neonatally treated CFLP mice. *Nat. Sci.*, ***2***, 11–18

Scherer, E. & Emmelot, P. (1975) Kinetics of induction and growth of precancerous liver-cell foci, and liver tumor formation by diethylnitrosamine in the rat. *Eur. J. Cancer,* ***11,*** 689–696

Seiler, J.P. (1977) Nitrosation *in vitro* and *in vivo* by sodium nitrite, and mutagenicity of nitrogenous pesticides. *Mutat. Res.,* ***48,*** 225–236

Sobti, R.C., Krishan, A. & Pfaffenberger, C.D. (1982) Cytokinetic and cytogenetic effects of some agricultural chemicals on human lymphoid cells *in vitro* organophosphates. *Mutat. Res.,* ***102,*** 89–102

Stott, W.T., Reitz, R.H., Schumann, A.M. & Watanabe, P.G. (1981) Genetic and nongenetic events in neoplasia. *Food Cosmet. Toxicol.,* ***19,*** 567–576

Uchiyama, M., Takeda, M., Suzuki, T. & Yoshikawa, K. (1975) Mutagenicity of nitroso derivatives of *N*-methylcarbamate insecticides in microbiological method. *Bull. environ. Contam. Toxicol.,* ***14,*** 389–394

Weisburger, J.H. & Horn, C. (1982) Nutrition and cancer: mechanisms of genotoxic and epigenetic carcinogens in nutritional carcinogenesis. *Bull. N.Y. Acad. Med.,* ***58,*** 296–312

Williams, G.M. (1981) Liver carcinogenesis: the role for some chemicals of an epigenetic mechanism of liver-tumor promotion involving modification of the cell membrane. *Food cosmet. Toxicol.,* ***19,*** 577–583

Worthing, C.R., ed. (1979) *The Pesticide Manual, A World Compendium,* British Crop Protection Council

Zweig, G., Selim, S., Hummel, R., Mittelman, A., Wright, D.P., Jr & Regelman, E. (1980) *Analytical survey of* N-*nitroso contaminants in pesticide products.* In: Walker, E.A., Castegnaro, M., Griciute, L. & Börzsönyi, M., eds, N-*Nitroso Compounds: Analysis, Formation and Occurrence (IARC Scientific Publications No. 31),* Lyon, International Agency for Research on Cancer, pp. 555–564

# DRUGS AND ENVIRONMENTAL CHEMICALS AS PROMOTERS

H. GREIM, E. DEML & D. OESTERLE

*Institute of Toxicology and Biochemistry, Society for Radiation and Environmental Studies, 8042 Neuherberg, Federal Republic of Germany*

## INTRODUCTION

The role of tumour promotion in the two-step model of experimental hepatocarcinogenesis has been the object of extensive investigation, and many drugs and environmental chemicals have been identified as promoters. Since humans are exposed to both groups of chemicals, over long periods of time and occasionally at high doses, the promoting effects of these substances in human carcinogenesis are worthy of concern.

Chemicals with promoting activity include persistent halogenated hydrocarbons, e.g., dichloro-diphenyl trichloroethane (DDT), polychlorinated biphenyls (PCBs), drugs such as phenobarbital and steroid hormones such as oestrogens (for review, see Pitot & Sirica, 1980). These substances are either environmental contaminants or frequently used drugs, and they reveal potent tumour-promoting capabilities in rodent experimental systems.

In ascertaining whether these experimental data are relevant to man, thus implying that the chemicals tested are also promoters in human carcinogenesis, several points must be considered: experimental procedure, dose-dependence, human exposure levels, parameters for diagnosis of tumour promotion in humans and epidemiology.

## EXPERIMENTAL PROCEDURES

### *Rat liver foci as a test system in promotion studies*

In experimental hepatocarcinogenesis in rats, liver tumour promoters enhance the occurrence of early preneoplastic foci, hyperplastic nodules and tumours. There are several systems, with different schedules, by which the promoting capability of a compound can be detected (for review, see Emmelot & Scherer, 1980).

Pitot *et al.* (1978) introduced a system involving partial hepatectomy before initiation, followed by promotion by phenobarbital. In the schedule of Peraino *et al.* (1971, 1978), partial hepatectomy is omitted, and phenobarbital is administered after initiation by 2-acetylaminofluorene (AAF). The same system is used by Kunz *et al.* (1978), by our group, using PCBs as promoters (Oesterle & Deml, 1983), and by Schulte Hermann *et al.* (1981), who administer hexachlorocyclohexane as a promoter, using *N*-nitrosodiethylamine (NDEA) or *N*-nitrosomorpholine (NMOR) for initiation.

The models that do not include partial hepatectomy or administration of hepatotoxic agents such as AAF or carbon tetrachloride (Tsuda *et al.,* 1980) obviously correspond more closely to the situation in man. This implies, however, that in human carcinogenesis the initiating event precedes exposure to the promoter. Experimental evidence indicates that application of the promoter before initiation diminishes or even abolishes tumour incidence (McLean & Marshall, 1971; Makiura *et al.,* 1974).

*Dose-dependence*

In order to extrapolate from animal experiments to the situation in man, a dose-effect relationship of the tumour-promoting capacity of a chemical is required. Such data show whether the promoting action is dose-dependent and may indicate whether a no-effect level exists. Furthermore, the effective dose in animal experiments can be compared with the concentrations present in the environment and with the actual uptake of the promoters by humans. The applicability of most such experimental data to human cancer risk assessment is therefore limited, because, for the most part, they do not include dose-effect curves. However, some available data reveal interesting aspects. The dose-dependency of the promoting effect of phenobarbital on preneoplastic islands in rat liver was studied by Kunz *et al.* (1982), who showed that daily oral administration of 75 mg/kg body weight phenobarbital for 18 weeks enhanced the number of preneoplastic islands, whereas 7.5 and 0.75 mg/kg did not (Table 1). These data indicate that promotion by chemicals is dose-dependent and that a no-effect level may exist.

Table 1. Dose dependence in the promotion of preneoplastic islands in rat liver[a]

| Initiating agent | Phenobarbital dose (mg/kg) | Preneoplastic areas (no./cm²) | |
|---|---|---|---|
| | | ATPase (−) | GGT[c] (+) |
| NNM[b] | water | 288 | 780 |
| NNM | 0.75 | 270 | 657 |
| NNM | 7.5 | 285 | 720 |
| NNM | 75 | 612 | 1 597 |
| water | 75 | 10 | 10 |
| water | water | 10 | 10 |

[a] From Kunz *et al.* (1982)
[b] *N*-Nitrosomorpholine
[c] γ-Glutamyltranspeptidase

Fig. 1. Dose-dependent enhancement of the number of ATPase-deficient islands in female Sprague-Dawley rats treated with a single dose of 8 mg *N*-nitrosodiethylamine/kg body weight and with various doses of Clophen A 50 three times a week for 11 consecutive weeks

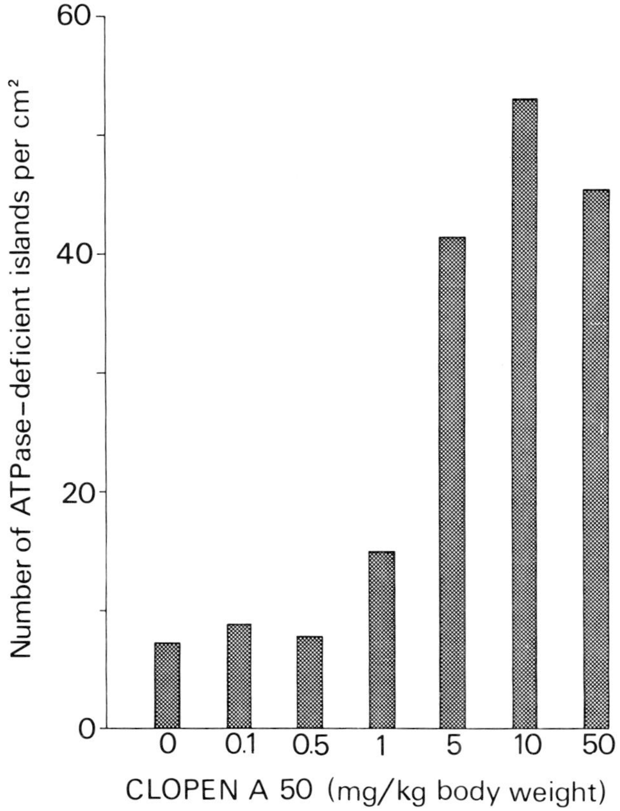


No-effect levels in phenobarbital promotion have been observed. After feeding 0.02% AAF for two weeks, Peraino *et al.* (1980) observed no increase in tumour incidence and only a slight enhancement of tumour frequency following administration of 0.002% phenobarbital in the diet, even after 84 weeks of treatment. The latter observation is particularly significant because most workers use short-term experiments to study the tumour-promoting effects of chemicals. The reliability of such short-term experiments for determining no-effect concentrations could be questioned on the basis that the experiments have been conducted for an insufficient period of time.

We observed recently a no-effect level in the promoting effect of PCBs in weanling female Sprague-Dawley rats (Deml & Oesterle, unpublished data), using NDEA for initiation and administration of different doses of Clophen A 50, a mixture of PCBs. Following initiation with a single oral dose of 8 mg/kg body weight of NDEA, 0.1–50 mg/kg body weight Clophen A 50 were given by gavage three times a week

Fig. 2. Dose-dependent enhancement of cytochrome P-450 content (▧) and aldrin epoxidase (□) activity in weanling female rats treated with a single dose of 8 mg *N*-nitrosodiethylamine/kg body weight and with various doses of Clophen A 50 three times a week for 11 consecutive weeks

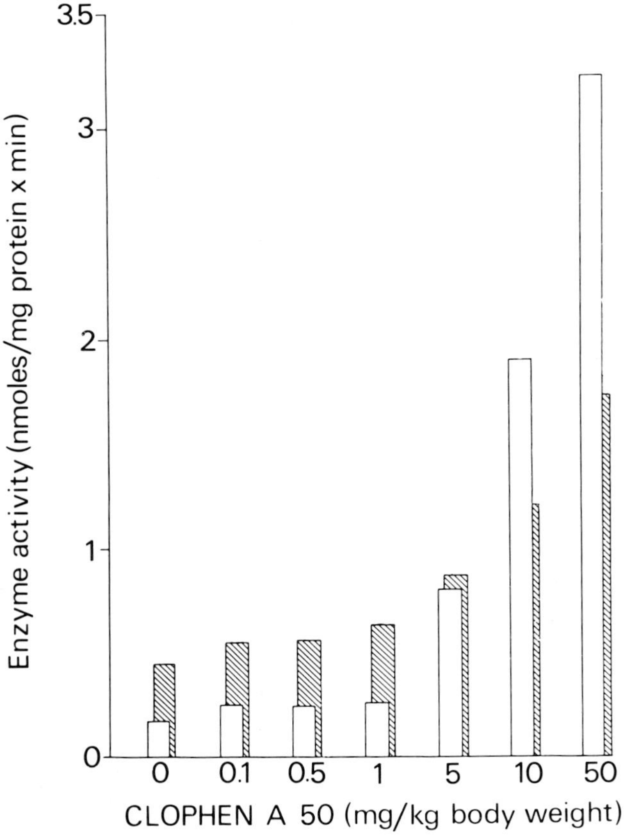


for 11 weeks. The animals were sacrificed 12 weeks after initiation in order to screen the livers for ATPase-deficient and γ-glutamyltranspeptidase (GGT)-positive islands.

Whereas the higher doses significantly increased the number of preneoplastic islands, no such effect was observed with doses of 1 mg/kg and below (Fig. 1). This again suggests a no-effect level in the promoting effect by chemicals.

The dose-dependent induction of a microsomal monooxygenase reaction, aldrin epoxidase activity (Wolff *et al.*, 1979) and cytochrome P-450 content were measured simultaneously. A positive correlation between enzyme induction, amount of cytochrome P-450 and promoting effect was found. No effect on enzyme induction was observed with 1–2 mg/kg body weight of Clophen A 50 applied three times a week (Fig. 2). These enzymatic activities can be determined readily in humans. Furthermore, in experimental animals and in man, microsomal enzyme induction is associated with a proliferation of the hepatic smooth endoplasmic reticulum, which can be diagnosed by electron microscopic examination of liver biopsies. Such a proliferation of the endoplasmic reticulum has been observed in the liver of a 'Yusho' patient (Kuratsune, 1980).

Thus, determination of the activity of hepatic microsomal enzymes can be used to establish effective promoting doses of environmental chemicals. Proliferation of the smooth endoplasmic reticulum may serve as a tool for diagnosing and evaluating the biological significance of exposure to tumour-promoting agents in humans.

In this respect, the potential roles of phenobarbital and PCBs as promoters in human carcinogenesis are evaluated.

*Phenobarbital*

Phenobarbital is a long-acting central nervous depressant. In antiepileptic therapy, it is given in daily doses of 50–200 mg, representing 0.7–3 mg/kg body weight. Generally, increased hepatic microsomal enzyme activity is observed in these patients, combined with a higher tolerance to other drugs that are metabolized by these enzymes (for review, see Greim, 1981).

Two epidemiological studies carried out on 9136 epileptic patients treated with anticonvulsant drugs, including phenobarbital (Clemmesen *et al.*, 1974), revealed that in patients treated for up to ten years the incidence of cancer at all sites, except for the liver, was the same or lower than that expected when compared with the incidence in the general population. Although in patients treated for more than ten years, four cases of liver cancer were observed in males, whereas 1.1 cases were expected, it was later revealed that three of the four patients had been treated previously with thorotrast (Clemmesen, 1975), which is known to induce liver tumours in man (Kiely *et al.*, 1973).

The apparently negative findings of these studies are supported by considerations of dose-effect. In promotion experiments, 0.05–0.1% phenobarbital is usually given in the drinking water or in the diet, corresponding to approximately 20–80 mg/kg body weight per day. According to Kunz *et al.* (1982), a dose of 7.5 mg/kg phenobarbital is ineffective in rats. The maximal therapeutic dose in epileptics of 4 mg/kg is even lower, and this dose is given for only short periods of time since it causes intensive sleepiness.

Although not substantiated by epidemiological studies, there is some indication of a reduced incidence of cancer at all sites in patients treated for up to ten years with phenobarbital. This would support the observation that phenobarbital reduces liver tumour incidence in rats when given prior to aflatoxin (McLean & Marshall, 1971).

Thus, present indications are that continuous therapeutic use of phenobarbital may have no tumour-promoting capacity in humans, although this finding may be related mainly to the low therapeutic doses used, as compared to those required for tumour promotion in experimental animals.

*Polychlorinated biphenyls*

From 1930 to 1970, PCBs were used in a wide variety of industrial applications; since then, their use has been voluntarily restricted to closed systems. This limitation reduced the extent of human exposure caused by environmental pollution and industrial accidents, as well as by migration from food packaging materials into food (Cordle *et al.*, 1978). The present intake by the general public is estimated to be 5–10 μg/day (0.07–0.14 μg/kg body weight per day) (Humphrey *et al.*, 1976). In fish-eating populations, a 5–30-fold higher intake has been suggested, since fish still contains significant amounts of these chemicals (Cordle *et al.*, 1978). Since, due to their lipophilicity, PCBs accumulate in adipose tissue, most human adipose tissue contains 1–2 mg/kg PCBs, with a range of 0.11–6.6 mg/kg in the Canadian population (Grant *et al.*, 1976). In spite of the relatively high exposure sustained by the Canadian population, no adverse effects have been observed.

In the Yusho food poisoning incident in western Japan in 1968, involving more than 1600 people, a commercial brand of rice oil was contaminated with PCBs, dibenzofurans and quarterphenyls (Kuratsune, 1980); the patients ingested an average of 633 mg of PCBs during a period of approximately ten weeks. The clinical signs of the disease persisted for approximately two years. Chloracne was the predominant symptom; other symptoms were pigmentation of the skin, visual disturbances, weakness, headaches and liver function disorders. The lowest dose producing overt effects was 500 mg total intake (Kuratsune *et al.*, 1976). Epidemiological data on the tumour incidence in this population and in other groups highly exposed to PCBs are incomplete. In the Yusho follow-up study at the end of 1977, 51 of the known patients had died, and neoplasms had accounted for 35.4% of the 31 classified deaths, representing a 21% higher mortality rate from neoplasms than in the unexposed population of that region (Urabe *et al.*, 1979). Although drug metabolism has not been studied in the Yusho patients, a liver biopsy from one patient revealed a marked proliferation of the endoplasmic reticulum (Kuratsune, 1980). Together with the observation of induced drug metabolism in workers exposed to high levels of PCBs (Alvares *et al.*, 1977), this finding suggests that Yusho patients were exposed to amounts with tumour-promoting capacity. Further epidemiological studies of this group of patients will be worthwhile.

With a daily intake of 5–10 μg of PCBs, the general population has a much lower exposure. Even highly exposed fishermen, who take up approximately 0.5–4 μg/kg body weight daily, do not receive the doses that have promoting effects in animal experiments. Thus, tumour-promotion by PCBs in the general population is unlikely, although highly exposed people may be at a certain risk.

## CONCLUSIONS

The currently available experimental models represent highly sophisticated methods for investigating the tumour-promoting effect of chemicals. They are designed preferentially for rapid and sensitive detection of this effect rather than for mimicking the way in which man is exposed to these chemicals. Furthermore, only a few studies provide data on the dose-effect relationship.

Consequently, only a limited number of experiments can be used to evaluate the significance of experimental tumour promotion for man. The experiments involving phenobarbital and PCBs, combined with very limited epidemiological data, do not permit the conclusion that chemicals that possess tumour-promoting capacities in animal experiments are relevant to human carcinogenesis. Human exposure to these compounds is within a dose range that does not seem to exert a promoting effect in animal experiments. It is to be expected, however, that the designs of future tumour-promoting experiments will include models that resemble the human mode of exposure and that they will take into account the need to establish dose-effect relationships and to ascertain whether no-effect levels do exist in the tumour-promoting effect of chemicals in the human environment.

## REFERENCES

Alvares, A.P., Fischbein, A., Anderson, K.E. & Kappas, A. (1977) Alterations in drug metabolism in workers exposed to polychlorinated biphenyls. *Clin. Pharmacol. Ther.*, ***22,*** 140–146

Clemmesen, J. (1975) Phenobarbitone, liver tumors and thorotrast. *Lancet*, ***i,*** 37–38

Clemmesen, J., Fuglsang-Frederiksen, V. & Plum, C.M. (1974) Are anticonvulsants oncogenic? *Lancet*, ***i,*** 705–707

Cordle, F., Corneliussen, P., Jelinek, C., Hackley, B., Lehman, R. & Shapiro, R. (1978) Human exposure to polychlorinated biphenyls and polybrominated biphenyls. *Environ. Health Perspect.*, ***24,*** 157–172

Emmelot, P. & Scherer, E. (1980) The first relevant cell stage in rat liver carcinogenesis. A quantitative approach. *Biochim. biophys. Acta*, ***605,*** 247–304

Grant, D.L., Mes, J. & Frank, R. (1976) *PCB residues in human adipose tissue and milk*. In: *Proceedings of National Conference on Polychlorinated Biphenyls, Chicago, 1975* (*EPA-560/6-75-04*), Washington DC, US Environmental Protection Agency

Greim, H.A. (1981) *An overview of the phenomena of enzyme induction and inhibition: their relevance to drug action and drug interactions*. In: Jenner, P. & Testa, B., eds, *Concepts in Drug Metabolism*, New York, Marcel Dekker, pp. 219–263

Humphrey, H.E.B., Price, H.A. & Budd, M.L. (1976) *Evaluation of Changes of the Level of Polychlorinated Biphenyls (PCBs) in Human Tissue* (*Final Report of FDA contract No. 223-73-2209*), Washington DC, US Government Printing Office

Kiely, J.M., Titus, J.L. & Orvis, A. (1973) Thorotrast-induced hepatoma presenting as hyperparathyroidism. *Cancer*, ***31,*** 1312–1314

Kunz, W., Appel, K.E., Rickart, R., Schwarz, M. & Stöckle, G. (1978) *Enhancement and inhibition of carcinogenic effectiveness of nitrosamines*. In: Remmer, H., Bolt, H.M., Bannasch, P. & Popper, H., eds, *Primary Liver Tumors*, Lancaster, MTP Press, pp. 287–302

Kunz, W., Schaude, G., Schwarz, M. & Tennekes, H. (1982) *Quantitative aspects of drug-mediated tumour promotion in liver and its toxicological implications*. In: Hecker, E., Fusenig, N.E., Kunz, W., Marks, F. & Thielmann, H.W., eds, *Carcinogenesis*, Vol. 7, *Cocarcinogenesis and Biological Effects of Tumor Promoters*, New York, Raven Press, pp. 111–126

Kuratsune, M. (1980) *Yusho*. In: Kimbrough, R.D., ed., *Halogenated Biphenyls, Terphenyls, Naphthalenes, Dibenzodioxins and Related Products*, Amsterdam, Elsevier/North-Holland Biomedical Press, pp. 287–302

Kuratsune, M., Masuda, Y. & Nagayama, J. (1976) *Some of the recent findings concerning Yusho*. In: *Proceedings of a National Conference on Polychlorinated Biphenyls, Chicago 1975* (*EPA-560/6-75-004*), Washington DC, US Environmental Protection Agency, pp. 14–29

Makiura, S., Aoe, H., Sugihara, S., Hirao, K., Arai, M. & Ito, N. (1974) Inhibitory effect of polychlorinated biphenyls on liver tumorigenesis in rats treated with 3-methyl-4-dimethylaminoazobenzene, N-2-fluorenylacetamide and diethynitrosamine. *J. natl Cancer Inst.*, ***53***, 1253–1257

McLean, A.E.M. & Marshall, A. (1971) Reduced carcinogenic effects of aflatoxin in rats given phenobarbitone. *Br. J. exp. Pathol.*, **52**, 322–329

Oesterle, D. & Deml, E. (1983) Promoting effect of polychlorinated biphenyls on development of enzyme-altered islands in livers of weanling and adult rats. *J. Cancer Res. clin. Oncol.*, ***105***, 141–147

Peraino, C., Fry, R.J.M. & Staffeldt, E.F. (1971) Reduction and enhancement by phenobarbital of hepatocarcinogenesis in the rat induced by 2-acetylaminofluorene. *Cancer Res.*, ***31***, 1506–1512

Peraino, C., Fry, R.J.M. & Grube, D.D. (1978) *Drug induced enhancement of hepatic tumorigenesis*. In: Slaga, T.J., Sivak, A. & Boutwell, R.K., eds, *Mechanisms of Tumor Promotion and Cocarcinogenesis*, New York, Raven Press, pp. 421–432

Peraino, C., Staffeldt, E.F., Haugen, D.A., Lombard, L.S., Stevens, F.J. & Fry, R.J.M. (1980) Effects of varying the dietary concentration of phenobarbital on its enhancement of 2-acetylaminofluorene-induced hepatic tumorigenesis. *Cancer Res.*, ***40***, 3268–3273

Pitot, H.C. & Sirica, A.E. (1980) The stages of initiation and promotion in hepatocarcinogenesis. *Biochim. biophys. Acta*, ***605***, 191–215

Pitot, H.C., Barsness, L., Goldsworthy, T. & Kitagawa, T. (1978) Biochemical characterization of stages of hepatocarcinogenesis after a single dose of diethylnitrosamine. *Nature*, ***271***, 456–458

Schulte Hermann, R., Ohde, G., Schuppler, J. & Timmermann-Trosiener, I. (1981) Enhanced proliferation of putative preneoplastic cells in rat liver following treatment with the tumor promoters phenobarbital, hexachlorocyclohexane, steroid compounds and nafenopin. *Cancer Res.*, ***41***, 2556–2562

Tsuda, H., Lee, G. & Farber, E. (1980) Induction of resistant hepatocytes as a new principle for a possible short-term *in vivo* test for carcinogens. *Cancer Res.*, ***40***, 1157–1164

Urabe, H., Koda, H. & Asahi, M. (1979) Present state of Yusho patients. *Ann. N.Y. Acad. Sci.*, ***320***, 273–276

Wolff, T., Deml, E. & Wanders, H. (1979) Aldrin epoxidation, a highly sensitive indicator specific for cytochrome P-450-dependent monooxygenase activities. *Drug Metab. Dispos.*, ***7***, 301–305

# INHIBITION OF TUMOUR PROMOTION

# CAN TUMOUR PROMOTION BE EFFECTIVELY INHIBITED?

T.J. SLAGA
*University of Texas System Cancer Center*
*Science Park – Research Division*
*Smithville, TX 78957, USA*

## INTRODUCTION

Research on tumour promotion has accelerated at an explosive rate during the past decade and continues to do so because of its importance in the understanding of the induction of human cancer. Furthermore, the promotion process is reversible for a relatively long period of time, which makes it possible to find very effective means of preventing the induction of cancer (Slaga, 1980). The extensive data available, as well as the multistage nature of tumour promotion, suggest that this process, which is now thought to occur in most tissues in which cancer can be induced or occurs spontaneously, may involve the interaction of a number of endogeneous chemicals at elevated levels, as well as environmental factors such as chemicals, radiation, viruses, and diet and nutrition. These concepts thus unify all the current areas of cancer research (Slaga, 1980). In terms of human cancer, smoking, asbestos, radiation, hormones and diet and nutrition, just to mention a few, are now thought to have more of a promotional influence in the multistage carcinogenesis process (Slaga, 1980). We discuss results obtained on various important aspects of promotion, inhibitors of skin tumour promotion and their specificity in multistage promotion. In addition, we present results that suggest that administration of a combination of certain inhibitors, at low and nontoxic doses, may be a rational and effective way of preventing the induction of cancer in man.

## INHIBITORS OF SKIN TUMOUR PROMOTION

A number of inhibitors of skin tumour promotion have been very useful to our understanding of the cellular events that are important in tumour promotion (Slaga *et al.,* 1982a). In general, as shown in Table 1, the majority of known inhibitors of skin tumour promotion are agents that inhibit the promoter-induced hyperplasia,

Table 1. Inhibitors of tumour promotion

| |
|---|
| 1. Agents that inhibit promoter-induced hyperplasia |
| 2. Agents that inhibit promoter-induced ornithine decarboxylase |
| 3. Agents that inhibit promoter-induced prostaglandins |
| 4. Agents that elevate cyclic adenosine monophosphate |
| 5. Agents that inhibit promoter-induced dark cells |
| 6. Antioxidants |

ornithine decarboxylase activity and subsequent polyamine levels, prostaglandins and dark basal keratinocytes (Slaga *et al.*, 1982a). In addition, skin tumour promotion can be counteracted by a number of antioxidants, vitamins and cyclic adenosine monophosphate (cAMP) or by agents that elevate endogenous levels of cAMP (Slaga *et al.*, 1982a). Table 2 lists a number of agents that have been shown to inhibit skin tumour promotion by 12-*O*-tetradecanoylphorbol-13-acetate (TPA). Since the last meeting on tumour promotion (Hecker *et al.*, 1982), a number of effective inhibitors of skin tumour promotion have been found (Slaga *et al.*, 1982b). Although, antioxidants have been shown to inhibit skin tumour initiation (Slaga *et al.*, 1982a), these agents have an even greater inhibitory effect on skin tumour promotion by TPA and benzoyl peroxide (Table 3). Selenium, anti-androgen cyproterone acetate and vitamins E and C have also been found to be effective inhibitors of skin tumour promotion (Table 2).

Although retinoic acid is an effective inhibitor of TPA promotion, it has no effect on benzoyl peroxide promotion or on complete carcinogenesis by 7,12-di-

Table 2. Inhibitors of phorbol ester skin tumour promotion

| |
|---|
| 1. Anti-inflammatory steroids; cortisol, dexamethasone and fluocinolone acetonide |
| 2. Vitamin A derivative |
| 3. Combination of retinoids and anti-inflammatory agents |
| 4. Protease inhibitors: tosyl lysine chloromethyl ketone; tosyl arginine methyl ester; tosyl phenylalanine chloromethyl ketone; antipain; and leupeptin |
| 5. Cyclic nucleotides |
| 6. Phosphodiesterase inhibitors; isobutylmethylxanthine |
| 7. Dimethylsulfoxide |
| 8. Butyrate, acetic acid |
| 9. Bacillus Calmette-Guerin |
| 10. Polyriboinosinic: polyribocytidylic acid |
| 11. Prostaglandin synthesis inhibitors 5,8,11,14-eicosatetraynoic acid and phenidone |
| 12. Thromboxane synthetase inhibitors; imidazolacetophenone and imidazolphenol |
| 13. Phospholipase $A_2$ inhibitor: dibromoacetophenone |
| 14. Arachidonic acid |
| 15. Polyamine synthesis inhibitor (difluoromethylornithine) |
| 16. Histamine |
| 17. Diphenhydramine ($H_1$ receptor inhibitor) |
| 18. Butylated hydroxyanisole and butylated hydroxytoluene |
| 19. Disulfiram and parahydroxyanisole |
| 20. Vitamins E and C |
| 21. Selenium |
| 22. Anti-androgen cyproterone acetate |

Table 3. Effects of antioxidants on skin tumour promotion after initiation with 7,12-dimethylbenz[a]anthracene

| Tumour promoter[a] | Antioxidant[b] (dose) | Tumour response (% of TPA controls) |
|---|---|---|
| TPA | | 100 |
| TPA | BHT (1 mg) | 54 |
| TPA | BHT (5 mg) | 23 |
| TPA | BHA (1 mg) | 42 |
| TPA | BHA (5 mg) | 18 |
| TPA | 2-TBHA (1 mg) | 44 |
| TPA | 2-TBHA (2 mg) | 23 |
| TPA | 3-TBHA (1 mg) | 5 |
| TPA | 3-TBHA (2 mg) | 4 |
| TPA | Disulfiran (1 mg) | 58 |
| TPA | Disulfiran (2 mg) | 16 |
| TPA | 4-*para*-Hydroxyanisole (1 mg) | 27 |
| TPA | 4-*para*-Hydroxyanisole (2 mg) | 10 |
| Benzoyl peroxide | | 100 |
| Benzoyl peroxide | BHT (1 mg) | 60 |
| Benzoyl peroxide | BHT (5 mg) | 23 |
| Benzoyl peroxide | BHA (1 mg) | 56 |
| Benzoyl peroxide | BHA (5 mg) | 35 |

[a] TPA, 12-*O*-tetradecanoylphorbol-13-acetate
[b] BHT, butylated hydroxytoluene; BHA, butylated hydroxyanisole

Table 4. Inhibitors of skin tumour promotion by 12-*O*-tetradecanoylphorbol-13-acetate (TPA) and benzoyl peroxide

1. Fluocinolone acetonide
2. Cyproterone acetate
3. Tosyl phenylalanine chlormethyl ketone
4. Selenium
5. Butylated hydroxyanisole, butylated hydroxytoluene and other antioxidants
6. Vitamin E
7. Vitamin C

Although retinoic acid inhibits TPA promotion, it has no inhibitory effect on benzoyl peroxide promotion or on complete carcinogenesis by 7,12-dimethylbenz[*a*]anthracene

methylbenz[*a*]anthracene. Table 4 lists the inhibitors that have been found to counteract both TPA and benzoyl peroxide promotion. It should be emphasized that not all the inhibitors listed in Table 2 have been tested on benzoyl peroxide promotion.

Skin tumour promoters bring about a number of important epigenetic changes in the skin, such as inflammation, epidermal hyperplasia, cell surface and membrane changes, and an increase in ornithine decarboxylase, polyamine, prostaglandins and protease activity, and dark basal keratinocytes, as well as other embryonic

Table 5. Effects of fluocinolone acetonide (FA), retinoic acid (RA), difluoromethylornithine (DFMO), tosyl phenylalanine chloromethyl ketone (TPCK), butylated hydroxyanisole (BHA) and cyproterone acetate (CPA) on tumour promotion and 12-*O*-tetradecanoylphorbol-13-acetate (TPA)-induced epidermal hyperplasia, dark basal keratinocytes and ornithine decarboxylase (ODC) and polyamine levels

| | Relative ability (%) to counteract | | | |
|---|---|---|---|---|
| Inhibitor | TPA promotion | TPA-induced hyperplasia | TPA-induced dark cells | TPA-induced ODC and polyamine levels |
| FA | 100 | 100 | 100 | 20 |
| RA | 80 | 0 | 0 | 85 |
| DFMO | 55 | 0 | 0 | 95 |
| TPCK | 70 | 0 | 70 | 10 |
| BHA | 95 | 0 | 0 | 85 |
| CPA | 90 | 60 | ? | 0 |

characteristics in adult skin (Slaga *et al.*, 1982a and references therein). In addition, skin tumour promoters cause a decrease in epidermal superoxide and catalase activities (Solanki *et al.*, 1981), as well as a decrease in the number of glucocorticoid receptors (Davidson & Slaga, 1983a) and a decreased response of $G_1$ chalone in adult skin (Kreig *et al.*, 1974). Table 5 summarizes the effects of fluocinolone acetonide, retinoic acid, tosyl phenylalanine chloromethylketone (TPCK), difluoromethylornithine, butylated hydroxyanisole and cyproterone acetate on TPA promotion and TPA-induced epidermal hyperplasia, dark basal keratinocytes and polyamine levels. Fluocinolone acetonide is effective in counteracting TPA-induced hyperplasia and dark basal keratinocytes but not the increased polyamine levels, whereas retinoic acid, butylated hydroxyanisole and difluoromethylornithine counteract only the TPA-induced increase in polyamine levels (Slaga *et al.*, 1980a). The antiandrogen cyproterone acetate has no effect on the TPA-induced ornithine decarboxylase or polyamines but it does decrease the TPA-induced hyperplasia (Davidson *et al.*, 1983). We are in the process of determining the effect of cyproterone acetate on TPA-induced dark basal keratinocytes. TPCK is a very interesting inhibitor of promotion, because it counteracts only the TPA-induced dark basal keratinocytes (Slaga *et al.*, 1980a).

## SPECIFICITY OF INHIBITORS IN MULTISTAGE SKIN TUMOUR PROMOTION

Before discussing the specificity of inhibitors in multistage skin tumour promotion, the important aspects of multistage promotion must be summarized. Skin tumour promotion can be operationally and mechanistically further divided into at least two stages (Slaga *et al.*, 1980a,b, 1982a,b). This classification was possible because we found that mezerein induced many of the cellular events that TPA does but was a weak or nonpromoting agent (Mufsan *et al.*, 1979). We rationalized that TPA must be inducing some additional cellular event(s) that mezerein could not effectively induce. If this is the case, then after limited TPA treatment mezerein should show a promoting activity that it would not have by itself. As reported previously (Slaga *et al.*, 1980a,b, 1982a,b), this regimen was an effective way of inducing tumours. Similar results were later found by Fürstenberger and coworkers (1981) using phorbol 12-retinoate-13-acetate as a stage II promoter.

Table 6 summarizes the known characteristics of the first and second stages of promotion. Both show a good dose-response relationship. It should be emphasized that only one application of a first-stage promoter is required, and this stage is irreversible for four to six weeks (Slaga *et al.*, 1982a; Slaga, unpublished data). Besides TPA and 12-deoxyphorbol-13-decanoate, which are known promoters, nonpromoters such as 4-*O*-methyl-TPA, calcium ionophore A 23187, hydrogen peroxide as well as wounding are effective stage I promoters (Slaga *et al.*, 1982a). These agents plus wounding increase the number of dark basal keratinocytes (stem cells?), which suggests that these cells are important in the first stage of promotion (Klein-Szanto & Slaga, 1981). Recent results also suggest that these dark cells are the critical target cells for skin tumour initiators (Slaga *et al.*, unpublished data).

Prostaglandin $E_2$ specifically enhances stage I of promotion, whereas putrescine specifically enhances stage II of promotion (Slaga *et al.*, 1982a). Stage I of promotion can be inhibited by fluocinolone acetonide and TPCK, which also counteracted TPA-induced dark basal keratinocytes (Slaga *et al.*, 1980a). Vitamin E also inhibits stage

Table 6. Characteristics of the first and second stages of tumour promotion

*Stage I*

1. A good dose-response exists for 12-*O*-tetradecanoylphorbol-13-acetate (TPA) and 12-deoxyphorbol-decanoate as first-stage promoters.
2. The nonpromoting agents, calcium ionophore A23187, 4-*O*-methyl-TPA, hydrogen peroxide and wounding can act as stage-I promoters.
3. Only one application of first-stage promoter is necessary.
4. Prostaglandins are important since prostaglandin $E_2$ can enhance stage I by TPA.
5. Partially irreversible
   (a) Four to six weeks can separate first and second stages of promotion without a decrease in tumour response.
   (b) There is an 80% decrease in tumour response if ten weeks separate stage I and II of promotion.
6. Increase in the number of dark basal keratinocytes (stem cells) is important. This occurs by direct stimulation of existing dark cells to divide, converting some basal cells to dark cells and increasing the differentiation of some basal cells and differentiated cells.
7. Decrease in glucocorticoid receptors by TPA may help in proliferation of dark cells.

*Stage II*

1. A good dose-response exists for mezerein as a second-stage promoter.
2. The nonpromoting agent 12-deoxyphorbol-13-2,4,6-decatri-enoate can act as a stage-II promoter.
3. Multiple applications are required.
4. Reversible for relatively long period, but later becomes irreversible.
5. Polyamines are important, since putrescine can enhance stage II by mezerein.
6. Most of the biochemical events shown to be important in promotion occur in this stage.
7. Mezerein can maintain dark-cell proliferation and decrease in glucocorticoid receptors but cannot induce these events by itself.

Fig. 1. Various stages of skin carcinogenesis showing the important events in Stages I and II of promotion and at which points the various inhibitors are effective
TPA, 12-*O*-tetradecanoylphorbol-13-acetate; A23187, calcium ionophore; DP-Tri-D, 12-deoxyphorbol-13-2,4,6-decatrienoate; FA, flucinolone acetonide; RA, retinoic acid; TPCK, tocyl phenylalanine chloromethyl ketone; DFMO, difluoromethylornithine; BHA, butylated hydroxyanisole; CPA, cyproterone acetate

| | STAGE I | STAGE II |
|---|---|---|
| INITIATION (1x) → | TPA (1x) → | MEZERIN |
| | | DP-Tri D |
| | A23187 (1x) | (multiple applications) |
| | $H_2O_2$ (1x) | |
| | 4-**O** METHYL TPA (1x) | |
| | WOUDING (1x) | |
| 1. DARK CELLS (STEM CELLS) ARE CRITICAL TARGET | 1. STIMULATION OF DARK CELL (PRIMITIVE SKIN STEM CELLS) | 1. POLYAMINES |
| | 2. PROSTAGLANDINS | 2. MAINTAINED CELL PROLIFERATION |
| | ↑ | ↑ |
| | ⊤ | ⊤ |
| | FA | RA |
| | TPCK | FA |
| | | DMFO |
| | | BHA |
| | | VITAMIN E |
| | | VITAMIN C |
| | | CPA |

I of promotion, but its effect on dark cells is not presently known (Slaga, unpublished data). These dark cells are normally present in high numbers in embryonic skin (20–50% of basal cells), but they are present in low numbers in adult skin (< 3% of basal cells). Papillomas and carcinomas also contain a large number of these dark cells (Slaga *et al.*, 1980b). As discussed earlier, the dark cells appear to be the critical target cells of the tumour initiator, and the first-stage promoters stimulate these cells to divide rapidly by both direct and indirect mechanisms (Slaga & Klein-Szanto, unpublished data).

The second stage of promotion is initially reversible but later becomes irreversible. A number of weak or nonpromoting agents, such as mezerein and 12-deoxyphorbol-13-2,4,6-decatrienoate, are effective second-stage promoters (Slaga *et al.,* 1982a). Although mezerein by itself is not able to increase the number of dark cells or to decrease the level of glucocorticoid receptors, it can effectively maintain these conditions after TPA treatment in a two-stage promotion protocol (Davidson & Slaga, 1983b). Stage II of promotion can be inhibited by fluocinolone acetonide, retinoic acid, difluoromethylornithine, butylated hydroxyanisole, cyproterone acetate and vitamins E and C, which counteract either the mezerein-induced ornithine decarboxylase, cell proliferation and/or as yet unidentified events (Slaga *et al.,* 1982a; Slaga, unpublished data). On the basis of these results with inhibitors, polyamines and epidermal cell proliferation, as well as some unidentified event(s), appear to be important events in stage II of promotion. Figure 1 depicts the various stages of promotion, the important events in each stage, and the points at which the various inhibitors are effective.

## COMBINATION OF INHIBITORS ON SKIN TUMOUR PROMOTION

Table 7 summarizes some recent studies on the combination of first- and second-stage inhibitors on skin tumour promotion. As reported previously (Weeks *et al.,* 1979), a combination of fluocinolone acetonide and retinoic acid was found to be effective in counteracting TPA promotion. A combination of TPCK (specific stage-I inhibitor) and difluoromethylornithine (specific stage-II inhibitor) was found to inhibit both TPA and benzoyl peroxide promotion in a synergistic manner (Slaga, unpublished data). Likewise, a combination of TPCK and butylated hydroxyanisole (stage-II inhibitor) was found effectively to counteract TPA and benzoyl peroxide promotion in a synergistic manner (Slaga, unpublished data). Although we do not know at present what stage(s) of promotion selenium can inhibit, a combination of selenium and vitamin E (stage-I and -II inhibitors) can inhibit TPA and benzoyl peroxide promotion in a synergistic manner (Slaga, unpublished data). Vitamin E and selenium have also been found to inhibit mammary carcinogenesis in a synergistic manner (Ip, 1982). In a preliminary experiment, we found that a combination of fluocinolone acetonide, TPCK, vitamin E, selenium and butylated hydroxyanisole, when applied topically at low nontoxic doses, completely counteracted skin tumour promotion. Extensive dose-response data with each inhibitor of tumour promotion is needed before combinations of inhibitors of tumour promotion can be properly studied and evaluated. Although this was not achieved in our preliminary experiment with a combination of a number of inhibitors, it was useful to see if such a treatment was effective in counteracting skin tumour promotion.

Numerous agents have been tested for their anti-carcinogenic activity in experimental animals (Waltenberg, 1978; Slaga & DiGiovanni, 1983; and references

Table 7. Effects of combinations of first- and second-stage inhibitors on skin tumour promotion

1. A combination of fluocinolone acetonide and retinoic acid inhibits skin tumour promotion by 12-*O*-tetradecanoylphorbol-13-acetate (TPA) in a synergistic manner.
2. A combination of tosyl phenylalanine chloromethyl ketone (TPCK) and difluoromethylornithine inhibits skin tumour promotion by TPA and benzoyl peroxide in a synergistic manner.
3. A combination of TPCK and butylated hydroxyanisole inhibits skin tumour promotion by TPA and benzoyl peroxide in a synergistic manner.
4. A combination of vitamin E and selenium inhibits TPA and benzoyl peroxide promotion in a synergistic manner.
5. A combination of fluocinolone acetonide, TPCK, vitamin E, selenium and butylated hydroxyanisole can completely counteract skin tumour promotion at low and nontoxic doses.

therein). However, many of these anti-carcinogenic agents have many side effects that would limit their usefulness in preventing cancer in man. For example, although, retinoic acid has been shown to inhibit the induction of cancer by a variety of carcinogens in a number of tissues, it also has been found to have no effect or an enhancing effect on others (Slaga & DiGiovanni, 1983). In addition, high doses of retinoic acid have been shown to have promoting activity after initiation by ultraviolet light and 7,12-dimethylbenz[*a*]anthracene (Forbes *et al.,* 1979; Slaga, unpublished data). Butylated hydroxytoluene can inhibit carcinogenesis and promotion in some carcinogenesis systems, but it can act as a promoter in others (Slaga & DiGiovanni, 1983). Furthermore, several inhibitors are very effective in counteracting the induction of cancer but are very toxic. Table 8 lists a number of anti-carcinogenic agents that may be useful in preventing the induction of cancer in man, for a number of reasons. Although, they may not be very useful individually, a combination of these agents at low and nontoxic doses may be a rational and effective means of preventing the induction of cancer in man.

Table 8. Anti-carcinogenic agents that may be useful in preventing the induction of cancer in man

Selenium
Vitamin E
Vitamin C
Butylated hydroxyanisole
Disulfiram
*para*-Hydroxyanisole
Protease inhibitors
Difluoromethylornithine

These agents may be important for the following reasons:
(1) Relatively nontoxic
(2) Inhibit carcinogenesis induced by different types of carcinogens and promoters in several tissues
(3) Can be easily given in the diet and/or drinking-water
(4) Some inhibit specific stages, whereas others inhibit multiple stages
(5) A combination of these agents at low and nontoxic doses may be the best approach, since all stages of the multistage carcinogenesis process would be inhibited.

## ACKNOWLEDGEMENT

Supported by Public Health Service grant, CA 34690 from the US National Cancer Institute.

## REFERENCES

Davidson, K.A. & Slaga, T.J. (1983a) Effects of phorbol ester tumor promoters and hyperplasiogenic agents on cytoplasmic glucocorticoid receptors in epidermis. *J. invest. Dermatol.*, ***79***, 378–383

Davidson, K.A. & Slaga, T.J. (1983b) Glucocorticoid receptor levels in mouse skin after repetitive applications of 12-*O*-tetradecanoylphorbol-13-acetate and mezerein. *Cancer Res.* (in press)

Davidson, K.A., Ewald, L., Hermann, A. & Slaga, T.J. (1983) Effects of the antiandrogen, cyproterone acetate, on tumor promotion, DNA synthesis and ornithine decarboxylase activity in mouse skin. *Carcinogenesis* (in press)

Forbes, P.D., Urbach, F. & Davies, R.E. (1979) Enhancement of experimental photocarcinogenesis by topical retinoic acid. *Cancer Lett.*, ***7***, 85–89

Fürstenberger, G., Berry, D.L., Sorg, B. & Marks, F. (1978) Skin tumor promotion by phorbol esters is a two-stage process. *Proc. natl Acad. Sci. USA*, ***78***, 772–775

Hecker, E., Fusenig, N.E., Kunz, W., Marks, F. & Thielmann, H.W., eds (1982) *Carcinogenesis*, Vol. 7, *Cocarcinogenesis and Biological Effects of Tumor Promoters*, New York, Raven Press

Ip, C. (1982) Vitamin E potentiates the prophylactic effect of selenium in chemically-induced mammary tumorigenesis. *Proc. Am. Assoc. Cancer Res.*, ***23***, 70

Klein-Szanto, A.J.P. & Slaga, T.J. (1981) Numerical variation of dark cells in normal and chemically induced hyperplasia epidermis with age of animal and efficiency of tumor promoter. *Cancer Res.*, ***41***, 4437–4440

Kreig, L., Kuhlmann, J. & Marks, F. (1974) Effects of tumor-promoting phorbol esters and of acetic acid on mechanisms controlling DNA synthesis and mitosis (chalones) and on the biosynthesis of histidine-rich protein in mouse epidermis. *Cancer Res.*, ***34***, 135–146

Mufsan, R.A., Fischer, S.M., Verma, A.K., Gleason, G.L., Slaga, T.J. & Boutwell, R.K. (1979) Effects of 12-*O*-tetradecanoylphorbol-13-acetate and mezerein on epidermal ornithine decarboxylase activity, isoproterenol-stimulated levels of cyclic adenosine 3′:5′-monophosphate and induction of mouse skin tumors. *Cancer Res.*, ***39***, 4791–4795

Slaga, T.J. (1980) *Cancer: etiology, mechanisms, and prevention – A summary*. In: Slaga, T.J., ed., *Carcinogenesis*, Vol. 5, *Modifiers of Chemical Carcinogenesis*, New York, Raven Press, pp. 243–262

Slaga, T.J. & DiGiovanni, J. (1983) Inhibition of chemical carcinogenesis. *Am. chem. Soc. Monogr.* (in press)

Slaga, T.J., Klein-Szanto, A.J.P., Fischer, S.M., Weeks, C.E., Nelson, K. & Major, S. (1980a) Studies on the mechanism of action of anti-tumor-promoting agents: their specificity in two-stage promotion. *Proc. natl. Acad. Sci. USA*, ***77***, 2251–2255

Slaga, T.J., Fischer, S.M., Nelson, K. & Gleason, G.L. (1980b) Studies on the mechanism of skin tumor promotion: evidence for several stages of promotion. *Proc. natl Acad. Sci. USA*, ***77***, 3659–3663

Slaga, T.J., Fischer, S.M., Weeks, C.E., Klein-Szanto, A.J.P. & Reiners, J. (1982a) Studies on the mechanisms involved in multistage carcinogenesis in mouse skin. *J. cell. Biochem.*, ***18***, 99–119

Slaga, T.J., Fischer, S.M., Weeks, C.E., Nelson, K., Mamrack, M. & Klein-Szanto, A.J.P. (1982b) *Specificity and mechanism(s) of promoter inhibitors in multistage promotion.* In: Hecker, E., Fusenig, N.E., Kunz, W., Marks, F. & Thielmann, H.W., eds, *Carcinogenesis*, Vol. 7, *Cocarcinogenesis and Biological Effects of Tumor Promoters*, New York, Raven Press, pp. 19–34

Solanki, V., Rana, R.S. & Slaga, T.J. (1981) Diminution of mouse epidermal superoxide dismutase and catalase activities by tumor promoters. *Carcinogenesis*, ***2***, 1141–1146

Waltenberg, L.W. (1978) Inhibition of chemical carcinogenesis. *J. natl Cancer Inst.*, ***60***, 11–18

Weeks, C.E., Slaga, T.J., Hennings, H., Gleason, G.L. & Bracken, W.M. (1979) Inhibition of phorbol ester-induced tumor promotion by vitamin A analog and anti-inflammatory steroid. *J. natl Cancer Inst.*, ***63***, 401–406

# CONCLUDING REMARKS

# CONCLUDING REMARKS AND FUTURE PERSPECTIVES

E. HECKER

*Institute of Biochemistry, German Cancer Research Center, 6900 Heidelberg, Federal Republic of Germany*

The Symposium on the role of cocarcinogens and promoters in human and experimental carcinogenesis, held in Budapest from 16–18 May 1983, is the fourth in the series of international symposia on this topic. It followed the third, convened in Cincinnati, Ohio, USA (October 1981), the second, in Elmau Castle, Bavaria, Federal Republic of Germany (October 1980) and the first, held in Gatlinburg, Tennessee, USA (March 1977) (for corresponding proceedings, see Pereira, 1983; Hecker *et al.*, 1982; Slaga *et al.*, 1978). In Budapest, altogether 84 presentations were delivered; of these, 30 were invited lectures, 14 were proffered papers, and 40 were posters. It is a challenging task to summarize and review some of the fascinating features of amplification of carcinogenesis by non-carcinogens, i.e., of cocarcinogenesis in its broadest possible sense. The intention is not just to repeat comprehensively the more important presentations of this Symposium; rather, I will try to pinpoint the highlights of the papers given orally, and to discuss future trends. Contributions existing only as abstracts which were not presented orally are not included. The following remarks necessarily have a personal touch, in that they reflect the facts coloured to a certain extent by my individual outlook on the background of the present state of the art. Some of my statements are certainly controversial, and some are made in a somewhat provocative manner, with the deliberate intention of stimulating discussion and uncovering new experimental challenges. The reader is invited to discover the identities of those responsible for new advances by examining the proceedings in detail. The references appended relate to the more general aspects of carcinogenesis, especially of initiation/promotion, and to general aspects of risk assessment.

## COCARCINOGENESIS AND INITIATION/PROMOTION IN EXPERIMENTAL MODELS

To my coworkers and myself, and perhaps also to many other participants of this Symposium, it was gratifying to see that of all the contributions presented, no less than about half dealt in one way or another with initiation (or tumour) promoters of the diterpene ester type, which are most frequently represented by 12-*O*-tetradecanoylphorbol-13-acetate (TPA), sometimes also called phorbol-myristate-acetate (PMA).

*Diterpene ester type and similar irritant promoters*

Diterpene ester irritants continue to be used on a wide scale as biochemical and biological tools in efforts to define operationally and to analyse in depth the complexity of the sequence of events of carcinogenesis, not only in stages such as initiation and promotion, but – as a recent trend – also in progression (see Hecker, this volume, especially Fig. 4).

*Skin as the target tissue:* Evidence was presented which revealed the appearance of skin tumours after TPA treatment of $F_1$ and $F_2$ descendants of mice exposed during pregnancy to a single intravenous dose of 7,12-dimethylbenz[*a*]anthracene (DMBA). These data show how the general idea that prenatal exposure to low doses of solitary carcinogens may result in an increase in the risk of cancer in the liters can be verified also in the initiation/promotion protocol by the use of an appropriate promoter.

In a report on the class of (complete) cocarcinogens of the diterpene ester type, structure/activity relations were extended by a set of semisynthetic 3-*O*-acylesters of ingenol. Of these, 3-*O*-tetradecanoylingenol (3-TI) was shown to be about as active as TPA, both as a mouse skin irritant and as an initiation-promoter. In a continuation of previous trials to subdivide the promotional stage of initiation/promotion in mouse skin (using croton oil combined with turpentine or, more recently, TPA combined with mezerein), a combination of TPA with its new semisynthetic and very labile retinoic acid analogue, 12-*O*-retinoylphorbol-13-acetate (RPA), was evaluated. It was already known from structure/activity investigations of many other esters of diterpenes carrying unsaturated acyl residues that irritant and hyperplasiogenic (mitogenic) properties are necessary yet insufficient prerequisites for a compound to be a complete promoter of initiation. The semisynthetic RPA is also highly irritant and hyperplasiogenic to the skin of NMRI mice but practically inactive as a promoter, whereas mezerein, which had been previously proposed as a so-called 'second stage promoter', is definitely a weak promoter. In the experimental protocol presented for NMRI mice (DMBA/TPA/RPA), it was shown that, following the initiator dose, only one (or at the most two) single dose(s) of TPA (promotional stage P I) is sufficient to elicit tumours when followed by multiple doses of RPA (promotional stage P II). When, in otherwise identical protocols, administration of TPA was omitted, very few tumours, if any, were elicited. RPA appears to be the best 'second stage' or 'stage P II promoter' known at present. In stage P I, evidently *specific* molecular event(s), which are necessary and sufficient for initiated cells to be promoted in P II by a less specific and, *per se,* insufficient irritant and hyperplasiogen such as RPA, take place. In experiments in which intervals of some weeks are inserted between the promotional stages P I and P II, the specific cellular (and molecular) events induced by TPA in P I were claimed to be slowly reversible ('memory effect'). Since the clinician Rudolf Virchow drew attention to a general etiological role of chronic inflammation in carcinogenesis, apparently on the basis of rather unspecific properties such as irritation and hyperplasiogenicity, a specific element, long-suspected but often denied, now appears to be established operationally in promotion. The $G_2$-inhibitor of the cell cycle, hydroxyurea, administered together with TPA during stage P I was shown to inhibit tumour formation in P II, i.e., by the subsequent protocol of RPA administration. Thus, it appears that critical interaction of the complete promoter TPA with initiated cells takes place in their S- or $G_1$-phases. It would be premature, however, to conclude from the 'memory effect' of TPA that the specific biological events induced in P I are qualitatively identical with the irreversible events induced by initiators (see also below).

Experimental data obtained *in vitro* on the new skin irritants and promoters of the indole type (dihydroteleocidin B, lyngbyatoxin A) and of the polyacetate type (debromoaplysiatoxin), which are not related structurally either to TPA or to its congeners, were reported in several presentations. Qualitatively, their actions appear to be identical with effects achieved under comparable conditions with diterpene ester type irritants and promoters; quantitative differences are obvious.

*Non-skin target tissue:* A number of papers reported systemic effects of diterpene ester-type promoters after topical administration to groups of mice, since this route of administration necessarily induces (mutual) licking activities as a (relatively undefined) means of systemic administration. It was previously shown that, in this way, a considerable dose of TPA enters the experimental animal by the oral route, although the actual dose of TPA taken up is not precisely known. It was therefore good to see, for the first time, that, besides the well-established administration of TPA by stomach tube or by intraperitoneal injection of low doses, it is also possible to administer TPA in drinking-water. In mice, uptake of TPA from drinking-water after initiation with 1,2-dimethylhydrazine revealed a new and important initiation/promotion model in which the colon is the target tissue.

*Host immune system, differentiating cells and viral genomes as targets:* It is important to investigate not only the target cells of any particular organ involved directly in carcinogenesis but also cells in additional compartments (e.g., blood, lymph), since they too may be involved indirectly in an extensive multistage process. Reports on activation and/or inhibition by diterpene ester-type promoters of macrophages, natural killer cells and B- and T-lymphocytes, which included some apparently conflicting data, ranged widely over this field. The doses of promoters used and/or the particular conditions under which target cells responded – either by activation or by inhibition – deserve further investigation, especially with regard to the corresponding situation *in vivo*. At first, stimulatory effects on the immune defense system of TPA and its congeners might theoretically appear to be incompatible with their promoting activity, in contrast to inhibition of macrophage and natural killer cell tumoricidal activities, also demonstrated *in vitro*. With respect to the adverse effects induced by diterpene ester-type promoters in immune competent cells, the present situation appears somewhat similar to that prevailing in certain other target cells with regard to induction or inhibition of differentiation. TPA and other diterpene esters may exhibit either one of these effects (e.g., induction of mitosis *versus* formation of differentiated 'dark cells' by TPA in basal cells of adult mouse epidermis; in contrast, epidermal cells of the baby mouse do not respond). These effects appear to depend on the properties and/or the status of the particular cells and/or tissues exposed.

Some years ago, the stimulation of virus synthesis *in vitro* by diterpene ester-type promoters in 'non-producer' lymphoblastoid cells carrying latent Epstein-Barr virus (EBV) genomes was reported. During the symposium, it was shown that a platelet-derived serum factor, not yet fully characterized, may induce expression of latent EBV information in a manner similar to TPA. In addition, a few other host-related endogenous factors that either mimic or inhibit TPA activity were described. It is tempting to speculate that such factors represent normal endogenous regulatory principles (e.g., certain hormones). Accordingly, these may become involved in the promotion of initiated cells; therefore, their investigation deserves special attention (see also below). In the skin of the multimammate mouse, *Mastomys natalensis,* the low spontaneous rate and yield of skin tumours may be increased by topical administration of TPA. In both spontaneous and TPA-induced tumours, expression of latent DNA-tumour viral genomes (papilloma virus) was detected. Such expression was not seen in normal parts of the skin of *Mastomys.* This is one of the first in-vivo tumour model systems that allows for a direct correlation of stimulation of expression of latent viral genomes by a diterpene ester-type promoter with an increase in tumour generation. While, until recently, latent RNA-tumour virus appeared to be largely refractory to stimulation by diterpene ester-type promoters, it was shown in three chronically-infected human cell types that TPA or teleocidin stimulates synthesis of primate retroviruses in a transient manner.

*Molecular mechanisms of action:* In mouse skin carcinogenesis, the stages of initiation and promotion (and, to a lesser extent, that of progression) are satisfactorily defined operationally (Hecker, this volume, Figs 2 and 4), and may be subdivided further (promotional stages P I, P II). Mechanistically, i.e., with respect to the relevant biochemical mechanisms involved, all the stages still have to be considered essentially as 'black boxes'. Information may be obtained by investigating target cell systems, primarily *in vitro,* while maintaining close connection with the situation *in vivo* (e.g., by using isogeneic cells *in vitro* and by controlling their capabilities *in vivo* by transplantation back into the whole organism). It was gratifying to see that close controls of this kind were carefully exercised by many of those who used cell cultures *in vitro* in mechanistic investigations.

*Initiation:* No doubt, the key to promotion is still held by the elusive 'initiated cell' or 'potential tumour cell' (Hecker, this volume, Fig. 4). In contrast with surrounding normal cells, the initiated cell must have acquired a unique susceptibility to promoters, i.e., it can grow preferentially and form tumours. A utopian goal of biochemists in the field, namely, to generate sufficient quantities of 'initiated' cells of identical properties *in vitro* by transformation of 'normal cells' with chemical carcinogens and to clone them, was achieved to some extent by the late Charles Heidelberger and his co-workers, using 3T3 and 10T ½ fibroblasts. Cultures of mouse epidermal cells are more closely related to the mouse skin model *in vivo.* A tedious period of trial and error has at last been rewarded by showing that these cells can be maintained and propagated by carefully controlling the calcium concentration of the medium. Manipulation of the media permits reliable exposure of the cultured cells to initiators and promoters when required. Yet the biochemical and molecular differences between 'initiated' epidermal cells and their 'normal' counterparts remain to be elucidated. First experiments towards the solution of this key problem were reported in C3H 10T½ cell lines using the oncogene approach. With a probe homologous to the long terminal repeat (LTR) sequence of Moloney murine sarcoma virus, it was found that cells transformed either by solitary chemical carcinogens or by radiation express a series of RNAs containing LTR sequences that are not present in untreated 10T½ cells. Similar RNA transcripts were also detected in tumour cells induced in intact rodents with solitary chemical carcinogens. Evidence was obtained suggesting that the expression of the RNAs of transformed cells reflects alterations in DNA methylation. Furthermore, in a cell line derived from a mouse myeloma (MOPC 21) originally induced by mineral oil, a sequence rearrangement and amplification of the cellular oncogene c-mos was detected. These and other findings suggest that *carcinogenesis* as a whole may involve diverse molecular changes in both cellular LTR and oncogene sequences. What correlation these and other similar molecular changes have with *initiation* (or, alternatively, with promotion) remains to be seen.

In all the in-vitro systems employing solitary chemical carcinogens as initiators, the metabolism of these compounds, and hence the chemical identity of the 'ultimate' initiator as the molecular entity interacting with the cellular genome, surprisingly has not been considered.

*Promotion:* The true target cells of promoters are 'initiated' cells surrounded by 'normal cells' of the target tissue. Because of their availability, normal cells are usually employed to answer basic questions regarding the biochemical mechanism of promotion. Interpretation of studies of this kind is, of course, burdened by the unproven postulate that both normal and initiated cells, in mechanistic terms, respond to promoters in a similar manner.

Primary molecular targets for diterpene ester-type promoters are membrane-associated specific binding sites, often called 'receptors'. Their existence was indicated by many structure/activity investigations *in vivo,* especially by the finding that phorbol-12,13-dipropionate, a non-promoter, can effectively inhibit promotion of mouse skin by TPA. In-vitro studies showed that a certain proportion of the overall binding to membrane fractions of phorbol-12,13-dipropionate, and likewise of the dibutyrate, is partly highly specific. Thus, inhibition of specific binding of labelled phorbol-12,13-dipropionate, -dibutyrate or TPA to membranes by diterpene ester-type promoters, and also by teleocidins, lyngbyatoxin and aplysiatoxin, may be used as a quick and quantitative measure of agonist-receptor affinity. However, an unequivocal and consistent correlation between biological activities *in vivo,* especially irritant and promoting activities, and inhibition of specific binding does not exist, e.g., the binding constant of RPA is only slightly lower than that of TPA. During the Symposium, evidence was presented that besides specific membrane-associated receptors for phorbol esters specific cytosolic receptors with similar binding characteristics also exist. The putative endogenous agonist(s) of these receptors (e.g., certain hormones, see above) have not yet been identified.

Various groups reported experiments aimed at clarifying the biochemical nature of specific membrane-associated receptors by photoaffinity labelling. Tritiated phorbol esters carrying diverse photoaffinity-labelled ester moieties were employed, as well as, in one report, direct photoactivation of [20-$^{3}$H]-TPA. Phosphatidyl serine and phosphatidyl ethanolamine, but no protein, were found to be mainly and most consistently labelled by the photoaffinity probes. These findings support the proposition that protein kinase C, known to require the presence of both phospholipid (phosphatidyl serine) and calcium for activity, is one of the most likely candidates for a membrane-associated promoter receptor. Supporting evidence may be adduced from the reported competitive inhibition of phorbol-12,13-dibutyrate binding to specific cytosolic receptors by diglycerides (e.g., 1,2-diolein), but at high doses corresponding to low affinity on the part of the diglyceride. Thus, phorbol esters might be considered exogenous analogues of diglycerides; this would not explain fully the specific component of their promoting activity. Further progress in this area obviously requires the isolation and characterization of the pure receptor protein(s) involved. It would be useful to see whether different receptors trigger the various biochemical cascades induced by phorbol esters (such as protein phosphorylation and prostaglandin synthesis), or whether they all have a common receptor. Furthermore, it remains to be seen if any one of the biochemical cascades triggered by phorbol esters is indeed associated with 'regulator gene amplification' and/or with 'gene transposition', as putative, and perhaps specific, key elements of promotion. Perhaps the stage P I in skin promotion is a good candidate for more detailed mechanistic investigations of this kind.

In this context, it was relevant that some lines of the mouse epidermal cell strain JB 6 respond to TPA and gain anchorage independence and malignancy (P+), while others fail to respond (P−). These lines can be used to search for biochemical membrane-associated differences: indeed (P+) cells were found to lack stimulated hexose transport, epidermal growth factor-receptor binding and susceptibility to mitogenic stimulation. Surprisingly, (P−) cells contained specific phorbol ester receptors; it was assumed that these do not control those biochemical functions required for manifestation of neoplastic transformation, but rather other basic cellular functions. In all (P+) cells tested, but in none of the (P−) cell lines, a decrease in the synthesis of plasma membrane trisialoganglioside is induced by TPA. Another event possibly involved in the promotion of in-vitro transformed cells appears to be a specific loss of collagen synthesis associated with a deficiency of translatable and hybridizable collagen m-RNA, as shown in (P−) cells. Most interestingly, it was shown that (P+) properties can be transfected into (P−) cells by isolated and purified (P+) DNA.

Previous metabolic and recent receptor binding studies of TPA have revealed that this molecule itself is most likely identical with what might be called an 'ultimate promoter'. Therefore, the problem of metabolic activation and deactivation of diterpene ester-type promoters, which is relevant in 'cryptic' promoters of this type, was neglected in the investigations reported.

*Progression:* In earlier trials, induction of progression *in vivo* was accomplished by administering a single small dose of an initiator at a late stage of skin tumour promotion (see Hecker, this volume, Fig. 4). It was noticed that similar effects can also be seen using epidermal cell cultures with controlled concentrations of calcium. The classical key problem of carcinogenesis at the cell level, i.e., whether the phenotype of the 'malignant' tumour (cancer) cell originates exclusively from cells of 'benign' tumour cells derived ultimately from a singular type of 'initiated cell', or whether there are two different types of 'initiated cells' from the outset with different genetic programmes expressing the benign or the malignant phenotype, respectively, could not be resolved against the background of controversial data presented during the Symposium.

It would be desirable if, in the epidermal model, biochemical markers could be established for initiation, for promotion (specifically for the operationally defined stages P I and P II) and for progression. The in-vitro and in-vivo data presently available on solitary carcinogen-induced initiation of epidermal cells and on their diterpene ester-induced promotion may suggest that critical biochemical events take place in both cases at the level of the gene(s). If this should be finally confirmed, it must be kept in mind that in-vivo initiation and promotion are clearly separable in time, and that chronic administration of a promoter alone does not produce tumours, always providing that the host target tissues have not previously been exposed to uncontrolled initiation (target tissue predisposition). Furthermore, metabolites of solitary carcinogens, e.g., of DMBA, considered to be 'proximate' or 'ultimate' initiators were shown to be mutagenic in bacteria and yeasts, whereas TPA and other diterpene ester-type 'ultimate promoters' (as well as other promoters of other organs; see below) are non-mutagenic in microorganisms. Therefore, if events critical for promotion take place at the gene level, in all likelihood they may be expected to be different *qualitatively* from those of initiators. In other words, initiators may cause irreversible alterations to genetic information contained in structural or regulatory genes, while promoters may alter the expression of genetic information by perhaps reversible alterations of regulatory genes such as activation, amplification or transposition. It would seem premature (e.g., IARC 1983) to separate genetic (initiation) from epigenetic (promotion) effects as principal mechanistic alternatives, and especially to draw up guidelines for legislatory action on such grounds, e.g., in environmental protection (Marshall, 1982; see also Albert, 1983; Benbrook, 1983; Todhunter, 1983; Weinstein, 1983).

### *Other promoters and their target tissues*

Some of the initiation/promotion/progression models that involve promoters other than those of the diterpene ester type and their target tissues still require definition of their operational stages. Progress in examining aspects of metabolism ('ultimate' initiators and promoters) and/or molecular mechanisms of action of 'ultimate forms' will necessarily follow. Yet, important conclusions relevant to risk assessment in human cancer can already be drawn. For example, several reports made during the Symposium further extended the list of environmental compounds with established promoting activity in liver and bladder. One report confirmed the role of alcohol in liver primarily as a stimulator rather than as a promoter of initiation, as already documented for other target tissues, e.g., oesophagus. (For typical alternative protocols of cocarcinogenesis illustrating such differences see Hecker, this volume, Fig. 2). Similarly, as already known in skin and in rat liver carcinogenesis, administration of initiators late in the promotional stage may give rise to an increase in the incidence of malignancy, as seen by the formation of secondary foci and microcarcinoma within precancerous liver lesions ('progressor'; see Hecker, this volume, Fig. 4). The problem of identifying unequivocally the existence of marker enzymes for the various stages of carcinogenesis in liver is being explored by extended measurements of enzyme patterns in liver foci and by examining the glycogen storage phenomenon. The identification of the 'ultimate molecular forms', i.e., of those molecular entities that undergo *critical* interaction with cellular targets in initiation, promotion and progression, and the targets themselves still needs more attention. Significant contributions to the metabolic aspects of the mechanism of action of promoters in liver included studies of the role of the cytochrome P-450 system.

The initiation/promotion/progression model classically of mouse skin has provided and continues to provide a most useful analogy for the experimental study of defined stages of carcinogenesis using initiators, promoters and progressors in non-epidermal tissues. However, it should be kept in mind that, by contrast with epidermal cells, other target cells such as hepatocytes represent stationary tissues. Therefore, the basic physiological machinery critical for carcinogenesis may be expected in these cells to show crucial differences from that, say, of epidermal cells. Hence, for analogous stages in the two different types of target cell, a simple common biochemical (molecular) denominator may not exist; most likely, the biochemical events underlying the operationally-defined stages of initiation, promotion and progression are more complicated than mere individual biochemical pathways. All in all, there is good reason to believe that different types of target cells need to take biochemically differing roads in order to become corresponding cancer cells, even if the individual roads can be divided up into apparently similar stretches.

It is gratifying that, after a lengthy descriptive period which started with skin and was followed by other target tissues, several experimental models now appear to be developed to the extent that the hitherto unsolved biochemical (mechanistic) issues of initiation, promotion and even perhaps of progression are becoming tractable. Although the hypothesis of somatic gene mutation was postulated by K.H. Bauer in 1926, it is only now that staging in experimental models and refinement of biochemical and molecular biological techniques are sufficiently developed that, looking to the future, experimental challenges at the gene level of this crucial hypothesis are becoming feasible.

## COCARCINOGENESIS AND INITIATION/PROMOTION IN RISK ASSESSMENT OF CANCER AND IN HUMAN CARCINOGENESIS

Established mechanisms of action of solitary carcinogens and cocarcinogens, especially promoters, will no doubt provide the *ultimate* criteria for assessment of the risk imposed on the human environment by these carcinogenic risk factors. Especially, such criteria will suggest leads also for appropriate short-term assays. However, risk assessment can hardly wait until the detailed mechanistic aspects of carcinogenesis at the cell and/or the molecular level have been explored. Therefore, at the present stage, it appears appropriate to use certain of the descriptive (empirical) criteria of dose/time-effect relationships in risk assessment that are already available, such as the putative irreversibility of action of solitary carcinogens *versus* the putative reversibility of action of cocarcinogens, especially promoters, as proposed and illustrated in a report during this Symposium.

*Experimental and epidemiological models and risk assessment*

Protocols of solitary carcinogenesis and of cocarcinogenesis in terms of initiation/promotion were analysed regarding the dose/time-effect relationships in focus formation of rat liver using the empirical log/log approach (see Hecker, this volume). Different relationships appear to exist for solitary carcinogenesis and for cocarcinogenesis of the initiation/promotion type, demonstrating the existence of thresholds for promoters. Similar relationships were shown to be valid for the classical initiation/promotion mouse skin model using DMBA/TPA. The proposed approach may turn out to be useful for distinguishing solitary carcinogens from cocarcinogens of the promoter type in whole animal assays. This possibility has still to be tested with many more promoters in various tissues and in combination with various initiators. Confirmation of the possibility would provide a sound basis for risk assessment of promoters in whole-animal testing. Short-term testing will have to await clarification of the mechanistic details of promotion (see below).

During the Symposium, the progress made in establishing stages in the development of human cancers was illustrated impressively by analyses of epidemiological data according to mathematical procedures. Reports were presented to suggest multiple stages in carcinogenesis involving exposure to cigarette smoking, ionizing radiation, asbestos, nickel, sunlight, sex hormones and unidentified endogenous risk factors (hereditary tumours). It was pointed out in many discussions that experimental models of carcinogenesis, primarily designed to answer mechanistic questions, cannot generally be considered optimal models also for risk assessments of carcinogenesis in comparable etiological situations for man. With this aim in mind, future experimental designs should allow more specifically for a particular etiological situation, for example, by employing non-conditioned experimental animals such as pets rather than conditioned (e.g., specific pathogen-free) experimental animals.

The epidemiological presentations stimulated discussion between epidemiologists and experimentalists on the precise meaning of the terminology they use: it was pointed out that the meanings of such terms as 'initiation', 'promotion' and 'progression' are not precisely the same when used in connection with epidemiological and with experimental models; only in the latter case do they reflect well-defined dose/time-effect relationships including mechanistic implications. In epidemiological models, which necessarily involve vague dose/time-effect relationships, it might be preferable to use terms that have merely descriptional (empirical) meanings, including etiological implications; e.g., instead of 'initiator', 'subcarcinogenic exposure to a solitary carcinogen', and instead of 'promoter', 'cocarcinogen' (see, for example, Higginson, 1979; Hecker, this volume). It was suggested that terms such as 'initiator', 'promoter' and 'progressor' be reserved exclusively for use in connection with experimental models with their well-defined dose/time-effect relationships. The problems dealt with in the discussion were reminiscent of considerations made several years ago and reflected in a proposal for a revised, concise terminology in carcinogenesis, which was made in response to a request from the Committee of International Collaborative Activities of the UICC (Hecker, 1976a–d, 1981, 1984a,b). In discussions during the Symposium, it became clear that the terminology problem raised is far more than one of pure semantics, and that its clarification would be of considerable heuristic value; efforts at a solution of the problem should be made at an international level, so as to promote better mutual understanding between epidemiologists and experimentalists, and also between scientists and legislators. It was considered a gratifying task for an international agency to stimulate and catalyse worldwide mutual understanding, active partnership and cooperation between experimentalists, epidemiologists and legislators for the improvement of standards of risk assessment in human cancers (see, for example, IARC, 1983).

Examples of mutual exchange between epidemiological and experimental investigations were given during the Symposium with regard to oesophageal cancers associated with 'lifestyle' high-risk areas of north-eastern Iran and of the Caribbean island of Curaçao.

In Iran, the high risk appears to be associated with the habit of smoking opium and with the ingestion of opium pyrolysates. These materials were shown to be mutagenic in bacteria. In long-term experiments using female $CD_1$ mice, no solitary carcinogenic activity was detected after administering high doses of pyrolysates of crude opium, of morphine and of '*sukhteh*' (extract of opium dross). However, in an initiation/promotion protocol with TPA as promoter, initiating activity was demonstrated by a relatively high dose of morphine. Transforming activity was observed for crude opium, morphine and *sukhteh* in Syrian hamster embryo cells but not in mouse C3H 10T½ cells.

In Curaçao, epidemiological investigations had revealed that the black and Creole population of the island habitually consumes a great variety of plant preparations and especially large amounts of a 'bush tea' made from the leaves of the indigenous bush *Croton flavens* L. (*welensali*). Also, persons at risk on Curaçao were most likely exposed at times to initiators of the polycyclic aromatic hydrocarbon type from a certain supply of drinking-water. The *welensali* leaves and the tea, the preparation used most frequently on Curaçao, were shown experimentally to contain a multitude of factors, F and F′ ('cryptic' forms of F), which were irritant and initiating-promoting in mouse skin. The compounds were isolated and characterized as diterpene esters of the tigliane type and turned out to be structurally related to, but not identical with, TPA. It was estimated that one cup of *welensali* tea contains a mixture of factors F in an amount equivalent to about ten times the irritant dose 50 of *welensali* factor F′ of leaves. The amount of *welensali* factors F′ present in one cup was estimated to be equivalent to slightly more than the irritant dose 50 of the F′-20-decanoate in the leaves. These amounts of *welensali* factors are more than sufficient to maintain chronic irritation of the human oesophagus. The pattern of events is illustrated by the following animal experiment: mice exposed to an initiation/promotion protocol by stomach tube with DMBA/TPA (and also with other initiators) have been shown to develop tumours of the forestomach. The investigation in Curaçao provides a strong case, and indeed the first of its kind, in which well-defined cocarcinogens of the promoter type are the principal carcinogenic risk factors in a particular form of human cancer.

## *Short-term assays in risk assessment* in vitro *and* in vivo

The detection of solitary carcinogenic activity and, hence, of initiators in the human environment by means of relatively inexpensive short-term tests of mutagenic activity, using a battery of appropriate target cells, from bacteria to man, with or without addition of activating enzymes, is widely considered to be a useful though by no means an ideal tool. At the least, such testing may help to select from the bulk of compounds those that give negative results in a relatively quick, inexpensive and fairly reliable first round. Compounds that react positively should be submitted to long-term animal testing for solitary carcinogenic activity in a second and more expensive round. This approach was illustrated during the Symposium by results of mutagenicity assays *in vitro* of agricultural chemicals and their possible contaminants (herbicides, pesticides, nitrite, nitrate). Yet, short-term assay systems related more directly to mammalian carcinogenesis, e.g., for testing initiation instead of mutation, are still very much needed. In this respect, an in-vivo initiation/promotion system using rat liver for detecting the initiators *N*-nitrosodiethylamine and benzo[*a*]pyrene, followed by a standard diet containing the promoter phenobarbital, was described. Hopes were expressed that this assay system would be capable of detecting *any* initiating and, hence, solitary carcinogenic activity within six to eight weeks, independent of the organotropy of the specific solitary carcinogen tested. The validity of this short-term assay system remains to be demonstrated in many more tests of solitary carcinogens.

As far as tests permit, the conclusion can be drawn that promoters are generally non-mutagenic. Yet, short-term testing for promoting activity of compounds occurring in the human environment is still at a trial-and-error phase, as a number of reports using various criteria, e.g., modulation of intracellular communication by promoters, show. Except in the case of diterpene ester-type promoters, it appears unclear at present whether or not promoters exhibit tissue specificity on their own, and to what extent organotropy is determined primarily by corresponding initiators. Moreover, it appears difficult at the present time to perceive a common cellular or biochemical denominator for all kinds of promoters, the chemical identities of which range from diterpene esters to phenobarbital and saccharin. At the present time, this area is a 'hot spot' in cancer research, because more information is urgently needed to indicate the criteria by which short-term assays should be set up in order to evaluate those environmental promoters that are already known (see, for example, Marshall, 1982; IARC, 1983).

## EPILOGUE

The Symposium has illustrated the availability of a number of experimental and epidemiological models, with which multistage carcinogenesis can be investigated on a broad scale. Studies on most experimental models have already made large contributions to the goals of defining and understanding component stages and, hence, etiologies and mechanism(s) of carcinogenesis. Some of the experimental and epidemiological findings reported may provide important clues for the identification of environmental risk factors and for the assessment of the corresponding risk of cancer in man.

Last but not least, and on behalf of all the participants, it is indeed a great pleasure to express our most sincere gratitude to all those who have made this remarkable

Symposium possible. Our thanks go not only to Professor Dr M. Börzsönyi and his many helpers of the congress secretariat, but also to the members of the international programme committee as well as to all the sponsors, especially to the International Agency for Research on Cancer (Dr L. Tomatis, Director) and to the Hungarian Cancer Society (Professor K. Lapis, President). They all did their best to make this, the fourth Symposium in the series of international symposia covering the topic of cocarcinogenesis and tumour promotion, another scientific and social success. Grateful thanks are due to everybody who contributed to this important event.

## REFERENCES

Albert, R.E. (1983) Carcinogen policy at EPA. *Science*, ***219***, 796–798

Benbrook, C.M. (1983) Carcinogen policy at EPA. *Science*, ***219***, 798

Hecker, E. (1976a) Definitions and terminology in cancer (tumor) etiology – an analysis aiming at proposals for a current internationally standardized terminology. *Int. J. Cancer*, ***18***, 122–129

Hecker, E. (1976b) Definitions and terminology in cancer (tumor) etiology – an analysis aiming at proposals for a current internationally standardized terminology. *Z. Krebsforsch.*, ***86***, 219–230

Hecker, E. (1976c) Definitions and terminology in cancer (tumor) etiology – an analysis aiming at proposals for a current internationally standardized terminology. *Gann*, ***67***, 471–481

Hecker, E. (1976d) Definitions and terminology in cancer (tumor) etiology – an analysis aiming at proposals for a current internationally standardized terminology. *Bull. World Health Organ.*, ***54***, 1–10

Hecker, E. (1981) Cocarcinogenesis and tumor promoters of the diterpene ester type as possible carcinogenic risk factors. *J. Cancer Res. clin. Oncol.*, ***99***, 103–124

Hecker, E. (1984a) Co-carcinogens of the initiation- (or tumor) promoter type as environmental risk factors of cancer in man — experimental analysis of an etiological model situation of life style cancer and current problems of assessment of cancer risk in multifactorial carcinogenesis. *Acta pharmacol. toxikol.*, Suppl. (in press)

Hecker, E. (1984b) *Multifaktorielle und Mehrstufen-Karzinogenese — Ätiologische und experimentelle Modelle sowie aktuelle Schlüsselprobleme für die Bewertung von Krebsrisikofactoren der Umwelt, Eröffnungsvortrag Expertengespräch 'Tumorpromotoren: Erkennung, Wirkungsmechanismen und Bedeutung'*. In: *Bundesgesundheitsamt, Max-von-Pettenkofer-Institut, 6–7 February 1984* (in press)

Hecker, E., Fusenig, N.E., Kunz, W., Marks, F. & Thielmann, H.W., eds (1982) *Carcinogenesis – A Comprehensive Survey*, Vol. 7, *Cocarcinogenesis and Biological Effects of Tumor Promoters*, New York, Raven Press

Higginson, J. (1979) *Environmental carcinogenesis: A global perspective*. In: Emmelot, P. & Kriek, E., eds, *Environmental Carcinogenesis: Occurrence, Risk Evaluation and Mechanisms*, Amsterdam, Elsevier/North-Holland Biomedical Press, pp. 9–22

IARC (1983) *Approaches to Classifying Chemical Carcinogens According to Mechanism of Action* (*IARC int. tech. Rep., No. 83/001*), Lyon, International Agency for Research on Cancer

Marshall, E. (1982) EPA's high risk carcinogen policy. *Science,* ***218,*** 975–978

Pereira, M.A., ed. (1983) Tumor Promotion. *Environ. Health Perspect.,* ***50***

Slaga, T.J., Sivak, A. & Boutwell, R.K., eds (1978) *Carcinogenesis,* Vol. 2, *Mechanisms of Tumor Promotion and Cocarcinogenesis,* New York, Raven Press

Todhunter, J.A. (1983) Carcinogen policy at EPA. *Science,* ***219,*** 794

Weinstein, I.B. (1983) Carcinogen policy at EPA. *Science,* ***219,*** 794–796

# AUTHOR INDEX

# SUBJECT INDEX

## IARC SCIENTIFIC PUBLICATIONS

Available from Oxford University Press, Walton Street, Oxford OX2 6DP, UK and in London, New York, Toronto, Delhi, Bombay, Calcutta, Madras, Karachi, Kuala Lumpur, Singapore, Hong Kong, Tokyo, Nairobi, Dar es Salaam, Cape Town, Melbourne, Auckland and associated companies in Beirut, Berlin, Ibadan, Mexico City, Nicosia.

| | |
|---|---|
| Liver Cancer | No. 1, 1971; 176 pages<br>£10 |
| Oncogenesis and Herpesviruses | No. 2, 1972; 515 pages<br>£30 |
| *N*-Nitroso Compounds, Analysis and Formation | No. 3, 1972; 140 pages<br>£8.50 |
| Transplacental Carcinogenesis | No. 4, 1973; 181 pages<br>£11.95 |
| Pathology of Tumours in Laboratory Animals—Volume I—Tumours of the Rat, Part 1 | No. 5, 1973; 214 pages<br>£17.50 |
| Pathology of Tumours in Laboratory Animals—Volume I—Tumours of the Rat, Part 2 | No. 6, 1976; 319 pages<br>(out of print) |
| Host Environment Interactions in the Etiology of Cancer in Man | No. 7, 1973; 464 pages<br>£30 |
| Biological Effects of Asbestos | No. 8, 1973; 346 pages<br>£25 |
| *N*-Nitroso Compounds in the Environment | No. 9, 1974; 243 pages<br>£15 |
| Chemical Carcinogenesis Essays | No. 10, 1974; 230 pages<br>£15 |
| Oncogenesis and Herpesviruses II | No. 11, 1975;<br>Part 1, 511 pages<br>£30<br>Part 2, 403 pages<br>£30 |
| Screening Tests in Chemical Carcinogenesis | No. 12, 1976; 666 pages<br>(out of print) |
| Environmental Pollution and Carcinogenic Risks | No. 13, 1976; 454 pages<br>£17.50 |
| Environmental *N*-Nitroso Compounds—Analysis and Formation | No. 14, 1976; 512 pages<br>£35 |
| Cancer Incidence in Five Continents—Volume III | No. 15, 1976; 584 pages<br>£35 |
| Air Pollution and Cancer in Man | No. 16, 1977; 331 pages<br>£30 |
| Directory of On-Going Research in Cancer Epidemiology 1977 | No. 17, 1977; 599 pages<br>(out of print) |
| Environmental Carcinogens—Selected Methods of Analysis, Vol. 1: Analysis of Volatile Nitrosamines in Food | No. 18, 1978; 212 pages<br>£30 |
| Environmental Aspects of *N*-Nitroso Compounds | No. 19, 1978; 566 pages<br>£35 |
| Nasopharyngeal Carcinoma: Etiology and Control | No. 20, 1978; 610 pages<br>£35 |
| Cancer Registration and Its Techniques | No. 21, 1978; 235 pages<br>£11.95 |
| Environmental Carcinogens—Selected Methods of Analysis, Vol. 2: Methods for the Measurement of Vinyl Chloride in Poly(vinyl chloride), Air, Water and Foodstuffs | No. 22, 1978; 142 pages<br>£35 |
| Pathology of Tumours in Laboratory Animals—Volume II—Tumours of the Mouse | No. 23, 1979; 669 pages<br>£35 |
| Oncogenesis and Herpesviruses III | No. 24, 1978;<br>Part 1, 580 pages<br>£20<br>Part 2, 522 pages<br>£20 |
| Carcinogenic Risks—Strategies for Intervention | No. 25, 1979; 283 pages<br>£20 |
| Directory of On-Going Research in Cancer Epidemiology 1978 | No. 26, 1978; 550 pages<br>£10 |
| Molecular and Cellular Aspects of Carcinogen Screening Tests | No. 27, 1980; 371 pages<br>£20 |
| Directory of On-Going Research in Cancer Epidemiology 1979 | No. 28, 1979; 672 pages<br>(out of print) |
| Environmental Carcinogens—Selected Methods of Analysis, Vol. 3: Analysis of Polycyclic Aromatic Hydrocarbons in Environmental Samples | No. 29, 1979; 240 pages<br>£17.50 |
| Biological Effects of Mineral Fibres | No. 30, 1980;<br>Volume 1, 494 pages<br>£25<br>Volume 2, 513 pages<br>£25 |
| *N*-Nitroso Compounds: Analysis, Formation and Occurrence | No. 31, 1980; 841 pages<br>£30 |
| Statistical Methods in Cancer Research, Vol. 1: The Analysis of Case-Control Studies | No. 32, 1980; 338 pages<br>£17.50 |
| Handling Chemical Carcinogens in the Laboratory—Problems of Safety | No. 33, 1979; 32 pages<br>£3.95 |
| Pathology of Tumours in Laboratory Animals—Volume III—Tumours of the Hamster | No. 34, 1982; 461 pages<br>£30 |
| Directory of On-Going Research in Cancer Epidemiology 1980 | No. 35, 1980; 660 pages<br>£10 |
| Cancer Mortality by Occupation and Social Class 1851–1971 | No. 36, 1982; 253 pages<br>£20 |
| Laboratory Decontamination and Destruction of Aflatoxins $B_1$, $B_2$, $G_1$, $G_2$ in Laboratory Wastes | No. 37, 1980; 59 pages<br>£5.95 |
| Directory of On-Going Research in Cancer Epidemiology 1981 | No. 38, 1981; 696 pages<br>£12.50 |
| Host Factors in Human Carcinogenesis | No. 39, 1982; 583 pages<br>£35 |
| Environmental Carcinogens—Selected Methods of Analysis, Vol. 4: Some Aromatic Amines and Azo Dyes in the General and Industrial Environment | No. 40, 1981; 347 pages<br>£20 |
| *N*-Nitroso Compounds: Occurrence and Biological Effects | No. 41, 1982; 755 pages<br>£35 |
| Cancer Incidence in Five Continents—Volume IV | No. 42, 1982; 811 pages<br>£35 |

| | |
|---|---|
| Laboratory Decontamination and Destruction of Carcinogens in Laboratory Wastes: Some *N*-Nitrosamines | No. 43, 1982; 73 pages £6.50 |
| Environmental Carcinogens—Selected Methods of Analysis, Vol. 5: Mycotoxins | No. 44, 1983; 455 pages £20 |
| Environmental Carcinogens—Selected Methods of Analysis, Vol. 6: *N*-Nitroso Compounds | No. 45, 1983; 508 pages £20 |
| Directory of On-Going Research in Cancer Epidemiology 1982 | No. 46, 1982; 722 pages £15 |
| Cancer Incidence in Singapore | No. 47, 1982; 174 pages £10 |
| Cancer Incidence in the USSR Second Revised Edition | No. 48, 1982; 75 pages £10 |
| Laboratory Decontamination and Destruction of Carcinogens in Laboratory Wastes: Some Polycyclic Aromatic Hydrocarbons | No. 49, 1983; 81 pages £7.95 |
| Directory of On-Going Research in Cancer Epidemiology 1983 | No. 50, 1983; 740 pages £15 |
| Modulators of Experimental Carcinogenesis | No. 51, 1983; 307 pages £25 |
| Second Cancers Following Radiation Treatment for Cancer of the Uterine Cervix: The Results of a Cancer Registry Collaborative Study | No. 52, 1984; 207 pages £17.50 |
| Nickel in the Human Environment | No. 53, 1984; 530 pages £30 |
| Laboratory Decontamination and Destruction of Carcinogens in Laboratory Wastes: Some Hydrazines | No. 54, 1983; 87 pages £6.95 |
| Laboratory Decontamination and Destruction of Carcinogens in Laboratory Wastes: Some *N*-Nitrosamides | No. 55, 1984; 65 pages £6.95 |
| Models, Mechanisms and Etiology of Tumour Promotion | No. 56, 1984; 532 pages £30 |

## NON-SERIAL PUBLICATIONS

Available from WHO Sales Agents

| | |
|---|---|
| Alcool et Cancer | 1978; 42 pages Fr. fr. 35.–; Sw. fr. 14.– |
| Information Bulletin on the Survey of Chemicals Being Tested for Carcinogenicity No. 8 | 1979, 604 pages US$ 20.00; Sw. fr. 40.– |
| Cancer Morbidity and Causes of Death Among Danish Brewery Workers | 1980, 145 pages US$ 25.00; Sw. fr. 45.– |
| Information Bulletin on the Survey of Chemicals Being Tested for Carcinogenicity No. 9 | 1981, 294 pages US$ 20.00; Sw. fr. 41.– |
| Information Bulletin on the Survey of Chemicals Being Tested for Carcinogenicity No. 10 | 1982, 326 pages US$ 20.00; Sw. fr. 42.– |

## IARC MONOGRAPHS ON THE EVALUATION OF THE CARCINOGENIC RISK OF CHEMICALS TO HUMANS

Available from WHO Sales Agents.

| | |
|---|---|
| Some Inorganic Substances, Chlorinated, Hydrocarbons, Aromatic Amines, *N*-Nitroso Compounds, and Natural Products | Volume 1, 1972; 184 pages (out of print) |
| Some Inorganic and Organometallic Compounds | Volume 2, 1973; 181 pages (out of print) |
| Certain Polycyclic Aromatic Hydrocarbons and Heterocyclic Compounds | Volume 3, 1973; 271 pages (out of print) |
| Some Aromatic Amines, Hydrazine and Related Substances, *N*-Nitroso Compounds and Miscellaneous Alkylating Agents | Volume 4, 1974; 286 pages US$ 7.20; Sw. fr. 18.– |
| Some Organochlorine Pesticides | Volume 5, 1974; 241 pages (out of print) |
| Sex Hormones | Volume 6, 1974; 243 pages US$ 7.20; Sw. fr. 18.– |
| Some Anti-thyroid and Related Substances, Nitrofurans and Industrial Chemicals | Volume 7, 1974; 326 pages US$ 12.80; Sw. fr. 32.– |
| Some Aromatic Azo Compounds | Volume 8, 1975; 357 pages US$ 14.40; Sw. fr. 36.– |
| Some Aziridines, *N*-, *S*- and *O*-Mustards and Selenium | Volume 9, 1975; 268 pages US$ 10.80; Sw. fr. 27.– |
| Some Naturally Occurring Substances | Volume 10, 1976; 353 pages US$ 15.00; Sw. fr. 38.– |
| Cadmium, Nickel, Some Epoxides, Miscellaneous Industrial Chemicals and General Considerations on Volatile Anaesthetics | Volume 11, 1976; 306 pages US$ 14.00; Sw. fr. 34.– |
| Some Carbamates, Thiocarbamates and Carbazides | Volume 12, 1976; 282 pages US$ 14.00; Sw. fr. 34.– |
| Some Miscellaneous Pharmaceutical Substances | Volume 13, 1977; 255 pages US$ 12.00; Sw. fr. 30.– |
| Asbestos | Volume 14, 1977; 106 pages US$ 6.00; Sw. fr. 14.– |
| Some Fumigants, the Herbicides 2,4-D and 2,4,5-T, Chlorinated Dibenzodioxins and Miscellaneous Industrial Chemicals | Volume 15, 1977; 354 pages US$ 20.00; Sw. fr. 50.– |
| Some Aromatic Amines and Related Nitro Compounds – Hair Dyes, Colouring Agents and Miscellaneous Industrial Chemicals | Volume 16, 1978; 400 pages US$ 20.00; Sw. fr. 50.– |
| Some *N*-Nitroso Compounds | Volume 17, 1978; 365 pages US$ 25.00; Sw. fr. 50.– |
| Polychlorinated Biphenyls and Polybrominated Biphenyls | Volume 18, 1978; 140 pages US$ 13.00; Sw. fr. 20.– |
| Some Monomers, Plastics and Synthetic Elastomers, and Acrolein | Volume 19, 1979; 513 pages US$ 35.00; Sw. fr. 60.– |
| Some Halogenated Hydrocarbons | Volume 20, 1979; 609 pages US$ 35.00; Sw. fr. 60.– |
| Sex Hormones (II) | Volume 21, 1979; 583 pages US$ 35.00; Sw. fr. 60.– |
| Some Non-nutritive Sweetening Agents | Volume 22, 1980; 208 pages US$ 15.00; Sw. fr. 25.– |
| Some Metals and Metallic Compounds | Volume 23, 1980; 438 pages US$ 30.00; Sw. fr. 50.– |
| Some Pharmaceutical Drugs | Volume 24, 1980; 337 pages US$ 25.00; Sw. fr. 40.– |
| Wood, Leather and Some Associated Industries | Volume 25, 1980; 412 pages US$ 30.00; Sw. fr. 60.– |
| Some Antineoplastic and Immunosuppressive Drugs | Volume 26, 1981; 411 pages US$ 30.00; Sw. fr. 62.– |
| Some Aromatic Amines, Anthraquinones and Nitroso Compounds and Inorganic Fluorides Used in Drinking-Water and Dental Preparations | Volume 27, 1982; 341 pages US$ 25.00; Sw. fr. 40.– |
| The Rubber Industry | Volume 28, 1982; 486 pages US$ 35.00; Sw. fr. 70.– |
| Some Industrial Chemicals and Dyestuffs | Volume 29, 1982; 416 pages US$ 30.00; Sw. fr. 60.– |
| Miscellaneous Pesticides | Volume 30, 1983; 424 pages US$ 30.00; Sw. fr. 60.– |
| Some Feed Additives, Food Additives and Naturally Occurring Substances | Volume 31, 1983; 314 pages US$ 30.00; Sw. fr. 60.– |
| Chemicals and Industrial Processes Associated with Cancer in Humans (IARC Monographs 1–20) | Supplement 1, 1979; 71 pages (out of print) |
| Long-term and Short-term Screening Assays for Carcinogens: A Critical Appraisal | Supplement 2, 1980; 426 pages US$ 25.00; Sw. fr. 40.– |
| Cross Index of Synonyms and Trade Names in Volumes 1 to 26 | Supplement 3, 1982; 199 pages US$ 30.00; Sw. fr. 60.– |
| Chemicals, Industrial Processes and Industries Associated with Cancer in Humans (IARC Monographs Volumes 1 to 29) | Supplement 4, 1982; 292 pages US$ 30.00; Sw. fr. 60.– |
| Polynuclear Aromatic Compounds, Part 1, Chemical, Environmental and Experimental Data | Volume 32, 1983; 477 pages US$ 35.00; Sw. fr. 70.– |
| Polynuclear Aromatic Compounds, Part 2, Carbon Blacks, Mineral Oils and Some Nitroarenes | Volume 33, 1984; 245 pages US$ 25.00; Sw. fr. 50.– |
| Polynuclear Aromatic Compounds, Part 3, Industrial Exposures in Aluminium Production, Coal Gasification, Coke Production, and Iron and Steel Founding | Volume 34, 1984; 219 pages US$ 20.00; Sw. fr. 48.– |